MANAGEMENT OF
SPINAL CORD INJURY

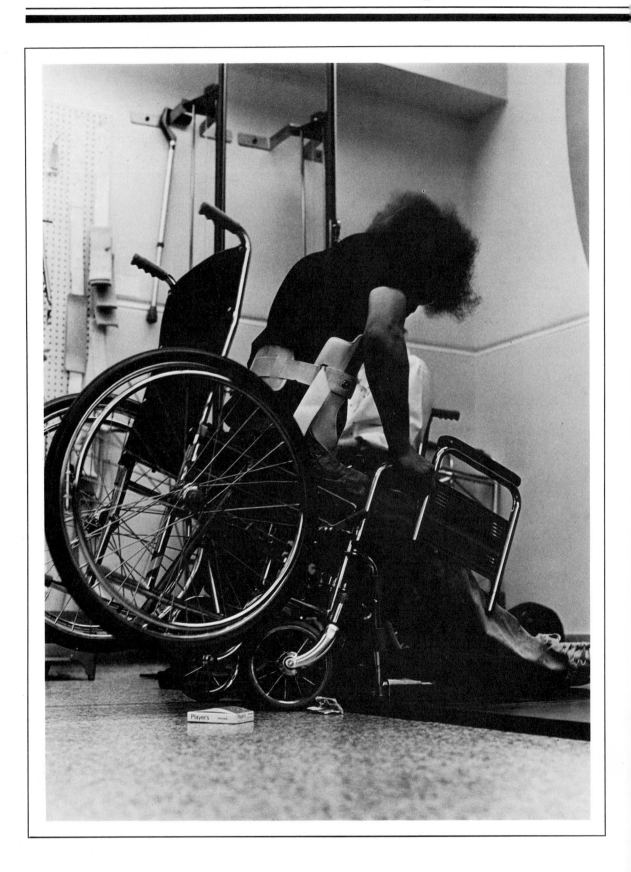

MANAGEMENT OF SPINAL CORD INJURY

Cynthia Perry Zejdlik, R.N.

Wadsworth Health Sciences Division
Monterey, California
A Division of Wadsworth, Inc.

Wadsworth Health Sciences Division
A Division of Wadsworth, Inc.

Printed in the United States of America
10 9 8 7 6 5 4 3 2 1

Library of Congress Cataloging in Publication Data

Zejdlik, Cynthia P.
  Management of spinal cord injury.

  Bibliography: p.
  Includes index.
  1. Spinal cord—Wounds and injuries—Nursing.
2. Physically handicapped—Rehabilitation.   I. Title.
RD594.3.Z44   1983   617′.482044   82-23904

ISBN 0-534-01339-2

Subject Editor: James Keating
Manuscript Editor: Loralee Windsor
Interior Design: Marilyn Langfeld/Julie Kranhold
Cover Design: Albert Burkhardt
Illustrations: Barbara Haynes
Typesetting: Typothetae, Palo Alto, California
Production Service Manager: Stacey C. Sawyer

Book Produced by Ex Libris Julie Kranhold

The thoughtful photographs have been provided courtesy of:

Joel Benard, Toronto, Ontario: pp. ii, xxiv, 42, 66, 98, 358, and 426

The Canadian Paraplegic Association, B.C. Division, Vancouver: pp. 164, 492, and 521

Lex Frieden and the Independent Living Research Project; Texas Institute for Rehabilitation and Research, Houston, Texas: pp. 124, 212, 330, 398, 473, 512, 515, 517, 519–521

Shaughnessy Hospital, Vancouver, B.C.: pp. 2, 28, 37, 56–59, 93, 152, 166, 184, 185, 186, 191, 225, 229, 233, 237, 255, 268, 345, 362, 363, 365, 366, 368, 369, 371, 372, 374, 378, 379, 380, 382, 383, 386, 387, 407, 409 (top), 410 (top), 412, 414, 415, 431 (top), 435–437, 439, 456 (top), and 494

G.F. Strong Rehabilitation Centre, Vancouver, B.C.: pp. 246, 263, 322, 384, 409 (bottom), 418, 438, 440–444 (top), 445–448, 453, 456 (bottom), and 458

Vancouver General Hospital, Vancouver, B.C.: p. 94

Vancouver Sun, Vancouver, B.C.: pp. 18, 30, 100, 356, 389, 390, and 431 (bottom)

Roger Zejdlik, Washington, D.C.: pp. 264, 265, 303, 304, 321, 410 (bottom), 444 (bottom), and 450–452

To all those who derive
benefit from this book
and
to Roger, Gina, and my parents

CONTENTS IN BRIEF

CONTENTS IN DETAIL

PART III ENHANCING FEELINGS OF SELF-WORTH

PART IV   MAINTAINING PHYSIOLOGICAL FUNCTIONS

Chapter 9   Promoting Optimal Respiratory Function   **167**

Chapter 10   Maintaining Cardio-vascular Function and Body Temperature Control   **213**

Chapter 11   Promoting Optimal Nutrition   **247**

PART V   REESTABLISHING MOBILITY AND INDEPENDENCE

Chapter 14   Maintaining Skeletal System Integrity   359

PART VI   PLANNING FOR THE FUTURE

LIST OF PROCEDURES

FOREWORD

How does one define a specialist in spinal cord injury? We, as health care professionals, are involved in the care of people with spinal cord injuries from the time they are hurt throughout the remainder of their lives. We are involved in the crises of the trauma. We serve at the center of the evolving process known as rehabilitation. We monitor and appropriately support the injured individual and his or her family as they cope in their community with the catastrophic medical, social, and psychological sequelae of spinal cord injury. Like experienced mountain guides, we must keep the rope taut during the ascent of the sheer cliffs, let it slacken on the rocky slopes, and remove it completely across the meadows.

Specialists in spinal cord injury are skilled medical/surgical/rehabilitation practitioners knowledgeable in the pathophysiological and the psychological ramifications and implications of spinal cord injury. We must be observant listeners and counselors. We must be teachers. We must be empathizers, but not sympathizers. We must be able to work confidently and comfortably with our peers from other professional disciplines to supply the comprehensive services required for people with spinal cord injuries.

Specialists in spinal cord injury are probably best defined by what they know and what they do. The philosophy, knowledge base, and professional skills required of those who provide nursing care to people with spinal cord injuries are competently and pragmatically documented by Cynthia Zejdlik in this book. Physicians, therapists, social workers, counselors, and other allied health professionals who share with nurses the philosophy and responsibilities of spinal cord injury care, will find *Management of Spinal Cord Injury* an outstanding and comprehensive source of information. The practitioner who masters its content and accepts its challenge can proceed with pride and confidence. Indeed *Management of Spinal Cord Injury* will make a major contribution to the quality of spinal cord injury care throughout the world.

JOHN S. YOUNG, M.D.
Medical Director
Spinal Cord Injury Consulting Service
Good Samaritan Hospital
Phoenix, Arizona

PREFACE

FEW INJURIES ARE as devastating to people as spinal cord injuries. To many, lay people and professionals alike, the magnitude of physical and emotional problems may well appear insoluble. But injured people themselves are not of that opinion. They have given their capabilities and life situations careful thought, and have formed very definite views about them—views that have been born of long years of suffering and hardship. Although not always recognized, these positive beliefs gradually infiltrated and significantly influenced the health care system. Today, the enlightened and combined efforts of people with spinal cord injuries and those who care for them have greatly improved the quality of care. This newer dimension is the foundation on which *Management of Spinal Cord Injury* is based.

Recent achievements of worldwide specialized facilities caring for people with spinal cord injuries have led to recognition that a skilled *interdisciplinary* approach is the only successful way to manage the diverse consequences of this complex injury. In North America alone, approximately 11,000 young men and women are injured each year and face a lifelong disability. The needs created are overwhelming, but, together, people with spinal cord injuries and interdisciplinary professionals have alleviated some of the major physical, psychological, social, and economic problems experienced by injured people, their families, and the communities in which they live.

Management of Spinal Cord Injury provides a unique resource for the entire interdisciplinary team. With the growth of the team concept, nurses' and other health professionals' roles have expanded in many challenging ways. Understanding the function of and collaborating with other disciplines to improve total patient care are complicated tasks. All disciplines interface with and rely on nurses to provide continuity with selected elements of patient care. The content herein summarizes, clarifies, and offers practical guidelines to enhance interprofessional services. Nurses, physicians, therapists, counselors, and others will find this information helpful to achieve interrelated care goals. College and university students of various disciplines and interests will find this an effective learning aid.

The content of *Management of Spinal Cord Injury* is coordinated in six interdependent parts.

Part I introduces current trends in and expresses a philosophical base for comprehensive care. The concept of prevention is emphasized as the best future management of spinal cord injuries.

Part II examines the priorities of life-saving techniques and concentrates on skilled assessment and management to prevent further neurological deficit.

Part III deals with the psychosocial, sexual, and educational aspects of injury. This is explored early in the book to stress the singular importance of creating a positive and constructive therapeutic environment. Without achieving this, patients and families will simply not be able to secure optimal benefits from other services provided.

Part IV describes specialized knowledge and skills essential to maintaining physiological well-being. It focuses on cardiopulmonary, gastrointestinal, and urinary function following injury.

Part V describes the momentum involved in regaining strength, reestablishing mobility, and achieving independence with activities of daily living. The special needs of those with respiratory quadriplegia are also included.

Part VI is devoted to the highly relevant processes of discharge and reintegration into the community. "Is there life after rehabilitation?" is a question posed and answered by people with spinal cord injuries. Their direct involvement will not merely effect immediate changes in the health care system, but will extend for the future a promise that a good life is possible.

Chapters are organized to include:

- Learning objectives to be achieved.
- Interdisciplinary goals of health care.
- Assessment guides. Assessment sections include a review of normal anatomy and physiology and highlight neural functions. Anticipated dysfunctions are then correlated to the levels of spinal cord injury, which enables better preparation for emergencies, specific directions for prevention of complications, and accuracy in planning future rehabilitation.
- Intervention guides. Intervention sections include preventive and restorative measures.
- Specific interventions for potential complications. In the event of complications, a problem-solving approach is utilized to present a statement of the problem, goals of care, implementation of selected treatment, and outcome criteria to facilitate evaluation.
- Procedures to make selected assessment and intervention techniques easily accessible. Each explains the purpose of the technique, details the recommended actions, and describes rationale to support those actions.
- Self-care skills. This plan provides guidelines for education of patients and families, an integral part of all care.
- Long-term implications. These conclusive sections consider the effects of permanent disability and give information to adjust assessment data, redefine goals, and make decisions about consultation and referral.
- Selected references and supplemental readings. All reference material is annotated to help direct further learning and research.

Management of Spinal Cord Injury offers a practical and theoretical guide to care from the moment of injury, through recovery, and toward independence. The focus on immediate and early management makes this book useful in prehospital care; emergency rooms; critical care units; specialty neurological, neurosurgical, and orthopedic areas; and general hospitals. Because acute and concurrent rehabilitative care is presented, concepts and techniques are of value in rehabilitation centers; services, such as urology and psychiatry, that provide ongoing and follow-up care; long-term facilities; and support services, such as home care, in the community.

Management of Spinal Cord Injury has many uses: as a reference for prevention of spinal cord injuries in the public sector; in planning and administration of health care facilities; in related fields of the medical-legal profession and health insurance industry; in community-based educational, vocational, and counseling services; in peer counseling; and in other resource and advocacy groups. In addition, sections of the book will be of interest to patients and families themselves.

Basically *Management of Spinal Cord Injury* considers each human need and examines the consequences that follow spinal cord injury. Management is detailed in a solid example of the uninterrupted continuance of care necessary from accident to home. The purpose of this approach—as opposed to presenting separate stages of acute, intermediate, and finally rehabilitative care as if isolated—is twofold:

- To enhance awareness of how personal contributions are both timely and relevant.
- To gain an appreciation of other disciplines' contributions, strengths, and limitations.

Objectivity, flexibility, and satisfaction of those who care for people with spinal cord injuries are of intrinsic importance to the rehabilitation process. *Management of Spinal Cord Injury* promotes such comprehension. Professionals with expertise, who are able to communicate these positive feelings and abilities, unify and strengthen the interdisciplinary approach and ultimately improve total patient care.

Cynthia Perry Zejdlik

Acknowledgments

I WISH TO ACKNOWLEDGE the patients, families, and interdisciplinary staff members of the *Acute Spinal Cord Injury Unit at Shaughnessy Hospital* in Vancouver, British Columbia, for their special contribution to an in-house manual on which *Management of Spinal Cord Injury* is based. Their interactions and willingness to share experiences led to an accumulation of skills, knowledge, and achievements that inspired the writing of this book. I express my sincere appreciation to the following people involved with the specialized unit at Shaughnessy Hospital:

- J. F. Schweigel, M.D., Director of Department of Surgery, whose wisdom and foresight helped initiate this project.
- Ferne Trout, B.A., R.N., B.Ap.Sc., D.H.A., former Director of Nursing, and her colleagues, nursing authors Barbara Kozier, B.S.N., R.N., M.N., and Glenora Erb, B.S.N., R.N., who helped to carefully guide this book off the ground.
- The staff nurses, both present and former, Mary Amos, R.N.; Rita Driscol, L.P.N.; Tricia Crimean, R.N.; Dianne Estreicher, R.N., B.S.N.; Judy Kelly, R.N., B.S.N.; Audrey McHattie, R.N.; and Donna Wilton, R.N. To these nurses, and those they represent, a tribute to their dedication, determination, and expertise in pioneering the care documented in this book is most fitting.
- Skender Adzijaj, Emergency Medical Assistant II, Emergency Health Services, Provincial Ambulance, British Columbia, and former nursing orderly, for sharing his unique combination of skills in prehospital care.
- G. Fred Pearson, Vice President of Staff Services, for his direction and support.
- Kathy Fukuyama, R.N., B.S.N., for her enthusiastic support with photographic direction, research, and annotation of the reference material.
- Sue Laughlin, B.S.R., for her wonderful way of communicating simply the intricacies of her specialty of occupational therapy and for her contributions to the self-care sections.
- Margaret McPhee, M.A., M.Sc., A.I.M.S.W., and Keith Wilkinson, M.Ed., Ph.D., for the diligent production of an in-house manual on which this book is based.

I am thankful to the consultants who have generously given time and expertise to contribute, revise, and clarify portions of this book:

- Gail Clements, R.N., B.S.N., Head Nurse at Shaughnessy Hospital, Vancouver.
- Cardiopulmonary specialists C. W. Fast, M.D., Shaughnessy Hospital, Vancouver; J. R. Ledsome, University of British Columbia, Vancouver; and Jeannie Sharp, R.N., Counselor, Vocational Rehabilitation Consultants, and Research Assistant, Department of Physiotherapy, University of British Columbia, Vancouver.
- Urologists Howard N. Fenster, M.D.; and Donald MacDonald, M.D., both of Shaughnessy Hospital, Vancouver.
- Norna Jolly, B.H.E., R.Dt., Nutritionist, Shaughnessy Hospital, Vancouver.
- Michael W. Jones, M.D., Neurologist, Shaughnessy Hospital, Vancouver.
- D. Duncan Murray, M.D., Department Head, Rehabilitation Medicine, Shaughnessy Hospital, Vancouver.
- Shirley McFeat,* M.S.W., Department of Social Services, Shaughnessy Hospital, Vancouver.

---

* Spinal cord injury person.

- Orthopedic Surgeons Kurt Van Peteghem, M.D.; and Peter Wing, M.D., both of Shaughnessy Hospital, Vancouver.
- Barrie Woodhurst, M.D., Neurosurgeon, Vancouver General Hospital, Vancouver.

I am also grateful to the patients and the interdisciplinary staff of *G.F. Strong Rehabilitation Centre* who, under the direction of Charles W. Grierson, Executive Director, made a wealth of information and services accessible:

- Edward J. Desjardins*, C.M. LL.D., Consultant, for stimulating creative thought on the many psychosocial implications surrounding people with spinal cord injuries. The impact of his continual challenges significantly influenced the direction of this book.
- Bridget Duckworth, M.A.O.T., O.T.R., Director of Occupational Therapy.
- Jack Ford, R.G., Director of Remedial Gymnastics, who finally taught me, among other things, how to transfer a patient in a Halo with ease!
- Marjorie L. Griffen, M.S.S.W., Department of Social Services.
- Kay Higgins, R.N., Discharge and Followup Coordinator.
- Pat Love, R.N., Inservice Education Instructor, and her nursing colleagues.

With respect and affection, I thank the *Canadian Paraplegic Association, British Columbia Division,* under the leadership of Douglas Mowat*, C.M., Executive Director, for graciously extending insight into many issues.

- Special thanks to Mary Lou Takasaki, Director of Administration.
- Norman Haw*, Director of Rehabilitation Services.
- Rehabilitation Counselors Diane Marshall*, R.N., and Colleen Smith*.

I am also appreciative to those who reviewed sections of the manuscript and made helpful suggestions to shape this book:

- June C. Abbey, R.N., Ph.D., F.A.A.N., formerly Professor and Director of Physiological Nursing Program, College of Nursing, University of Utah, Salt Lake City.
- Christine Sorok Benvenuti, R.N., I.C.P., Head Nurse, Spinal Cord Injury Service, Veterans Administration Medical Center, Long Beach, California.
- Nancy Meyer Holloway, B.S.N., M.S.N., Critical Care Specialist, San Francisco, California.
- Roberta Treischmann, Ph.D., Consulting Psychologist, Scottsdale, Arizona.
- George Szasz, M.D., and Lex Frieden*, Ph.D., M.S.P., for their active support, willingness, and ability to blend their contributions with the overall feeling of this book.
- John S. Young, M.D., Medical Director, Spinal Cord Injury Consulting Service, Good Samaritan Hospital, Phoenix, Arizona, for his sincerity and enthusiasm in supporting this book.

Appreciation is also extended to those involved in the production services. Their orchestrated efforts resulted in the fine quality of this book:

- My typists Alenka Goldie of Vancouver, British Columbia, and Kathy Sasser of Bakersfield, California, who cheerfully assisted with countless details.
- Jim Keating, Executive Editor of Wadsworth Health Sciences, who had faith in me as a new author and nurtured me along in the business of writing; and to his associates Robert V. Wilson and Stacey Sawyer.
- Julie Kranhold of Ex Libris Production Service for her infinite patience, good humor, and skillful direction with design and editing; Loralee Windsor for amazing jobs as copy editor; and illustrator Barbara Haynes for her explicit and creative interpretations.

To my family and friends, who have repeatedly juggled their schedules to provide the impossible, I am deeply grateful. I especially thank my husband, Roger, who has carted this manuscript from the mountaintops of Italy to the shores of Hawaii! As a family, we travel extensively with his work as a geodesist, tracking (or should I say chasing) satellites all over the world. Roger has served variously as Xeroxer, photographer, consultant, babysitter, and full-time homemaker. Without his constant support, I simply could not have endured the five long years of writing *Management of Spinal Cord Injury.*

C.P.Z.

CONTRIBUTORS

Lex Frieden, Ph.D.

Director
Independent Living Research Utilization Project
Texas Institute for Rehabilitation and Research
Houston, Texas

George Szasz, M.D.

Director
Sexual Health Services
Acute Spinal Cord Injury Unit, Shaughnessy
Hospital, and G.F. Strong Rehabilitation Centre
Vancouver, British Columbia

Jane Andrew, Dip, P.T., O.T., M.Ed.
Patient and Family Health Coordinator
G.F. Strong Rehabilitation Centre
Vancouver, British Columbia

Mary Beth Berkoff

Director
Accident Prevention
Chicago Rehabilitation Institute of Chicago
Chicago, Illinois

Kathy Fukuyama, R.N., B.S.N.

Former Clinical Nurse Specialist
Acute Spinal Cord Injury Unit
Shaughnessy Hospital
Vancouver, British Columbia

Judy Little, R.N.

Critical Care Coordinator
Acute Spinal Cord Injury Unit
Shaughnessy Hospital
Vancouver, British Columbia

Susan Laughlin, B.S.R.
Director
Rehabilitation Services
Shaughnessy Hospital
Vancouver, British Columbia

Linda MacNutt, R.P.N., B.S.W., M.S.W.

University of British Columbia and
Pearson Hospital
Vancouver, British Columbia

Dierdre Webster, B.S.R.

School of Physiotherapy
University of British Columbia
Vancouver, British Columbia

MANAGEMENT OF
SPINAL CORD INJURY

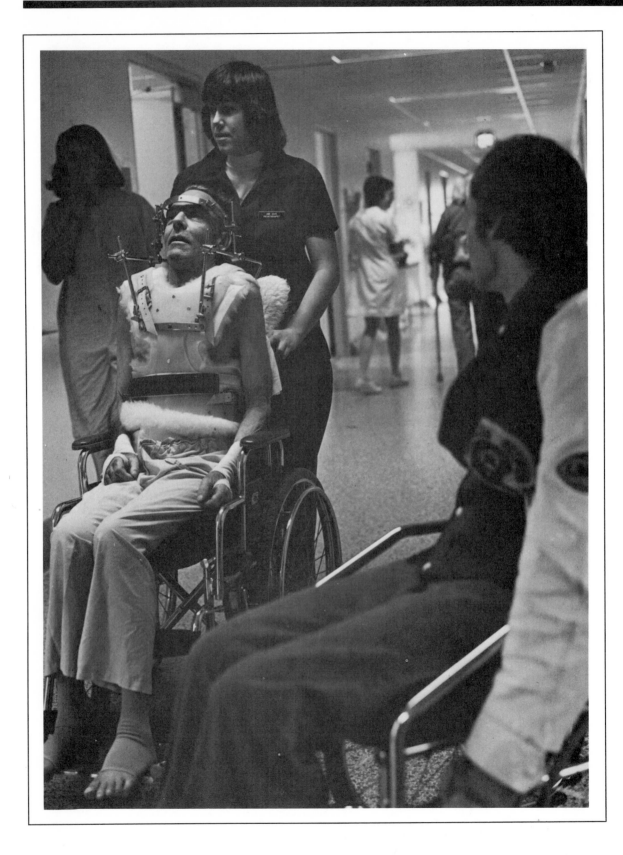

PART I

PERSPECTIVES ON SPINAL CORD INJURY

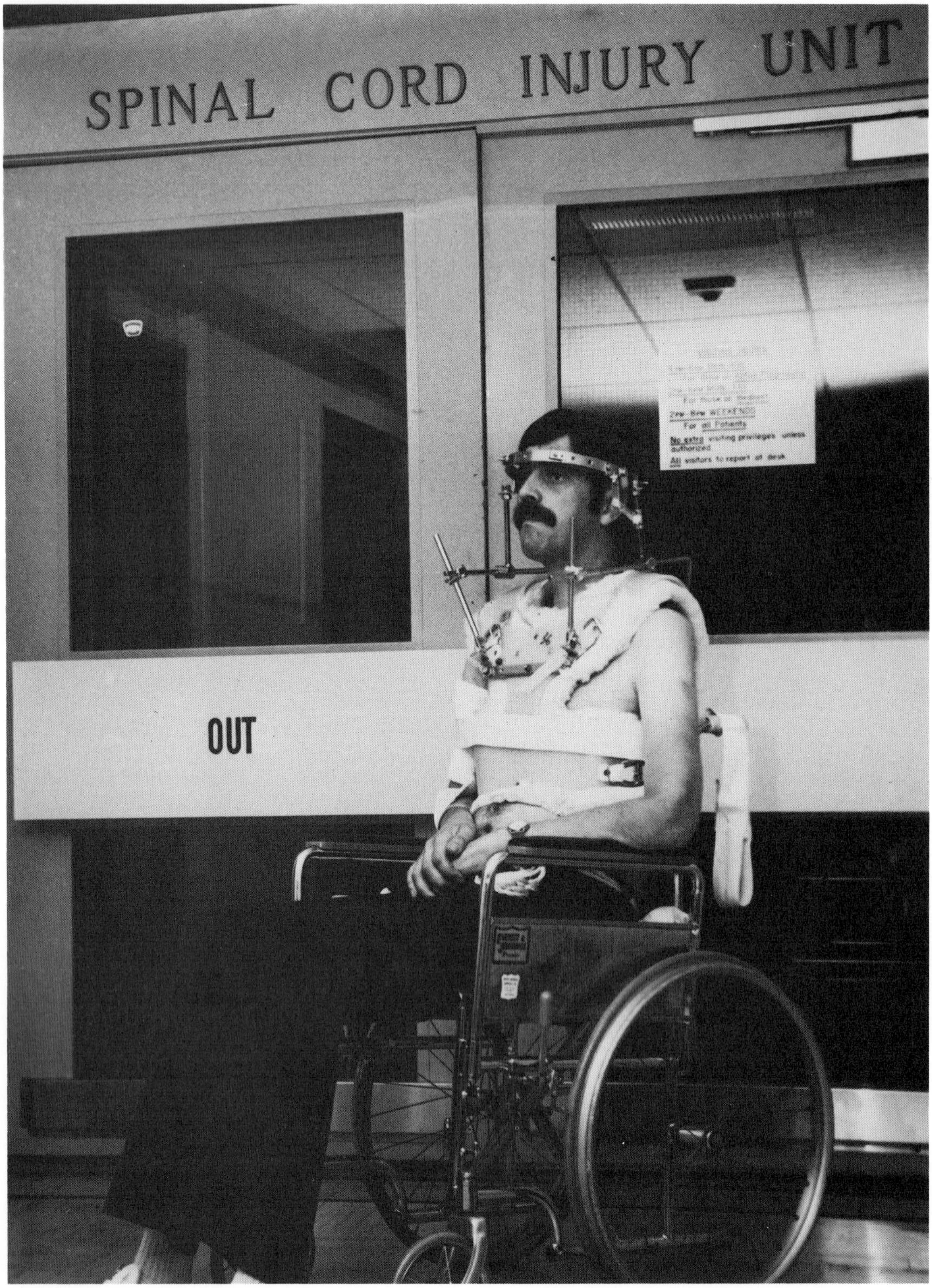
SPINAL CORD INJURY UNIT
2pm-8pm WEEKENDS
For all Patients
No extra visiting privileges unless authorized
All visitors to report at desk
OUT

Chapter 1

Health Care Concepts and Spinal Cord Injury

OBJECTIVES

- To define spinal cord injury and describe implications of severe physical disability
- To gain perspective on the impact of spinal cord injury and its meaning to individuals, families, the health care system, and the community at large
- To identify steps of the nursing process and apply to goal-oriented rehabilitative care

Spinal injury with paralysis has been recorded throughout civilization as one of the most debilitating afflictions known to humanity. The descriptions in ancient Greek and Egyptian medical records; the accounts of historical figures, such as Lord Nelson, who suffered spinal cord injuries; and the horrific tales from the battlefields of World War I consistently depict the victims of spinal cord injury as doomed to death. The picture of those who survived—wracked with infections, contractures, bedsores, and mental anguish—is surely one of the most depressing in medicine. Only very recently has this gloomy picture begun to brighten.

HISTORICAL BACKGROUND

Throughout history there has been little change in health care concepts of spinal cord injuries. In the twentieth century, however, great strides have been made. The major turning point in the care of people with spinal cord injuries occurred when great numbers of World War II veterans returned to their homes in various parts of the world. Although combat injuries cause a relatively small percentage of spinal cord injuries, veterans have historically been highly influential in inspiring worldwide movements to improve comprehensive health care. For the first time in history the health sciences were sufficiently advanced and public attitudes sufficiently receptive to allow appropriate attention to the total rehabilitative needs of people with spinal cord injuries.

During the aftermath of World War II, Sir Ludwig Guttman, working at Stoke-Mandeville Hospital in England, virtually revolutionized the concept of health care for people with spinal cord injuries (1976). Guttman's philosophy emphasized centralized, comprehensive services for the *total spinal person*, as opposed to institutionalized custodial care for *cripples*. To achieve the goals of his philosophy, he developed an integrated, interprofessional team; improved and interrelated acute and long-term care facilities; and social and vocational counseling and after-

care services. This model inspired other countries to adopt a similar approach: the belief that the spinal cord injured individual is a physically disabled but healthy person, with a productive future in society, is now a fundamental concept of health care in most modern nations.

In support of specialized treatment, Schweigel and Peerless (1971: 2–4) write:

It is generally agreed that intensive medical/rehabilitative care must begin as soon as possible after the spinal cord injury. The dramatic improvement in the morbidity and mortality statistics in countries where centers were established years ago, for example, in Great Britain in the 1940s, Australia in the 1950s, and South Africa in the 1960s, has clearly shown the desirability for such centers for the management of the spinal injured. . . . However, with the declining numbers of military personnel and the sharply rising incidence of civilian spinal cord injured, a fragmentary and haphazard approach to this problem currently exists.

It is sometimes said that a patient with spinal cord injury is too ill to be moved to a major center. Actually those individuals are too sick to be safely managed in small hospitals or in large hospitals where fragmentation of services and specialty groups prevent the overall view of their complex problems. The care of these severely disabled patients includes the prevention of the complicating manifestations; as well, the psychological, physical, social, and vocational rehabilitative measures require a highly sophisticated team approach in which each team member contributes within the realm of their expertise. Over and above the humane factor, favorable prognosis as to the life expectancy and stability of neuromuscular disability justifies a considerable investment of time, money, and effort required to rehabilitate the patient with a spinal cord injury.

The complexity of the many intrinsic and extrinsic factors encountered in the care and rehabilitation process of these patients demands the full cooperation of a large number of medical, paramedical, and nonmedical personnel, ranging from the ambulance driver to the future employer of the patient, characteristically exemplifying the so-called team approach. The core medical team may well be composed of a neurosurgeon, an orthopedic surgeon, a neurologist, a urologist, a respiratory consultant, an anesthetist, an internist, a psychiatrist, and quite possibly a plastic surgeon and a pediatrician. Clinical and counseling professionals likewise belong to the team and so do the patient and family.

As stated in a report on the current status of the care of the spinal cord injured patient (Committee on the Skeletal System 1967: 6–7), "if total effective care is the goal, it is essential that centers be provided for the treatment of spinal cord injuries, where the condition itself, rather than the medical complications, is the focal point."

CURRENT DEVELOPMENTS IN THE UNITED STATES*

In the United States, health care for people with spinal cord injuries is currently delivered in three distinct treatment systems: those using the model systems concept; Veteran's Administration spinal cord injury centers; and community facilities.

The Model Systems Concept

Since 1970, the Rehabilitation Services Administration (RSA) of the Department of Health, Education and Welfare, has supported a growing number of model demonstration projects for Regional SCI (spinal cord injury) Systems. These are strategically located throughout the country in Birmingham, Ala; Phoenix, Ariz; San Jose, Northern Calif; Northridge, Central Calif; Downey, Southern Calif; Englewood (Denver), Colo; Miami, Fla; Chicago, Ill; New Orleans, La; Boston, Mass; Columbia, Mo; Rochester, NY; New York, NY; Philadelphia, Pa; Houston, Tex; Fisherville, Va; and Seattle, Wash.

As indicated in *Guidelines for Facility Categorization and Standards of Care* (1981:5),

> A spinal cord injury system of care must provide an integration and continuum of treatment services for the spinal cord injured victim from the

moment of injury through lifetime follow-up and community integration. . . . Each separate component must be developed to maximum efficiency and be tied together by strong, functional interrelationships. The major components are:

1. An organized emergency medical service.
2. Trauma centers with a spinal cord injury trauma unit.
3. Rehabilitation facilities with an identifiable spinal cord injury care area or beds, to include all medical, surgical and rehabilitation services.
4. Long-term comprehensive follow-up (to include medical, social, psychological and vocational).
5. Community integration.

The model systems concept embodies the following objectives:

- To establish, within a catchment area or region of natural patient flow, a multidisciplinary system of providing comprehensive rehabilitation services to meet the patient needs from point of injury (emergency treatment and transportation) through acute care; rehabilitation, including vocational and educational preparation; community and job placement; and long-term follow-up.
- To achieve new knowledge through research in reducing disability and treating the spinal cord injury and its complications.
- To demonstrate and evaluate the development and application of improved methods and equipment essential to the care, management, and rehabilitation of the spinal cord injured patient.
- To demonstrate methods of community outreach and education for the spinal cord injured in housing, transportation, recreation, employment, and other community activities.

In an extensive research project supported by the National Spinal Cord Injury Foundation to determine cost-effectiveness of specialized treatment centers, Matlack (1974) powerfully summarizes information meaningful not only to the economic, but also to the clinical, issues surrounding comprehensive care for spinal cord injured persons. Rather than debating the issue, worldwide leaders unanimously prefer coordinated, comprehensive, concurrent care by all the related health care professionals from the onset of injury, through rehabilitation, to discharge

---

* This section and the next section are based on the skillful interpretation of facts by Roberta Treischmann in *Spinal Cord Injuries; Psychological, Social, and Vocational Adjustments,* New York: Pergamon Press, 1980.

■ *What Is Spinal Cord Injury?*

Spinal cord injury is a lesion of the cord that if complete, causes permanent motor paralysis below the level of the lesion with corresponding loss of sensation. However, as emphasized by the National Spinal Cord Injury Foundation (1981: 26):

The catastrophic nature of spinal cord injury is much more complex than loss of feeling and inability to move. Individuals who experience damage to their spinal cords also contend with impairment of bladder, bowel, and sexual function. Added to this are the psychological effects of adjustments that must be made to social, economic, and emotional ramifications of spinal cord injury.

Paraplegia refers to paralysis of the lower portion of the body, which includes the legs and may include the trunk. Paraplegia occurs with injury to the second thoracic segment or below. Because upper body strength is preserved, a paraplegic person has the potential physical ability to become independent in all aspects of personal care and wheelchair mobility. For those receiving injury to the lower thoracic cord (T_9 and below) ambulation with long leg braces and crutches may be possible; for those receiving injury to the sacral cord, ambulation, with or without short leg braces, is possible.*

Quadriplegia, or *tetraplegia,* refers to paralysis of the lower and upper portions of the body including partial or complete involvement of the arms and hands. Quadriplegia occurs with injury to the first thoracic segment or above. Rehabilitation is much more complex. Physical abilities and independence potential for personal care and wheelchair mobility are dramatically affected by the level of lesion. Acute quadriplegia also poses a significant threat of respiratory insufficiency. In addition, the autonomic nervous system, controlled by coordination from higher centers, does not function normally.

Pentaplegia is a term used for extremely high cord injury in which paralysis extends to the muscles of the neck and the back of the head and the breathing muscles, primarily the diaphragm. A patient with pentaplegia will require a lifelong respiratory support system and total assistance with personal care. Mobility may be aided by the use of environmental control systems.

---

* Chapter 16 (Table 16–5) gives an overview of levels of functioning for people with paraplegia, quadriplegia, and pentaplegia.

---

with ongoing specialized services for the disabled person in the community. As a federal government representative notes,

Despite the fact that there is every reason to believe that the RSA model systems approach to spinal cord injury care is appropriate, beneficial in rehabilitation outcomes, and significantly cost-effective over all other alternatives; and that alternatively, there is every likelihood that there will be unsatisfactory patient–client outcomes, catastrophic medical complications, incredibly high costs for hospital and nursing home care, and a tremendous drain on personal, private, and public resources; *only about 15 percent of all newly injured patients receive care under this concept.* [Humphreys 1978: 3–5]

If this concept is superior, why has it not been more widely adopted in North America? Matlack and others concluded that medical apathy, characterized by parochialism and institutional rigidity, is one problem but that financial concerns are probably the main reason. However, the conclusions of Matlack's cost-effectiveness study invalidate these concerns. Analyzing direct costs (primarily those of hospitalization and lifelong nursing and medical costs) and indirect costs (primarily those of lost earnings) and comparing the costs for patients who were cared for in specialized centers with the costs for those were not, he writes:

> there are no competing economic or medical costs to compare—all are on the side of spinal cord injury center treatment. . . . The parameters of the model suggest norms for the length of hospitalization and treatment outcomes. Since prolonged treatment is often due to preventable complications, cost control and quality control reinforce each other. At least in the case of spinal cord injury, the best quality treatment is also the least costly for the patient, for third party payers, and for society. [Matlack 1974: 20]

Veterans Administration Spinal Cord Injury Centers

The Vietnam War caused a sudden and disproportionate increase in the incidence of spinal cord injury among young Americans. Not only has this group significantly contributed to increasing public awareness, they and the health care professionals caring for them have strengthened and advanced the interdisciplinary concept to improve comprehensive health care within the general medical–rehabilitative community.

Specialized spinal cord injury centers are located in Veterans Administration hospitals in Long Beach and Palo Alto, Calif; Miami and Tampa, Fla; Brockton and West Roxbury, Mass; Hines, Ill; East Orange, NJ; Bronx and Castle Point, NY; St. Louis, Mo; Cleveland, Ohio; San Juan, Puerto Rico; Memphis, Tenn; Houston, Tex; Hampton and Richmond, Va; and Wood, Wisc.

Military veterans who are injured, either while in active service or during inactive duty, qualify for care at a specialized center within a Veterans Administration hospital. However, this is a relatively small percentage of the total spinal cord injured population; the majority of patients receive care in community facilities.

Community Facilities

Although estimates vary, between 50% and 70% of the people with new spinal cord injuries

probably receive their acute management and rehabilitation training at a local facility. Only those with complicated cases of high quadriplegia are likely to be referred to a model systems center (Trieschmann 1980).

The decision to refer people with spinal cord injuries to a specialized center depends largely on the consulting physician and, one would like to think, the preference of the patient and family. However, it is doubtful that most individuals get appropriate or adequate information about the health care delivery options available, both from a clinical and economic point of view. Therefore, it is quite possible that in the emotional turmoil surrounding the initial injury, neither patients nor families are able to make a well-informed choice from the alternatives currently available.

This difficult situation challenges the nurse's role as patient advocate in terms of informing patients and families of the newer options available in spinal cord injury care. Giving this information often directly conflicts with the consulting physician's wishes. The nurse must exercise professional judgment in weighing the timing and the relevance of the information against threatening patient and family confidence in the consulting physician. Sometimes the solution to this problem lies in collaboration with a third party, such as the patient's family physician.

SOME STATISTICAL INFORMATION ABOUT PEOPLE WITH SPINAL CORD INJURIES

In a collaborative project with the model systems concept, the RSA established the National Spinal Cord Injury Data Research Center in Phoenix, Ariz., to collect, analyze, and disseminate common data. The Director of the Center, Dr. John S. Young (1978: 9–12), writes:

> The purpose of the project is to acquire sufficient data and develop information which will lead to the upgrading of the quality and availability of health care for the spinal cord injured. Also, it will help define the most cost-effective method of supplying this care.

The National Data Research Center will direct its ongoing study to supplying answers to questions pertaining to the care and treatment of spinal cord injured persons. Many of those questions are epidemiological in nature, relating not only to the injury but also to the disability created by the injury.

We need to know specifically what type of person gets hurt? What is the etiology of their injury? What is the specific nature of their injuries? What associated injuries do they have? Are there psychological and social components associated with the etiology of the accident?

In Table 1–1, Dr. Young presents further factors that affect care and treatment of people with spinal cord injuries.

The following statistics and comments (Young and Northrup 1979) are based on accumulated data from 1973 through 1977. It must be remembered that they represent only those patients cared for at model systems centers and are therefore not a fully valid representation of the nation's spinal cord injured population. For example, there appears to be a fairly equal distribution of paraplegia and quadriplegia, but other international studies indicate there is usually a higher incidence of paraplegia. The anomaly is probably caused by the fact that local facilities are more likely to refer quadriplegic rather than paraplegic people to a regional center.

Trieschmann (1980) notes that spinal cord injury is a low-incidence but high-cost disability that usually makes tremendous changes in the person's life-style. About 150,000 people in the United States today have traumatic spinal cord injuries, and from 7000 to 10,000 people are newly injured each year. Spinal cord injury occurs most frequently in the younger age groups—80% under the age of 40 and 50% between the ages of 15 and 25. See Figure 1–1. Average lifetime care costs are conservatively estimated at $325,000 to $400,000 for a person with quadriplegia and $180,000 to $225,000 for a person with paraplegia (Humphreys 1978). The combination of early onset of severe disability coupled with achievements in medical science that allow almost a full life expectancy yields a catastrophe in terms of human disability and social economics. Considering these two factors, lifetime care costs might be more realistically estimated as ranging from $350,000 to $600,000.

TABLE 1–1 ■ FACTORS THAT ARE OF CONCERN TO THE NATIONAL SPINAL CORD INJURY DATA RESEARCH CENTER

Nature of Disability

We need information pertaining to the nature of the disability in its broadest sense: medical, psychological and social. We must be interested not only in what happens to the individual but also to members of his family.

We need to know what compounds the disability. What is contributed by the attitudes of the family and friends, the attitudes of society and such things as architectural barriers limiting function of the spinal cord injured person in his environment?

We are also interested in negative motivational factors compounding disability. Included in these are the effects of benefits and awards given to handicapped persons which may tend to perpetuate their disability.

Health Service Delivery

Of paramount interest to the project is the identification of present methods for delivery of health services to the spinal cord injured. What services are given? What is the time sequence of delivery? What is the pattern of delivery? Is it a systematized approach? Lastly, what is the Optimal System?

Medical Care

We will investigate ongoing spinal cord injury medical care. What recurrent medical complications do spinal cord injured people have? What is their life expectancy? What are the causes of death? In addition to the medical end product, we must define the social end product. How well do spinal cord injured people live? What should society expect from them and what should they expect and receive from society? What is the cost of medical treatment, rehabilitation, health maintenance and loss of productivity? Lastly, to what extent can the cost of spinal cord injury be offset by containment of personal cost and productive employment?

Questions such as these require multivariate analysis and correlation for they represent the summated effects of many variables. As a consequence, large numbers of cases are required to produce meaningful information.

Source: Young 1978: 8.

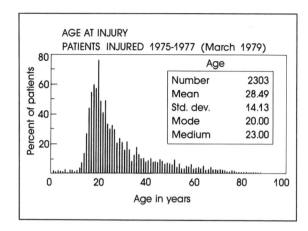

FIGURE 1–1 ■ Age at injury. Patients injured, 1975–1977 (Young and Northrup 1979:4).

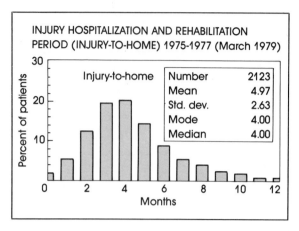

FIGURE 1–2 ■ Initial hospitalization and rehabilitation period (injury-to-home), 1975–1977 (Young and Northrup 1979:13).

The most striking information reveals that spinal cord injury occurs predominately in the young male population (82% male versus 18% female) and is most frequently caused by motor vehicle accidents. Further analysis reveals that 57% of the victims possess high school education or more and that most either were working (58%) or were full-time students (24%) at the onset of injury. As can be expected with a predominately young age group, over half the injured were single.

People with spinal cord injuries usually spend between two and six months in the hospital for initial treatment and rehabilitation and at a substantial cost. The amounts shown in Figures 1–2 and 1–3 include hospitalization costs (primarily), physicians' fees, equipment, and other expenses, such as evaluation, environmental modification, and vocational counseling.

As shown in Table 1–2, motor vehicle accidents account for 46% of injuries, followed by falls and sports accidents with 16% each. Causes vary in different groups depending on such characteristics as age of onset, sex, and racial or ethnic background. For example, motor vehicle accidents and sports injuries had a high occurrence in the 15 to 29 group, whereas older people (over 60) were more likely to be injured by falls. And surprisingly, children (0 to 14) experienced a high percentage of penetrating wounds.

In terms of neurological impairment, the same percentage of quadriplegia and paraplegia resulted from motor vehicle accidents. However,

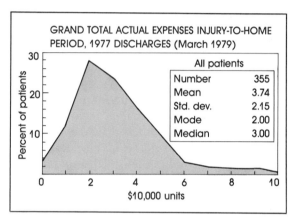

FIGURE 1–3 ■ Grand total actual expenses of injury-to-home period, 1977 discharges (Young and Northrup 1979:17).

paraplegia occurs more with penetrating wounds (which are more likely to be received in the back than in the small area of the neck) and quadriplegia occurs more with sports injuries. Contact sports and diving accidents are the main sports causes of quadriplegia. (These accidents account for approximately 10% of all injuries.)

The causes of injury in different racial or ethnic groups are shown in Table 1–3. Sports injuries occur most frequently among white people, whereas penetrating wounds are the greatest cause of injury among black people. American Indians are most often injured in motor vehicle accidents.

TABLE 1–2 ■ ETIOLOGY BY GROUPED CATEGORIES (March 1979)

Etiology (Grouped)	Reported Cases	
	N	%
Vehicular Accidents	1058	46
Penetrating Wounds	276	12
Sports	357	16
Falls	364	16
Other	241	10
ALL	2296	

Source: Young and Northrup 1979:8.

Among given communities, there are likely to be differences in etiology of injury. For example, in British Columbia, although motor vehicle accidents are the major cause of spinal cord injuries, there is a relatively high number caused by falls in the province's major logging industry and by water- and mountain-related sports. Spinal injuries from gunshot wounds seldom occur in Canada but cause 11.6% of the total spinal cord injuries in the United States. This is probably related to the difference in handgun legislation. The climate also exerts a major influence on frequency of injury: in the summer industrial productivity and recreational activities rise sharply, increasing the number of spinal cord injuries.

Statistics clarify that the spinal cord injured population is predominantly a young, male one, typically at a critical juncture in planning for adult life. Analysis of statistical information can be particularly helpful to nurses involved with planning comprehensive care to meet the unique needs of this group, staff allocation, and preventive programs. For example, staffing requirements based on an average patient occupancy rate calculated on a yearly basis do not take into account the peak periods of spinal cord injuries, usually during the summer months. This can create alternate periods of understaffing and overstaffing. Calculating an average amount of care for all the spinal cord injury patients in a center does not provide sufficient information. If most of the patients are quadriplegic at a particular time, an average staffing pattern will be inadequate. Nurses must be aware that incorrect or insufficient analysis of statistical data can misdirect many efforts.

TABLE 1–3 ■ RACE BY ETIOLOGY CATEGORY (N = 2296; March 1979)

Race	Etiology				
	Vehicular Accidents %	Penetrating Wounds %	Sports %	Falls %	Other %
White	49	7	18	16	11
Black	27	39	7	17	10
American Indian	74	8	4	8	8
Spanish	36	24	11	18	11
Other	50	23	5	23	0
ALL	46	12	16	16	11

Source: Young and Northrup 1979:11.

A PHILOSOPHICAL APPROACH TO NURSING PEOPLE WITH SPINAL CORD INJURIES

Just as patients adapt physically following spinal cord injury, so they must adapt to disability as total people. Nurses can facilitate this process by recognizing that all human needs are interwoven and that people fulfill their needs in highly individual ways.

> Focusing on one need to exclusion of others ignores the totality of the person and diminishes the effect of nursing intervention. . . . Rehabilitation nursing demonstrates the belief that every client is unique, is a member of a family constellation, and has needs that must be met to attain and maintain his full potential for rehabilitation. . . . Since the philosophy of rehabilitation nursing espouses a belief in the fundamental needs of humans interacting with their environment to achieve maximum potential, it seems unnecessary to search further for a more appropriate universal philosophy for nursing care. The real need, then, is to articulate this philosophy throughout nursing practice and education. [Mahoney 1979: 28–29]

In 1975 the United Nations Assembly published a *Declaration on the Rights of Disabled Persons* and now continuously calls for national and international action to ensure that it will be used as a basis for protection of the human rights of disabled people. The following rights, among others in the declaration, have specific implications for nursing practice in caring for people with spinal cord injuries:

- The term *disabled person* means any person unable to ensure by himself or herself, wholly or partly, the necessities of a normal individual and/or social life, as a result of a deficiency, either congenital or not, in his or her physical or mental capabilities.

- Disabled persons shall enjoy all the rights set forth in this Declaration. These rights shall be granted to all disabled persons without any exception whatsoever and without distinction or discrimination on the basis of race, color, sex, language, religion, political or other opinions, national or social origin, state of wealth, birth, or any other situation applying either to the disabled person himself or herself or to his or her family.

- Disabled persons have the inherent right to respect for their human dignity. Disabled persons, whatever the origin, nature, and seriousness of their handicaps and disabilities, have the same fundamental rights as their fellow citizens of the same age, which implies first and foremost the right to enjoy a decent life, as normal and full as possible.

- Disabled persons are entitled to the measures designed to enable them to become as self-reliant as possible.

- Disabled persons have the right to medical, psychological, and functional treatment, including prosthetic and orthotic appliances, to medical and social rehabilitation, education, vocational training and rehabilitation, aid, counseling, placement services, and other services which will enable them to develop their capabilities and skills to the maximum and will hasten the process of their social integration or reintegration.

- Organizations of disabled persons may be usefully consulted in all matters regarding the rights of disabled persons.

- Disabled persons, their families, and communities shall be fully informed, by all appropriate means, of the rights contained in this Declaration.

An expressed philosophy or statement of beliefs is the foundation on which the goals of nursing practice are based. To attain the goals of nursing practice in rehabilitation requires the nurse to fulfill a multifaceted role, including direct-care coordination, education, counseling, and advocacy. The philosophy of nursing practiced at the Acute Spinal Cord Injury Unit at Shaughnessy Hospital in Vancouver, BC, closely parallels the beliefs expressed by Mahoney and those proclaimed by the United Nations. The unit's nursing philosophy emphasizes acute and concurrent rehabilitative care for the catastrophically injured. Although life-saving techniques take priority during the earliest phases of care, preventive and restorative measures must also begin on admission.

A correlation between philosophical beliefs and goal setting for nursing practice is outlined

TABLE 1–4 ■ CORRELATING AN EXPRESSED PHILOSOPHY WITH GOALS OF NURSING CARE FOR SPINAL CORD INJURED PATIENTS

Philosophy	Goals Are:	Nurse's Role Emphasized
1. Patients suffering from spinal cord injuries present a complex picture from a clinical, psychosocial, and economic point of view and are entitled to receive optimum care to meet their needs.	To provide or secure the best health care possible for patients suffering from spinal cord injuries.	Practitioner/advocate
2. Patients should be assisted to achieve and maintain an optimal level of physical and mental health and retain a sense of spiritual and social well-being.	To ensure that patients are cared for with respect as individuals and to help them reestablish their autonomy.	Counselor
3. Families (or significant others) constitute an integral part of patients' lives and should be included in comprehensive health care for spinal cord injured patients.	To provide psychosocial support to families and include them in assessing and meeting patients' rehabilitative needs.	Counselor
4. The nurse should develop expertise to apply the nursing process (assessment, goal setting, implementation, and evaluation) skillfully and systematically to ensure individualized total patient care.	To promote physical and psychological well-being by minimizing risk factors, practicing preventive measures when possible, recognizing onset of complications early, initiating immediate action within the scope of nursing practice and hospital policies, and evaluating care given.	Practitioner
5. Patient and family health education is an integral part of rehabilitation and must begin the moment of injury. Provision of an environment in which patients, families, and nurses can use their education, judgment, and individuality (creativity) is most conducive to a successful rehabilitation experience.	To provide a teaching/learning rehabilitation experience that actively involves patients (and families when appropriate) as participants and resource persons in the decision-making process, through which they can experience personal growth and independence.	Educator

(Table continues)

in Table 1–4. The table also identifies the aspect of the nurse's role emphasized by each goal.

Providing or securing optimal health care challenges the nurse's role as expert practitioner, coordinator, counselor, educator, and advocate. Frequently this involves defense of the rights of the disabled person: always it demands personal professional growth and development. The interdisciplinary conceptual approach to nursing people with spinal cord injuries is becoming a distinctive specialty in its own right. These concepts are, of course, part of general nursing practice; but they are of essence when hospitalization will profoundly affect the remainder of a person's life.

As advanced prehospital and medicosurgical techniques save people with greater and greater degrees of disability, undoubtedly the demands on the health care profession as a whole will proliferate. Nurses who specialize in rehabil-

TABLE 1–4 (continued)

Philosophy	Goals Are:	Nurse's Role Emphasized
6. Acute and concurrent rehabilitative care requires a skilled, well-integrated, interdisciplinary team. Nurses should cooperate and communicate with other team members to correlate treatment goals so that patients receive the maximum benefits from the interdisciplinary approach.	To provide coordinated care in a helpful, tolerable sequence for patients and families.	Coordinator
7. Nurses should assume major responsibility for coordination and continuity of health care to facilitate transition (relocation) periods, especially from an institution to the community.	To determine patients' readiness for discharge and to initiate appropriate follow-up health services.	Coordinator/practitioner
8. Nurses should take responsibility for assessing and improving personal knowledge, attitude, and skills and should maintain awareness of current developments in the health care field.	To plan and participate in ongoing educational activities on a regular basis.	Practitioner

■ PERSONAL VIEWPOINT

I was injured in a parachuting accident (my first jump) at age 23 and received a T_{12} spinal cord injury. This resulted in complete paralysis below that level, but I still have some preserved sensation. That was six years ago. Now I attend the university and live in an apartment in Vancouver's West Side. I am able to walk with the aid of bilateral short leg braces and arm crutches but use my wheelchair most of the time around home, on campus, and when shopping.

On looking back, the nurses at the Acute Spinal Cord Injury Unit at Shaughnessy Hospital played the most important role of all in helping me maintain my self-esteem and regain my independence.

During the early days when I depended on them for everything, they were never patronizing. Since many of them were my own age, they treated me like one of their peers. They related to the part of me that was whole and like them, not the part of me that had changed. They reassured me about my future by portraying their own positive attitude. At the same time they educated me about my body. They allowed me to participate in my care—first as an informed observer, then as a guided participant—until finally I was independent.

I will always remember the sensitivity that was used to help me accept my bowel and bladder routines. (We spent many long hours locked in the bathroom together!) The warmth and understanding that was shown to me by these special nurses will always be a treasured memory.

Colleen Smith

itation, be it in an acute or long-term setting, have much to contribute toward meeting this challenge. Sharing expertise as practitioners, researchers, change agents, and educators is an important part of our role. With our unique body of knowledge, skills, and caring we as nurses have a responsibility to present and future disabled people and their families: a responsibility that demands projection of ourselves at a personal, local, and national level to defend the rights of disabled people and to help secure the resources they require to fulfill their potential.

THE NURSING PROCESS

Goal-oriented rehabilitative care requires skillfull application of the nursing process. This continuous process involves the interrelated steps of assessment, goal setting, implementation, and evaluation. According to Andreoli and Thompson (1977):

> nurses must possess intellectual skills for problem-solving, critical thinking, and nursing judgments; interpersonal skills for the ability to communicate, listen, inform, and obtain necessary data in a manner that enhances the individuality of the client as a person; and finally technical skills to relate methods, procedures, and machines used to bring about specific results or the desired behavioral responses of the client.

A myriad of factors affect the quality of nursing care delivered, not the least of which are the personal attributes of each nurse. Caring for patients with severe physical disability demands a unique kind of interest and dedication and an openness to develop a positive attitude toward severe physical disability. The work is hard both physically and mentally, but the rewards are unquestionable, not depressing as many tend to think. Desirable qualities in any team member include: sound professional judgment, knowledge, and skills; ability to work enthusiastically and relate continually with others in a variety of situations in a close setting; willingness to learn from and to teach others; endless patience for exacting work; and a good sense of humor!

Assessment

Comprehensive assessment is the cornerstone on which to plan, implement, and evaluate nursing care. Developing expertise in assessment is a continual learning process because the consequences of spinal cord injury are so diverse, often subtle yet still devastating. To manage the vast potential of complications following spinal cord injury, the nurse must acquire specialized knowledge; adapt skills; and develop a helpful, positive attitude. A major premise of this book is *that many complications are entirely preventable or can be minimized if recognized early*. Prevention and early recognition of problems directly depend on astute nursing assessment. The quality of assessment is a pivotal component of the nursing process, directly enhancing or limiting the delivery of total patient care.

Assessment focuses on the patient's current health status and on collective background information that will also give direction to individualized care. Data pertaining to physical and psychological health are obtained from numerous sources: direct patient observation and contact; the medical record; diagnostic tests; monitoring devices; communication with other health team members; and consultation with significant people in the patient's life. The patient's health history is of vital importance. Factors such as associated injury, preexisting health and illness (both from a physical and a psychological viewpoint), and age profoundly influence how and to what extent each individual will experience the effects of spinal cord injury. Although the urgency of the situation will dictate priorities, an in-depth assessment is meaningful and quite possible, as the length of stay in any one setting for people with spinal cord injuries is usually extensive.

Goal Setting and Implementation

Planning and implementing goal-oriented care are progressive or building steps in the nursing process, which in rehabilitation must lead patients to take responsibility for managing the effects of their disability and maintaining optimal health care. Patients must participate in personal care, initially as informed observers and gradually as active performers.

■ *PERSONAL VIEWPOINT*

My first experience with the spinal cord injured patient was as Special Nurse in the Acute Spinal Cord Injury Unit at Vancouver's Shaughnessy Hospital. I was assigned to an acutely ill respirator-dependent young man, who had been involved in a motorcycle accident. His body was unmarked externally, but an instantaneous fracture (flexion type) of the fourth cervical vertebra had rendered him paralyzed. An innocent drive around the block and a reckless car driver would drastically alter the life of a young father and physical education teacher.

Six years after this dramatic entrance into the world of the spinal cord injured patient I am working at G. F. Strong Rehabilitation Centre in Vancouver with patients who have sustained a spinal cord injury and are anywhere from 3 to 18 months into their rehabilitation.

Certainly the person who has become disabled in this way has definite needs specific to his injury and future life-style.

The nurse's role within the rehabilitation setting is a relational one in terms of the patient working through the adjustment process. What I have realized is that quality of life is not so much external and circumstantial as it is conditional to the heart and the sense of purpose.

People who have been put into a situation where they no longer have control over some of their circumstances are acutely aware of how fragile physical life really is. They are the same people they were before the tragedy that changed their physical lives. Circumstances have really not changed who they are. They are brought face to face with questions about the deeper meaning and value of life, questions we all share. As a nurse relating to people in various stages of adjustment to their physical condition, it is a privilege to work with people looking for and sometimes finding answers to the questions we have all asked.

Deborah Good, RN

A major premise of this book is that *rehabilitation is a process that begins at the moment of injury.* Health care goals, from an interdisciplinary perspective, are presented in each chapter to facilitate care planning.

Evaluation

In the nursing process evaluation is necessary to determine the effectiveness of all the previous steps. Evaluation should be thought of as a continuous process, not a final step. Such continuous evaluation will ensure flexibility and give direction to care planning. To facilitate evaluation, most chapters list ideal outcome criteria for specific potential problems.

SELECTED REFERENCES

Andreoli, K., and Thompson, C. 1977. The nature of science in nursing. *Image* 9:32–37. *Exploration of the relationship between science and nursing, suggesting that although science does exist in nursing, the science of nursing is still at a very young stage.*

Committee on the Skeletal System, Division of Medical Sciences, National Research Council. 1967. *Report of a Conference on the Current Status of the Care of the Spinal Cord Injured Patient.* National Academy of Sciences, Washington, DC *Cited in Matlack* (1974).

Guidelines for Facility Categorization and Standards of Care: Spinal Cord Injury. 1981. Copyright American Spinal Injury Association and American Spinal Injury Association Foundation, Chicago, Ill. *Clearly presents purposes and requirements of the five major components of care; emergency medical services, trauma centers, specialized acute care and rehabilitation facilities, and follow-up community care.*

Guttman, L. 1976. *Spinal Cord Injuries Comprehensive Management and Research.* 2d ed. London: Blackwell Scientific Publications. *A classic, multifaceted reference text on spinal cord injuries. Includes historical background information; general statistics; legal aspects; detailed anatomy and neuropathology of cord trauma and resulting effects on all body systems; regeneration; fractures and dislocations, gunshot injuries and stab wounds; and neurophysiological and clinical management aspects. Extensive bibliography.*

Humphreys, R. R. 1978. *Role of Rehabilitation Services Administration in the Improvement of Spinal Cord Injury Services.* Proceedings of the National Spinal Cord Injury Model Systems Conference, Phoenix, Ariz: April 1978, pp. 3–5. *Overview of federal government concerns.*

Mahoney, K. E. 1979. A philosophical approach to nursing education. In *Current Perspectives in Rehabilitation Nursing,* Eds. R. Murray and J. L. Kijeck. St. Louis: C. V. Mosby, pp. 27–31. *Presents philosophical principles of rehabilitation, to help meet the ever-changing needs in society and thus in health care.*

Matlack, D. R. 1974. *Cost-effectiveness of Spinal Cord Injury Center Treatment.* National Spinal Cord Injury Foundation, Chicago, Ill. *Careful and specific documentation of financial savings to society when comprehensive and system care programs are made available. Cost savings analysis presented to stimulate expansion of other spinal cord systems throughout the United States. Highly recommended.*

National Spinal Cord Injury Foundation. What is spinal cord injury? And what can we do about it? 1981. *National Spinal Cord Injury Foundation Convention Journal,* Chicago, Ill. *Defines spinal cord injury and goals of the foundation. Includes implications for both health professionals and the general public.*

Perry, C., and Dever, P. 1976. *Acute Spinal Cord Injury Unit—A Successful Comprehensive Approach.* Proceedings of Annual Meeting of Canadian Association of Neurological and Neurosurgical Nurses. Winnipeg, Manitoba: 1976. *Overview of acute services for spinal cord injured persons and their families.*

Schweigel, J., and Peerless, S. 1971. A proposal for a spinal cord injury unit at Shaughnessy Hospital. Preliminary research review for Canadian Paraplegic Association, Vancouver, BC. *Summary of historical developments and current local developments to stimulate development of specialized services.*

Trieschmann, R. 1980. *Spinal Cord Injuries, Psychological, Social and Vocational Adjustment.* New York: Pergamon Press. *Only existing work exclusively devoted to the psychosocial impact of spinal cord injuries on both disabled people and their families. Includes an exhaustive critique of the literature with a view to dispelling myths and stimulating research.*

Young, J. S. 1978. *National Spinal Cord Injury Data Research Center.* Proceedings of the National Spinal Cord Injury Model Systems Conference, Phoenix, Ariz: April, pp. 9–12. *Statement of objectives and services.*

Young, J. S., and Northrup, N. E. 1979. *Statistical Information Pertaining to Some of the Most Commonly Asked Questions About Spinal Cord Injury.* National Spinal Cord Injury Data Research Center, Phoenix, Ariz. *Data collected from 1973 through 1978. Analyzes etiology, hospitalization time and costs, and some post-discharge factors. Ready reference in question/answer format, for example, what is the life expectancy of persons with spinal cord injury? Subheadings include demography, etiology, length of hospital stay, cost of hospitalization, use of ongoing services, social and vocational achievements, and life expectancy.*

SUPPLEMENTAL READING

Arndt, K.; Teterycz, P.; and Valentin, L. 1978. Interdisciplinary rehabilitation modules. *Supervisor Nurse* 9: 18–19. *A formal structure presented to enhance coordination of patient-focused rather than discipline-centered care.*

Bedbrook, G. 1979. Spinal injuries; an opportunity. *Australian and New Zealand Journal of Surgery* 49: 173–175. *An international perspective focusing on the need for development of spinal cord injury services.*

Byl, N. N. 1979. Teaching the concepts of rehabilitation in a primary care setting. *Archives of Physical Medicine and Rehabilitation* 60: 230–236. *Encourages daily chart reviews as a means to develop sensitivity among staff members to the problems of dys-*

function and to the rehabilitation resources available, thus promoting primary care staff's responsibility for problem solving.

Fine, P., et al. 1979. Spinal cord injury: an epidemiologic perspective. *International Journal of Paraplegia* 17: 237–250. *Select psychosocial characteristics indicate a high proportion of preinjury productivity, findings contrary to many previous beliefs.*

Gunley, P. 1981. From regeneration to prosthesis: research on spinal cord injury. *Journal of the American Medical Association* 245: 1293–1297. *Review of current American research in regeneration, old and new therapies, and prosthesis. Concise and clear.*

———. 1981. New focus on spinal cord injury. *Journal of the American Medical Association* 245: 1201–1206. *Updated overview of spinal cord injury centers in the United States. Also presents general overview of the care in the centers.*

Guttman, L. 1979. Past, present and future of the specialized service for spinal cord sufferers. *International Journal of Paraplegia* 17: 122–127. *Defends continuation of specialized services. An international perspective.*

Hassard, G. H., et al. 1978. The rehabilitation team. *Journal of Practical Nursing* 28: 23–25. *An overview of interdisciplinary interaction to achieve goal-oriented care. Directed toward the licensed practical nurse.*

Hendriksen, J. D. 1976. Specialized care of the spinal cord injured patient. *Journal of Practical Nursing* 26: 21, 34. *Focus on significance of preexisting health problems such as obesity, heart disease, and hypertension and advanced age.*

Koehler, M. L. 1981. Continuity of care for spinal cord injury—a reality. *Rehabilitation Nursing,* January–February, pp. 16–18. *Focus on continuing education for nurses in the expanded role; calls for specialization of nurses at each phase of care.*

Kowalsky, E. L. 1979. The nurse's role in health maintenance of the physically disabled client. *American Rehabilitation Nurses Journal* 4: 12–15. *A wellness-oriented approach to promotion of general health, which may be affected by limitations of disability; includes particularly helpful sections on dental care and nutrition.*

Kreger, S. M., and Whealon, R. 1981. A procedure for goal-setting: a method for formulating goals and treatment plans. *Rehabilitation Nursing* 6: 22–25, 30–31. *Describes role of primary nursing in ensuring collaborative, interdisciplinary goal setting; focuses on patient and family input and involvement.*

Kurtzke, J. F. 1975. Epidemiology of spinal cord injury. *Experimental Neurology* 48: 163–236. *A detailed overview of international data with concise summary as it applies to the United States.*

McKibbin, B. 1976. The clinical team in action—the management of spinal injuries: Part 1. *Nursing Mirror,* 25 November, pp. 47–58. *A British perspective of interdisciplinary care.*

Shea, J. D. 1979. Spinal cord injury—state of the art in Florida. *Journal of the Florida Medical Association* 66: 68–70. *Model for initiating comprehensive care that looks beyond the medical-surgical problems to total rehabilitation and community reentry.*

Starck, P. L. 1978. A model for emphasizing rehabilitation in the nursing process. *American Rehabilitation Nurses Journal* (March–April): 10–15. *Presents a model to incorporate the principles of rehabilitation into the nursing process in any care setting. Includes valuable comprehensive assessment tools and correlates intervention and evaluation guidelines. Highly recommended.*

Tator, C., and Edmonds, V. 1979. Acute spinal cord injury: analysis of epidemiological factors. *Canadian Journal of Surgery* 22: 575–578. *A Canadian perspective with particular reference to age and cause with future implications for preventive care.*

Thomas, J. P. 1978. *Rehabilitation Services Administration Model Systems Concept.* Proceedings of the National Spinal Cord Injury Model Systems Conference, Phoenix, Ariz: April, pp. 5–9. *Overview of components, from emergency to community care.*

Tretick, G. 1978. The rehabilitation nurse as a vital member of the rehabilitation team. *Journal of Practical Nursing* 28: 26–28. *Valuable introductory reading for the licensed practical nurse in an interdisciplinary care team.*

Walsh, A. 1980. *The Expanded Role of the Rehabilitation Nurse.* Thorofare, NJ: Charles B. Slack. *Based on a three-day symposium held in California, the book defines new roles, discusses specific educational preparations, and explores ways to contribute nursing expertise to the severely disabled.*

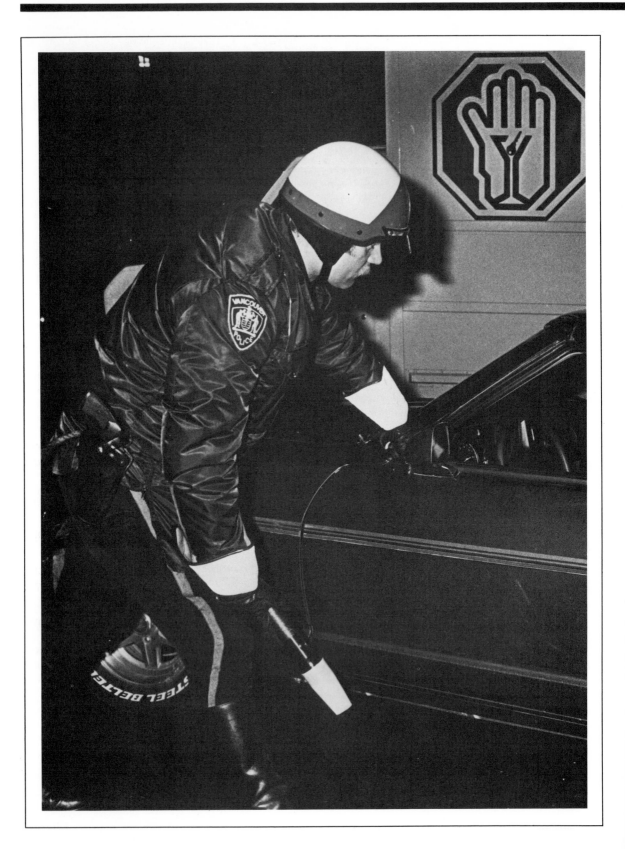

Chapter 2

Prevention

OBJECTIVES

- To increase nurses' awareness of the scope of known precautions to minimize risk of spinal cord injury
- To help health care professionals realize their responsibilities in preventive health care
- To recognize and use opportunities for participation
- To indicate the significance of such forces as the media and legislative bodies in mass communication of preventive messages
- To describe components of accident prevention programs

Prevention, in its broadest sense, is a fundamental concept of this book. Three levels of prevention are of concern (Fleshman and Jacobson 1979: 4):

- *Primary prevention deals with health promotion and specific protection against disease.* Or as is the case with spinal cord injury, accident. Public education regarding the consequences of actions involving alcohol and drug abuse combined with driving and other high-risk activities is an example of health promotion. Specific protection includes law enforcement for usage of passenger restraint systems (seat belts and car seats) and against traffic violators and drunk drivers.
- *Secondary prevention focuses on early diagnosis and prompt intervention in the disease process.* Professional specialization in emergency health services and public education in first aid are examples of secondary prevention. Indeed, recognizing accident victims who have received or who are at risk of receiving a spinal cord injury will ensure appropriate treatment is begun. Most primary care services are aimed at prevention of secondary complications.
- *Tertiary prevention uses rehabilitation activities to prevent further complications and to restore as much as possible in the way of optimal functioning.* For example, development and utilization of spinal cord injury centers would significantly help more spinal cord injury victims to achieve their fullest potential of returning to the community as persons of independence and worth.

This chapter will concern itself with primary prevention.

GOALS OF PREVENTION

Accident and injury prevention is a public health issue. Health care professionals must become active in accident prevention; we must probe how organizations can develop media, educational, and legislative programs; and we must explore ways in which public health groups and the government can work together to develop strong, nationwide accident prevention programs. Goals of health care in primary prevention are:

- To act as a motivating resource for preventive health care activities
- To communicate preventive measures to the general public
- To motivate the general public to take responsibility for practicing safety precautions
- To participate with others in protecting children and developing safety-conscious behavior at an early age

In many ways primary prevention of disease demands little effort on the part of the general public. Health care professionals do most of the work, requiring beneficiaries to do little more than show up and take their medicine. For example, immunization programs against polio have virtually eradicated this disease, which in the past accounted for a large proportion of people with paraplegia and quadriplegia. Programs designed to prevent the new major causes of spinal cord injury—motor vehicle accidents, penetrating wounds, sports accidents, and falls—will require more active participation by members of the public. The problem is that we have not yet learned how to make information available to people in ways that will motivate them to take responsibility for their own health and safety (Fleshman and Jacobson 1979). Programs to enhance primary prevention extend well beyond nursing and other health care professions to include such forces as the media, educators, the legal profession, and legislative bodies. However, health care professionals and those who are disabled or have suffered personal loss tend to initiate preventive actions as exemplified in the accompanying personal viewpoints. People who deal with the daily realities of disability provide a credible resource and a strong motivating influence for prevention. The last section of this chapter presents a model plan for developing primary prevention programs.

ASSESSMENT AND INTERVENTIONS IN PREVENTION

Epidemiological factors give direction to preventive activities. Assessment of cause, incidence and prevalence of age, racial background, sex, and other subgroups, especially in relation to risk-taking behavior, helps indicate to whom and how teaching would be most effective.

Currently, major preventive activities are directed toward motor vehicle accident prevention. Lack of protection from adult or child passenger restraint systems, alcohol and drug abuse problems, and unsafe motorcycle practices pose significant threats to public safety. Widespread public education, specific legislation to enforce mandatory use of restraint systems, and continued research to improve or design alternatives for restraint systems will help reduce these risks. The combination of alcohol or drug abuse with driving presents more complex problems.

> Against accidents, the attack is education, manufacturing with safety of employees and customers in mind, safety legislation, and continued research. [DHEW 1971: 8]

■ *PERSONAL VIEWPOINT*

Recently a group of victims, survivors, and concerned citizens formed Mothers Against Drunken Drivers (MADD). The group is committed to preventing the tragic consequences of alcohol-related accidents by mounting a strong consumer voice in educational and civic affairs. Representatives of MADD provide service and consultation to community, business, and educational groups, including medical facilities and driver education programs. Their efforts have resulted in the development of several state task forces to study the problem of drunk driving. They also work on a national level to support legislation for reform of laws on drunk driving.

In Washington, D.C., preventive activities of the National Highway Traffic Safety Administration continue to include investigation into results of trauma to the spinal cord during accident simulations with lifelike figures. This administration uses the information gathered to support

---

■ *PERSONAL VIEWPOINT*

The Canadian Paraplegic Association is an example of an organized group of disabled persons in the community who include preventive activities among their services. For example, with the help of health care professionals, the B.C. Division was instrumental in securing mandatory seat belt legislation in the province. Every summer the following radio messages are aired regularly, and more frequently during holiday weekends, to increase safety awareness.

"It's tragic the number of young people who become permanently paralyzed each year in accidents. Last year alone, 134 people were admitted to the Spinal Cord Injury Unit in our province. Most of these people will be in wheelchairs for the rest of their lives. More than half of these injuries occurred in motor vehicle accidents. The Canadian Paraplegic Association wants to remind you to buckle up, drive sober, and drive safely. We're not fooling. It can happen to you."

"Have you heard the story about the fellow that dove into the empty swimming pool? Well, to us it's not a joke because every summer there are a number of people who do just that and end up in a wheelchair for the rest of their lives. We're the Canadian Paraplegic Association, and we're reminding you to be careful this summer. Be sure the water is deep enough before you dive—otherwise, you can be plunging into more than you bargained for."

Source: Canadian Paraplegic Association, B.C. Division (1981).

lower speed limits and passenger restraint systems.

There is also national interest in data collection to determine causes of sporting injuries and to develop guidelines to help prevent them. The National Athletic Trainers Association and the Center for Sports Medicine at Temple University School of Medicine, Philadelphia, have established a national head and neck injury registry, for example.

Indisputably, today's challenge, in terms of preventing spinal cord injury, is to motivate the general public to apply what is already known and to realize the possible consequences of their actions. However, practicing safety precautions and minimizing risk situations may be viewed as inconvenient at best, or as an impingement on personal life-style. For example, some people consider mandatory seat belt legislation a violation of human rights and some refuse to accept responsibility for the consequences of their actions while under the influence of alcohol or drugs. Ultimately, however, real primary prevention rests with personal control of life-styles. This is not meant to imply that all spinal cord injuries are directly or indirectly self-induced; some are associated with risk taking but many are innocent victims.

■ A Model Plan for Rehabilitation Hospitals/Spinal Cord Injury Treatment Centers to Develop Accident Prevention Programs

The Rehabilitation Institute of Chicago (RIC) and the Midwest Regional Spinal Cord Injury Care System have developed a preventive medicine program which could serve as a blueprint for other institutions interested in stemming the epidemic of disabling accidents which they treat. Begun in September 1978 as the result of a citywide conference entitled "Youth and Driving, the Road to Death," *Accident Prevention/Chicago* was initially designed to impact on teenage accidents. It has been expanded, however, to include other areas that often cause disabling accidents in the young; diving and handgun mishaps are two examples.

The program is directed by an RIC staff member in collaboration with an advisory council and steering committee of educators, business people, health care professionals, and representatives of Chicago government, law enforcement, and the media.

Accident Prevention/Chicago has two phases; one phase is immediate and media oriented; the other phase is long range and educational.

Immediate and Media-Oriented Prevention

As part of the first phase, the program was instrumental in effecting legislation to raise the drinking age in Illinois from 18 to 21. Research studies show that when the drinking age was lowered to 18 from 21, the number of teenage driving accidents soared. Accordingly, a staunch stand in support of legislation to reverse the move was appropriate. To this end, a videotape was sent to the Illinois Legislature dramatically showing the disabilities and difficulties of four young men, all former RIC patients who were disabled by alcohol-related accidents. The media reacted most favorably to an institution of RIC's stature taking a stand on such an issue.

Currently *Accident Prevention/Chicago* is active in both state and national initiatives to tighten legislation dealing with those who drive while intoxicated. Because we see the tragic results of this type of behavior, our efforts to strengthen laws are very credible.

(Box continues)

■ *Model Plan (continued)*

As well as being an office that can lend support to lobbying efforts, *Accident Prevention/Chicago* is working in other visual areas to encourage the use of seat belts and the practice of safe driving techniques. Because it is known that we live in a media society, we are attempting to creatively use the media in a variety of ways to further our goals. *Accident Prevention/Chicago* has been assisted by the creative staff of a large advertising agency, for example, to produce Public Service Advertising spots aimed at children to encourage the use of seat belts.

One of our most visible (and audible) areas of endeavor is our 60-second radio public service announcement series produced by CBS Radio Network. The series was designed to encourage safety in driving over the Labor Day Weekend and throughout the year. The tapes, produced locally and aired nationally, incorporated testimonials from five former RIC patients all talking about the events leading up to their accident and the resulting physical disabilities. This was not done as a "scare" technique, but rather to deeply impress the general public with how dramatically one's life changes in one, brief, irretrievable moment. This series was made in cooperation with the National Safety Council, which provided us with fatality and serious injury statistics. The tapes were given cross-country attention, not only on the radio but on network and local television news shows and in newspapers everywhere. It is our plan that a series of radio spots will be aired each major holiday period.

We also address disabilities resulting from diving accidents and handgun mishaps. In addition to helping with public information on stories on diving accidents, diving safety is being promoted by a comical poster nicknamed "Mr. Clunk." This poster has been distributed by RIC and the Midwest Regional Spinal Cord Injury Care System staff to the Chicago and Regional Transit Authorities, major motel chains, the YMCA, academic institutions, and park districts. We are hoping that "Mr. Clunk" will be to hazardous actions what "Mr. Yuk" has been to poisonous substances. With respect to handguns, we are a reference/resource center for the Committee for Handgun Control in the city, and for interested, responsible media people.

In a collaborative effort with the Women's Board of the RIC, a film entitled *Consequences: Spinal Cord Injury* (produced under the sponsorship of the Northwest Regional Spinal Cord Injury Center at the University of Washington in Seattle) has been disseminated to school groups throughout the Chicago area. It is used as a springboard for discussion about safety and the notion that wheelchairs are "not just for grownups."

Consequences: Spinal Cord Injury is a powerful but sensitive presentation showing young people involved in high-velocity, high-risk activities. The message is NOT *don't do it,* BUT *if you're going to do it, do it well, and know your limitations.* The consequences are described by young people who have broken their necks, "telling it like it is." The film runs 9 minutes and was produced to have great appeal to young audiences. Of particular value to the nurse-educator involved with school or young teenage groups is a study guide developed for use with the film. The study guide, presented on the next page, could be improved by including statistics, a set of definitions, and suggestions for different age groups.

■ *Model Plan (continued)*

STUDY GUIDE FOR THE FILM "CONSEQUENCES"

Time Frame	This teaching module is also designed to fit into a 40–45 minute class session. Make this clear when presenting the idea initially to teachers and principals. The space and timing of the film showing is extremely important. This film should *never* be shown in a large assembly fashion.
Level	Junior High School through High School (Grades 6–12/Ages 12–18).
Structure	The presentation should be divided into three segments: prediscussion, film showing, and postdiscussion. Each of these segments is equal in importance, and should not be skipped.
Subject Area Where Film Might be Shown	Health, Physical Education, Physical Science, Psychology, and Drivers Education. It is a good idea to have the teacher remain in the room to intervene when necessary. Thought should be given to involving the physical education departments when possible. The student population we are focusing on generally respects the coaching staff as strong role models and thus would be influenced positively by them.
Calendar Time When Film Can Be Shown	Eighth graders and seniors in high school are usually very busy in late spring, so when targeting these groups especially attempt to schedule the presentation in the fall: October or November. The fall or early spring are good times to show the film.
Before the Film	Lead the class in an opening discussion about the film. The instructor should make a few remarks about the film and its purpose. Ask students to pose the following questions to themselves as they watch the film. Who are the people in the film? In what ways are they like me? How are they different from me? What are the requirements of a skilled sportsperson? The teacher should stress that the purpose of the film is not to scare the students or tell them what to do, but to make them aware of some of the causes of physical disability and ways to prevent these types of problems from occurring. Also stress the positive aspects of the message: that they have control over their lives, that all of this goes hand in hand with health and taking care of yourself. Students in this age bracket will tend to deny anything which reminds them they are less than invulnerable or capable of anything they wish. Presenters are encouraged to expand prediscussion ideas; try to maximize group involvement. Ask the students if they are familiar with local rehabilitation facilities and initiate discussion about people they know with spinal cord injury.
After the Film	Again stress that this film was not meant to scare them, but to present some additional information about high-risk activities. REDEFINE clearly the following: spinal cord injury quadriplegia paraplegia

(Box continues)

■ *Model Plan (continued)*

Writing or Discussion Activities

Ask students to trace their daily activities: think about all those same things if they were in a wheelchair or could not use their hands. How would their personal and social life be changed?

Ask students how they would deal with possible lifelong dependency.

Ask them to think about what causes them to lose control: lead into drugs and alcohol. (This particular aspect possibly should be written as opposed to discussed due to peer group feelings making it a delicate issue.) Discuss how peer group pressure affects risk-taking behavior.

Ask students for the key words. There are key words which may be used again and again:

"hellraiser"

"new life"

"born again" (what this really means)

Ask them how they might lessen risk in each of their lives. Try to relate the film to local sports, situations, and interests. Work in the concept of limit setting and that a set of reliable values/goals can preserve your life.

Source: Mary Beth Berkoff, Director, Accident Prevention/Chicago Rehabilitation Institute of Chicago, Ill.

Long-Range and Educational Activities

As previously stated, it is important to influence children's behavior to encourage them to begin safe behaviors at an early age. In regard to this long-range educational phase of our program we have approached major television programmers requesting them to include coherent, consistent safety messages in basic children's programming. For example, we have encouraged them to show people buckling up when getting into a car, checking the depth before they dive into unknown waters, wearing adequate protection when involved in sports or riding a motorcycle. We believe that positive role modeling in this most influential format will augment our other educational endeavors.

Everybody wears a seat belt—even clowns and gorillas—in a series of innovative, new public service announcements

aired on nationwide network and local children's television programs. Announcements were funded by the Illinois Department of Transportation. Because of their quality and because they fill a void in public service advertising, these spots, titled *Belt Someone*, have received incredibly widespread airing.

Similar to our approach with television programmers, we have been developing a strategy to encourage textbook manufacturers to include basic safety messages in their earliest learning materials. In order for them to be effective, we believe that safety messages must not be extra; they must be fully integrated into a person's education from the earliest years.

Consistent with the belief that behaviors are formed at an early age, *Accident Prevention/Chicago* has addressed and been actively involved in providing adequate child passenger protection. This activity resulted

(Box continues)

■ *Model Plan (continued)*

in our organizing a workshop and giving public testimony at a Child Passenger Protection Conference sponsored by the National Highway Traffic Safety Administration in December 1979. We addressed the need for media support of our efforts, both by including positive safety messages in their programming and by eliminating unsafe messages from their existing shows.

At the present time we are engaged most actively in this type of legislation. Following a child passenger safety conference here at the Institute, the Illinois Child Passenger Safety Association was formed to educate the people of Illinois about the importance of restraining small children in cars. Building on the experience of Tennessee, where the first child passenger law was passed in 1978; where child restraint usage has tripled; and fatalities of children under the age of five in cars has been cut in half, we are attempting to see that this type of law is passed in Illinois.

Most recently, a new series of commercials, called *The Cure,* are designed to convince adults that to protect their children adequately in cars, they must put them in seat belts or car seats. This idea is also being ex-

panded to extend the campaign into other media areas.

Using the resources of this office, this institution, in fact the whole medical center, we have been able to provide a unique service to the entire community. By supplying information to the media, to the schools, and lending our support to legislative efforts consistent with our goals we are attempting to prevent the types of disabling accidents we treat.

We see *Accident Prevention/Chicago* as a functioning and active resource for the community. It may be a model for other such programs in similar health care facilities. If there were a network of these programs throughout the country, the strength of the individual programs would increase geometrically. Our goals include a continuation and expansion of ongoing projects and evaluation followed by possible entry into areas where our influence would cause change in our society.

Source: Mary Beth Berkoff, Director, *Accident Prevention/Chicago* Rehabilitation Institute of Chicago, Ill.

End

SELECTED REFERENCES

DHEW. 1971. *Spinal Cord Injury, Hope Through Research.* DHEW Publication No. (NIH) 72–160. Public Health Service Publication No. 1747, Health Information Series No. 143. *Presents overview of definitions, economic factors, and care requirements; focuses on status of spinal cord regeneration research.*

Fleshman, R. P., and Jacobson, M. J. 1979. An introduction to community health nursing. In *Community Health Nursing.* 2d ed. Eds. S. E. Archer and R. P. Fleshman. North Scituate, Mass: Duxbury Press. *Chapter 1 describes roles, preventive concepts, and challenges in community health nursing.*

Lechman, B. C., and Bonwich, E. B. 1981. Evaluation of an education program for spinal cord injury prevention: some preliminary findings. *Spinal Cord Injury Digest* 3: 27–34. *The Missouri Regional Spinal Cord Injury System undertook a spinal cord injury prevention campaign in the spring of 1980. This program was directed at the most accessible high-risk population—local high school students. Preliminary analysis suggests that the program does have a positive effect.*

SUPPLEMENTAL READING

Betts, H. 1977. An interdisciplinary congress in disability prevention, community involvement and consumer concern. *Archives of Physical Medicine Rehabilitation* 48: 191–195. *A multifaceted overview of the concept of prevention and suggestions for development.*

Gunley, P. 1981. From regeneration to prosthesis: research on spinal cord injury. *Journal of the American Medical Association* 245: 1293–1297. *The complexities and unknown factors encountered in research clearly emphasizes the paramount importance of prevention of injury.*

Selzer, M. L., and Payne, C. E. 1962. Automobile accidents, suicide and unconscious motivation. *American Journal of Psychiatry* 119: 237–240. *Increases awareness of how to recognize people with this problem and thus gives direction to prevention.*

Smart, R. G., 1980. *The New Drinkers.* 2d ed. Toronto, Canada: Addiction Research Foundation. *An informative source drawn from current Canadian and American research; explores problems of young people and alcohol abuse and emphasizes prevention. Describes possible roles and activities of parents, young people, schools, health professionals, and governments.*

Tator, C. H.; Edmonds, V. E.; and New, M. L. 1981. Diving: a frequent and potentially preventable cause of spinal cord injury. *Canadian Medical Association Journal* 124:1323–1324. *A retrospective study of 358 patients in Toronto with acute spinal cord injury showed 11% of the 358 injuries were due to diving accidents. The authors suggest education about the hazards of diving.*

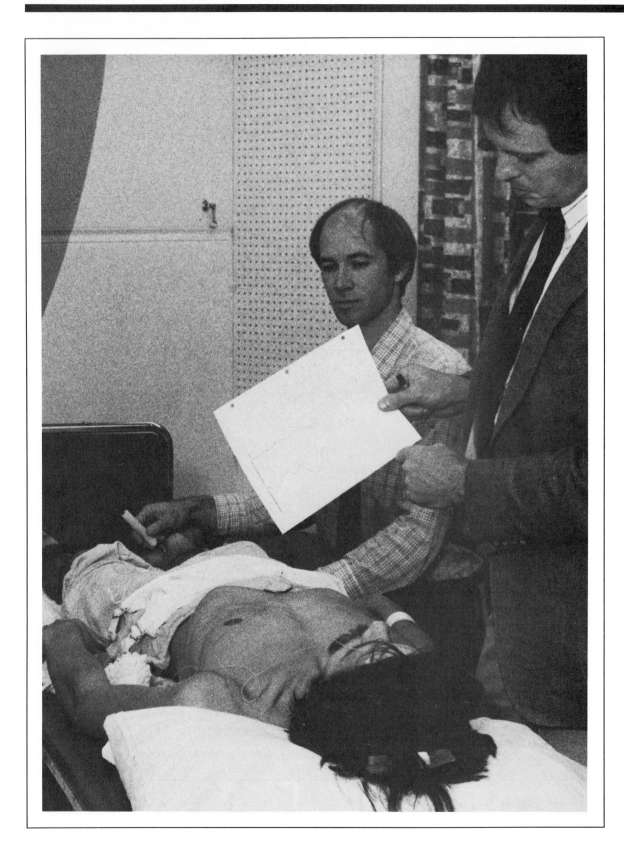

PART II

PROVIDING
EARLY ASSESSMENT
AND CARE

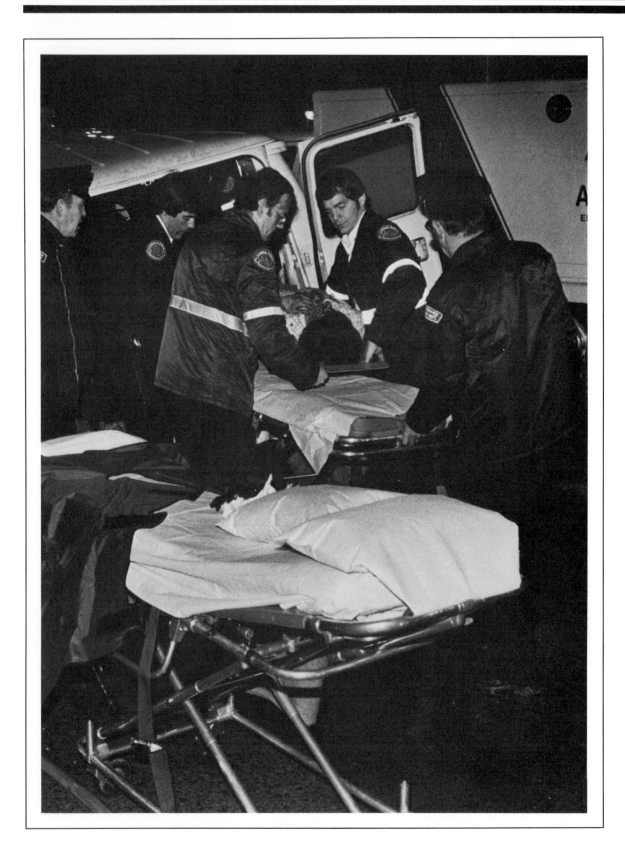

Chapter 3

Prehospital Care for People with Spinal Injuries*

CHAPTER OUTLINE

OBJECTIVES

- To explain the significance of anticipating a spinal injury in a trauma victim
- To recognize mechanisms of injury and describe their significance
- To describe priorities of prehospital care
- To explain jaw thrust and chin lift maneuvers to open the airway
- To describe how to immobilize the spine
- To describe history taking and physical examination in prehospital care
- To describe care during transport and identify potential problems

---

* Modified from *Acute Care of the Spinal Cord Injured at the Site of Injury.* Courtesy of R. Rimel, R. Eldich, H. Winn, A. Butler, and J. John. Copyright the Rector and Visitors of the University of Virginia, 1978.

The ultimate outcome of only a few injuries is as dependent on prehospital care as spinal cord injury. Expert rescue, rapid transport, and coordination with trauma facilities are essential components of management.

GOALS OF PREHOSPITAL CARE

The key to prehospital management is to anticipate the possibility of a spinal cord injury in the trauma victim before an attempt is made to move the patient. *The type of accident is the key factor in identifying trauma victims also at risk of spinal injury. In a victim with a head injury or an unconscious victim, assume that there may be a spinal injury present.* If in doubt, always assume there is a spinal cord injury and treat accordingly.

The goals of prehospital care are:

- To anticipate the possibility of a spinal cord injury in the trauma victim and initiate appropriate treatment
- To administer life-saving priority techniques oriented toward the possibility of spinal cord injury
- To prevent further neurological damage in the patient with a spinal cord injury

ASSESSMENT AND INTERVENTIONS IN PREHOSPITAL CARE

In addition to anticipating a spinal cord injury, emergency personnel must complete a primary survey of the patient to determine (1) if the patient is responsive and breathing or breathing without difficulty, and (2) if the patient is bleeding. When these priorities are stabilized, a secondary survey including history taking and a physical and neurological assessment can then be carried out.

Stabilizing the Patient

Airway and breathing

Care to establish an airway and breathing must be adapted to the possibility of spinal cord injury. Respiratory depression can be caused by several factors. In the unconscious patient major problems are aspiration and the tongue falling back, occluding the airway. In a patient with a neck fracture, the nerve control to the muscles of breathing may be impaired. Patients sustaining injury to the higher portion of the cervical cord (C_4 and above) cannot breathe spontaneously because innervations to the diaphragm and other chest muscles needed for breathing are immediately lost. Injury sustained to the lower portion of the cervical cord (C_5 and below) render the diaphragm as the only driving force for breathing. With diaphragmatic breathing, the chest does not rise and fall with respiration. Instead, there is a more exaggerated movement of the abdominal muscles. Fatigue and possible increasing neurological impairment pose significant hazards to sustained breathing. (Chapter 9 details assessment and management of respiratory depression.)

If the patient is unresponsive, determine whether the patient is breathing. Without moving the patient's neck, face the patient's chest, place your cheek near the patient's mouth, and

- *look* for rise and fall of the chest
- *listen* for breath sounds
- *feel* for the patient's carotid pulse

Patients are found in many awkward positions. Return the patient to the supine position. If the neck is twisted, when placed supine, apply *very gentle* traction to the head while straightening the neck and body. If breathing is not restored by this maneuver, open the airway by using the modified jaw thrust maneuver. This procedure lifts the tongue off the back of the throat without moving the neck. See Procedure 3–1.

If the patient is still not breathing, continue with airway management. If the chest does not rise use the chin lift maneuver in conjunction with as much extension of the neck as is required to open the airway. See Procedure 3–2. After an

PROCEDURE 3–1 ■ THE JAW THRUST MANEUVER

Purpose

The jaw thrust maneuver, or forward displacement of the jaw, is a technique designed to minimize neck movement when opening the upper airway, rather than the standard maneuver, which is to hyperextend the neck. This maneuver is indicated for a patient with a fractured cervical spine.

Action	Rationale
1. Stand or kneel behind the patient's head if possible; place hands on either side of the patient's head.	To maintain the head and neck in a fixed, neutral position without hyperextension or tilting from side to side.
2. Support elbows on the surface on which the patient is lying.	To provide an anchor point to gain momentum for the maneuver.
3. Grasp the angles of the patient's lower jaw with fingers, place thumbs carefully on patient's cheekbones.	Positioning of thumbs also provides an opposing point to gain momentum with lifting movement.
4. Using the thumbs to provide a focal point for opposing pressure, thrust (displace) the jaw forward with a lifting movement.	This thrust unlocks the jaw and avoids inadvertent movement of the head.

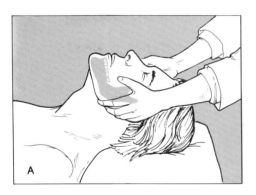 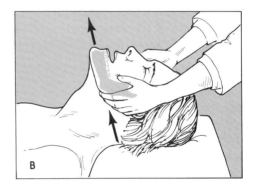

5. If the lips close, quickly move one thumb to retract the lower lip.	
6. If this is unsuccessful, tilt the head slightly backward and make another attempt to open the airway.	Establishing an open airway takes priority over treatment of the spinal cord injury.

airway is established begin to assist ventilation. Deliver two breaths every five seconds. This ventilatory rate is approximately twice that of normal. Ideally, 100% humidified oxygen should be delivered by a bag-mask resuscitator. Pay careful attention to the accumulation of fluid in the throat of the unconscious patient. Insert a plastic catheter along the oral airway to suction the nasopharynx as needed. When the patient regains consciousness, remove the oral airway immediately.

In the unconscious spinal cord injured patient establishing an airway and assisting ventilation is usually sufficient to revive the patient. For example, a patient with C_5 quadriplegia was found unresponsive and not breathing but had a

PROCEDURE 3–2 ■ THE CHIN LIFT MANEUVER

Purpose

To open the airway with minimal extension of the neck. This maneuver is indicated if the jaw thrust maneuver is unsuccessful.

Action	Rationale
1. Using one hand, place your thumb in the patient's mouth with the thumbnail between the patient's teeth; grasp the patient under the chin with your fingers.	If the patient's mouth closes, the teeth will strike your thumbnail.
2. Lift the patient's chin.	
3. Observe for elevation of the chest to indicate air entry.	
4. If unsuccessful, repeat maneuver using as much extension of the neck as required.	Establishing an open airway takes priority over treatment of the spinal cord injury.

carotid pulse. Hyperventilation with an oxygenated bag-mask resuscitator was successful in relieving hypoxia and reviving the patient. If these techniques are not successful, intubation, by those who have had advanced training, is then necessary.

In the conscious patient who is breathing, administer humidified oxygen (10 liters/min) via a reservoir mask to protect the cord from oxygen deprivation, especially if the patient is hypotensive.

If a spine and chest injury both occur (and this is not uncommon with fractures of the thoracic spine), stabilize the patient on a *scoop* stretcher secured to a long backboard for maximum lateral support. Tip toward the affected side of the chest. This allows for greater expansion of the unaffected lung.

Circulation

Low blood pressure occurs with cord injury because the autonomic nervous system that controls the size and tone of blood vessels throughout the body is disrupted. Also hypovolemic shock from blood loss can occur in any trauma victim. The hypotensive state caused by loss of peripheral vascular resistance with blood pooling in the extremities differs from hypovolemic shock in that the patients have warm, dry skin with full veins and a more regular, not rapid, pulse. Rapid transport is indicated for medical management. (See Chapter 10 for discussion of this complication.)

History and physical examination

The types of trauma most likely to result in spinal fracture and instability are (1) automobile and motorcycle accidents (particularly accidents that involve violent forces), (2) gunshot wounds, (3) diving injuries, (4) cave-ins, and (5) falls (from heights, in the home, and from falling objects). The type of accident will give direction to the steps involved in prehospital history taking and physical examination. See Procedures 3–3 and 3–4.

The forces or stresses imposed by the accident that produces spinal cord injury are described as *mechanisms of injury* and detailed in Chapter 5 (Table 5–1). Describing the accident as accurately as possible aids in diagnosis and early hospital management.

Immobilizing the Patient Before Transport

The cardinal principle in moving a patient with a suspected spinal injury is to prevent any motion of the spine that can further damage the cord or nerve roots. Immobilizing the patient's head, neck, and back before and during transport protects the patient from further injury. See Procedure 3–5.

PROCEDURE 3–3 ■ TAKING A HISTORY IN PREHOSPITAL CARE

Purpose

The purpose of taking a history in prehospital care is to determine how the injury was sustained (mechanism of injury) and if any other medical factors require emergency intervention. This information has implications for management.

Action	Rationale
If the patient is conscious:	
1. Ask what bothers him or her the most (*isolation of chief complaint*).	Isolation of chief complaint gives direction to further questioning. If, for example, patient complains of difficulty in breathing, the nature of the complaint must be clarified. Checking medical history for such problems as cardiac insufficiency or asthma helps determine whether difficult breathing is a direct result of cord injury or not.
2. Ask if there is any neck or back pain.	Patient will likely have severe pain in the affected area, which will localize level of injury.
3. Ask if patient has any medical problems, is on any medication, has taken any alcohol or drugs.	
If the patient is unconscious or unable to provide reliable information:	
4. Ask a witness (a relative if possible) these same questions.	

To stabilize the neck, one rescuer must apply traction to the head, while another applies a cervical collar and secures it. Backboards are used to stabilize the head, neck, and torso. Victims found lying on the ground should be transported on a long backboard, but victims in a sitting position should be immobilized on a short backboard before being transferred to the long backboard. See Procedures 3–6 and 3–7 for using long and short backboards.

The Robinson orthopedic stretcher, sometimes described as a *scoop* or *split-away* stretcher, is an ideal adjunct to the long backboard and is carried on an increasing number of emergency vehicles. This apparatus divides longitudinally for ease in lifting the patient with minimal risk of moving the unstable spine. It provides a rigid surface suitable for transport and greatly simplifies subsequent transfers on admission to the hospital. Procedure 3–6 also describes the combined use of the scoop stretcher with the long backboard.

Nongravitational dependent systems are recommended for cervical traction. In this method, a traction or extension force is secured or tied on to the carrying apparatus, avoiding use of weights that become hazardous with the movement of the plane or vehicle. Particular care is necessary to secure the patient's head, trunk, and limbs to the carrying apparatus so that movement of the patient's body weight will not add stress on the tensioning device.

In handling victims sustaining possible spinal injury from water-related accidents, such as diving or boating mishaps, remove them from the water *only* after the neck or back has been splinted properly. See Procedure 3–8.

Transporting the Patient to Appropriate Medical Facility

After stabilizing, a patient should be quickly transported to an appropriate medical facility, ideally a trauma center. If this distance is greater

PROCEDURE 3-4 ■ PERFORMING A PREHOSPITAL PHYSICAL ASSESSMENT

Purpose

The purpose of performing an immediate physical assessment is to detect injury to the spinal cord.

Action	Rationale
1. Measure and record vital signs (pulse, respirations, and blood pressure).	Abnormalities in vital signs due to spinal cord injury are discussed in Chapters 4 and 10.
2. Assess motor strength in upper and lower extremities: • Ask if there is any weakness in arms or legs.	Spinal cord injury must be suspected if the patient has any difficulty in moving extremities on command. If patient shows any obvious weakness, assume there is injury to the spinal cord.
• Ask patient to wiggle fingers of both hands. If this is achieved, have patient raise arms, one at a time. Now, ask patient to squeeze your fingers with both hands. • Ask patient to wiggles toes. If toes of both feet can wiggle, ask patient to raise legs slightly, one at a time.	Movement of the upper extremity is undertaken if no obvious fractures are present. The strength of patient's grasp should be similar in both hands. If patient cannot move fingers and arms, or has obvious weakness, he or she probably has spinal cord damage in the neck, whereas failure of only the lower extremities to respond indicates injury to the back.
3. Perform sensory examination: • Ask if there is any numbness in arms or legs. • Touch patient's ankles and wrists and ask if your touch is felt.	The presence of a sensory deficit confirms the suspicion of cord injury. If your touch is felt, spinal cord damage is not probable. If your touch is not felt in one or more places, or if there is numbness or tingling, spinal cord damage is likely.
4. Check the condition of the spinal cord in the unconscious patient who is a victim of trauma:	The unconscious patient who is a victim of trauma should be suspected of having a spinal cord injury because the forces necessary to produce a brain injury are also in the range of those that cause spinal injuries.
• Observe for *diaphragmatic breathing.*	The presence of diaphragmatic breathing in an unconscious patient is the most obvious sign that a spinal cord injury exists.
• Prick the fingertips of each hand and soles of the feet or skin of the ankles with a sharp object, such as a pin.	If there is no spinal cord damage, the painful stimulus triggers an involuntary muscular reflex and the extremity will move. If the cord is damaged, there will be no reflex reaction. Lack of response to a pinprick in the upper extremities indicates damage to the spinal cord in the neck, whereas failure of only the lower extremities to respond indicates injury in the spinal cord of the back.

than 60 miles (97 kilometers) air evacuation is indicated; if less than 60 miles use ground transportation. During transport, monitor the patient's vital signs every 15 minutes.

When contacting the hospital base station, communicate such pertinent information as:

• Patient's age
• Patient's sex
• Mechanism of injury
• Vital signs
• Intake and output
• Brief history
• Neurological exam
• Other injuries
• Treatment
• Information about contact of family members

PROCEDURE 3–5 ■ IMMOBILIZING THE NECK

Purpose

When a cervical injury is suspected, the neck, the most vulnerable area, must be immobilized before turning or positioning the patient. Stabilizing the fractured neck will protect the spinal cord and nerves from further damage. This procedure requires two rescuers.

Action	Rationale
First Rescuer	
1. Return the patient's head to neutral position. If possible, approach victim found in the sitting position from behind and use your elbows stabilized on the victim's upper back to achieve this maneuver.	
2. Hold the patient's head firmly, pushing up slightly on hands to create a gentle traction on the cervical spine.	
Second Rescuer	
3. Apply cervical collar and secure with tape or velcro closures.	The collar must fit snugly to immobilize the neck adequately.

PROCEDURE 3–6 ■ USE OF THE LONG BACKBOARD

Purpose

To completely immobilize the victim's spine in preparation for transport. Patients are secured in such a manner that they may be positioned laterally, turned to the side to facilitate vomiting or drainage of secretions, or rotated or raised vertically without experiencing any significant movement. Unless the scoop is available, this procedure requires four or five people. If necessary, bystanders may need to be recruited.

Equipment Needed

- Scoop stretcher (ideal adjunct but optional)
- Long backboard
- Two 7-8 foot (2.5 meter) straps
- Two sandbags (or rolled blanket substitutes)
- Rolled blankets (optional)
- Bandaging materials

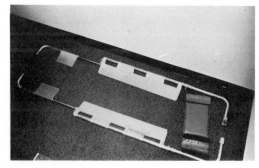

Scoop stretcher

Action	Rationale
If a scoop stretcher is available:	
1. Ensure the cervical injured patient has a collar on. Position the patient supine. Apply gentle traction to straighten the neck, if necessary. Then place patient on the scoop stretcher.	To immobilize the neck before moving.
	(Procedure continues)

PROCEDURE 3–6 ■ USE OF THE LONG BACKBOARD (*continued*)

Action	Rationale

Action

2. Place the patient, in the scoop stretcher, on top of a long backboard.

3. Proceed to secure the patient to the long backboard with straps and implement steps 9–12.

If the long backboard is available:

1. Position the long backboard alongside the patient.

2. Place padding on the backboard for the small of the back, the knees, and the ankles.

3. Position one rescuer at the patient's head, one at the chest, one at the hip, and one at the lower leg.

4. While the first rescuer supports the head, the others reach across the patient's body. On a signal from the first rescuer at the patient's head they logroll the patient, as a unit, toward themselves.

5. Instruct another rescuer to slide the backboard under the patient. Tilt the backboard upward to center the patient on the backboard as it is lowered.

6. On a signal from the first rescuer at the patient's head, lower the patient onto the backboard.

7. Place sandbags on each side of the patient's head and tape into place. Alternatively use rolled towels, blankets, or improvise with clothing.

8. If the patient is smaller than the backboard, add extra padding between the patient's legs and along each side of the body.

9. Secure the patient to the backboard with straps:
- Place strap over the patient's chest, midsternum above the nipple line, and attach under axillae and secure shoulders (A).
- Place additional straps in a criss-cross manner over the iliac crests, lower abdomen, pelvic region (B), and below the patient's knees (C).

10. Immobilize the patient's head to the board with bandages. Do not wrap too tightly.

11. Immobilize the arms by tying wrists together. Do not place the arms under a strap.

12. Pad areas where pressure may cause a problem at any point during this procedure.

Rationale

The rescuer positioned at head leads the transfer.

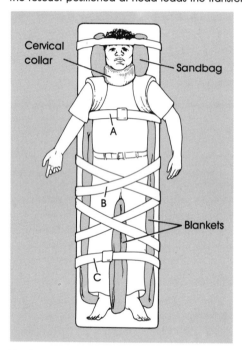

The lower chest and upper abdomen are left free of restrictive straps to facilitate impaired breathing. Also the chest is accessible for resuscitation.
Diagonal straps best minimize the momentum of body movement in any direction. Movement of the body can cause a dragging or a compression force on the neck.

The chin is left free to facilitate drainage of vomitus or secretions.

The arms are left free to monitor blood pressure and to start intravenous therapy, if necessary.

PROCEDURE 3–7 ■ USE OF THE SHORT BACKBOARD

Purpose

The purpose of the short backboard is to immobilize the spine of a victim who is found in an automobile or in a sitting position. The use of the short backboard requires two rescuers and a third rescuer to position the long backboard in preparation for transport.

Equipment Needed

- Short backboard
- Straps to secure head, neck, torso, groin, and legs and arms
- Two sandbags (or substitutes)
- Padding

Action

First Rescuer

1. Stabilize the patient's head, neck, and shoulders, and continue to do so throughout the procedure.

Second Rescuer

2. Slide the short backboard behind the patient at a 45-degree angle; squeeze the bottom end of the backboard in place between the lower back and the car seat.

3. Pivot backboard to its normal upright position.

4. Once in place, tilt forward against the patient's back, centering the patient's head on the headpiece.

5. As a unit tilt victim and the backboard back to rest on the seat of the car.

6. Secure the patient to backboard with straps:
- Attach across forehead and across the collar.
- Attach diagonally across torso, across chest under axillae, and across abdomen.
- Attach around each thigh, as close to the groin as possible, and tie to lower corners of backboard.
- Immobilize legs with straps around the knees and ankles.
- Immobilize arms with a strap at the wrists.

Both Rescuers

7. With one hand under the patient's hip and one hand behind the short backboard, raise the patient sufficiently to permit another person to slide the foot of the long backboard under the patient.

Rationale

Ensure that the patient has a collar to immobilize the neck before using the short backboard.

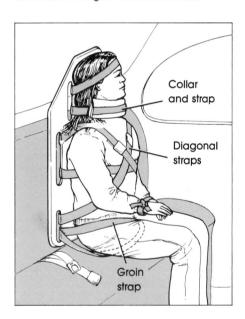

Collar and strap

Diagonal straps

Groin strap

The chin is left free to protect the airway.
This prevents the patient from slipping sideways.

This anchors patient to the backboard and prevents slipping down and out of head straps.
Padding between the legs may also be added for protection from pressure.
This prevents arms from slipping, becoming trapped, or being injured.

This prepares the patient for transport.

(Procedure continues)

PROCEDURE 3–7 ■ USE OF THE SHORT BACKBOARD (*continued*)

Action	Rationale
8. With the patient sitting on the long backboard, pivot and tilt the patient to the supine position. Then slide the patient as a unit onto the upper part of the long backboard.	The priority is to maintain alignment from the head to the hips. The legs can be bent and moved with caution.
9. Place the patient on backboards on the ground. Secure the short backboard to the long one with straps across upper chest and lower abdomen. Untie the legs, and place flat on the long backboard; resecure them.	

PROCEDURE 3–8 ■ EXTRICATION OF A PATIENT FROM THE WATER

Purpose

The purpose is to establish an airway and adequate ventilation while immobilizing the spine. The procedure requires at least two rescuers before removing the victim from the water.

Equipment Needed

Long backboard or substitute, such as a door or any object that provides a rigid, flat surface.

Action	Rationale
1. If the patient is found floating face up in the water, maintain in straight position.	
First Rescuer	
• Position yourself at patient's head. Grasp shoulders and stabilize the neck and head between your arms.	
Second Rescuer	
• Start mouth-to-mouth ventilation, if necessary, or assist the patient's breathing.	
2. If the patient is found floating face down in the water, support the head and neck while turning victim over.	
3. Position patient on a long backboard (or substitute) before removing victim from water.	
First Rescuer	
Hold head, neck, and shoulders firmly in alignment.	
Second Rescuer	
Slide long backboard under the patient. Float the board to the edge of the water and gently lift the patient and the board out of the water.	Attempt to carry patient from water only when there are enough people to provide proper handling.
4. Proceed to secure patient to long backboard in preparation for transport.	

Potential problems encountered during transport

Airway obstructions   Watch for signs of airway obstruction, which will result in accumulation of carbon dioxide (CO_2) in the blood. Elevation of the level of carbon dioxide in the blood is extremely dangerous, as it results in increased intracerebral and intraspinal pressures that may intensify the spinal cord injury. In the unconscious patient, hyperventilation is often beneficial since it reduces the level of CO_2 in the blood.

Aspiration pneumonia   Frequently the patient with traumatic injuries becomes nauseated and vomits. Serious pneumonia ensues when a patient aspirates the vomitus into his lungs. Keep a portable suction apparatus at the patient's side at all times and be prepared to suction all vomitus. Another helpful maneuver is to turn the entire backboard on its side so that the vomitus can drain from the mouth. In the unconscious patient, an esophageal airway frequently can protect the patient's airway from aspiration of gastric juices.

Spinal cord edema   Spinal cord edema may be reduced by an intravenous injection of methylprednisolone (Solumedrol). The following regimen is recommended:

- 15 years and older — 2 grams IV
- 5 to 15 years — 1 gram IV
- Under 5 years — 0.5 gram IV

This complication is described further in Chapter 4 under nursing interventions.

Lowered body temperature   A degree of hypothermia may exist due to an autonomic nervous system dysfunction secondary to the cord injury. Be sure the patient is adequately covered for warmth and comfort. (See Chapter 10.)

Pressure areas on skin   Pressure areas on the skin can develop over longer transports (over one hour in duration) and add complications in treatment and recovery. Vulnerable areas are the sacrum and backs of heels. Adequate padding, tilting the immobilized victim on the backboards lightly every 15 minutes, and inserting a hand under the patient for gental massage of the area minimize this risk.

SELECTED REFERENCES

Emergency Health Services Academy, Justice Institute of British Columbia. Undated publication. Instructional notes on care of spinal cord injuries. Vancouver, BC. *Updated handout materials, the content of which is based on highly coordinated rescue, transport, and immediate admission services to a specialized provincial spinal injury center.*

Rimel, R., et al. 1978. *Acute Care of the Spinal Cord Injured at the Site of Injury.* Rector and Visitors of the University of Virginia.

Meyer, P., et al. 1976. Fracture dislocation of the cervical spine: transportation, assessment, and immediate management. In *Instructional Course Lectures*, vol. 25. St. Louis, Mo: Mosby. *Comprehensive overview of the major concepts of care for quadriplegic patients; focuses on increasing chances of neurological recovery by injury recognition, skilled extrication, and transportation to specialized facilities.*

Meyer, P. R. 1978. The Illinois emergency medical service. *Model Systems Conference*, April, pp. 1–4. *Presents concise criteria for transfer protocols.*

———. 1979. Development of transfer and triage protocols. In *Management of Acute Trauma.* Chicago: Year Book Medical Publishers, pp. 61–67. *Introduces concept of multistate spinal centers and examines transfers agreements, transfers, and pitfalls. Includes self-evaluation quiz.*

SUPPLEMENTAL READING

Grant, H. E., and Murray, R. H., Jr., 1978. *Emergency Care.* 2d ed. Englewood Cliffs, NJ: R. J. Brady/Prentice-Hall, pp. 201–203, 475–483. *Well-illustrated, comprehensive guide to extrication of the possible spinal cord injured victim.*

Patient Handling Manual. 1972. U.S. Department of Transportation, National Highway Traffic Safety Administration, August, pp. 10–14 and 89–91. *Deals extensively with scoop type emergency stretcher: includes use, transport, and safety precautions.*

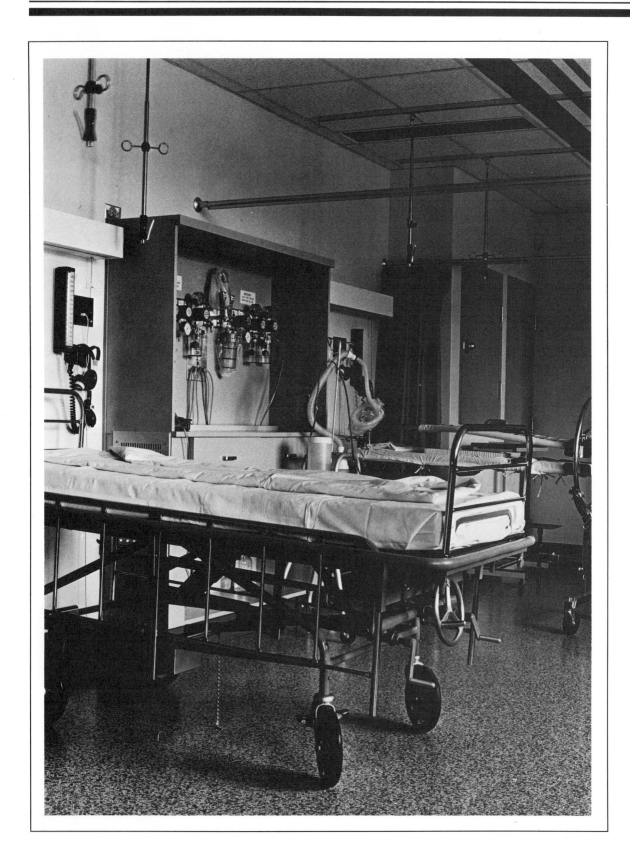

Chapter 4

Beginning Rehabilitation During Critical Care

CHAPTER OUTLINE

OBJECTIVES

- To increase awareness of rehabilitative aspects of goal-oriented critical care
- To clarify the significance of the critical care nurse's role in beginning a positive rehabilitation process
- To expand awareness of the value of an interdisciplinary approach
- To summarize the consequences of spinal cord injury

Practicing rehabilitative concepts to provide goal-oriented care emphasizes how similar components of the nursing process are for the nurse engaged in critical, acute, or long-term care of people with spinal cord injuries.

If critical care and concurrent rehabilitative expertise are not combined, patients with spinal cord injuries and their families are subject to any number of preventable consequences. These consequences present grave concerns with clinical, professional, and economical implications. The critical care nurse is in a unique position to influence the entire rehabilitation process, in either a positive or a negative direction.

The concept of rehabilitation is a continuous process beginning the moment of injury and not "something that happens to the patient down the line." The summarized information in this chapter will focus on potential rehabilitative aspects of immediate management. This chapter also serves as an overview to the events of spinal cord injury.

GOALS OF HEALTH CARE

Only the collective expertise of an interdisciplinary team during the critically ill period can meet the challenge of preventing physical and psychological deterioration, minimizing suffering, and successfully engaging patients and families in progressive rehabilitation. The goals of critical care are:

- To provide optimal critical and concurrent rehabilitative care
- To prevent or control secondary complications
- To establish a trusting relationship between the health care team and patients and their families

Use of the interdisciplinary approach makes it possible to begin dealing with all these components simultaneously. Patients and families both benefit from an interdisciplinary approach. If this ideal is not a reality, nurses must examine the implications in their role as patient advocates. For a discussion of the delicate issue of informing patients and families about alternate health care options, see Chapter 1.

ASSESSMENT AND INTERVENTIONS TO BEGIN REHABILITATION IN A CRITICAL CARE SETTING

In the immediate aftermath of spinal cord injury, hypotension, hypoxemia, and anemia may not only threaten life but also increase the impairment of the surviving patient (Tyson et al. 1978: 34). Cardiopulmonary resuscitation and exclusion of life-threatening hemorrhagic injuries take priority. At the same time, the utmost care to protect the spinal cord from further damage to preserve the patient's physical integrity, and promote psychological well-being is essential.

Table 4-1 serves to summarize major aspects of early hospital care. This poster is distributed as a guide for emergency facilities and includes preparation for transport to a specialized center.

History

Once the patient has been observed for acute distress and appropriate interventions have been taken, it is important to collaborate with transferring personnel to obtain and record pertinent information. (See Procedure 4–1.)

Summarized information obtained within a few days of injury, as shown in the sample nursing history in Figure 4–1, is a valuable, readily available resource for the entire interdisciplinary team to begin comprehensive assessment. This and other information can be transposed to a large interdisciplinary Kardex, which is easily accessible to each team member. See Figure 4–2.

Sections devoted to history taking in subsequent chapters explain the significance of such factors as age, associated injuries, and pre-existing health and disease. This information will help the team determine the extent of the effects of spinal cord injury on an individual basis.

PROCEDURE 4-1 ■ TAKING AN ADMISSION HISTORY

Purpose

The major clinical purpose for collecting this information is to establish baseline data to compare with present neurological and physical status. Such comparisons help determine if the patient has deteriorated, remained unchanged, or improved neurologically.

Action	Rationale
1. Assemble medical records provided (including ambulance company records), any previous emergency or hospital admission notes, records kept during transport, and any initial radiographic studies.	
2. Obtain a comprehensive report from transferring personnel to confirm or clarify preadmission information and describe: • Mechanism of injury. • Respiratory status and management. • General condition, vital signs, and tolerance to transport. • Neurological status. • Type of immobilization measures used. • Medications.	
3. Check for indwelling catheter and inquire about any previous catheterizations. Note amount and type of IV fluids absorbed and amount and nature of urinary output. Check oral fluid intake, if any. Examine intake (oral and IV) and output.	If there is no indwelling catheter, there will likely be bladder overdistension. Also be alert for possible fluid overload. Often increased fluids are mistakenly given to compensate for neurogenic hypotension. Oral fluid intake is extremely hazardous for people with spinal cord injuries due to the risk of aspiration from paralytic ileus. Insertion of a nasogastric tube for decompression of the stomach can reduce the risk.
4. Note psychological response manifestations and previous psychological or psychiatric problems.	
5. Include other helpful information from or about family members or friends accompanying the patient, such as details about the accident or other significant events.	

Promoting Optimal Cardiopulmonary Function

Progressive cardiopulmonary dysfunction is a constant and critical danger throughout the initial 72-hour postinjury period, especially for the patient with quadriplegia. Although many patients with quadriplegia are not in severe or even obvious respiratory distress on admission, there is a high risk of deterioration because of accumulative fatigue (increased demand on fewer muscles to maintain respiration and clear lung secretions) and potential expansion of cord edema or hemorrhage to higher segments that may involve diaphragmatic function. Aspiration (due to unconsciousness or water-related injuries), preexisting pulmonary conditions, associated injuries, or advanced age also increase the risk of respiratory dysfunction. (A specialized respiratory team should always be involved in

TABLE 4–1 ■ INITIAL CARE OF SPINAL CORD INJURY

1. Prepare Equipment for Patient's Arrival

2. Prevent Further Injury to Cord

Rx—Immobilize neck and back on long backboard

3. Treat Breathing Difficulty First

- Obstructed Airway with Suspected Cervical Spine Injury

Rx—Straighten neck without hyperextension

Rx—Insert oral airway

Rx—Bag mask ventilation with oxygen (10-12 liters/min)

- Hypoventilation (Neural Control of Intercostal and Diaphragmatic Muscles May Be Impaired in Cervical Spine Injuries)

Dx—Obtain arterial blood gas 3 min after breathing room air

Rx—If $Po_2 < 80$ mmHg + signs of respiratory failure, provide ventilatory support via nasotracheal intubation. Hyperventilate patient maintaining arterial Pco_2 between 22 and 30 mmHg.

Dx—Monitor adequacy of ventilation with serial blood gases

4. Establish Circulation

- Absent Pulse

Rx—CPR

- Arterial Hypotension

Rx—Establish IV line with #18 percutaneous plastic catheter using 5% dextrose in Ringer's Lactate

Rx—Elevate foot of backboard

Rx—Humidified oxygen (10-12 liters/min)

5. Perform History and Physical Examination

Dx—Establish level of consciousness (Glasgow Coma Scale)

Dx—Check for *changes* in symptomology since injury

Dx—Identify level of neurological deficit by checking sensation, muscular strength and reflexes of the right and left arms and legs (anesthesia, numbness, paralysis, paresis)

Dx—Search for other injuries

Rx—Remove clothing and jewelry with minimal manipulation

6. Relieve Bladder Distension

Rx—Foley Catheter

7. Obtain Appropriate X-Rays

- Cervical Vertebrae

Dx—Order cross-table lateral x-ray first. If normal, obtain AP view of vertebrae

Dx—Order open mouth view of atlantoaxial articulation in conscious patient

View all 7 cervical vertebrae. If necessary, depress shoulders by pulling upper extremities toward feet. Visualize odontoid process in conscious patient.

- Thoracic Vertebrae

Dx—Order AP and lateral views of thoracic vertebrae. View all 12 thoracic vertebrae

- Lumbar Vertebrae

Dx—Order AP and lateral views. Check all 5 lumbar vertebrae. Send all X-Rays with Patient When Transferred to Spinal Cord Center

8. Reduce Spinal Cord Edema

Rx—Methylprednisolone (Solumedrol)
2 grams IV push (>15 y.o.)
1 gram IV push (5–15 y.o.)
0.5 gram IV push (<5 y.o.)

9. Stabilize in Neutral Position the Head of a Patient with a Neck Injury

Rx—Apply cervical collar or preferably Gardner-Wells tongs attached to 5 lb weight. If tongs are not available, staff from Spinal Cord Center will apply skeletal traction before transport.

10. Treat Ileus

Rx—# 18 Sump Nasogastric Tube

11. Tetanus Prophylaxis

12. Transfer to Spinal Cord Treatment Center

Indications
Any *suspected* cervical, thoracic or lumbar spinal injury with or without neurological deficit and/or fracture

13. Expedite Transfer

Air if > 60 miles from trauma center
Ground if < 60 miles from trauma center

14. Contact Spinal Cord Treatment Center before Transfer

Ask for Neurosurgeon on duty

Courtesy of Regional Spinal Cord Injury System, University of Virginia, Charlottesville, Virginia.

CLINICAL NOTES

DATE	TIME	EACH NOTE MUST BE SIGNED WITH A LEGAL SIGNATURE
		Source of Hx *Patient*
		Diagnosis *#C4-5 Complete quadriplegia (C5 on right; C4 on left) MVA*
		1. Appearance first sight *healthy looking Caucasian male*
		appears stated-age, Co-operative, Friendly
		(Estimated on admission) (Lost 16 lbs since then)
		Weight: *155 lbs* ∧ Height: *6' 1"*
		2. Patient's understanding of condition/acceptance of limitations *Understands neck fracture*
		and motor and sensory loss over most of his body. Does not
		expect to recover the same as before, but hopes to gain
		more movement in upper extremities and maybe to walk again
		3. Previous hospital admissions/illnesses
1969		*Bladder surgery for enlarged ureter*
1975		*Wisdom tooth removed at Children's Hospital*
		Experience of family or friends *nothing significant*
		4. Expectations/fears of hospitalization *Expects his condition will get better*
		following hospitalization. Dislikes lack of information
		and too many procedures happening all at once. Sharp
		pain in left arm that is aggravated by sudden
		movement or prolonged immobility
		5. Sociocultural Hx
		Language spoken *English*
		Occupational/Educational Hx *Completed high school-academic program*
		Attended college for one year-general arts. Worked
		as logger for summer
		Religious Affiliation *Protestant (has strong faith)*
		Family/Significant Persons
		Parents (father-businessman, mother-homemaker)
		Older married brother, three younger brothers at home
		Met girlfriend last summer but she has returned
		to England.
		(Notes continue)

FIGURE 4–1 ■ A sample nursing history obtained 6 days after the injury. The patient
was rendered quadriplegic from a motor vehicle accident. (From the Acute Spinal Cord
Injury Unit, Shaughnessy Hospital, Vancouver, B.C.)

CLINICAL NOTES

DATE	TIME	EACH NOTE MUST BE SIGNED WITH A LEGAL SIGNATURE
		Change in family arrangements due to hospitalization:
		Parents live in Vancouver. Visit daily. Father comes in after work, Mother comes in early afternoon Several friends also visit.
		Visitors expected Yes ✓ No Restrictions *routine hours 4-8 pm*
		6. Habits of Daily Living
		(a) Usual bedtime *1030* Waking time *0630* Nap *no*
		Usual Px for restlessness *To pray whenever he is restless or has difficulty sleeping. Sports.*
		(b) Elimination Patterns
		Bowels - Regular *Everyday*
		Irregular *no*
		Laxatives *none*
		Urinary irregularities *No problems after 11 years of age (previous medical history to be obtained)*
		(c) Respiratory
		Smoker Yes ✓ No Amount *1/2 pack/day*
		Cough Describe *coughed occasionally (nonproductive)*
		Sputum Describe *no*
		Shortness of Breath Describe *no*
		(d) Nutrition: Diet *Eats three regular meals/snacks no special diet*
		significant weight Likes *meat and potatoes*
		loss since admission Dislikes *liver* Allergies *no*
		(e) Significant Skin Conditions *Raised, reddened pimply rash on face, neck and shoulders (side effect of Dexamethazone therapy). Otherwise skin condition good*
		(f) Personal Hygiene Bath Time *after work*
		Shower ✓ *daily*

FIGURE 4–1 ■ *(continued)*

CLINICAL NOTES

DATE	TIME	EACH NOTE MUST BE SIGNED WITH A LEGAL SIGNATURE
		Menstrual Hx Date of last period *not applicable*
		Regular Irregular
		Usual Cycle Contraception Oral
		(g) Activity
		Mobility *good prior to injury. Presently beginning to get up*
		Limitations *Undergoing assessment*
		Recreation *hockey, hand ball, skiing several times a*
		week. Was saving money for a trip to Europe
		Plays church piano and organ
		(h) Senses Glasses/Contacts *glasses (short-sighted)*
		Hearing Aid
		Dentures Prosthesis *no*
		Other
		(i) Medication At home *Multivitamins, iron*
		Brought to Hospital *none*
		Allergies *none known*
		(j) Special Fears *Fear of being physically helpless. Described*
		bad dream of overhead bar falling on him and he
		couldn't move his arms to save himself.
		(k) Sexual Concerns *Has given much thought to his*
		inability to father children. Feels he will not
		marry because he can't take care of himself.
		Advised of Sexual Health Care Service.
		(l) Description of Temperament *Describes himself as calm*
		individual. Relieves tension by physical activity.
		Doesn't like to "lose his temper."
		(m) Interpersonal and Communicative Patterns
		Patient's point of view
		Not very talkative but can make friends easily
		if both parties express the same interest.
		(Notes continue)

CLINICAL NOTES

DATE	TIME	EACH NOTE MUST BE SIGNED WITH A LEGAL SIGNATURE
		(m) Con't.
		Nursing point of view
		Nonverbal behavior during interview Good eye-contact. Moves left forearm and wrist occasionally.
		Verbal behavior during interview Gives simple, direct answers Co-operative, shows interest in interview. Asks questions Has difficulty remembering past events about accident.
		(n) Patterns of Dependency/Independency
		Patient's description of self - Independent person. Lives at home because it is cheaper but pays room and board. Cares for own bedroom and car.
		7. Sources or security/comfort Small amount of savings in the bank. Plans to live at home for a year or so. Father has agreed to support him while he returns to vocational school. Active church member. Likes to have someone sit down and talk with him.
		8. Problems Identified Additional Comments
		1. C4-5 quadriplegia
		2. To gain back appropriate weight and maintain good eating habits
		3. Aggravation of potential chest complications by smoking.
		4. Painful left arm
		5. Potential aggravated condition of upper urinary tract from previous surgery and present neurogenic bladder.
		6. Concern over sexually related problems
		7. Skin rash
		8. To help patient adjust to disability. Somewhat unrealistic at this time but generally shows many strengths.
		9. Poor memory at this time.
		10. Short-sightedness (potential problem)
		Signature Rowanne Vivoda R.N.

FIGURE 4–1 ■ *(continued)*

the initial management of patients with quadriplegia or those with associated chest trauma.) The nurse must watch for progressive changes in vital signs to detect neurogenic and/or hypovolemic shock. Skillful application of the nursing process is essential to promote optimal cardiopulmonary function and detect complications, which tend to progress rapidly and appear insidious to the unskilled observer.

Assessing and managing the airway

After spinal cord injury, airway management is of continuous vital importance to ensure adequate ventilation and tissue perfusion.

Aspiration of vomitus is a potentially fatal complication for the patient with quadriplegia. Burke and Murray (1975) emphasize that unrecognized paralytic ileus is probably the most common cause of sudden death in the quadriplegic patient during the first 48 hours, when decreased coughing ability leads to aspiration of stomach contents and respiratory arrest. In addition, abdominal distension caused by paralytic ileus will significantly inhibit diaphragmatic movement.

Head injury can also be associated with high velocity accidents and most frequently is associated with trauma to the cervical spine. Resultant increased intercranial pressure will depress the neural drive controlling respiration rate. It is important to note whether the patient experienced any period of unconsciousness.

Airway obstruction is also common with injuries to the cervical spine due to associated head and facial trauma. Soft tissue swelling may cause progressive difficulties with breathing. Occlusion of the airway is aggravated when the patient is immobilized in the supine position.

Maintaining a patent airway may require any or all of the following:

- Prophylactic use of nasogastric drainage to evacuate stomach contents
- Nasopharyngeal and oral suction
- Placement of an oral airway
- Side positioning (which may involve emergency logrolling the patient with manual cervical immobilization when an unstable spinal fracture is not yet protected with traction)
- Bag ventilation
- Intubation and ventilatory support

Resuscitation techniques must be modified to avoid unnecessary manipulation and hyperextension of the fractured neck, which could compromise vascular supply to the cord or further compromise the nerve roots or the cord itself, resulting in progressive neurological damage. For nasal or oral airway insertion and endotracheal intubation use the jaw thrust maneuver (see detailed procedure in Chapter 3). Most people with cervical spinal cord injuries experience progressive deterioration of pulmonary function before recovery. Tracheal intubation is by far the most commonly selected artificial airway, because long-term intubation is predicted.

Assessing and promoting ventilation

For the patient with quadriplegia, paralysis of the intercostal and abdominal musculature leaves the diaphragm as the sole remaining muscle responsible for ventilation (with minimal assistance from the accessory muscles in the neck and shoulders). Furthermore, limited chest expansion reduces the ability to cough and mobilize secretions. The major muscles involved in expiration are the abdominal muscles innervated by the lower thoracic cord (T_{6-12}). Therefore, patients with cervical cord injuries and those with thoracic cord injuries must be assessed closely for retention of pulmonary secretions.

Although uncomplicated injuries to the thoracic spine seldom cause respiratory failure, they are commonly associated with pulmonary and chest wall injuries. In these instances, a chest X ray will give more information for immediate management than a spinal X ray.

Increased rapid shallow respirations are a classic sign of progressive respiratory dysfunction for the spinal cord injured patient. A moist-sounding but unproductive cough is the first clinical sign to indicate problematic retention of secretions.

Determination of arterial blood gases is an essential part of initial management for patients with cervical and thoracic cord injuries. It may be necessary to establish an arterial line for repeated blood-gas analysis. Be alert for signs of respiratory acidosis from ineffectual respirations. Vital capacity, which can be easily obtained

FIGURE 4–2 ■ A large interdisciplinary Kardex form developed from the nursing history shown in Figure 4–1. Note: each discipline directly enters and updates pertinent information. (From Acute Spinal Cord Injury Unit, Shaughnessy Hospital, Vancouver, B.C.)

ALLERGIES: None known

NAME:	Q. Smith
S.I.N. NO:	202-139-049
X-RAY NO:	TL 12394
DATE OF INJURY:	Feb 1, 1982
ADMISSION DATE:	Feb 1, 1982

DIAGNOSIS:
Fracture dislocation C4-5
with complete quadriplegia
C5 on right
C6 on left
M.V.A.

OPERATIONS:

DATE	
Feb 1	Halo ring with 10 lbs traction
7	Application of halo – thoracic vest

CONSULTANTS:

NEURO SURGERY:	G.B. Thompson
ORTHOPEDICS:	P. Kokan
UROLOGY:	Z. Perler
FAMILY PRACTITIONER:	P. Taylor

TREATMENTS:

DATE	
Feb 7	Pinsite care q8h for halo-ring
7	Physiother washes to face, neck and shoulders B.i.D. for rash (am care and qhs)

SPECIMENS:

Feb 1	Urinalysis / Urine C+S weekly

SPECIAL PROCEDURES/X-RAYS:

Feb 1	Cervical spine, A/P & Lateral Chest X-ray
Feb 2	Cervical spine, chest X-ray Intravenous pyelogram
7	Cervical spine (post halo application) chest X-ray

MEDICATIONS:

DATE	REORDER	DISC.	MEDICATIONS
Feb 7			Darvon plain i̅ - ii̅ po q4h for neck or arm pain

BOWEL ROUTINE:
Fruit lax 1 tbsp.
Glycermid tabs i̅ } 0800
Glycerine supp q 2 days

H.S. SEDATION:

52

Nursing Care Plan

PROBLEMS	GOALS	SPECIAL NEEDS/APPROACH	OCCUPATIONAL THERAPY: TIME 0900–1045 Individual / 1400–1500 Hand class
• Painful (L) arm	Reduce pain & Maintain range.	a) Avoid sudden movement & prolonged elevated position. Assess need for analgesic prior to physical therapy.	SPLINTING: Wear at night only. Long opponens splint for (L) hand. Short opponens splint for (R) hand
• Poor memory.	Regain orientation	a) Use direct simple explanations. Repeat when necessary for teaching.	
• Unrealistic hope of recovery.	Develop realistic expectations	Be realistic & honest. Avoid giving false hope. Support strengths.	
• Potential chest complications	Minimize risk conditions that aggravate quadriplegia	Complete patient health education. Encourage to stop smoking.	A.D.L. Feeding–sit-up. Uses grooming–uncap, squeeze toothpaste. Needs assistance in bed. Dressing–dependent
			A.D.L. splint and spoon. Able to use cup and eat finger foods with minimal assistance.

I.V. THERAPY:

INTAKE	q4h	
OUTPUT	q4h	
T.P.R.	9 am	
B.P.	9 am	

DIET: Full diet High pro/cho drink T.I.D. Regulate intake = 2000 ml. Teach drinking pattern.

PHYSIOTHERAPY: TIME 1045

Daily Program Schedule
0745–0830 Breakfast
0900–1045 O.T. introducing — Dressing in bed, grooming individual treatment at sink next week
1045 Physical therapy (individual) 1330
1145 Lounge for lunch
1230 Rest — Introduction to mat & floor exercise
1330 Physical therapy (group)
400 Occupational therapy (hand class) 1500
Mon,Thurs/Sat 1500 Physical therapy (individual treatment)
1700 Dinner

TURNING/POSITIONING:
Side to side q2h
Introduce proning in afternoon
Night splints

BATH:	Bed & Showed/Tub q3 days	DAY: Mon, Thurs	TIME: 0900

INTERMEDIATE PLAN:
1. Mobilize as tolerated
2. Guilford brace/soft collar in early May

BLADDER CARE: Intermittent catheterization q4h. If residual urine greater than 500 ml Contact resident.
TIME: 0200–0600–1000–1400–1800–2206

BOWEL CARE: Check manually — daily. Glycerine supp. q2 days (odd). Position in bed.
TIME: 9 am

DISCHARGE PLAN:
• G.F. Strong Rehabilitation Center mid-May as in-patient.
• Eventually home with parents
• Vocational Counselling

SOCIAL SERVICE:
FINANCIAL RESPONSIBILITY: Insurance Corporation of B.C. providing full coverage. Canadian Paraplegic Association. CPA J. Parker, Peer Counsellor
ADDRESS: 1234- W. 14 Ave. Vancouver

NEXT OF KIN: Mr. and Mrs. R. Smith
RELATIONSHIP: Parents | TELEPHONE NO.: 224-0896 | RELIGION: Protestant | MARITAL STATUS: S☑ M☐ W☐ D☐

ROOM: 315-4 | NAME: J. Smith | AGE: 20 | BIRTHDATE: MOD. 3/59 at the bedside with a spirometer, is the most useful pulmonary function study to indicate deep breathing capacity and ability to cough effectively.

An admission chest X ray helps to assess the patient's current pulmonary status, detect associated trauma, and/or rule out preexisting conditions. However, chest X rays are less likely to show deterioration, unless it is advanced. For example, microatelectasis, which readily occurs with early retention of secretions, is not visible on X ray.

Skilled assessment is really skilled intervention because it will prevent a host of pulmonary complications that may be life threatening or contribute to further neurological deficit. If pulmonary dysfunction progresses to respiratory arrest, emergency intubation poses a major hazard. In addition, research data suggest that systemic hypoxemia increases severity of spinal cord injury. In experimental paraplegia, inflicted on animals for research purposes, bruised or edematous cord tissue surrounding the injury site is especially sensitive to low oxygen tension. The extreme sensitivity of all neurological tissue to oxygen deprivation allows irreversible damage to the threatened cord tissue to progress rapidly, even in the absence of clinical signs of hypoxemia (Tyson et al. 1978).

Interdisciplinary and nursing goals are to maintain a PaO_2 of 80 mmHg; to assist the patient to free the respiratory system of retained secretions; and to prevent or recognize early major complications, such as atelectasis, hypostatic pneumonia, or pulmonary edema.

Preventive measures to promote air entry and combat retention of secretions include avoiding upper airway obstruction; turning every two hours and correct positioning; employing manual techniques of deep breathing, assisted (diaphragmatic) coughing, and vibration and clapping in conjunction with postural drainage; and possible prophylactic use of intermittent positive pressure breathing (IPPB), ultrasonic nebulization, and carbon dioxide rebreathing therapy. These measures should be employed before clinical signs of retained secretions become evident. Immediate physical therapy consultation on admission is essential to implement these and other measures (primarily active exercises for unaffected limb musculature) to maintain cardiopulmonary reserve.

Restorative measures include oxygen therapy, tracheal intubation, and mechanical ventilation. Chapter 9 details how to identify the need and choose and implement the correct respiratory care for patients with spinal cord injuries.

Interpreting vital signs

Neural control of blood pressure, pulse, and temperature (cardiovascular function) is affected by autonomic nervous system dysfunction secondary to spinal cord injury. Below the level of lesion, passive vasodilation of the powerful vascular network significantly compromises venous return to the heart. With the diminished volume of blood circulating, cardiac output decreases. Lack of vasomotor control also hampers the body's ability to conserve (by vasoconstriction) or dissipate (by ability to perspire and vasodilation) body heat; therefore the body tends to assume the temperature of the immediate environment. Generally the higher the level of lesion, the greater the body area affected and the more profound the effects.

Cardiopulmonary assessment includes blood work to indicate abnormal blood composition, inadequate oxygenation, hemorrhage, and fluid and electrolyte imbalances. Adequate baseline data include a complete blood count with differential, coagulation studies, and type and crossmatch.

For the patient with quadriplegia anticipate hypotension (around 100/60 mmHg); bradycardia (a low pulse rate around 60 beats per minute); and some hypothermia (body heat lost through the passively dilated cutaneous vascular bed when environmental temperatures are generally lower than normal body temperature). The patient with a high thoracic lesion (T_{1-4}) may experience these signs to a lesser degree. The patient with a lower thoracolumbar lesion should not demonstrate these signs because the peripheral sympathetic nervous system remains intact.

Neurogenic and hypovolemic shock Hypotension and bradycardia following spinal cord injury constitute neurogenic shock. In the multiple traumatized patient, however, neurogenic shock and hypovolemic shock can, and often do, occur together. As a lowered blood pressure is a common factor in both, the rate and volume of the pulse become the key diagnostic factors. A slow bounding pulse and warm dry skin are symptoms of neurogenic shock. Tachycardia—characterized by a rapid, weak, and thready pulse—and pallor and thirst are symptoms of hypovolemic shock. In the patient with a lower thoracolumbar injury, deteriorations in vital signs are more indicative of hypovolemic shock.

Internal and external bleeding If tachycardia is evident, look for signs of internal or external bleeding. At greatest risk are patients who have been involved in high-velocity accidents, such as motor vehicle or industrial accidents, or severe falls. Common results of such accidents are abdominal injuries and fractures of the pelvis or long bones that can cause significant blood loss. Diagnosis is made more difficult by the lack of sensation below the level of lesion. There is no pain—an early localizing symptom—or guarding of an area for protection. Therefore acute *clinical* assessment becomes crucial.

To detect abdominal injury closely observe the patient with superficial abdominal bruising, swelling, or lacerations. Also remember that the patient with a thoracolumbar injury is more susceptible to internal complications as thoracolumbar trauma is associated with particularly violent force.

To further assess and treat abdominal trauma, the physician will likely order an indwelling catheter and a nasogastric tube if they are not already present. Observe and test for hematuria or blood in the gastric returns. Techniques used for assessment of the abdomen are detailed in Chapter 11.

The physician may do a rectal examination and order an anteroposterior abdominal X ray to identify misplaced abdominal structures or determine structural changes, such as fractured lower ribs or pelvis. (Whenever possible, position the X-ray cassette with the patient prone on a Stryker frame, then turn the frame before the X ray is taken. Otherwise, use a cautious three-person lift.) An emergency intravenous pyelogram (IVP) can also be taken at the bedside. Remember that if the patient's general condition is not stable, prolonged radiologic investigation in a main department is hazardous.

To observe for fractures in the extremities always compare limbs bilaterally for localized areas of heat, redness, or swelling. Obvious misalignment or joint instability may be present with gross fractures.

Stabilizing vital signs

Management of associated trauma involves integration of priorities of care in a life-threatening situation. Goals are early detection and control of hemorrhage and restoration of function. Surgical exploration and repair may be necessary.

Bradycardia secondary to quadriplegia does not require specific treatment. However, definitive treatment is needed for any cardiac arrhythmias. Patients with preexisting disease or multiple trauma, especially patients of advanced age, are at greater risk and should be continuously observed with a cardiac monitor until stable.

To combat hypothermia cover the patient to conserve body heat, using a warmed blanket if necessary. Never use heating devices such as electric heating pads or hot water bottles for patients without sensation. If the patient develops an elevated temperature, suspect infection.

To ensure stabilization of vital signs take measures to prevent or manage hypoxia, help the physician maintain desirable blood volume and composition, and promote blood flow in paralyzed limbs.

To maintain a systolic pressure around 100 mmHg and to avoid overcompensating for a low blood pressure from neurogenic shock, the physician generally orders intravenous therapy at an infusion rate of 75–100 cc/hour. A recommended solution is 5% dextrose in Ringer's solution (Tyson et al. 1978). Whole blood should be used for replacing blood loss. Dextran may be used as a plasma expander to provide a margin of safety to spinal cord blood vessels around the traumatized area of the cord that may otherwise remain dangerously hypotensive (Meyer and Me-

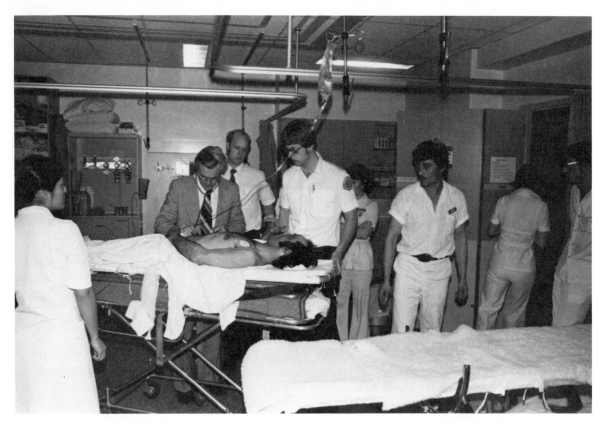

FIGURE 4–3 ■ The physician performs a cursory physical examination before moving the patient.

yer 1979). Pressor agents are used with caution only when an unsatisfactory intravascular volume exists.

Although previous measures take priority, an important adjunct is promotion of blood flow in paralyzed limbs. Tissue perfusion when the vascular bed is passively dilated is enhanced by regular turning; correct positioning to prevent gravitational edema (including elevation of limbs); passive range of motion exercises, especially ankle-pumping exercises; application of antiembolitic stockings; and protection of blood vessels from localized trauma. These measures must be implemented for the patient on a variety of immobilization beds. To minimize risk factors, identify the need, and initiate appropriate interventions to promote optimal cardiovascular function in the spinal cord injured patient, refer to Chapter 10.

Preventing Further Neurological Damage

Before moving the patient from the ambulance stretcher to an immobilization bed, the physician will make a cursory examination to assess the patient's current cardiopulmonary status and confirm the approximate level of the lesion. See Figure 4–3.

Neurological assessment

After life-threatening effects have been managed, the team will do an in-depth neurological assessment. Nurses will assist the physician to complete a physical assessment by providing examination equipment and helping to position or turn the patient as required. It is important to understand the physician's in-depth findings. This may involve direct discussion or joint examination to clarify baseline data with which all future nursing observations will be compared.

Nursing assessment of neurological status is generally completed every one to two hours during the initial 24- to 72-hour postinjury period and then as specifically required. Neurological assessment includes examination of motor power, sensory level, and reflex activity. To detect deterioration or improvement in the neurological level of injury assessment data are compared to baseline data.

Critical care nurses are not usually responsible for performing in-depth assessments of motor function, which involve detailed systematic muscle testing and grading power on an internationally based scale from 0 to 5. (For more information on muscle testing as it is used throughout the rehabilitation process, see Chapter 5.) However, it is helpful to become familiar with certain movements of the limbs that can be used for determining motor power to detect changes in neurological status.

Sensory testing is a more exact skill and takes considerably less practice to perfect than testing for motor power. Critical care nurses will also want to be aware of the presence or absence of general reflex activity below the level of lesion and in particular the status of the perineal reflexes. This information will help clarify the significance of physicians' and therapists' findings in terms of prognosis and diagnosis. Most significantly, the return of reflex activity indicates the passing of spinal shock and has specific implications for managing bowel, bladder, and sexual dysfunctions.

The nursing techniques generally used to test sensorimotor function of the extremities are not exact enough to detect neurological changes in patients with spinal cord injuries. For example, if a patient has been diagnosed as having a fracture dislocation of T_3 with a T_4 paraplegia (complete), then testing handgrasps (which will remain strong), leg movements, or foot plantar flexion and dorsiflexion (which will remain absent) gives little information about any neurological level changes at the injury site, which is the most important area. Chapter 5 describes neurological assessment in greater detail including assessment techniques, methods of recording, and understanding the significance of findings.

In both complete and incomplete cord injury, neurological deterioration characterized by additional loss of function may be due to spinal cord edema (just as a fractured ankle swells, so does the cord following trauma), cord hemorrhage, a compromised cord blood supply, possibly further necrosis of susceptible cord tissue from low systemic oxygenation, or further neurological damage from an unstable fracture. The first 72 hours after injury are considered critical in terms of possible interventions to enhance remaining spinal cord function. Astute nursing observation can help the physician to promptly adjust immobilization techniques, prescribe appropriate medications, proceed with special diagnostic procedures, alter medical management, or possibly intervene with surgery.

Assessment of spinal column injury

Assessment of vertebral column injury is closely related to neurological assessment. Be prepared to help the physician and X-ray personnel position the patient for initial portable spinal and chest films. If neurological deficit is increasing, anticipate more sophisticated diagnostic procedures to follow. Assessment techniques, radiographic, neuroradiographic, and neurophysiological procedures, including patient preparation and postprocedure care, are discussed in Chapter 5.

Nursing interventions

Nursing interventions are directed toward immediate and constant spinal immobilization and minimizing the effects of neurological edema. This may include assisting with a number of experimental procedures in specialized centers. To ensure immediate immobilization of the patient's spine, carefully plan the initial transfer from the ambulance stretcher to the immobilization bed.

Spinal immobilization A number of precautions must be taken when initially transferring the patient from the transport stretcher to the immobilization bed selected (see Procedure 4–2). If a *scoop* stretcher is used in transport this procedure is not necessary.

PROCEDURE 4–2 ■ TRANSFERRING A PATIENT (A FOUR-PERSON LIFT)

Purpose

The primary purpose of this technique is to maintain alignment of the spinal column by ensuring a safe transfer for the patient with an unstable fracture. Any movement at an unstable fracture site can damage the cord further, either by direct trauma or by compromising the vital blood supply to the cord.

Action	Rationale
1. Assess strength and experience of four assistants. Select five assistants for taller, heavier patients.	A typical critical care unit is cramped for space. Clearing the area, except for those directly involved with the actual transfer, will eliminate confusion.
2. Assign one assistant to manage the head and neck and three assistants, standing on the same side of the patient, to lift the body. Assign the strongest assistant to lift the heavier midsection of the patient.	
3. Prepare the patient by explaining the planned procedure.	Patients feel tense and fear pain on movement.
4. Instruct the patient to fold arms on chest if possible. Secure or tie paralyzed arms together.	It is important for the patient not to attempt to hold on to the assistants and cause twisting of the spine.
5. Try to maintain direct eye contact throughout.	This will reassure the patient and ensure relaxation during the transfer. Remember neck immobility restricts the visual field so eye contact is usually best maintained by the person situated at the patient's head.
6. Whenever possible, plan to relocate the stretcher and bed, not the patient. Allow ample space to move beds quickly (perhaps most convenient in the hallway); remove any obstacles on the floor; and remove armboards and footboards from the bed. When the lift is performed, have other assistants remove the stretcher and then position an immobilization bed directly underneath the patient. See Figure A.	This eliminates those lifting the patient from actually walking while trying to maintain skeletal alignment.

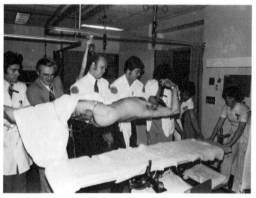

A

Action	Rationale
7. Have the person at the patient's head immobilize the neck by placing the inner forearms against the side of the head and firmly grasping the patient's shoulders. See Figure B.	This helps avoid inadvertent flexion of the head while lifting and is possible with a neck collar or skull tongs in place.

(Procedure continues)

PROCEDURE 4–2 ■ **(continued)**

Action

8. Clearly communicate the plan of action:

• Delegate "positions" for lifting.
• Assign additional duties, such as managing intravenous or respiratory equipment.
• Clarify any questions.

9. Instruct the assistant at the head to count "1, 2, 3" when ready.

10. Move the patient on the count of "3."

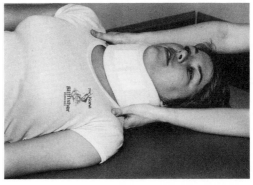

B

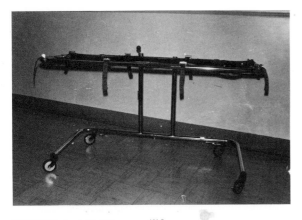

FIGURE 4–4 ■ The surgilift.

It may be possible to use special devices for initial and subsequent transfers. The *surgilift* (Figure 4–4) has a removable canvas sheet and adjustable frame. The patient should not be wheeled any distance on a surgilift, because the soft canvas does not provide enough support for an unstable spine. The electrically controlled *mobilizer stretcher* (Figure 4–5) is designed to facilitate transferring patients from one flat surface to another. While the stretcher base remains stable, the narrow, flat supporting surface is extended by roller mechanisms to slip underneath the patient. The patient is gradually returned to the stretcher base, which provides a firm surface ideal for transferring patients between departments.

Cervical traction Continuous cervical traction may be applied by using a variety of skull tongs or the Halo-ring. The Halo-ring is being used increasingly for initial management with the vest apparatus applied later when the fracture is reduced and the chest condition stabilized (see Chapter 14). Although this eliminates the tong insertion procedure, it can be difficult to release excess pressure when the patient is immobilized on a mattress or turning frame.

The application of skull traction can be particularly frightening for the acutely traumatized patient and can cause side effects of nausea and vomiting. Insertion of a nasogastric tube can

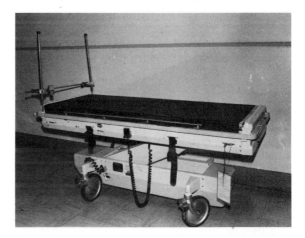

FIGURE 4–5 ■ The electrically controlled mobilizer stretcher.

help prevent these effects. Request pre-medication for the patient, and provide continuous monitoring of vital signs and possibly cardiac monitoring for the multiple traumatized or older patient. For nursing care of the patient, including criteria for selection of immobilization beds and application of cervical traction and the Halo device, see Chapter 14.

Minimizing effects of cord edema To minimize the effects of spinal cord edema, the physician may order dexamethasone therapy. Corticosteroids are potent anti-inflammatory drugs that reduce edema and also seem capable of providing some protection for cells near the trauma site that are susceptible to destructive autoimmune forces after trauma (Meyer and Meyer 1979). Initial dosages vary from 10 to 20 mg IV and are followed by gradually reduced dosages for five to seven days.

The continuous infusion of intrathecal cooled normal saline is an experimental method sometimes used to combat cord edema. In order to be effective local hypothermia must be done within eight hours of injury (Isaacs 1978). To enhance the effects, steroid therapy must also begin during this time, preferably during transport. Intrathecal cooling involves a surgical procedure to expose the dura and allow epidural placement of the cooling device for periods of up to four hours. Temperatures as low as 6°C (43°F) are reached before the cord is allowed to resume normal temperature. The possibilities of local hypothermia promise far-reaching positive effects in the future.

Caring for Physiological Needs

Caring for physiological needs to preserve or enhance existing function and to maintain existing muscular tone is a tangible way to incorporate rehabilitation concepts into critical care.

In addition to compromise of cardiopulmonary function, patients are likely to suffer impaired neural control of urinary function, gastrointestinal function, and the integumentary system. Loss of voluntary motor control and lack of sensation over much of the body will require nursing actions that maintain musculoskeletal system integrity and reestablish physical activity.

Bladder dysfunction

Almost all patients with spinal cord injuries will experience partial or complete, temporary or permanent loss of bladder function due to impaired neural control. Hypotension, secondary to neurogenic spinal shock or possibly hypovolemic shock, compromises urinary output. To maintain adequate renal function, a systolic pressure of 80 mmHg is needed. Frequent monitoring of vital signs and hourly urinary output measurement are indicated. The poorly understood phenomenon of posttraumatic diuresis is likely to arise within the first ten days of injury.

Neurogenic bladder management is of paramount importance as development of severe renal problems is still a major cause of death for the spinal cord injured. Prevention of complications begins on admission. Initially, neurogenic bladder management involves insertion of an indwelling catheter to prevent overdistension and ureterovesical reflux; to monitor diuresis and renal function and fluid management; and to detect hematuria, which indicates urinary system trauma. Early commencement of an intermittent catheterization regime is universally recommended to maintain optimal functioning of the urinary system. Under certain conditions it is possible to initiate intermittent catheterizations within hours after injury. On these and other nursing measures essential to neurogenic bladder care, see Chapter 12.

Gastrointestinal dysfunction

The nature and extent of gastrointestinal dysfunction is directly related to the level of lesion. The patient with a cervical cord injury, often with respiratory insufficiency and multiple trauma, runs the greatest risk of developing gastrointestinal difficulties that can progress to fatal complications. When a patient is without sensory warning mechanisms, the traditional signs of pain or abdominal guarding are absent, and the patient being mechanically ventilated may be further compromised by inability to communicate. Therefore, nursing actions must focus on specific preventive measures and modified assessment techniques, including recognition of abnormal laboratory results and identification of referred pain.

Paralytic ileus is a likely consequence of spinal cord injury. Onset tends to be immediate for those with thoracolumbar lesions; delayed 24 hours for those with high thoracic lesions; and delayed 48 hours for those with cervical lesions. If unchecked, paralytic ileus can lead to aspiration of vomitus and subsequent respiratory arrest. This is also true of acute gastric dilatation from any cause. Initial management involves withholding all oral fluids and inserting a nasogastric tube to decompress the stomach, prevent aspiration of stomach contents, and minimize the effects of abdominal distension. Continuous low-pressure nasogastric suction (approximately 20 mmHg) is often needed for patients with paralytic ileus.

Acute peptic ulceration is another potential complication during the initial seven- to ten-day postinjury period and often presents as an acute gastrointestinal bleed. The problem of malnutrition and significant weight loss during the critical period contributes to fatigue, poor wound healing, and skin breakdown and generally prolongs the rehabilitation period. Specific metabolic support is a meaningful adjunct during the critical phase of spinal cord injury. Chapter 11 describes these potential complications and nursing actions that promote optimal gastrointestinal function. It also identifies risk factors, preventive measures, and signs and symptoms that are made more difficult by spinal cord injury.

Bowel dysfunction

Neurogenic bowel care is another paramount concern for people with spinal cord injuries. Although impairment of gastrointestinal motility subsides with the passing of spinal shock, almost all patients will experience partial or complete loss of voluntary bowel control on a permanent basis. Correct techniques for evacuating the bowel during the acute period contribute to maintenance of bowel tone, regularity, and ease in developing a reliable bowel program. Poor bowel management techniques lead to further destruction of bowel tone and significantly prolong and complicate bowel retraining. The correct techniques of bowel care are given in Chapter 13.

Skin breakdown

Lack of sensation, inability to move freely, and circulatory changes predispose patients with spinal cord injuries to potential problems of skin breakdown. During *spinal shock* capillary pressure is greatly reduced, and this reduction is increased by likely hypotension, hypoxia, and/or anemia. These factors render the integumentary system even more susceptible to the effects of pressure during the immediate postinjury period. It is important to remember that once skin has broken down, even though it heals, it never regains its full resistance to the effects of pressure. Successful nursing interventions to manage the immobilized, acutely ill patient involve understanding the effects of pressure as a primary cause of skin breakdown; determining secondary factors contributing to skin breakdown; and integrating astute assessment with numerous manual skills to prevent development of pressure areas. Chapter 15 deals with how a patient's history, physical examination, and psychosocial status contribute to assessment data and then focuses on preventive nursing care measures. Note the specific section on management of pressure areas if trauma to the skin is associated with the initial injury.

Musculoskeletal integrity and physical activity

The entire philosophy of physical rehabilitation rests on preventing further neurological damage, facilitating return of potentially weak musculature, and promoting maximum activity of unaffected muscles. An admission consultation with both physical and occupational therapists will help the critical care nurse concurrently maintain musculoskeletal system integrity and begin to reestablish physical activity. All care is directed toward functional mobility, that is, developing useful movements that will eventually help the disabled with everyday living.

A program of active and passive exercises strengthens existing muscles, improves circulation, prevents contractures, and contributes to the patient's general well-being. Early upper extremity splinting for the patient with quadriplegia will help maintain a functional hand position essential for future rehabilitation activities and self-care. Therapists can also develop positions of ease for feeding, bathing, and personal hygiene and initiate self-care activities on a Stryker frame or other immobilization bed. (Part V details these aspects of care.)

Providing Psychological Support

Just as shared interdisciplinary knowledge and skills enhance physical rehabilitation, so shared philosophical approaches provide optimal psychological support. A critical care nurse is in a unique position to establish rapport with the newly injured person and to facilitate interdisciplinary interventions designed to make coping with this highly traumatic time more effective for all concerned.

Within the first few hours of injury many patients are in a state of severe mental and physical shock. Management of anxiety is complex but of the utmost importance regardless of how much physical care is required (Weller and Miller 1977a, b). Families also need emotional support. At this stage the nurse has vital concrete tasks to perform that will afford some relief of anxiety:

- Demonstrating knowledge and skill in an organized and confident manner.
- Careful control of pain by analgesics and muscle relaxants. As many treatments as possible (including those of other disciplines) should be done when medications are at their most effective.
- Calm and simple explanations of the many procedures required. The patient may seem to understand what is said, but information and instructions may have to be repeated again and again.

Although the patient may be seriously ill, the critical care nurse can promote an early trusting relationship between the interdisciplinary team and the patient and family. It is most important to include patients and families in order to minimize their feelings of helplessness and loss of control.

An honest, open relationship without false hope is a fundamental concept of nursing patients with spinal cord injuries. Part III presents general guidelines for enhancing self-concept and self-esteem; deals with personal feelings; and specifically discusses the nurse's role in giving information during the early stages, which includes revealing the prognosis. Even at this early stage, an overly sympathetic nonobjective attitude can convey feelings of hopelessness to patients and families. Sympathy is a natural human reaction, but the coping nurse will acknowledge these feelings and move on to develop more positive attitudes about the quality of life remaining for the spinal cord injured. This may be more difficult for critical care nurses because they don't see the recovery and rehabilitation of patients with spinal cord injuries. But it is crucial for critical care nurses to develop positive attitudes, because they can set the tone for the rehabilitation experience.

Nurse–patient rapport can best be developed if the nurse is supported by counseling professionals. For example, the nurse will be in a better position to meet the physical *and* emotional needs of the patient while a social worker intervenes with the family. This will give the family a formal, uninterrupted opportunity to express their grief and concerns. The social worker can provide early supportive care, detect any misconceptions, clarify concerns, and illicit information about the patient's preinjury personality and previous coping abilities. This valuable information can then be interpreted to the interdisciplinary team to the ultimate benefit of patients and families.

SELECTED REFERENCES

Burke, D. C., and Murray, D. D. 1975. *Handbook of Spinal Cord Medicine.* London and Basingstoke: Macmillan. *Concise presentation of acute management in Chapter 6.*

Isaacs, N. M. 1978. The treatment of acute spinal cord injury using local hypothermia. *Journal of Neurosurgical Nursing* 10(3): 95–101. *Describes combined steroid and hypothermia treatment of a young paraplegic male; includes thorough overview of experimental development, preoperative care, operative technique, wonderful clinical results, and related nursing care.*

Meyer, E. C., and Meyer, P. R. 1979. Initial management of the client with acute spinal cord injury. In *Current Perspectives in Rehabilitation Nursing.* Eds. R. Murray and J. C. Kijeck. St. Louis, Mo: C.V. Mosby, pp. 55–75. *Discusses transport, neurological assessment, drug administration, principles of management, and related nursing care.*

Tyson, G. W., et al. 1978. *Acute Care of the Head and Spinal Cord Injured Patient in the Emergency Department.* Charlottesville, Va: Dept. of Neurosurgery, University of Virginia. *A well-prepared booklet for emergency personnel. Major concepts and principles of resuscitation, detecting associated injuries that may be masked by neurological deficit, initial and repeated neurological assessment, and preparation of the patient for transport. Highly recommended.*

Weller, D. J., and Miller, P. M. 1977(a). Emotional reactions of patient, family and staff in acute care period of spinal cord injury: Part I. *Social Work Health Care* 2: 369–377. *Analyzes psychosocial implications in the acute period and describes their significance in later rehabilitation. Part I focuses on introductory material and patient responses.*

———. 1977(b). Emotional reactions of patient, family and staff in acute care period of spinal cord injury: Part II. *Social Work Health Care* 3:7–17. *Part II considers emotional reaction of family members and staff with further implications for treatment.*

SUPPLEMENTAL READING

Burgess, C. S., and Murphy, M. M. 1979. Rehabilitation nursing in the intensive care unit. In *Current Perspectives in Rehabilitation Nursing.* Eds. R. Murray and J. Kijeck. St. Louis, Mo: C. V. Mosby, pp. 76–83. *Incorporating interdisciplinary expertise in critical care; focus on spinal cord injury.*

Caldwell, E. 1978. The psychologic impact of trauma. *Nursing Clinics of North America* 13(2): 247–253. *Presents a crisis intervention model to deal with psychological conflicts surrounding trauma; explores nurses' roles and feelings.*

Church, C. S. 1981. Social work involvement with families at the acute stage of spinal cord injury. *Model Systems' Spinal Cord Injury Digest* 3(Winter): 49–53. *Describes function of the social worker at the acute stage of spinal cord injury: to help families deal with their own feelings and then to assist in providing support to the patient.*

Davis, J. E., and Mason, C. B. 1979. *Neurologic Critical Care.* New York: Van Nostrand Reinhold. *Section on general neurological trauma includes information on admission to a critical care unit, history taking, neurological assessment, establishing priorities of care, indications for surgical intervention, and some psychological aspects of care.*

DeJesus-Greenberg, D. A. 1980. Acute spinal cord injury and hyperbaric oxygen therapy: a new adjunct in management. *Journal of Neurosurgical Nursing* 12(3): 155–160. *Reviews the pathophysiology of spinal cord injury, experimental and clinical studies of animals and humans with hyperbaric oxygen therapy, and nursing care of patients during administration of hyperbaric oxygen therapy.*

Dossey, B. 1979. Perfecting your skills for systemic patient assessments. *Nursing '79,* February, pp. 42–45. *Presents guidelines for the head-to-toe physical assessment and for the major systems physical assessment; emphasizes need to practice and perfect whatever system you prefer for total patient care.*

Gilroy, A., and Caldwell, E. 1978. Initial assessment of the multiple injured patient. *Nursing Clinics of North America* 13(2): 177–190. *Comprehensive overview encouraging integration of skills to maintain integrity of vital systems; includes implications for spinal cord injury.*

Gunley, P. 1981. New focus on spinal cord injury. *Journal of the American Medical Association* 245(12): 1201–1206. *General overview of spinal cord injury centers in the United States. Also presents general overview of the care in the centers.*

Guttman, L. 1973. *Spinal Cord Injuries Comprehensive Management and Research.* Oxford: Blackwell Scientific Publications. *A classic, multifaceted reference text on spinal cord injuries. Includes historical background information; general statistics; legal aspects; detailed anatomy and neuropathology of cord trauma and resultant effects on all body systems; regeneration; fractures, dislocations, gunshot injuries, and stab wounds; and neurophysiological and clinical management aspects. Extensive bibliography.*

Hahn, H. R. 1977. Emergency management of the patient with spinal cord injury. *Resident and Staff Physician,* 23 February, pp. 50–57. *A comprehensive overview of acute management stressing the coordinated actions of a specialized interdisciplinary team. Highly recommended.*

Halstead, L.; Claus-Walker, J.; Herna, D. 1978. Neurologically active drugs in spinal cord injury; a clinical coding system. *Archives of Physical Medicine and Rehabilitation* 59(Aug.): 358–362. *Presentation of drugs commonly prescribed for the spinal cord injured; includes drugs used to compensate for neurological dysfunction and neurological side effects of drugs used to treat other problems. Focuses on actual and potential interactions with implications for physicians, pharmacists, and nurses. Darvon, Demerol, Talwin, Urecholine, and Valium are among those discussed.*

Hart, G. 1981. Spinal cord injury: impact on clients' significant others. *Rehabilitation Nursing,* January–February, pp. 11–15. *Findings from interviews, beginning within hours after injury, suggest that significant others need to feel adequately informed, to feel helpful to the client, and to feel the client is getting good care. The nurse must listen and react to the concerns and needs of significant others as part of the rehabilitation approach.*

Hussey, R. W., and Rossier, A. B. 1977. Problem oriented medical record: a predetermined problem list for spinal cord injury. *Archives of Physical Medicine and Rehabilitation* 58(July): 314–320. *Explains how the problem-oriented medical record facilitates documentation and management, with the complexities of physical and psychological involvement and long-term follow-up. Selects eight problem areas and presents two case studies, one of a newly injured patient and one of a long-term patient, to illustrate applications of this approach.*

Jackson, F. E. 1979. Vulnerable vertebrae. *Emergency Medicine,* 15 March, pp. 33–43. *Review of initial emergency room management in an easy-to-read style.*

King, B., and Dudas, S. 1980. Rehabilitation of the patient with a spinal cord injury. *Nursing Clinics of North America* 15(2): 225–243. *Comprehensive overview of aftereffects from spinal cord injury and related nursing care; includes introductory comments on acute management, focuses on later rehabilitation. Highly recommended.*

Larrabee, J. H. 1977. The person with spinal cord injury: physical care during early recovery. *American Journal of Nursing:* August 1320–1329. *Strong implications for concurrent rehabilitation focus in acute care period.*

Meyer, P. R., et al. 1976. *Fracture Dislocation of the Cervical Spine: Transportation, Assessment, and Immediate Management.* Instructional Course Lectures, vol. 25. The American Academy of Orthopaedic Surgeons, St. Louis, Mo: C. V. Mosby. *Comprehensive overview of the major concepts of care for quadriplegic patients; focuses on increasing chances of neurological recovery by injury recognition, skilled extrication, and transportation to specialized facilities.*

Meyer, P. R., et al. 1980. *Spinal Cord Injury: A Guide for Patients and Their Families.* Chicago, Ill: Midwest Regional Spinal Cord Injury Care System, Northwest Memorial Hospital, The McGraw Medical Center of Northwest University. *Excellent introductory guide for acute care period: includes goals, objectives, and medical definitions; describes initial care, physiological changes, psychological adjustments, and surgical interventions; and outlines the roles of team members and patient's family.*

Molter, N. C. 1979. Needs of relatives of critically ill patients: a descriptive study. *Heart Lung* 8(2): 332–339. *Focuses on crisis intervention with families to improve total patient care.*

Munro, D. 1964. Management of patients with traumatic paraplegia. *New England Journal of Medicine* 270(22): 1167–1171. *Concise overview of early care.*

Ng, P. K. 1979. Compatibility guide for combining IV medications. *American Journal of Nursing* —: 1292. *An easy-to-use, pull-out drug interaction chart. Note drugs commonly used with spinal cord injury: Dexamethasone NaPO$_4$, diazepam, dopamine HCL, furosemide (Lasix), Meperadine, and Morphine SO$_4$.*

Schnaper, N., and Cowley, R. A. 1976. Overview: psychiatric sequelae to multiple trauma. *American Journal of Psychiatry* 133(8): 883–889. *Focus on the roles of the psychiatrist in the critical care setting. Specifically includes some concerns about people with spinal cord injuries.*

Selecki, B. R. 1979. Severe injuries to the cervic cord and spine: neurosurgical management in the acute and early stage. *Australian and New Zealand Journal of Surgery* 49(2): 267–274. *An Australian viewpoint of comprehensive acute care in specialized centers. Highly recommended.*

Singletary, Y. 1977. More than skin deep. *Journal of Psychiatric Nursing and Mental Health Services* 15 (Feb.): 7–13. *Describes the role of a clinical nurse specialist in the critically ill and acute phase of a young man with extensive burns. Applicable to the psychosocial trauma experienced by people with spinal cord injuries.*

Tator, H., and Rowed, W. 1979. Current concepts in the immediate management of acute spinal cord injuries. *Canadian Medical Association Journal* 121: 1453–1464. *Excellent review of updated care describes sophisticated diagnostic tests, treatment methods, and related nursing care to minimize secondary pathological processes following initial trauma. Extensive bibliography. Highly recommended.*

Wiley, L., Ed. 1978. Family centered conferences for better trauma care. *Nursing '78*, August, pp. 71–77. *Nursing grand rounds format reviews a series of interdisciplinary conferences for a quadriplegic patient during acute care, emphasizing and explaining how to enhance independence, help face reality, and prepare for the future. Highly recommended.*

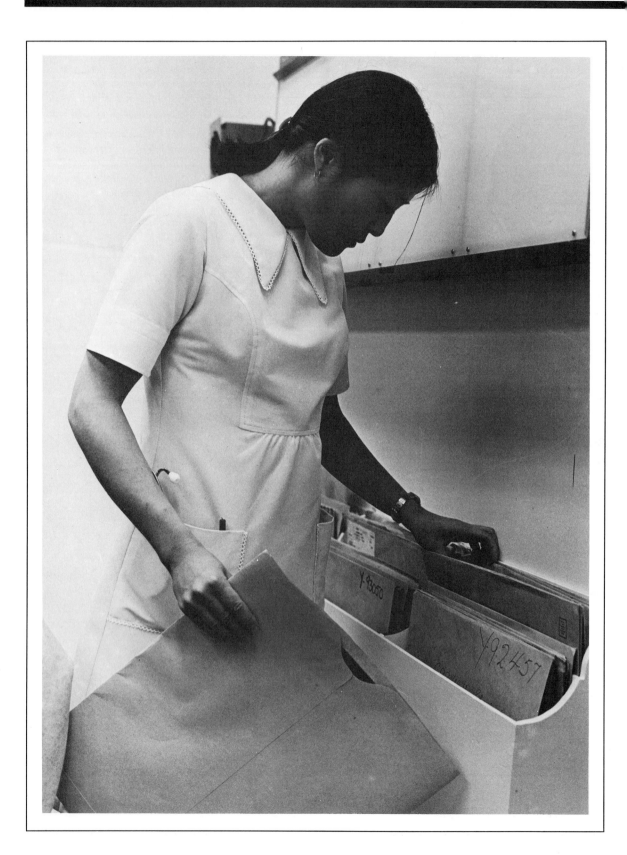

Chapter 5

Assessing Vertebral Column and Spinal Cord Injury

CHAPTER OUTLINE

OBJECTIVES

- To define health care goals when assessing the patient with an injured spine and spinal cord
- To describe the spine and factors that govern stability
- To explain the significance of stable versus unstable vertebral column injury and complete versus incomplete neurological injury
- To describe how mechanisms of injury damage the vertebral column
- To describe the structure and function of the spinal cord and nerves
- To describe the structural and functional differences between the sympathetic and parasympathetic nervous systems
- To explain dysfunctions of the nervous system following spinal cord injury and to describe sensorimotor loss and altered reflex activity as they relate to the level of lesion diagnosed

- To define paraplegia, quadriplegia (tetraplegia), and pentaplegia; complete transverse syndrome, Brown-Séquard syndrome, anterior artery syndrome, conus and cauda equina injuries, and sacral sparing
- To explain the significance of and how to obtain a pertinent medical history
- To describe a physical examination of the spine and assessment of neurological dysfunction following spinal cord injury
- To explain the procedure for and significance of radiologic examination, computerized axial tomography, tomography, myelography, somatosensory evoked potentials, and spinal cord monitoring, including patient preparation and post-procedural care when applicable

In order to competently deliver specialized care to the spinal cord injured patient, it is essential for the nurse to understand the significance of the neurological examination. Understanding is based on gaining an appreciation of the spinal cord and its role in the integration of body function and movement, rather than memorizing complex neuroanatomical terms. Closely related to neurological assessment is assessment of vertebral column injury. This chapter will help you sharpen assessment skills; recognize immediate and potential problems; participate in establishing realistic goals for physical rehabilitation; and offer reassurance, guidance, and health education for patients and families.

GOALS OF HEALTH CARE

A correct and accurate diagnosis of paraplegia or quadriplegia due to spinal cord injury is the first fundamental step in delivery of compre-

hensive health care. Goals of health care are:

- To provide a correct and accurate diagnosis on which to initiate appropriate management
- To establish reliable baseline data with which all future physical assessments can be compared to determine improvement or deterioration and to evaluate progress
- To develop realistic goals for physical rehabilitation

THE SPINE

The Skeletal System

The spinal column is composed of individual vertebrae, sharing certain common characteristics but grouped according to site and function. See Figure 5–1. There are generally 7 cervical, 12 thoracic, and 5 lumbar vertebrae; the sacral and coccygeal vertebrae are fused in the adult to form the sacrum and coccyx or "tail bone." The

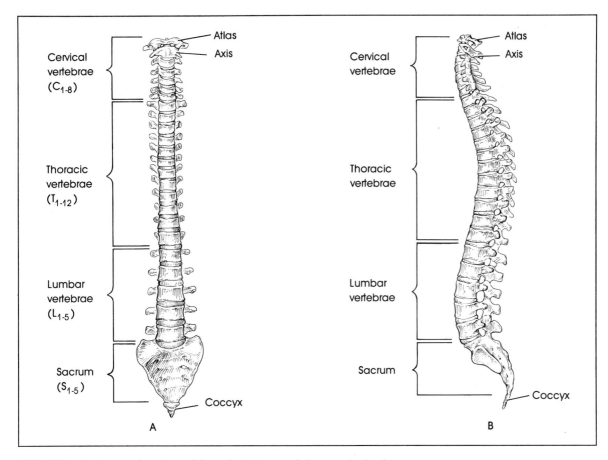

FIGURE 5–1 ■ Anterior (**A**) and lateral (**B**) views of the vertebral column.

vertebral column is strong and flexible, because it is composed of separate bones connected by tough, fibrous tissues called ligaments and cushioned by cartilaginous discs. Contributing to control and balance of the spinal column are the stabilizing rib cage, the superficial and deep trunk muscles, and the natural curvatures of the spine.

Vertebrae

All the vertebrae, with the exception of the first cervical vertebrae, share general features but differ slightly according to their function and level in the body. Each vertebra consists of a body (anterior) and an arch (posterior). See Figure 5–2.

Each arch is composed of two paired *pedicles,* which attach the arch to the disc body; two paired *laminae,* which form the roof of the arch to complete the structure; and seven *processes* or bony protusions—two above and two below

(*superior* and *inferior facets*), two at the sides (*transverse processes*), and one behind (*spinous process*). These articulating surfaces form the *neural arch.* The vertebrae provide bony protection for the cord by forming the *spinal canal.* See Figure 5–3.

The vertebrae in different portions of the spine have different sizes and shapes and directions of processes. For example, the transverse processes in the lumbar area are large to accommodate the attachment of lower limb muscles; in the thoracic area they possess tubercles or "stumps" for rib attachments; and in the cervical area they have openings to admit the generous arterial blood supply.

Different vertebrae also have functional differences. The lumbar vertebrae allow for powerful flexion and some extension; the thoracic vertebrae limit movement, and, at the cervical level, the atlas (C_1) and the axis (C_2) are so formed as to allow flexion, extension, and rotation of the head. Vertebral bodies generally in-

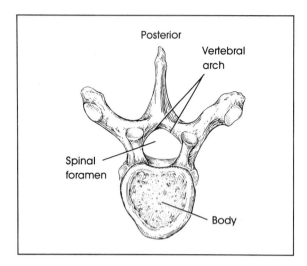

FIGURE 5–2 ■ A simple cross-section of vertebra outlining the neural (vertebral) arch.

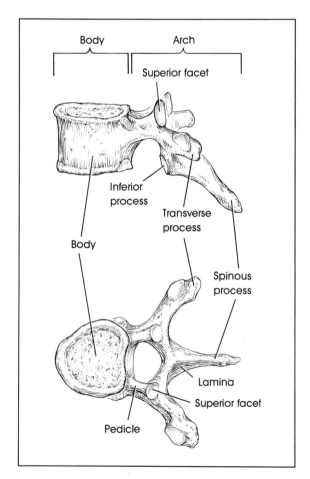

FIGURE 5–3 ■ A lateral view and cross-section of a vertebra detailing the vertebral arch.

crease in size to bear additional weight as they descend.

Discs and ligaments

Vertebral bodies are joined by intervertebral cartilaginous discs. These discs are made of a tough outer "shell" and a soft, gelatinous center that acts as a "shock absorber" and weight-bearing structure.

Two major ligaments run from the atlas to the sacrum on the front and back surfaces of the bodies and discs, holding them in alignment. See Figure 5–4.

Vertebral arches are joined to each other up and down the spinal column by short, dense ligaments. Ligamenta flava run between laminae, supraspinous and interspinal ligaments run between spinous processes, and the intertransverse ligaments run between the transverse processes. See Figure 5–5. These ligaments protect the spine against undesirable movement such as severe hyperextension or extreme flexion.

The Nervous System

The *central nervous system* is composed of the brain and spinal cord. The spinal cord is essentially an extension or elongation of brain tissue, sharing similar functions and protective structures of bone, meninges (coverings), and cerebrospinal fluid.

The *peripheral nervous system* is composed of the cranial and spinal nerves, which extend from the brain and spinal cord to branch out into many free nerve endings over the entire body.

A *neuron* is the basic unit or cell of the nervous system. As Liebman (1979) explains, the main properties that distinguish neurons from other types of cells are:

- Their specialization for conduction of impulses
- Their great sensitivity to oxygen deprivation
- Their importance for many vital functions
- The fact that they don't multiply or regenerate once destroyed (as would a broken bone or damaged skin)

This last fact is responsible for the irreversible damage caused by spinal cord injury.

The spinal cord

The spinal cord runs through the hollow canal in the center of the vertebral column. It acts as a two-way communication cable, carrying motor messages from the brain to the peripheral nervous system and carrying sensory messages from the peripheral nervous system back to the brain.

The spinal cord is a cylindrical, pliable structure that extends from the brain, starting at the foramen magnum and ending at the first or second lumbar vertebra. The cord is divided into cervical, thoracic, lumbar, and sacral segments. The cord enlarges in the cervical and lumbar areas to receive additional nerves from the upper and lower limbs. Because the cervical and lumbar areas of the spine are most mobile, these areas of the cord are most vulnerable to injury. The cord terminates in a tapered cone shape called the conus medullaris. This area contains major reflex centers for bowel, bladder, and sexual functions.

The main blood supply for the spinal cord is provided by two major vessels:

1. The anterior spinal artery supplies the front two thirds of the cord.
2. The posterior spinal arteries supply the back one third of the cord.

In addition, many smaller vessels (radicular arteries) supply the outer circumference of the cord at various levels. See Figure 5–6. Interruption of this vital blood supply can cause necrosis and permanent cord damage, which can result in specific clinical patterns of pathophysiology.

Throughout the central nervous system, *cell bodies* of neurons group together to form gray matter. Nerve fibers of neurons that are insulated or myelinated group together to form white matter.

Gray matter In the spinal cord, gray matter is composed of groups of cell bodies in a centrally located **H** or butterfly shape. This shape varies at different levels of the cord:

• *Anterior columns* or *horns* compose the front portion or legs of the **H** and contain motor cells to transmit messages of movement from the brain out through the anterior root.
• *Posterior (dorsal) columns* or *horns* compose the back portion or legs of the **H** and contain sen-

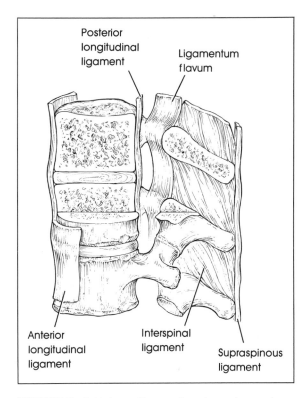

FIGURE 5–4 ■ A median section through vertebrae illustrating the supporting ligaments.

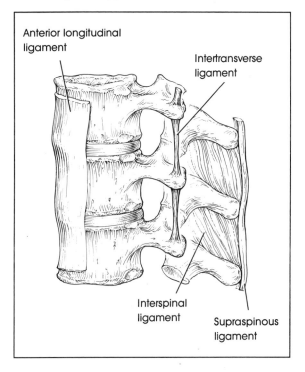

FIGURE 5–5 ■ A lateral view of vertebrae illustrating the supporting ligaments.

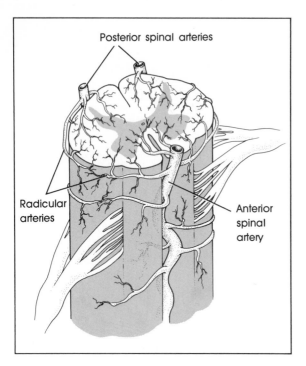

Posterior spinal arteries

Radicular
arteries

Anterior
spinal
artery

FIGURE 5–6 ■ The blood supply to the spinal cord.

sory "relay cells" to transmit incoming messages received through the posterior root, from the body to the brain.

- *Intermediate* or *lateral columns* contain a number of intermediate cell bodies, and in the thoracic section give rise to the sympathetic nervous system.

White matter   White matter is composed of ascending and descending nerve fibers that are insulated or myelinated and surround the central gray matter. Tracts, or bundles, of these nerve fibers are organized within the spinal cord according to function and act as transmission cables, sharing a common origin and common destination. For example, all fibers carrying motor messages travel together, as do all fibers carrying pain messages. See Figure 5–7.

Tracts have specific and complicated names, but the beginning of the word usually describes the origin; and the ending, the destination. All tracts are bilateral for control of each side of the body. There are three major tracts:

1. The *corticospinal tract* or *voluntary motor pathway* originates in the motor cortex of the brain and descends through the brain stem (where it crosses over to innervate the opposite side of the body), to the spinal cord. The corticospinal tract is contained in the posterolateral quadrant of the cord.
2. The *spinothalamic tract* originates in the spinal cord and ascends to the thalamus in the brain. Sensations of pain and temperature enter the cord from the opposite side of the body. The spinothalamic tract is located in the anterolateral portion of the cord.
3. The *posterior columns* are composed of sensory pathways for touch, vibration, and position sense. They are composed of several tracts located in the posterior portion of the cord.

The spinal nerves

The *spinal nerves* provide pathways for automatic reactions or involuntary movements in response to stimuli. *Efferent fibers* carry outgoing motor messages from the brain through the cord to various parts of the body. *Afferent fibers* carry incoming sensory messages to the cord where they are relayed to the brain.

The spinal nerves occur in pairs and correspond to the 31 segments or divisions of the cord and the 31 vertebrae. See Figure 5–8. Each nerve is attached to the cord by an anterior and posterior root. The two roots join in a common sleeve before exiting through openings at each vertebral level to branch out to almost all parts of the body. See Figure 5–9. The *anterior (ventral) root* is attached to the front portion of the cord. The *posterior (dorsal) root* is larger and thicker and attached to the back portion of the cord.

Some of the spinal nerves join in complex networks outside the spinal cord to form a *plexus* to innervate certain body parts. For example, the brachial plexus controls most of the arm and hand. Some spinal nerves have important functions and are given specific names. For example, the phrenic nerve innervates the diaphragm.

The *cauda equina*, which literally translated means the "horse's tail," is so named because of its appearance and is formed from the lowest

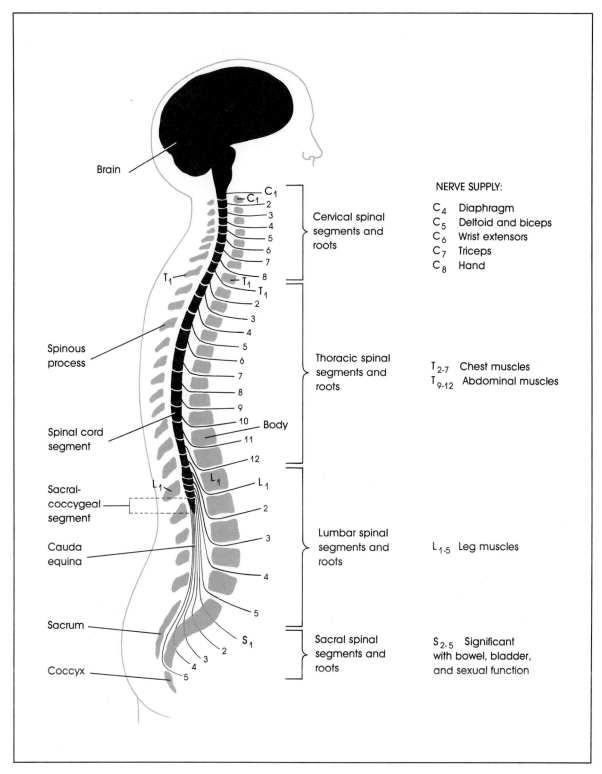

FIGURE 5–7 ■ The spinal cord and spinal nerves.

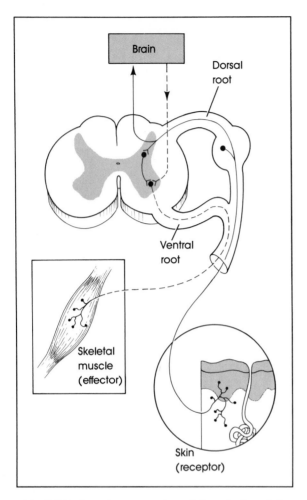

FIGURE 5–8 ■ A cross-section of the spinal cord detailing the attached spinal nerve.

nerve roots fanning out from the end of the cord. It is important to remember that injury to this area has some potential for recovery.

CONSEQUENCES OF INJURY

Vertebral Column Injuries

Injury to the vertebral column may be in the form of a fracture to the vertebrae or of a sprain or rupture to the supporting ligaments or a combination of both. Vertebral column injuries are described as *stable* or *unstable*. An unstable situation exists when vertebral and ligamentous structures are not able to support or protect the injured area. Inexpert movement can cause increased pressure with resultant damage to the spinal cord from displacement of the bony structures at the injury site. A spinal column injury is considered stable when the bony and/or ligamentous structures support the injured area sufficiently to prevent progression of neurological deficit and prevent bony deformity. If the posterior supporting complex—consisting of the ligaments that run between the neural arches and the articulating facet joints—survive, the spinal injury is considered stable.

The distinction between stable and unstable injuries cannot be made without clinical expertise and radiological diagnosis. *Thus, all injuries even suspected of causing spinal trauma must be treated as unstable until proven otherwise.* This principle applies during rescue, transport, and early hospital care.

Loss of Sensorimotor Function

Neurological injuries are described as either *complete* or *incomplete*. A complete injury is loss of all conscious motor and/or sensory function below the level of lesion. An incomplete injury preserves (or spares) some motor or sensory function. This includes several particular syndromes or distinct patterns of neurological deficit. Incomplete injury is very significant, because there is potential for recovery. Sometimes, however, preserved sensory functions are not very helpful to the patient; they may cause feelings of painful nerve irritation or build false hopes. Sometimes a patient can feel an unpleasant sensation of "pins and needles" or numbness in a limb. This is referred to as *paresthesia*. Even more painful is *hyperesthesia* when touch is grossly exaggerated. For example, when a bed sheet touches a patient's limb, the patient may describe it as "nails driving into the skin." Unpleasant sensations may be caused by root irritation. At other times, preserved sensation can be helpful in alerting the patient to a full bladder or to the position of legs in the wheelchair.

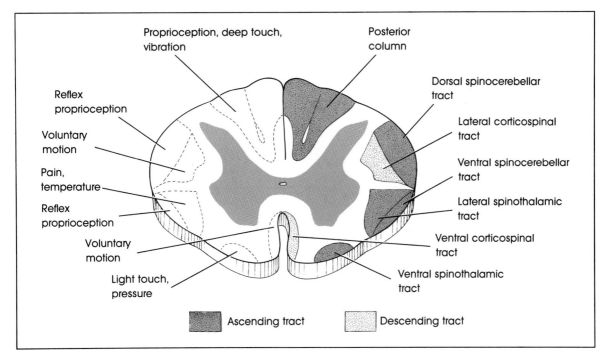

FIGURE 5–9 ■ A cross-section of the spinal cord detailing major motor and sensory tracts and their functions.

Complete syndrome

Complete transverse syndrome This syndrome causes loss of all nerve transmission to areas below the level of the lesion. See Figure 5–10. Complete paraplegia or quadriplegia occurs. Causes are:

- Complete severance of the cord.
- Complete breakage of nerve fibers by stretching of the cord. Coverings may still be intact and the cord may still look normal.
- Complete ischemia of the cord by interruption of the total blood supply.

Incomplete syndromes

Central cord syndrome Central cord syndrome is caused by damage to the central portion of the cord only. This occurs with cervical injury. See Figure 5–11.

Some distal nerve transmission is still intact. Lower segments are supplied by outer white matter. For example, corticospinal tract fibers are organized with those controlling the arms located most centrally, the trunk intermediately,

and the legs laterally. Fibers located most centrally are damaged and fibers located most laterally are spared. Therefore, arm movement is affected, but leg movement may not be.

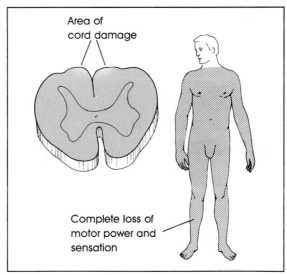

FIGURE 5–10 ■ Spinal cord damage causing a complete transverse syndrome.

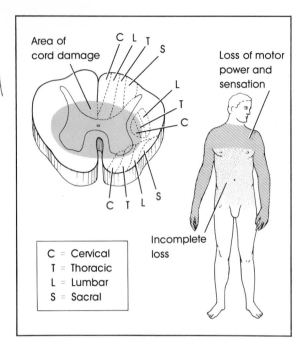

FIGURE 5–11 ■ A cross-section of the spinal cord depicting damage that causes a central cord syndrome.

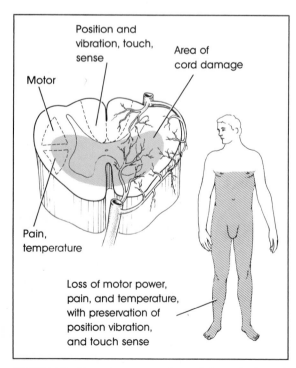

FIGURE 5–12 ■ A cross-section of the spinal cord showing damage that causes an anterior artery syndrome (or sparing of the posterior columns).

Anterior artery syndrome or sparing of posterior columns Anterior artery syndrome is usually caused by damage due to infarction from the main anterior artery; the resulting loss of blood supply damages the anterior two thirds of the cord. The posterior third of the cord is unaffected. See Figure 5–12.

The effects include:

- Loss of function below the level of lesion of the portion of the cord that controls voluntary motor pathways and major sensory tracts
- Sparing of the posterior columns as the vascular supply is obtained from a different source
- Preservation of position, vibration, and touch sense

Brown-Séquard's syndrome This syndrome is caused by damage to one side of the cord only. See Figure 5–13.

The effect is loss of function below the level of the lesion of the portion of the cord that controls voluntary motor pathways on the same side of the body and pain and temperature on the opposite side of the body.

Conus and cauda equina injuries These injuries involve damage to the conus medullaris or spinal nerves forming the cauda equina (see Figure 5–14). Common effects are:

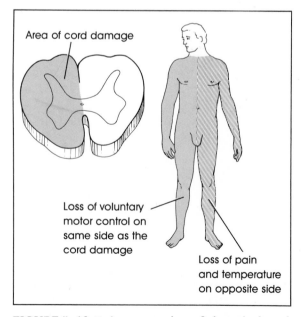

FIGURE 5–13 ■ A cross-section of the spinal cord showing damage that causes a Brown-Séquard syndrome.

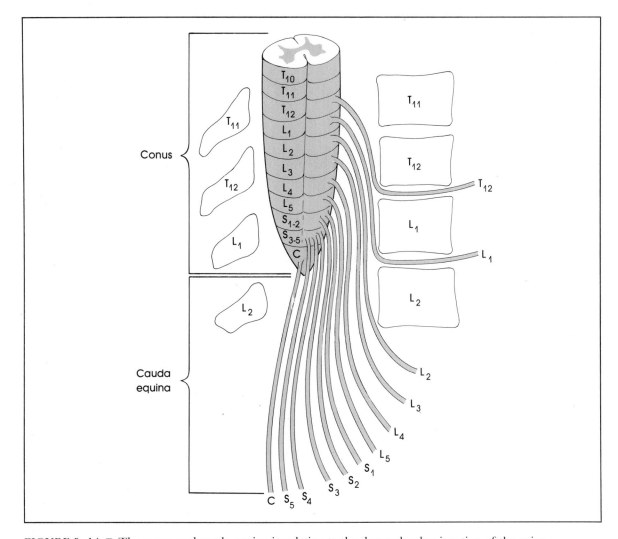

FIGURE 5–14 ■ The conus and cauda equina in relation to the thoracolumbar junction of the spine.

- Loss of motor function (leaving sensory function not markedly impaired).
- An extremely variable pattern with asymmetrical involvement. Roots have some recovery potential, so outlook is often favorable.
- Lower motor neuron (flaccid) involvement of bowel, bladder, and sexual functioning because those reflex centers are located in the conus.

Sacral sparing In this syndrome there is damage to the major part of the cord and/or blood supply, but radicular arteries preserve the outer circumference of the cord. See Figure 5–15. Therefore, sensation of the sacral area is preserved in an otherwise paralyzed patient.

Upper Motor Neuron and Lower Motor Neuron Lesions

To understand the many neurological aspects of rehabilitation, it is essential to grasp the concept of upper motor neuron and lower motor neuron lesions. Spinal cord injury can result in damage to upper motor neurons, lower motor neurons, or a combination of both. Particularly when the sacral portion of the cord is injured, differentiating between upper motor neuron and lower motor neuron involvement is essential to determine the nature and extent of bladder, bowel, and sexual dysfunction. Understanding spinal shock, spasticity, and hyperactive reflexes is also based on this concept.

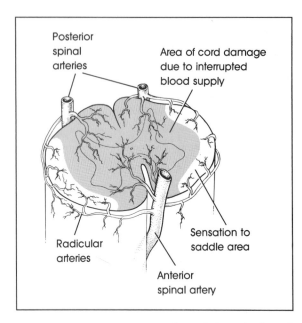

FIGURE 5–15 ■ A cross-section of the spinal cord illustrating damage that allows sacral sparing.

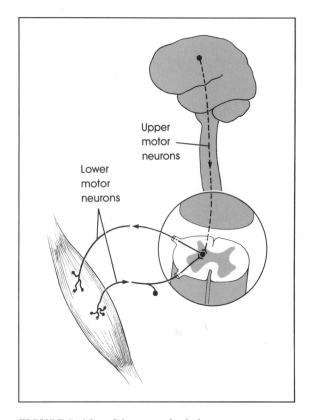

FIGURE 5–16 ■ Diagram depicting upper motor neuron and lower motor neuron pathways.

Upper motor neurons

Upper motor neurons are long neurons that originate in the brain and travel in bundles or tracts within the spinal cord. The cell bodies of these neurons are located in the motor strip of the cerebral cortex and the brain stem with the axons extending down through the spinal cord. These ascending and descending tracts resemble transmission cables. Upper motor neurons terminate at each segmental level throughout the entire length of the spinal cord to synapse (transmit a nerve impulse) with lower motor neurons, which arise in the spinal cord and connect to a muscle or organ. See Figure 5–16. The brain, via the upper motor neurons, suppresses or inhibits the lower motor neurons so that they do not become hyperactive to local stimuli. Any injury that damages upper motor neurons destroys cerebral influence or control over lower motor neurons and is termed an *upper motor neuron lesion.*

An *upper motor neuron* or *spastic paralysis* results when damage to the upper motor neuron pathways causes loss of coordinated and integrated cerebral control over all reflex activity below the level of lesion. Patients experience spasticity of limbs and of bowel and bladder functioning. Male patients experience reflex erections. However, spasticity is not all undesirable, and rehabilitation includes training these abnormal movements to assist patient mobility and management of body functions.

Lower motor neurons

Lower motor neurons originate in the spinal cord and travel outside the central nervous system to form the spinal nerves and subsequent branches of the peripheral nervous system. The cell bodies of these neurons are located in the central gray matter throughout the entire length of the spinal cord. The axons extend out through the spinal nerve roots and peripheral nerve branches to muscle fibers throughout the body. A lower motor neuron may be thought of as a wishbone, with the joint inserted into the spinal cord. A lower motor neuron may transmit stimulation from a muscle or organ to the spinal cord where it synapses with another lower motor neuron, which carries the response back to the muscle or organ. This pathway is known as a *reflex arc* and must be intact to create an involuntary response, such as jerking a finger away from a hot stove. See Figure 5–17. Although simultaneously the painful sensation is appreciated, the reflex action is innervated by the spinal cord and not controlled by the brain. Any damage to the lower motor neuron is termed a *lower motor neuron lesion.*

A *lower motor neuron* or *flaccid paralysis* results when damage to the lower motor neuron pathways causes destruction of the reflex arc and breaks pathways of communication to the intact upper motor neurons. Although lower motor neuron damage can occur at any segment of the cord, significant clinical manifestations only result from damage to the sacral portion of the cord. When injuries occur to the sacral portion of the cord where lower motor neurons have a vital role in controlling major body functions (such as bowel, bladder, and sexual responses), the implications are very obvious and serious. Patients experience "floppy" paralysis of lower limbs, loss of bowel and bladder tone, and eventual muscle atrophy or wasting. Reflex erections are not possible. Circulatory problems tend to be more serious due to chronic passive vasodilation and lack of muscle tone.

The sacral segments of the cord correspond to the T_{12} vertebrae. Fractures at or above this level usually cause a general spastic paralysis. However, many injuries near this level can result in a *mixed* upper motor neuron/lower motor neuron picture that particularly presents very difficult bladder management problems. See Chapter 12.

The Autonomic Nervous System

The *autonomic nervous system* is composed of complex peripheral nerves that can be severely affected by spinal cord injury. The autonomic nervous system provides automatic control, at a subconscious or involuntary level, of such vital functions as blood pressure, heart rate, body temperature control, appetite, fluid balance, bladder emptying, gastrointestinal motility, carbohydrate and fat metabolism, sleep, and sexual functioning.

Governing the autonomic nervous system is a function of the hypothalamus, located deep within the brain, and, to a certain extent, of local

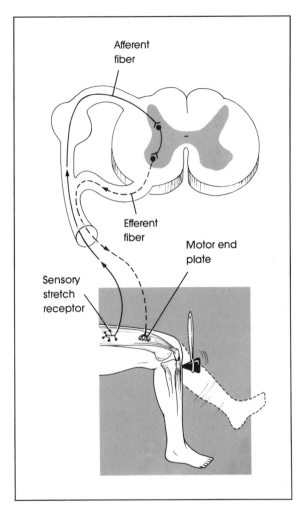

FIGURE 5–17 ■ Pathway of the lower motor neuron or reflex arc.

reflex activity. This is an *action* nervous system composed almost entirely of outflowing motor fibers. Impulses are conducted out of but seldom back to the central nervous system. From the hypothalamus, neurons descend through the brain stem and spinal cord to terminate in three groups:

1. One group clustered near certain cranial nerve roots in the brain stem (cranial outflow).
2. Another group located between the first thoracic and first lumbar segments of the spinal cord (thoracolumbar outflow).
3. A group centered between the second and fourth sacral segments of the cord (sacral outflow).

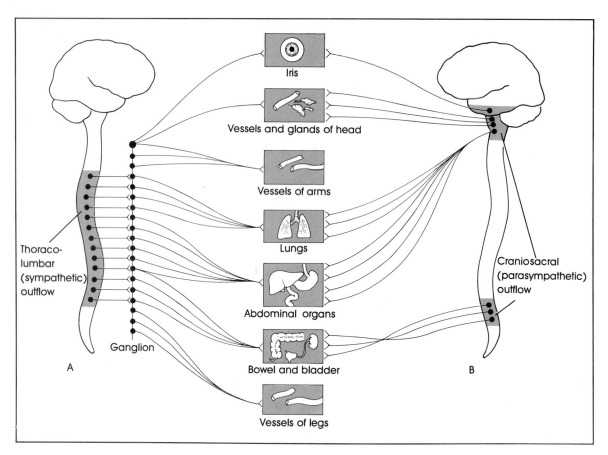

FIGURE 5–18 ■ A symbolic diagram of the sympathetic nervous system, composed from the thoracolumbar outflow (**A**), and of the parasympathetic nervous system, composed from the craniosacral outflow (**B**).

The *thoracolumbar outflow* gives rise to the *sympathetic* division of the autonomic nervous system (see Figure 5–18a), and the *craniosacral outflow* gives rise to the *parasympathetic* division (see Figure 5–18b). These autonomic nerve fibers then share various common pathways with cranial and spinal nerves and blood vessels to arrive at their destination in muscles, organs, and glands.

The division of the autonomic nervous system into *sympathetic* and *parasympathetic* sections is based on differences not only in ana-tomical structure but also in function. The sympathetic and parasympathetic systems are functional opposites, thus maintaining a stable internal environment. Most muscles and organs receive stimulation from both systems. For example, the sympathetic system will speed the heart rate, whereas the parasympathetic will slow it down.

The balance can be changed in two ways: by increasing the amount of stimulus to either division or by decreasing (blocking) the amount of discharge from either division. This very important principle, which is explained by Liebman (1979), forms the basis for many neurologically active drugs.

The sympathetic division

Function   The sympathetic division allows for maximum energy expenditure for stress defense. Stimulation to this system provides a generalized response from the body because of the widespread network of nerves to the entire body. See Figure 5–19. It is important for the nurse to know the body's *fight or flight* mechanism in order to observe for the most subtle changes when caring for patients under severe physical and emotional stress, especially when control from higher centers may be impaired.

To prepare the body for violent action, the sympathetic nervous system will:

- Increase heart rate and respirations and shunt blood from less-important areas to cardio-pulmonary circulation
- Decrease gastrointestinal, urinary, and other less-important functions
- Release red blood cells from storage in the spleen for additional energy
- Stimulate the adrenal gland above the kidney to release adrenalin

Structure   The dorsal and ventral roots attach each spinal nerve to the spinal cord. At the point where these roots join in a common sleeve, nerve fibers extend both upward and downward to establish communication with a sympathetic ganglion. A sympathetic ganglion is simply a mass of sympathetic nervous tissue previously described as clustered or grouped around each side of the thoracic and lumbar cord. These ganglia are then linked together to form a chainlike structure, which extends bilaterally from the base of the cranium to the coccyx just outside the vertebral column and innervates the entire body.

The chemical transmitter between the sympathetic fibers and the structures they innervate is *adrenalin* (or *noradrenalin*). Drugs that mimic this effect are known as *adrenergic* or *sympathomimetic* agents. In patients with spinal cord injuries a drug like ephedrine may be used to combat severe and prolonged effects of postural (orthostatic) hypotension by raising the blood pressure. To block effects of the sympathetic system, such as is necessary in uncontrolled autonomic dysreflexia, hydralazine hydrochloride (Apresoline) may be used to lower the blood pressure.

The parasympathetic division

Function   The parasympathetic division controls everyday body functioning. See Figure 5–20. It initiates such functions as digestion or elimination and conserves body energy. Stimulation to this system produces more specific responses than are produced in the sympathetic system, for example, increased intestinal motility

to aid elimination or increased contractions of the bladder wall to accomplish voiding.

Structure   Long nerve fibers extend from their craniosacral origin in a direct pathway to reach the muscle or organ innervated by the parasympathetic nervous system. Stimulation is most abundant in the head and abdominal area. Parasympathetic stimulation is not extended to certain muscles and organs, which allows the sympathetic influence complete control in stressful situations. Receiving sympathetic stimulation only are the voluntary muscles, skin, sweat glands, adrenal gland, and spleen.

The chemical transmitter between the parasympathetic fibers and the structures they innervate is *acetylcholine*. Drugs that mimic this effect are known as *cholinergic* or *parasympathomimetic* agents; thus such a drug's reaction resembles parasympathetic discharge. Drugs such as bethanecol chloride (Urecholine) may be used to stimulate bladder emptying and combat urinary retention in patients with spinal cord injuries. To minimize the effects of parasympathetic stimulation a drug such as Pro-Banthine may be selected to achieve dryness when incontinence is caused by hyperactivity of the detrusor muscle due to parasympathetic stimulation.

Dysfunctions after injury

Because maintaining homeostasis within the body is largely a function of the autonomic nervous system, internal stability is threatened when intricate communications with the central nervous system are interrupted. Generally, the higher the level of lesion, the more profound the effects become, as a greater portion of the body is involved.

Instability of the cardiovascular system and inability to regulate body temperature can be a particular problem for the patient with quadriplegia. A lowered pulse, a lowered blood pressure, postural hypotension, and a tendency to assume the temperature of the environment are obvious symptoms. One phenomenon unique to the spinal cord injured is the dangerous condition of *autonomic dysreflexia (hyperreflexia)*, which is created when the sympathetic division of the autonomic nervous system responds in an unin-

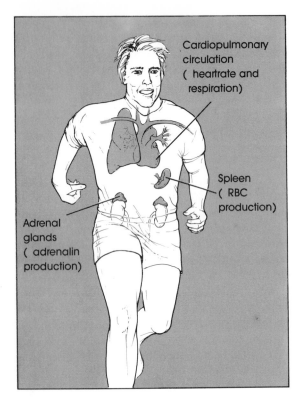

FIGURE 5–19 ■ The sympathetic division activates the entire body for stress defense. Major responses to stress include an increase in cardiopulmonary blood supply; a release of more red blood cells from the spleen; and an increased production of adrenalin from the adrenal glands.

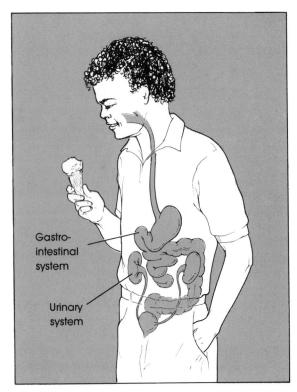

FIGURE 5–20 ■ The parasympathetic division initiates such bodily functions as digestion and elimination to create an internal homeostasis.

hibited manner due to lack of control from higher centers. See Chapter 10 for assessment, specific nursing interventions, and criteria for evaluating care for a patient with autonomic hyperreflexia, other instabilities of the cardiovascular system, and lack of body temperature control.

Spinal shock is a collective term meaning physiological disorganization of cord function. It occurs immediately following spinal cord injury and is characterized by a temporary flaccid paralysis caused by loss of all reflex activity below the level of lesion. It is a poorly understood phenomenon that may take hours, days, weeks, or months to subside, depending on the individual. Recovery of reflex activity usually occurs in an ascending pattern.

ASSESSMENT OF INJURY

Taking a History

Facts in the history that affect a diagnosis include mechanisms of injury, preexisting conditions or disease, and advanced age.

Mechanisms of injury

The forces or stresses producing injury are referred to as *mechanisms of injury*. Knowledge of their nature assists the physician with diagnosis and treatment, and they are recorded in the admission history. A detailed account of the accident is needed to describe these mechanisms.

These forces often occur in combination. The most common mechanisms of injury that result in spinal cord injury include:

- Forced flexion, or flexion with rotation
- Forced extension (hyperextension)
- Vertical compression ·

Open wounds, such as gunshot or knife injuries, may also cause spinal cord injury and are also referred to as mechanisms of injury.

The common sites of injury are the most mobile parts of the spine: the cervical area and the thoracolumbar junction. The severity of bony injury does not always correspond with the extent of neurological damage. Gross fractures may cause little motor or sensory loss, and minor fractures may result in extensive paralysis. Table 5–1 outlines some common mechanisms of injury and the vertebral column injury that may result.

Preexisting conditions or disease

A number of preexisting conditions or diseases that directly affect the spine may have predisposed the patient to the initial cord injury. These high-risk patients are susceptible to cord damage from relatively minor trauma; a bedridden patient may even incur a spontaneous dislocation. If the spine is grossly unstable, the physician may order surgical intervention to prevent neurological damage.

Ankalosing spondylitis is a disease affecting the spinal column, characterized by calcification and ossification of soft tissue and ligamentous structures. The spinal column is converted into a rigid structure when the shock-absorbing qualities of the spine are lost. Relatively minor trauma, particularly in the cervical area, can result in severe cord damage. Rheumatoid arthritis, a chronic inflammatory condition, may attack the spine and cause osteoporosis and ligamentous damage, which cause abnormal mobility of the spine and vulnerability to injury. Space-occupying lesions or infective processes may also cause disc degeneration or collapse, direct pressure on the cord, or interruption of cord blood supply (venous infarction). Examples of these include an epidural abscess secondary to a distant infection and tuberculosis or cancer of

the spine. Despite the cause, the onset of paralysis demands the same comprehensive management as other spinal cord trauma.

Any past conditions that would limit movement or impair sensation must be noted to complete a neuromuscular assessment. Certainly the patient's general health before injury will significantly influence the effects of spinal cord dysfunction on that individual.

Advanced age

In the course of normal aging, muscles, bones, and articulations undergo changes that affect their physiological function and physical appearance. Degenerative and osteoporotic changes in the spine are referred to collectively as *cervical lordosis of aging*. In the elderly the back may be rounded, the shoulders stooped, and the head tilted backward to compensate. The elderly become particularly prone to hyperextension injuries of the cervical spine due to a blow to the face or forehead, often caused by a simple fall. This type of injury results in the classic central cord syndrome with minimal or no bony damage and accounts for up to 30% of all cervical spine injuries (Burke and Murray 1975).

Physical Examination of the Spine

In-depth physical examination of the spine is the responsibility of the physician. The physical examination should include general observation of the neck and back and examination of the fracture site.

The neck and back

The spine is the main axial support of the body and functions with the skin, major muscles and muscle groups, and supporting bony structures to hold the head erect and the body in an upright position. Natural slight curvatures of the vertebral column—the cervical curve (convex anteriorly), the thoracic curve (concave anteriorly), and the lumbar curve (convex anteriorly)—enhance this strength. Any exaggeration of these curves or lateral deviations are abnormal. For example, if the thoracic curve is excessive, it is called a *kyphosis* (hunchback); if a lum-

**TABLE 5–1 ■ SOME COMMON MECHANISMS OF INJURY
AND EXAMPLES OF RESULTANT TRAUMA TO THE VERTEBRAL COLUMN AND SPINAL CORD**

Flexion

Flexion injuries to the cervical spine may result from a motor vehicle accident, typically a head-on collision, when the victim's head is first hyperextended then thrown violently forward from the arrested momentum. Similar flexion injuries can result when the head is struck from behind or the victim falls and strikes the back of the head. In the cervical region extensive tearing of the posterior ligamentous complex may result in severe forward dislocation.

In the thoracic or lumbar region flexion injuries can be caused by a fall onto the buttocks. Typically the vertebral bodies are wedged and compressed as a result of a pure flexion injury.

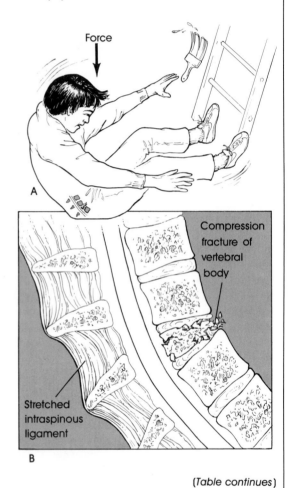

(Table continues)

---

bar curve is excessive, it is called a *lordosis* (swayback); and if a lateral curve exists, it is called a *scoliosis*. Abnormal shape of the back or unusual bony protuberances or prominences may be caused by congenital deformity or disease or the initial trauma. Spinal curvatures may also be postinjury complications associated with inadequate early immobilization and stabilization.

The fracture site

The fracture site is examined for surrounding edema, open areas, or entry wounds in gunshot or stabbing cases. Compound spinal fractures are rare. A *gibbous* deformity—a humped protuberance or sharp angulation of the spine—may occur immediately as a result of vertebral injury. When there is any abnormality in the shape of the neck or back or at the fracture

TABLE 5–1 *(continued)*

Flexion with Rotation

Flexion and rotational forces occurring concurrently are particularly potent and are associated with fracture dislocations at any level of the spinal column. Typically the posterior ligamentous complex is ruptured accompanied by vertebral body fracture(s) rendering this injury highly unstable. Causes may be related to any number of accidents.

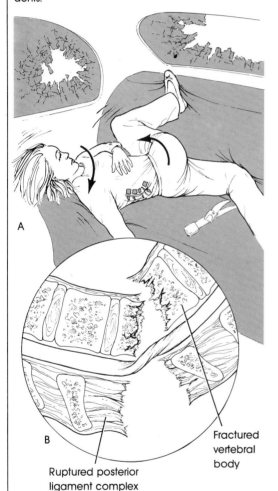

Fractured vertebral body

Ruptured posterior ligament complex

Forced Extension (Hyperextension)

Forced extension (hyperextension) injuries are typically seen in elderly persons, when degenerative changes have narrowed the spinal canal. Injuries, usually at the cervical level, are often related to falls in which chin or face is struck, causing violent extension of the neck.

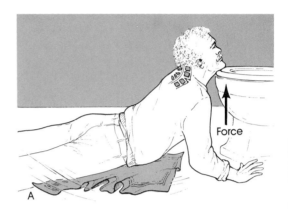

Force

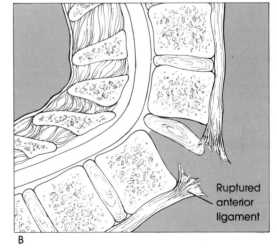

Ruptured anterior ligament

(Table continues)

site, nurses should anticipate modifications to turning, positioning, and skin care measures.

Physical Examination of Neurological Function

Physical examination of neurological function involves examination of *movement, sensation,* and *reflex activity.* The key to neurological assessment is using consistent methods and terms to define the level and nature of the lesion and comparison of serial data to detect any deterioration or improvement.

When describing the vertebrae or cord segments, abbreviations of letters and numbers are used for convenience. For example, the fourth cervical vertebra and segment are labeled C_4; the

TABLE 5–1 *(continued)* ■ SOME COMMON MECHANISMS OF INJURY AND EXAMPLES OF RESULTANT TRAUMA TO THE VERTEBRAL COLUMN AND SPINAL CORD

Vertical Compression

Fractures resulting from vertical compression typically occur at the cervical and sometimes thoracolumbar areas of the spine. A high-velocity blow to the top of the head can cause a shattered vertebral body to burst into the spinal cord.

seventh thoracic vertebra and segment are labeled T_7; and so on.

The number of the vertebra does not necessarily correspond to the number of the adjacent cord segment. In the cervical region the spinal roots extend almost laterally, and there is little difference between the cord segments and the vertebral body levels. From C_8 down, the spinal roots travel varying distances in the spinal canal before exiting through the vertebral column. In the fetus, the cord extends the full length of the vertebral canal, but later the canal grows longer than the cord, thus causing the appearance of cord shrinkage and the downward projections of roots into the canal. This can become confusing when trying to relate the vertebral fracture level to the injured spinal cord segment. For example, a T_{12} fracture may cause S_2 cord damage.

Diagnosis describes both the bony involvement, sometimes referred to as the *level of injury,* and the extent of neurological deficit, called the *level of lesion.* The level of lesion refers to the last normal functioning segment of the spinal cord. For example, the diagnosis "fractured C_5 with C_5 quadriplegia complete" means that the C_5 segment and nerve root are functioning normally, and C_6 and below are damaged. If the injury is incomplete, it is described in more detail such as "incomplete below C_5" and "complete below C_7." Involvement may differ between the right and left sides. This would also be described.

This section on neurological function focuses on some key observations particularly useful for early neurological assessment of the spinal cord injured patient. As rehabilitation progresses, skilled assessment remains essential to evaluate progress and to determine realistic physiological and mobility goals. As such, further neurological assessment techniques have been integrated throughout the text. (Table 16–7, for example, correlates neurological status with functional expectations.)

Motor function

Examination of functional movements is used to determine motor power. In-depth assessment detailing motor power in all major muscle groups is not generally within the scope of nursing practice, but it is important to recognize the significance of other team members' findings.

Nursing assessment of motor function focuses on the detection of gross neurological changes once the level of lesion has been diagnosed. Assessment of motor function is a prime concern of the nurse providing continuous observation in a critical care area.

Motor power can be described as strong (normal), good (only slightly impaired), moderate, weak, or absent. A visible or palpable muscle contraction without actual movement of the limb may be described as a flicker or trace of movement. These terms are included in an international five-point scale used for grading muscle power or strength. Table 5–2 presents this manual muscle-testing and grading system. To test and grade motor power the examiner first asks the patient to follow a number of commands; often the examiner must provide resistance to determine the strength of the movement re-

quested. To allow for observation of a very weak muscle contraction the examiner must support the limb. For example, a patient with quadriplegia asked to flex an arm may not be able to do so, but if the arm is supported at the elbow and wrist, the examiner may observe a flicker of movement in the biceps.

Figure 5–21 presents a motor scale scoring system based on muscle testing. The representative muscle groups on this scale were chosen on the basis of functional significance as it correlates to the level of injury.

When examining patients with quadriplegia, nurses should test whether patients can:

- Shrug shoulders
- Elevate arms
- Flex elbows
- Extend elbows
- Flex wrists
- Extend wrists
- Flex, extend, and spread fingers

As the most common sight of cervical injury is C_{5-6}, most patients with quadriplegia are able to flex but not extend their arms. In addition, the examiner should closely monitor the respiratory function of the patient with quadriplegia. Progressive difficulty breathing and subsequent retention of pulmonary secretions may be due to fatigue but may also be due to an increasing

TABLE 5–2 ■ A MANUAL MUSCLE-TESTING GRADING SYSTEM

Grade	Movement	Amount
0	No movement or evidence of muscle contraction.	Absent
1	Visible or palpable evidence of muscle contraction but no joint movement.	Trace, flicker
2	Strength sufficient to move the adjacent joint through the complete range of motion in gravity-eliminated position. (Examiner would support the limb.)	Poor, weak
3	Strength to move the joint through the complete range of motion against gravity (move freely).	Fair, moderate
4	Ability to move the joint and overcome some resistance as well. (Resistance is offered by the examiner, weights, or equipment.)	Good, only slightly impaired
5	Normal movement and power.	Normal, strong

Adapted from Burke and Murray (1975).

Part A ■ MOTOR EVALUATION FORM

The Motor Scale scoring system is based on muscle testing. There is general agreement in the literature that certain muscle groups are innervated by specific anatomical portions of the spinal cord. The representative muscle groups were chosen on the basis of functional significance as it correlates to level of injury. Since 44 muscle groups are tested on a 5-point basis, the total Motor Scores range from 0 to 220.

Patient Name: _____   Test Performed By: _____

Patient # _____   Date of Test: _____

Date of Admission: _____   Level of Injury: _____

	LEFT SCORE	RIGHT SCORE	TOTAL SCORE
SHOULDER ELEVATION			
ARM ELEVATION			
ARM HORIZONTAL ADDUCTION			
ELBOW FLEXORS			
ELBOW EXTENSORS			
WRIST FLEXORS			
WRIST EXTENSORS			
EXTRINSIC FLEXORS			
EXTRINSIC EXTENSORS			
THUMB OPPOSITION			
FINGER ABDUCTION			
UPPER ABDOMINALS			
LOWER ABDOMINALS			
HIP FLEXORS			
HIP EXTENSORS			
HIP ABDUCTION			
KNEE FLEXOR			
KNEE EXTENSORS			
FOOT DORSI-FLEXION			
FOOT FLEXOR			
TOE EXTENSOR			
		Grand Total	

CODE:

0 = No Function

1 = A visible or palpable flicker of contraction, but no resultant movement of limb or joint.

2 = The muscle can only move normally when the limb is so positioned that gravity is eliminated.

3 = The muscle is able to move normally against gravity, but not against additional resistance.

4 = The muscle, though able to move normally, is overcome by resistance.

5 = Normal muscle power.

FIGURE 5–21 ■ Neurospinal functional capacity rating. The Motor and Sensory subscale scores can be added together to yield an overall neurospinal functional capacity rating. These assessments are made at stated intervals and can be used to chart progression or regression for individuals or groups of patients over a given time period. Additionally, individual assessments are sensitive to small changes, thus the effect of specific interventions can be monitored in an ongoing fashion. Differential changes of any of the subscales can indicate the area affected by that intervention. Tests are performed by experienced physical therapists. (Reprinted from Klose and Goldberg, 1980, with permission from the copyright owner, National Spinal Cord Injury Data Research Center, Good Samaritan Hospital, Phoenix, Arizona.)

Part B ■ UNIVERSITY OF MIAMI NEURO-SPINAL INDEX (UMNI)
SENSORY EVALUATION FORM

The Sensory Scale score is a measure of total body sensation. Within the spinal cord, two major spatially separated tracts carry information from different sensory modalities. The lateral spinothalamic tracts are assessed by pin prick, while the dorsal columns are assessed with vibration. The rationale for testing both columns is that it provided a more sensitive measure of completeness of injury. Since different skin areas or dermatomes of the body are innervated by specific levels of the spinal cord, this test also determines the level of injury for that modality. Pain sense is determined by pin prick and vibration sense with a 256 hz tuning fork. Each stimulus is presented bilaterally to each of the dermatome areas innervated by the 30 levels of the spinal cord. Item scores are assigned as follows: 0 = absent; 1 = present, but abnormal; 2 = normal. Sensory indices range from 0 = no detectable sensation to 240 = total normal body sensation.

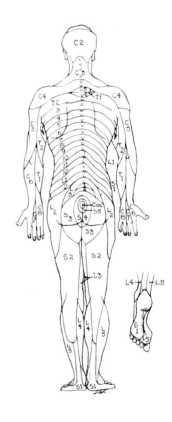

DORSAL COLUMN FUNCTIONS (DCF): vibration
LATERAL SPINOTHALAMIC TRACT FUNCTIONS (LSTF): Pain

Code:
2 = present/normal
1 = present/abnormal
0 = absent

LEFT	DCF	LSTF	CERVICAL	DCF	LSTF	RIGHT
			2			
			3			
			4			
			5			
			6			
			7			
			8			
			THORACIC			
			1			
			2			
			3			
			4			
			5			
			6			
			7			
			8			
			9			
			10			
			11			
			12			
			LUMBAR			
			1			
			2			
			3			
			4			
			5			
			SACRAL			
			1			
			2			
			3			
			4			
			5			
			COCCYGEAL			
			1			

TOTAL _____

GRAND TOTAL: ___ Test performed by: ___ Date of test:___

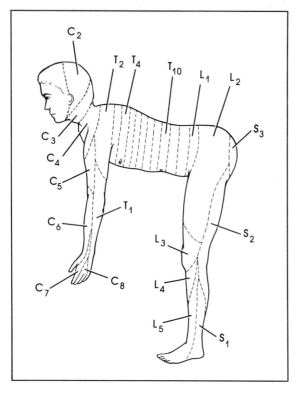

FIGURE 5-22 ■ Arrangement of dermatomes is more easily understood when an individual is considered in the quadruped (crouched) position. It is important to correlate the level of injury with the area of the body surface that is affected (dermatome).

neurological deficit. The examiner should note any changes in the power of coughing ability, a decreased vital capacity, or increasingly limited chest expansion.

When examining the patient with paraplegia, nurses should test whether patients can:

- Move hips
- Flex knees
- Extend knees
- Flex feet
- Extend feet
- Wiggle toes

Sensory function

Detailed sensory testing—a more exact skill, which is easier to perfect than muscle testing—is used to detect changes in neurological function. Sensation may be described as simple or "crude," such as appreciation of light touch, pain, or tem-

perature, or as more sophisticated or discriminative, such as position sense, or appreciating where limbs are in space, and vibration sense. For ease of examination sensory testing can be confined to testing for pain with pinprick and for light touch with the aid of a cotton swab. General appreciation of basic touch by placing hands on the patient and asking for a verbal response can also be used. Patients must close their eyes to reduce the chances that "wishful" thinking will lead to inappropriate responses. Always compare sensation bilaterally. It is important to correlate the level of lesion to the actual body surface area that is without sensation or has impaired sensation. Again, the most important clinical aspect is to know the exact point or level on the patient where normal sensation is present. The best way to ensure continuity and accuracy of comparing serial data is to mark the patient's skin lightly and ensure that if the mark is washed it is replaced.

Sensory distribution to the entire skin surface of the body is organized in dermatomes. A *dermatome* is simply a section or area of cutaneous distribution innervated by a cranial or spinal nerve. Arrangement of dermatomes is more easily understood if an individual is first considered in the quadruped (crouched) position (Figure 5-22).

The examiner should systematically test dermatomes, working upward on the body from areas of impaired sensation to normal zones. See Procedure 5-1. Examination of the trunk should always begin in the midaxillary line and progress to the arms and then the hands where the C_{6-8} dermatomes are represented (without inclusion of the arms, T_2 borders C_4 on the anterior chest). Sensation may be described as normal, impaired, or absent. Sometimes the terms *anesthesia* (sensation of touch absent); *analgesia* (sensation of pain absent); *hypoaesthesia* (reduced sensation) or *hyperaesthesia* (exaggerated sensation) are used. Figure 5-21 presents a detailed sensory evaluation form.

Reflex activity

Formal testing of reflex activity is not generally within the scope of nursing practice. However, it is helpful to beware of the presence or absence of general reflex activity below the level

PROCEDURE 5–1 ■ SENSORY TESTING

Purpose

The primary purpose of this technique is to detect changes in neurological function. Sensory testing is a more exact skill that is easier to perfect than detailed muscle testing and is particularly valuable to nurses during the critical 48–72 hour postinjury period.

Action	Rationale
1. Explain procedure and ask patient to close eyes.	Reduces chances of "wishful thinking" that might lead to an inappropriate response.
2. Position in basic anatomical alignment.	
3. Select pin, cotton swab, or light touch of hand for examination.	
4. Systematically test dermatomes, working upward on the body from area of impaired sensation to normal zones.	Easier for patient to first concentrate and then give exact verbal response.
5. Conduct testing in the midaxillary line, progress to the arms, and then to the hands.	Without inclusion of the arms, T_2 borders on C_4 on the anterior chest; C_{6-8} dermatomes are represented on the hands.
6. Lightly mark patient's skin where normal sensation is present.	Ensures continuity and accuracy of comparing serial data.
7. Compare data bilaterally.	
8. Draw on sensory chart.	

of lesion, particularly the perineal reflexes. For example, during nursing care, nurses may notice the beginning of reflex penile erections or extremity spasms. Knowing the status of reflex activity will help the physician formulate diagnosis and prognosis and help nurses plan interventions, specifically bladder and bowel management.

Useful reflexes the physician will test are the *deep tendon reflexes* of the biceps (C_5), supinator (C_6), and triceps (C_7) in the upper extremities; and the knee (L_3) and the ankle (S_1) in the lower extremities. If a patient presents soon after injury with deep tendon reflexes below the level of lesion, it can be a good prognostic sign of an incomplete neurological injury (Burke 1979). However, following acute trauma to the spinal cord, most patients experience temporary physiological disorganization of cord function (spinal shock) characterized by a flaccid paralysis with depressed or no reflex activity below the level of

the lesion. The presence of the bulbocavernosus reflex and the anal wink reflex is the first indication that cord function reorganization is occurring. The presence or absence of these reflexes helps differentiate between an upper motor neuron lesion and a lower motor neuron lesion involving the conus or cauda equina. The presence of these reflexes suggests upper motor neuron dysfunction; their absence suggests lower motor neuron dysfunction. The status of these reflexes becomes the main indicator of the physiological basis for bladder, bowel, and sexual dysfunction.

The *bulbocavernosus* reflex can be elicited by placing a gloved finger in the patient's rectum and squeezing the glans penis in the male or clitoris in the female or by tugging on the Foley catheter. A positive reflex will cause a sharp, distinct rectal sphincter contraction. The *anal wink* is another cord reflex. A pinprick in the perianal skin will cause a visual external anal sphincter contraction.

DIAGNOSTIC PROCEDURES

Neuroradiologic and neurophysiological techniques are becoming increasingly sophisticated and are enhancing the accuracy of diagnosis and prognosis, especially in the acute phase of spinal cord injury. However, many diagnostic procedures still require turning or manipulation of the patient, so skilled supervision is essential to ensure that spinal alignment is maintained. If procedures are completed within hours after injury, provision must also be made for constant nursing observation of the patient's general tolerance to the procedure, particularly if respiratory and cardiovascular instability is a potential problem.

Radiologic Examination

Extreme caution must be exercised when positioning the patient for initial radiologic examination. Any movement of an unstable vertebral column may cause further neurological damage. All patients should be managed as if their injuries were unstable until proven otherwise. To reduce risk, minimal movement of the patient is indicated rather than excessive movement for the purpose of obtaining "good" X rays.

The physician will initially examine the spinal X rays for malalignment; fractures or compressions of the vertebral bodies; fractures or dislocations of the neural arches; and evidence of ligamentous injury. Ligamentous rupture may be indicated by widening of disc spaces or spreading of the spinous processes at the level of injury. Neurological deficit may well occur without radiographic evidence of damage to the vertebral column, particularly in children and the elderly. Also radiologic examination does not necessarily show the extent of bony displacement at the moment of injury. The injured vertebrae may have returned to normal alignment.

Basic investigation includes *lateral* and *anteroposterior* views of the spine. Particularly with cervical injury, a *lateral* view is usually taken first,

before the patient is moved. For this a portable machine is necessary. A physician should supervise removal and replacement of a cervical collar. To ensure that all seven cervical vertebrae are well visualized, the physician may gently pull the patient's wrists down to lower the shoulders. The patient must be carefully lifted to position the film cassette for *anteroposterior* views. If the patient is on a turning frame, turn the patient prone to position the cassette and return to the supine position to take the X ray.

If further investigation is needed to determine ligamentous damage, the physician may order flexion/extension or other special views of the cervical spine. These are high-risk procedures and must be supervised by a skilled physician. Tomography and computerized axial tomography (CAT) have replaced some of these procedures and present less risk to the patient.

In some cases, radiologic examination is used to evaluate treatment. For example, during closed reduction attempts, when additional weights (progressive traction) are added to increase the traction pull on the cervical spine, serial X rays are ordered to determine if satisfactory reduction has been achieved (Figure 5–23). And postoperative films may be taken to determine whether proper alignment has been achieved.

Computerized Axial Tomography (CAT) Scanning

Computerized axial tomography (CAT) scanning has made possible great advancements in the field of neurodiagnosis. CAT scanning of the spine and spinal cord outlines the spine and perispinal structures clearly. This technique improves assessment of bony stability and helps clarify diagnoses. For example, if a patient is deteriorating neurologically, there may be pressure on the cord. CAT scanning makes it possible to investigate the exact cause of that pressure. It is also possible to view fractures and contents of the spinal canal and to differentiate hematomes and bony fragments from cord edema.

CAT scanning uses computer-reconstructed images from multiple X-ray absorption measurements. The technique uses a thin, concentrated X-ray beam rather than the diffuse or scattered radiation used in conventional X rays. As the thin beam is emitted from the scanner, the computer measures the radiation intensity before the beam enters the patient and after it emerges from the patient. The X-ray tube makes a 180-degree arc around the patient, obtaining numerous scans in 1-degree steps.

The amount of absorption is measured according to density and is expressed in Hounsfield units (named after the British physicist who researched the technique). Water is arbitrarily given a density of 0, bone + 500, air − 500, cerebral spinal fluid 0–10, clotted blood 50–75, and so on. The actual density numbers of each structure are recorded on a matrix (computer printout) and then converted to a visual picture on a television screen or photograph. The denser the structure, the higher the number on the computer printout, and the lighter or whiter the image on the picture. The less dense the structure, the lower the number on the computer printout, and the darker or blacker the image on the picture.

CAT scanning equipment is very sophisticated and expensive. The major components consist of the scanner itself, which houses the X-ray tubes and radiation detectors and is a large, cylindrical object surrounding a motorized patient table; the computer necessary for data processing, computer printouts, and visual displays; and a controller's console and monitor. See Figure 5–24.

To prepare the patient, describe the rather awesome equipment and explain the procedure. This is a noninvasive, painless procedure lasting about 30 minutes. Contrast enhancement, administered via spinal puncture, may occasionally be required. If contrast material is used, preparation and postprocedure care is similar to that for a myelogram.

Tomography

Although rapidly being replaced by CAT scanning, tomography or polytomography may be used to evaluate the extent of bony injury. Tomography is particularly useful for obtaining

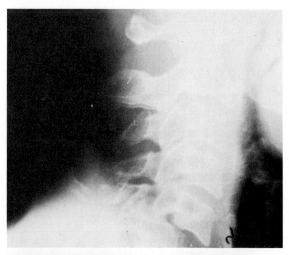
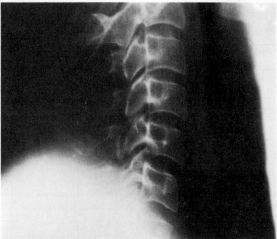
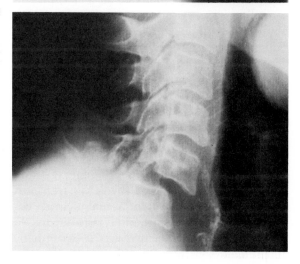

FIGURE 5–23 ■ Series of films taken to monitor results of progressive traction. Successful reduction of a C_6 bilateral facet dislocation is shown.

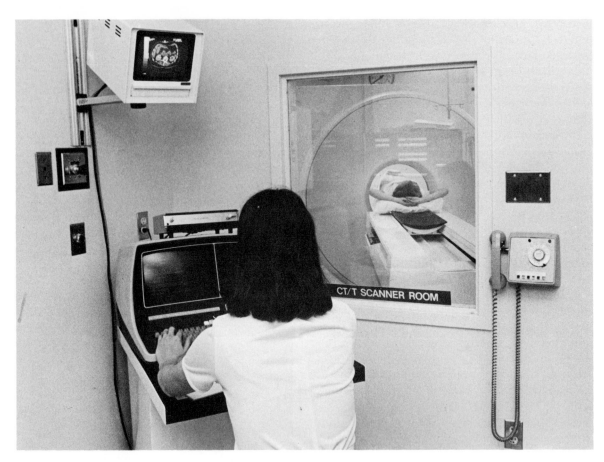

FIGURE 5–24 ■ Computerized axial tomography: the CAT scanner.

longitudinal cross-sections of the vertebral column. Special X rays are taken at different levels, or *cuts,* of the injured site and are arranged to outline more extensive, poorly visualized, or hidden fractures that may be overshadowed by other structures.

Equipment that can take anteroposterior and lateral tomograms while the patient remains supine is particularly desirable for patients with spinal cord injuries.

Tomography is usually completed within 24 hours after injury. The patient's general condition must be stable enough to tolerate transport to and endure a stay in a main X-ray department. The procedure often lasts one to two hours. Nurses should be prepared to accompany and remain with patients throughout the procedure. Assemble needed equipment such as the medical chart, previous X-ray films, IV solutions, blood pressure cuff, stethoscope, and medications that may be due within the next two-hour period. Prepare the patient by describing the equipment used, especially the cumbersome, large X-ray arm that swings back and forth overhead; explaining the reason for the examination; and administering preanalgesia as ordered. To protect the skin and make the patient comfortable, pad the X-ray table with a foam sheet or synthetic sheepskin. It may also be convenient to obtain an intravenous pyelogram for baseline urological data at this time, since the patient will be delayed in the main X-ray department for some time.

Myelography

The physician may order myelography if there is any evidence of pressure or impingement on the spinal cord or a nerve root. Such evidence would consist of an increasing neurological deficit. Diagnosis of persistent cord compression is especially important for the patient with an incomplete injury. Myelography may also be indicated when bony and neurological lesions differ or when neurological deficit occurs without bony injury. If surgical intervention is being considered to decompress the spinal cord, evidence of cord compression or compromise of the spinal canal on a myelogram or CAT scan constitutes an essential part of the preoperative assessment.

Myelography is an invasive procedure. An oil-based radiopaque dye is injected into the subarachnoid space via lumbar puncture. The patient is positioned prone and tilted in various directions to exert gravitational forces on the dye while serial X rays are taken to visualize the spinal canal. Because of the inherent danger in manipulating a patient with an unstable spinal fracture, myelography is considered a high-risk procedure for the acute spinal cord injured patient. To minimize the risk of excessive neck movement, a traction unit, consisting of two side poles with a cross-bar and pulley device, can be clamped to the myelogram table. A hospital maintenance department could construct such a device.

The newer water-soluble, rather than oil-based, contrast material mixes with cerebrolspinal fluid and can be checked fluoroscopically, therefore minimizing the hazards of turning and tilting involved with the conventional myelogram. (For the cervical injured patient a spinal puncture is made at the C_{1-2} interspace. For the thoracolumbar injured patient a lumbar puncture is carried out; however, the thoracic spine cannot be viewed very well.) Moreover, water-soluble contrast material does not have to be removed and does not react with blood. This reduces the incidence of postprocedure arachnoiditis.

Preparation of the patient includes explanation of the procedure and reason for examination; early completion of routine bladder and bowel procedures before examination; and administration of preanalgesia as ordered. Assemble equipment as if preparing for tomography and be prepared to accompany the patient for a two-hour period to monitor general condition and tolerance of procedure.

Following the procedure, nursing care is directed by the type of contrast medium used. If an oil-based contrast material is used, the patient must remain flat for 24 hours to minimize post-procedure headache. If water-soluble contrast material is used, the patient should either be up in the wheelchair or have the head of the bed elevated 30 degrees to 45 degrees if possible to exert gravitational forces on the unremoved contrast material and thus minimize cerebral irritation. To dilute the contrast material, increase fluid intake for a 12-hour period. Analgesics and antiemetics may be required.

Somatosensory-Evoked Potentials

Recording of somatosensory-evoked potentials is done mainly to establish a prognosis. The test is done by stimulating a peripheral nerve in the arm or leg (below the level of lesion) and recording the neurological response (evoked potential) from the cerebral cortex through scalp electrodes (similar to those used in electroencephalography). This is a noninvasive procedure and can be done in the emergency or operating room, because a small portable computer is used to summate the responses.

When the injury is complete, somatosensory-evoked potentials are absent; when the injury is incomplete, a marked alteration in response is noted. The test has been valuable in the assessment of prognosis and response to treatment (Tator and Rowed 1979). Early persistence and progressive normalization of evoked potentials precedes the clinical evidence of improvement and is therefore a favorable prognostic sign.

HOPE FOR THE FUTURE THROUGH RESEARCH

Among researchers investigating spinal cord injury, there is a quest to stimulate a means for the regrowth or rejoining of human central nervous system tissue. But is this regeneration possible? At the National Institute of Neurological and Communicative Disorders and Stroke many scientists now agree that central nervous system nerve regeneration in humans may be possible. Such regeneration is evident in some lower vertebrates, such as the lizard and the lamprey, which serve as models for research into cellular factors linked to recovery and regrowth. In higher vertebrates there is a suggestion of regeneration of nerve buds, but the process soon stops. Until this process of sprouting can be encouraged, it is unknown if the regenerated nerve fibers could find or be directed to the right target—that is, would a regenerated bladder nerve find its way to the bladder or would it end up in the big toe (Gunley 1981)?

There are numerous conflicting and confusing reports on interventions that minimize the effects of spinal cord injury. Perhaps one of the most alarming claims involved Russian experiments describing recovery in some patients following enzyme therapy; American investigators were unable to reproduce these results in laboratory animals. Spinal cord cooling and administration of corticosteroids to combat spinal cord edema have some clinical application immediately after injury. Use of dimethyl sulfoxide (DMSO) and opiate antagonists to minimize spinal shock is still experimental.

Patients and their families often seek clarification of the status of research. While it is worthwhile to hope for a cure in our lifetime, persistent "shopping around" for solutions that are not yet available can be costly and psychologically detrimental. The nurse can help minimize such problems by interpreting the current status of research.

SELECTED REFERENCES

Burke, D. C. 1979. The neurological examination (spinal). *Australian Family Physician* 8 (Feb.): 119–128. *Excellent guide to accurate diagnosis of spinal cord injury; simplified guide to some traps and subtleties of diagnosis. Highly recommended.*

Burke, D. L., and Murray, D. D. 1975. *Handbook of Spinal Cord Medicine.* London and Basingstoke: MacMillan Press. *Concise review of functional anatomy and injuries to the spinal column and spinal cord in Chapters 2, 3, and 4.*

Gunley, P. 1981. From regeneration to prosthesis: research on spinal cord injury. *Journal of the American Medical Association* 245(13): 1293–1297. *Review of current American research in regeneration, old and new therapies, and prosthesis. Concise and clear.*

Klose, K. J., and Goldberg, M. L. 1980. Neurological change following spinal cord injury: an assessment technique and preliminary results. *Spinal Cord Injury Digest* 2 (Summer): 35–42. *Description of a quantitative tool: the University of Miami Neuro-Spinal Index (UMNI), which consists of the sensory scale and the motor scale. Scale scores are indicators of overall spinal cord functional capacity within the sensory and motor modalities.*

Liebman, M. 1979. *Neuroanatomy Made Easy and Understandable.* Baltimore: University Park Press. *Presents fundamental basis for neuroanatomy, neurophysiology, neuropharmacology, physical diagnosis, and neurology. Helpful sections on spinal pathways and the autonomic nervous system. Valuable glossary relating Latin origins to everyday language.*

SUPPLEMENTAL READING

Tator, C. H., and Rowed, D. W. 1979. Current concepts in the immediate management of acute spinal cord injuries. *Canadian Medical Association Journal* 121 (Dec.): 1453–1464. *Excellent review of updated care; describes sophisticated diagnostic tests, treatment methods, and related nursing care to minimize secondary pathological processes following initial trauma. Extensive bibliography. Highly recommended.*

Charlton, O. P. 1979. Roentgenographic evaluation of cervical spinal trauma. *Journal of the American Medical Association* 242(10): 1073. *The authors detail their approach to radiographic assessment used with 400 patients and interpret common findings.*

Claus-Walker, J., and Halstead, L. 1978. Autonomic drugs in spinal cord injury: temporal prescription profile. *Archives of Physical Medicine and Rehabilitation* 59 (Aug.): 363–367. *Examines drugs used to modify the effects of acute hyperactive gastrointestinal irritability (related to peptic ulceration), bradycardia, orthostatic hypotension, neurogenic bladder dysfunction, and autonomic dysreflexia and derives a clearer understanding of the progressive recovery and adaptation process of the autonomic nervous system.*

Gunley, P. 1981. New focus on spinal cord injury. *Journal of the American Medical Association* 245(12): 1201–1206. *General overview of spinal cord injury centers in the United States. Also presents general overview of the care in the centers.*

Halstead, L.; Claus-Walker, J.; Herna, D. 1978. Neurologically active drugs in spinal cord injury; a clinical coding system. *Archives of Physical Medicine and Rehabilitation* 59(Aug.): 358–362. *Presentation of drugs commonly prescribed for the spinal cord injured; includes drugs used to compensate for neurological dysfunction and neurological side effects of drugs used to treat other problems. Focuses on actual and potential interactions with implications for physicians, pharmacists, and nurses. Darvon, Demerol, Talwin, Urecholine, and Valium are discussed.*

Hardy, A. G. 1977. Cervical spinal cord injury without bony injury. *International Journal of Paraplegia* 14: 296–305. *Detailed review of incidence, causes, predisposing factors, illustrated neuropathology, and prognosis of central cord injury.*

Hoppenfeld, S. 1977. *Orthopedic Neurology—A Diagnostic Guide to Neurologic Levels.* Philadelphia: J. B. Lippincott. *Excellent, clinically relevant, clearly illustrated guide to neurological assessment, particularly motor function. Chapters 3 and 4 devoted to spinal cord injury. Highly recommended.*

Mechner, F., and Mahoney, P. 1976. Patient assessment: neurological examination, Part III. *American Journal of Nursing* 76 (4): programmed instruction page 1–25. *Particularly helpful for assessment of sensory function.*

Netter, F. H. 1975. *The Nervous System. The CIBA Collection of Medical Illustrations, Vol. I.* New York: CIBA Pharmaceutical Co. *Colorful lifelike art detailing the central nervous system and protective (bony) structures.*

Hemmy, D. C., and Larson, S. J. 1979. Gas myelography in spinal cord injury. *The Journal of Trauma* 19(3): 145–148. *Technical but well-illustrated article.*

Holdsworth, F. 1970. Fractures, dislocations, and fracture-dislocations of the spine. *Journal of Bone and Joint Surgery* 52–A(8): 1534–1551. *Based on studies of 1000 cord injury patients. The author describes characteristics of resultant bony and neurological sequelae.*

Kewalramanii, L. S., and Jorge, A. T. 1980. Spinal cord trauma in children. *Spine* 5(1): 11–15. *Presents the incidence of radiologic abnormalities prognosis and pathomechanics of cord injury in children, based on 97 cases. Also includes an extensive literature review and discusses implications for management.*

Locke, G. E., et al. 1977. Myelography during craniocervical traction in the early management of acute cervical cord injuries. *Spine* 2(3): 173–175. *Describes technique of Pantopaque myelography using a C_{1-2} spinal puncture site while the patient is immobilized on a Stryker frame; focuses on advantages of minimal neck manipulation for maximum safety.*

Madeja, C. 1977. Computerised tomography: an introduction. *Journal of Neurosurgical Nursing* 9(2): 87–89. *Basic introduction to technical procedure.*

Munro, D. 1965. Factors that govern the stability of the spine. *International Journal of Paraplegia* 3: 219–228. *Examines motions in the normal spine and results of pathology: explains principles of wiring, spinal instrumentation, and fusion.*

Oberson, R., and Azam, F. 1978. CAT of the spine and spinal cord. *Neuroradiology* 16: 369–370. *Brief summary of standard and contrast enhancement, myelography used in conjunction with computerized axial tomography.*

O'Reilly, B. J. 1979. Preparing the patient for computerized tomography. *Journal of Neurosurgical Nursing* 11: 42–43. *Reviews mechanics and description of scan procedure; includes patient preparation and postprocedure care when contrast material is used.*

Roub, L. W., and Drayer, B. P. 1979. Spinal computed tomography: limitations and applications. *American Journal of Roentography* 133: 267–273. *Advanced, well-illustrated article discussing diagnostic usefulness of CAT.*

Stauffer, E. S. 1975. Diagnosis and prognosis of spinal cord injury. *Clinical Orthopaedics* 112 (Oct.): 9–15. *Describes assessment and significance of perineal reflexes, motor and sensory function in planning rehabilitation from the onset of injury.*

Taylor, J. W., and Ballenger, S. 1980. *Neurological Dysfunctions and Nursing Interventions.* New York: McGraw-Hill. *Presents chapters on motor, sensory, and autonomic dysfunction followed by related nursing management; includes review of anatomy and physiology correlated to clinical manifestations.*

Williamson-Kirkland, T., and Berni, R. 1980. Neurological aspects of rehabilitation, Part 2: spinal cord injury. *Rehabilitation Nursing*, July–August, pp. 8–13. *Presents overview of neurological basis for common rehabilitation problems: includes pathological basis for bladder, bowel, and sexual dysfunction and autonomic hyperreflexia.*

Yashon, D. 1978. Pathogenesis of spinal cord injury. *Orthopedic Clinics of North America* 9(2): 247–289. *Detailed review of vascular damage, edema, and actions of catecholamines; includes rationale for corticosteroid therapy.*

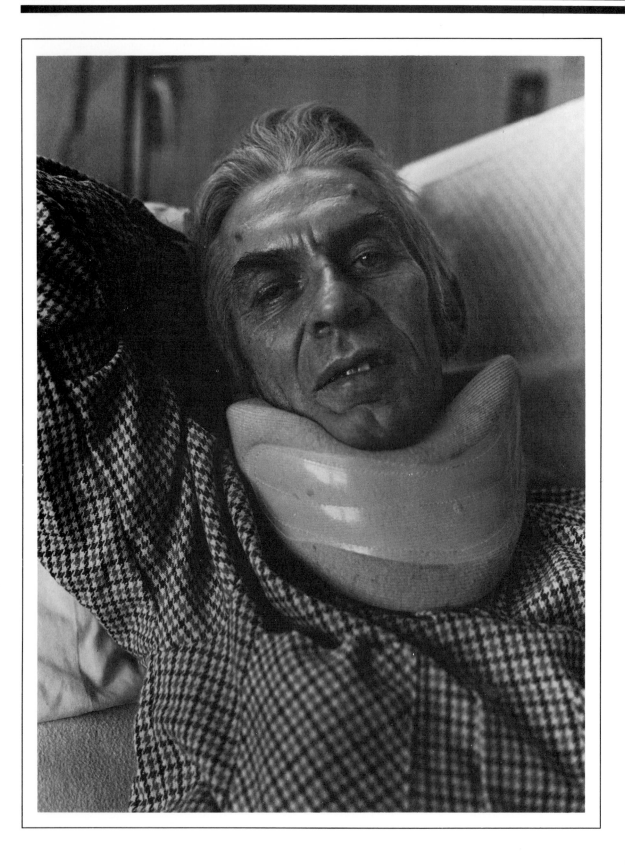

PART III

ENHANCING FEELINGS OF SELF-WORTH

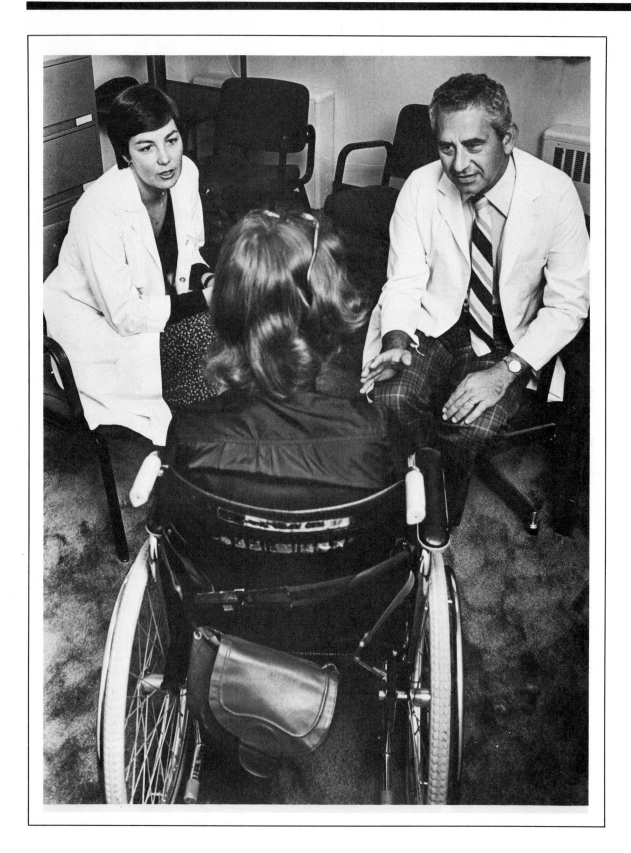

Chapter 6

Psychosocial Adjustment Following Spinal Cord Injury

CHAPTER OUTLINE

OBJECTIVES

- To describe health care goals that enhance psychosocial adjustment following spinal cord injury
- To identify possible patient and family concerns
- To describe the role of counseling professionals in interdisciplinary care
- To develop awareness of attitudes toward disabled patients, impact of nursing behavior on patients, and families, and the personal limitations need to seek assistance when required
- To describe signs of stress in others, including fellow staff members, and to demonstrate supportive responses

- To explain how experiencing loss applies to physical disability and how these feelings can be manifested
- To explain how feelings of guilt, helplessness, low self-esteem, role dysfunctions, and physical illness can threaten self-concept
- To explain the significance of the patient's preinjury personality and family support systems on the rehabilitation process
- To indicate how crisis intervention techniques apply to rehabilitation and how nurses can react appropriately in crisis situations
- To develop awareness of long-term implications of living with spinal cord injury

In relation to physical illness and disability, trends in contemporary medical knowledge frequently demonstrate that psychosocial aspects are an integral part of medical well-being. Consequently, nurses are constantly made aware of and must deal with the psychosocial implications of spinal cord injury.

Psychological support—from caring for newly injured people in an intensive care unit to helping people cope with the devastating realities of physical disability—is a dramatic challenge to all health care professionals. Although it is not possible to protect patients and families from the psychosocial implications of spinal cord injury, it is possible to help people resume productive lives despite physical disability.

GOALS OF HEALTH CARE

The goals of psychosocial rehabilitation are:
- To recognize and understand the significance of patient and family concerns
- To obtain and interpret a preinjury psychosocial profile of the patient and family, and appreciate how the preinjury situation will influence the adjustment process

- To develop an individualized approach that will help patients and families capitalize on previous strengths to reach their fullest potential
- To include the patient and family as integral members of the rehabilitation team
- To recognize psychosocial problems that will require additional professional help and refer them to appropriate resource persons
- To create a therapeutic rehabilitative environment conducive to psychological growth for patients and families adjusting to the effects of spinal cord injury

FACTORS THAT AFFECT THE THERAPEUTIC ENVIRONMENT

The Philosophy of Rehabilitation Practice

The National Council on Rehabilitation defines *rehabilitation* as the restoration of individuals to the fullest physical, mental, social, vocational, and economic capacity of which each is capable. To achieve this overall objective, rehabilitation must begin at the moment of injury to prevent deterioration and promote restoration.

A rehabilitative philosophy provides vital concepts to believe in or strive for and a structure for rehabilitation practice.

If an institution's philosophy is simply that rehabilitation consists of learning self-care and mobility techniques, rehabilitation programs may become very rigid and not be directed to patients' *total* needs. If the philosophy includes the belief that patients should be taught to apply these techniques to the business of living, rehabilitation programs will become more flexible. To illustrate this point let us consider a patient who is having difficulty with a bowel management program. To help the patient it may be necessary to alter therapy times. In a flexible situation the nurses would feel comfortable making the change, but in a rigid situation therapists might resent this intrusion on their time. From the patient's point of view, however, bowel irregularity and difficulty with bowel control is a major factor influencing participation in any number of events, from therapy to a family outing. Indeed, one study demonstrated that bowel accidents were rated the most uncomfortable of twenty socially embarrassing situations (Dunn 1977). Thus, the philosophy of rehabilitation practiced within any one institution significantly affects the scope of personal interactions among the interdisciplinary team, patients and families.

The Interdisciplinary Team

To ensure that the definition of rehabilitation is not altogether physical, counseling professionals trained in the behavioral sciences are becoming increasingly involved in interdisciplinary treatment. There are other team members whose primary role is to assist with the psychosocial aspects of rehabilitation. Sexual health counselors with varied professional backgrounds, leisure therapists, and people with spinal cord injuries engaged in peer counseling are some examples.

The social worker

Social workers are an integral part of the treatment team, whose involvement encompasses the patient, the family, the interdisciplinary team, and the community at large. Social workers gather and interpret personal, family, financial, and environmental resource data to help patients and families cope with the many stressful psychosocial problems that sudden, severely disabling injuries bring. Their services include help with family and marital concerns, accident and medical insurance, and income difficulties. They also provide links with ongoing and community resources, particularly those related to the discharge process.

The clinical psychologist

Clinical psychologists play a significant role as behavioral consultants, as researchers into the rehabilitation process, as evaluators of the psychological strengths and assets of the person with a spinal cord injury, and as therapists and counselors (Treischmann 1980). Treischmann goes on to explain that when rehabilitation is considered a learning process and when the person with a spinal cord injury is considered not as having psychological problems per se but as having problems coping in a world designed for the nondisabled, psychologists can make unique contributions to the rehabilitation process. Psychologists are trained in the principles of behavior, in particular the principles of learning. For example, if a patient is unreliable about taking regulated amounts of fluid or performing catheterizations on time, the psychologist might focus on the patient's cooperation and interaction with the nurse. Thus, as a behavioral consultant, the psychologist can help the patient learn the tasks at hand and gain maximum benefit from the rehabilitation opportunities offered.

Psychosocial implications for the team

The impact of catastrophic injuries on the entire health team can never be underestimated. All staff members who come into contact with the patient must examine their beliefs about the quality of life remaining for the physically disabled person, and their role in it.

Because of the nature of accidents causing spinal cord injury and the physical demands of patient care, staff and patients are often in the same young-adult age range. The closer in age and life circumstances the staff member is to the patient, the closer and more threatening the identification. Those beginning to care for patients with spinal cord injuries, may especially need the support of other staff, since many must work through somewhat the same psychological processes as patients and families. It is important for them to verbalize feelings of disbelief, anger, and depression appropriately if they are to have the psychic energy to help others in turmoil.

Conflicts within the team can lead to each discipline feeling poorly understood, ineffectual, and frustrated. If, for example, counseling professionals cannot convey a feeling of empathy for nurses, who may be faced with some outrageous behavioral situations, nurses feel unsupported and isolated. By the same token, if nurses become so emotionally entangled in the situation that they lose professional objectivity, they may develop unrealistic expectations of what counseling professionals can and cannot do. It is important to dispel the myth of "magical cures" by behavioral scientists.

Each member of the interdisciplinary team possesses a unique personality, a specialized body of skills and knowledge, a variety of professional experiences, and different personal and professional assets and expectations. To develop a truly skilled interdisciplinary team, it is necessary to create a warm and respectful atmosphere in which the significance, expectations, and limitations of each team member's role are recognized and understood.

Ongoing education and support for the team

Preparation and ongoing education for nurses is a multifaceted issue. A comprehensive orientation, ideally including participation from other disciplines, can ease the nurse into the intricate care needed by the catastrophically injured and help develop harmonious interdisciplinary relationships.

Patients' anger, among other reactions frequently encountered, may cause frustration in staff who are trying very hard to help. This may cause displacement of anger on other staff members. In addition, veteran staff members require support and ongoing educational opportunities to avert the problems of "burnout." Educational activities and moral support can best be built around ongoing, informal meetings of small groups to discuss problems with self, patients, families, and fellow staff members (Gunther

1980). These groups are best led by an accepted member of the staff, who is aware of both the rehabilitative and the psychological implications of staff problems. The most beneficial techniques include eliciting feedback from more experienced staff members, facilitating peer support, and sharing of suggestions or coping techniques being employed by other staff members (Roglitz 1978).

The clinical nurse specialist is particularly valuable in providing comprehensive health care for patients who, in addition to the complexities of physical care, must incorporate vast and permanent changes in life-style to maintain optimal health.

One issue that inevitably arises is whether staff should accompany patients on various outings. Outings with staff may be very positive experiences for patients, stimulating them and helping them feel "normal" rather than "disabled." However, staff must remain objective about the patients for their own well-being. Some specialized units discourage these outings, but this may create hidden resentment toward the policy makers. Much can be learned when negative experiences are worked through appropriately. To help maintain objectivity, staff members need to maintain if not increase outside activities and friends.

A very special issue is that of emotional attachments. While these feelings may be very real for the nurse and the patient, there may be confusion about the role of the nurse as a care giver rather than a partner. A similar situation occurs if a nurse and patient become "good buddies." Maintaining an appropriate nurse–patient relationship in these situations is almost impossible. Orientation should inform a nurse of the potential difficulties of close personal relationships and why such relationships are best discouraged until the patient is discharged, when the two adults involved are, of course, free to make their own choices.

Often nurses feel obligated to patients, feeling that refusal to meet a request or arrange an outing may contribute to feelings of rejection or lowering of self-esteem. They may simply need help in explaining the nurse's role in order to avert complicated emotional situations in the future.

The pressures of this work demand a strong supportive structure and personal stability and maturity. These circumstances require a strong working collaboration with professionals trained in the behavioral sciences and recognition that staff must support each other and often need help with their feelings. Nursing leaders must recognize staff needs and learn how to deal with them, seeking appropriate help from others when necessary.

The Nurse

The nature of nursing and significance of attitudes

The very nature of nursing presents some unique difficulties that are not always given the thoughtful consideration or recognition they deserve, either by nurses or other members of an interdisciplinary team. The basic essentials of eating, bathing, getting up in the morning, and going to bed at night take place in the ward setting as they do in the home. The ward environment also provides opportunities to establish acceptable behavioral patterns and social skills. Finally, the ward is the place where patients return when they become too fatigued, too upset, or too "something" to function elsewhere in the therapeutic environment (Gunther 1980). Thus, the nursing service provides a combination of home base, school or workplace, and retreat from burdensome activities of the day. For these reasons, patients often direct their feelings of hostility, frustration, and exhaustion toward nurses.

Furthermore, nursing functions frequently involve exposing the patient for bathing and handling of intimate areas of the body for bladder and bowel procedures. The nature of these activities tends to heighten the patient's feelings of embarrassment, helplessness, dependence, and asexuality. Even self-care for these procedures tends to create rather than relieve frustration, because it involves fine motor activity.

Nurses, unlike those specifically trained in the behavioral sciences, are less prepared to deal with behavioral problems. This is particularly true of the large numbers of nursing assistants, such as practical nurses, aides, and orderlies, who spend a great deal of time engaged in direct patient care. But persons engaged in direct daily care are of paramount importance to the disabled person's socialization process. Therefore, so are their values and attitudes. As studies by Leinart (1979) and Sadlick and Penta (1975) point out, a positive attitude toward the rehabilitation outcome is essential to the success of the process.

Nurses, especially in an acute setting, may never see patients who adapt well to their disability. When nurses continually care for patients in the "middle" stages of adjustment and seldom see a patient and family coping well and enjoying life, they may well perceive their efforts as futile and experience feelings of hopelessness themselves. It is very rewarding when staff are able to see patients after their rehabilitation course. Former patients could be encouraged to drop in to visit a unit or keep in touch by telephone or mail. Christmas time is a favorite time for patients to write in about the year's progress and events. This type of contact and information is invaluable.

The well-rehabilitated person is one of the most valuable, but most poorly used resources that health care professionals have. Disabled people could be of great help in developing positive attitudes in nurses and others to enhance the goals of rehabilitation. More and more, innovative facilities are inviting disabled persons not only to serve as positive role models for patients but also to serve as resource persons to health care professionals. However, particularly in acute care settings, their presence is often considered too "upsetting" for everyone or has simply never been considered at all.

Lack of positive feelings can and do block communication, and patients can begin to perceive themselves as helpless and less worthwhile. In addition, overly sympathetic, nonobjective attitudes can easily communicate feelings of hopelessness to the patient and family. To overcome these feelings it is important to understand the human potential for adjustment to disability—an understanding appreciated on an emotional level rather than an intellectual one. Unfortunately, health care professionals often fail to recognize the importance of this fundamental concept.

FACTORS THAT AFFECT PSYCHOSOCIAL ADJUSTMENTS

Patient Concerns

A spinal cord injury affects all aspects of the individual's life. It instantly imposes an overwhelming complex of losses: of mobility, control, virility, independence, pleasure sensations, wholeness, and, immediately, of life (Weller and Miller 1977a). The person must face a loss of life as it was yet still live. There may also be a temporary loss of future life expectations, such as marriage, parenthood, employment or career, and one's general place in the community. In addition, many patients are separated from families and loved ones when they are transported to and rehabilitated in a major center. Concerns about their families' reaction to disability, their ability to cope at home, and economic pressures may also be a burden.

Following injury most people find themselves reevaluating their lives in terms of this significant event that will affect their future. Some thoughts and concerns (Virginia Manual 1980) include:

- Am I a valuable person?
- Am I sexually attractive?
- Can I be a good parent?
- Am I a burden to my family?
- Will my old friends accept me?
- Will I be able to make new friends?
- Will I be able to support myself or my family?
- Would it be better if I had died?
- Will I be able physically to protect myself and my family?
- What will I do if I have a bowel or bladder accident in public?
- Will I ever be able to work again?
- Can I enjoy life again?

Family Concerns

Family concerns closely reflect those of the patient. Initially families are concerned about the patient's survival, relief from pain, and adequate medical care. They are deeply aware of shattered dreams or life expectations for a spouse, son or daughter, or other relative. Reactions to this loss include anger, disbelief, helplessness, and guilt. Overprotectiveness is a common reaction (Weller and Miller 1977b). Some questions families may ask include:

- Will they live?
- Will they be crippled for life?
- Why did this happen to us?
- What can we do to help?
- How will they ever manage their lives?
- Will they always be depressed?
- Can they have sex again?
- How can we look after them at home?
- How will our friends react?
- Can they get a job?
- Will there be enough money?
- How can we protect them?
- How will we cope?

Theoretical Considerations

In addition to the medical situation, the individual with spinal cord injury experiences psychological stresses fraught with acute anxieties. When faced with sudden disability, patients must absorb the traumatic effect of injury, physical shock, hospitalization, severe motor and sensory loss, and changes in body image and self-identity. They will experience interactional changes within both their families and the community.

How can they deal with these changes? Much of the literature attempts to answer this question within the realm of mastering adaptation, adjustment, and coping techniques.

Shontz (1975) views severe physical disability as a crisis, and adjustment to crisis as *a succession of approach–avoidance cycles*. In the early stages, cycles recur rapidly with high levels of emotional intensity. Later the cycles become less frequent, less intense, and gradually fade out. Shontz believes it is essential to go through the sequence of two phases: the impact phase (shock and encounter) and the postimpact phase (retreat and acknowledgment). Shock is described as a depersonalized emergency reaction; the characteristics of encounter are panic, disorganization, and helplessness as shock wears off. Because encounter is too intense the stage of retreat begins. Denial and isolation can be forms of retreat. Acknowledgment is the final stage in adaptation and consists of cycles of approach and avoidance. This cyclical approach denotes a dynamic and lengthy adaptation process through which patients must encounter and be forced to face different crises. Consequently they are permitted to get a feeling of themselves in new terms at their own pace.

Thompson and Lott (1980) relate the sequences of psychosocial events following spinal cord injury to the descriptions of Erikson's life span development stages. The most relevant concept is that people must continually *reprocess* past stages to deal with ordinary life development.

> Think of the severity, the intensity, the psychosocial trauma that is present when a person starts to reprocess these stages after intense body changes brought about by spinal cord injury. . . . To regain the balance in a positive direction means a redevelopment of trust, autonomy, initiative, industry, and identity, versus mistrust, shame, guilt, inferiority, and diffusion. [Thompson and Lott 1980: 43]

Hohmann (1975) postulates that a person experiences a number of feelings and attitudes similar to those that may be experienced with any severe loss—in other words "normal reactions to an abnormal situation." The first reaction is denial, which, when relinquished, allows depression to set in. The depressive phase may be characterized by withdrawal and internalized hostility, which is then externalized. After these reactions have been worked through, there will usually be a reconstitution of the person's preinjury personality. The stages of grieving are likened to phases of adjustment to disability and are often described as feelings of shock, denial, anger, depression, and finally adjustment. These feelings may also be thought of as periods of disorganization, reorganization, and resolution. However, the most striking observation is the variability of each individual's response.

While the concept of stages of grieving, which denotes a static sense of adjustment, may not be wholly applicable to the individual experiencing the effects of a spinal cord injury, behavioral aspects of various stages are still apparent while nursing the patient. Observation of behavioral responses provides information relevant to assessing the patient and family's psychosocial status, and it gives invaluable direction to nursing care.

While there are theoretical and descriptive differences among the various events or phases of grieving that follow a major life-changing or life-threatening event, one notable similarity is that adaptation to a loss such as that incurred as a result of a spinal cord injury is a process that occurs over time. The time interval since injury is a significant factor in the adjustment process to disability, particularly with regard to patients' ability to solve problems, to make decisions about their care, and to set realistic goals for themselves (MacLean 1981).

Adjustment to disability is highly individualized. It seldom progresses smoothly from beginning to end but is more like a series of encounters and reencounters with any number of events or setbacks that occur over time. This significant observation suggests that problems have to be faced again and again in different situations and with different degrees of intensity, rather than "worked through" once and for all.

It is important to realize that while the rehabilitation process has a beginning and an end, the process of adjustment to disability may not. However, as most disabled people attest, it is possible to adapt to or cope with the effects of spinal cord injury even though some people and some families are never able to mobilize the strength to attain this capability. As one person with respiratory quadriplegia explains,

> I still get depressed but manage to keep it within working bounds. Personally, I believe that a disabled person never really accepts being the way they are. After all, every day you are working against nature. We are not meant to be like this. However, I know that with maturity and understanding one can work around it and live a constructive, meaningful life.

Self-Concept and Self-Esteem

Self-concept is a combination of feelings and beliefs that people hold in regard to themselves. Both the physical and the personal are included in self-concept. Self-esteem is one's feeling of personal value or worth (Kozier and Erb 1983). Self-esteem is largely developed on feedback from others in our lives. The way in which we deal with feelings and expressions of anger and aggression, in particular, stems from the limitations imposed by others during our upbringing. Without such limitations we cannot learn the consequences of various behaviors and as adults may have difficulty setting limits or controlling our behavior.

Psychosocial development is a natural part of the maturational process. In past decades the original works of psychologists such as Erickson and Maslow stressed the ability to learn and to grow psychologically throughout life. Learning is a continual process that helps us adapt to new roles in life: intimate partner, parent, or leader, for example. Psychological growth also helps us adapt to crises such as injury leading to disability.

The way people feel about themselves affects the way in which they deal with their environment. People with high self-esteem will deal more actively with their environment and feel secure. People with low self-esteem will view the environment as negative and threatening (Roy et al. 1976: 233).

Some common manifestations of low self-esteem include (Roy et al. 1976: 236–237):

- Expressions of self-depreciation or self-dislike
- Sensitivity to criticism; self-consciousness
- Anorexia or overeating
- Tendency to be a listener rather than a participant
- Difficulty sleeping or oversleeping
- Withdrawal from activities
- Decreased motivation, interest, and concentration
- Seeing self as burden to others

Through assessment of a patient's self-concept, it is possible to predict potential problems the patient will have in reacting to and coping with a spinal cord injury. Moreover, the health care team can promote the patient's adaptation to disability by capitalizing on strengths of self-concept and self-esteem.

In the aftermath of spinal cord injury, both patients and families are subject to a magnitude of psychosocial influences during and after the rehabilitation period. Strong psychosocial support from a variety of sources is essential to enhance all other aspects of the rehabilitation program and prepare for discharge.

Helplessness

Patients may feel powerless if they fail to realize the connection between behavior and control of environment. Initially patients are generally aroused by this threat to their freedom, but some patients gradually stop trying when they feel complete loss of control (Treischmann 1980: 61). The person may then become apathetic, anxious, and depressed. The theory of *learned helplessness* states that uncontrollable failure leads to depression and feelings of helplessness, while self-controlled success fosters feelings of competence and industriousness.

> Although not generally diagnosed as having a learned helplessness syndrome by rehabilitation counsellors, many spinal cord injured patients seem to demonstrate a learned helplessness response to their paralysis. Often these emotions, natural reactions to the initial trauma and early recovery period following spinal cord injury, become ingrained and, as with learned helplessness effects among other patient populations, they begin to influence the spinal cord patient's general life orientation. [Wool et al. 1980: 321]

Age

The age of onset of disability is an important factor affecting psychological adjustment. Individuals born with a disability, or who acquire one early in life, learn behavioral patterns appropriate to their degree of impairment while growing up; there is essentially no interruption or lack of congruence between old behaviors and new. Disabilities acquired later in life generally have a sudden onset, which precipitates a basic incongruence between old and expected new behaviors and initial difficulty to perform the new and different behaviors.

During young adulthood, for example, we strive to demonstrate to the community and ourselves that we are socially and physically acceptable as an adult. Developmental tasks for this maturational period can include establishing a home, getting started in a career, marrying and starting a family, and finding a congenial social group. The young adult with a spinal cord injury is faced not only with achieving physical independence, but also with finding alternate ways to achieve appropriate maturational goals. The nature of the goals that have been interrupted and the extent to which the individual is able to set new goals that are congruent with an altered reality are important factors to consider in the rehabilitation process.

Acquisition of New Roles

There is some evidence that rehabilitation is a process of socialization during which people with spinal cord injuries learn new roles. Furthermore, the extent to which disabled individuals successfully perform their roles will be determined by their attitude and stage in the adjustment process and the degree to which they are able to adapt to their disability.

Thomas (1966) described some characteristic roles for disabled people. The first of these, the "disabled patient role," is characterized by sick role expectations extended and made enduring. The "helped person role" involves being on the receiving end of helping acts and adaptation to being an object of aid. The "disability comanager role" is a role characterized by active participation of the disabled person in decisions attending impairment and rehabilitation. Finally, the "role of the public relations person" places a burden of explanation and interpretation of impairment on the disabled person. Learning these new roles is viewed as a resocialization process whereby new behaviors are learned and other behaviors no longer possible or appropriate are unlearned.

Adaptation to disability is an important intervening variable influencing role performance of the disabled person. The essence of acquiring these new behaviors is to enhance "normal" interactions with others. When disabled people feel comfortable with themselves they will communicate the feeling to others. In turn, when others feel more at ease, they will respond with more valid or "normal" behaviors.

Physical disability is potentially stigmatizing, particularly when visibility is high as is the case with paraplegia and quadriplegia. In the sheltered social environment of the hospital, patients are somewhat protected from the stigma of disability. In the world outside the hospital, however, the social stigma becomes readily apparent. Although the situation is improving, a disabled person can still be devalued in our society. To become successfully rehabilitated, people with spinal cord injuries must learn the physical and social skills necessary to project positive feelings of self-worth to reduce stigmatizing effects (MacLean 1981).

Physical Health

Psychological health cannot be considered in isolation from physical health, mobility, and independence. In general, if physical health is poor or if methods to control body functions are unreliable, ability to deal with psychological adjustments is lowered. Therefore, throughout the rehabilitation period, physical needs must be assessed and managed carefully. We should *never* underestimate how irritable or depressed a patient can be if suffering from chills, fever, nausea, pain, or spasms.

During the immediate postinjury period, the patient in a critical care setting may experience severe sensory and perceptual deprivation, especially if the stay is prolonged. On meeting his surgeon again several years after the injury, a young man with quadriplegia was astounded to see that the man was of average height and build. The patient had perceived the physician as one of several towering figures looking down at him on the Stryker frame. The patient's position flat in bed; movement restrictions that limit the field of vision; loss of sensation over large body surfaces; and medications are some physiological factors that cause general disorientation and cloud thought processes for weeks.

USING THE NURSING PROCESS TO PROMOTE PSYCHOSOCIAL ADJUSTMENT

Assessment

Psychosocial assessment of the patient and family encompasses two major components: comprehensive history taking and continuous observation of psychosocial status.

History

Understanding the patient's and family's background will provide a basis on which to plan and offer psychosocial support. The patient is the same person after the spinal cord injury as before. Therefore, if patient and family were harmonious, industrious, and satisfied before the disability, they are likely to resume that pattern. If there were major difficulties, however, the disability is likely to make the threatened situation worse.

Counseling professionals make an in-depth assessment of the patient's preinjury personality and family support structures. They assess the strengths and resources of both patient and family and interpret them to the interdisciplinary team. For example, they explore previous ways of dealing with frustration or coping with responsibilities. Cultural influences, position or role in the family, interpersonal relationships, educational and vocational background, and socioeconomic status must all be assessed with insight and expertise.

People with spinal cord injuries comprise a truly heterogeneous population whose personalities and adjustment capabilities vary widely. However, factors that seem to aid in adjustment are emotional maturity, good self-esteem, intact family supports, higher levels of education, and financial and job security. People whose work

and leisure activities are more physical might find the onset of spinal cord injury more disruptive than people who are less physically inclined (Treischmann 1980).

Unfortunately, many people with spinal cord injuries are young. According to the National Spinal Cord Injury Data Research Center (Young and Northrup 1979), approximately 50% of all injuries occur in the 15 to 25 age group. Therefore a most complex and delicate problem facing health care delivery systems is this core group of youth.

Immature and usually at an age when confusion about identity and developing intimate relationships can threaten and lower self-esteem and confidence, young people are also at a crossroad where they must make the choice between employment and further education and are at a peak of physical prowess, which tends to outweigh intellectual interest (Weller and Miller 1977). This critical juncture in the lives of individuals who are severely injured obviously has a profound impact on their reaction to disability and to their ability to plan for their future. The problems of this group are compounded by all the ramifications of a society rapidly departing from traditional values about morality, work, family life, and spiritual beliefs, many of which seem to help people adjust to disability. Moreover, this group's tendencies toward impulsive, aggressive, and verbally abusive behavior make such patients difficult to deal with on a day-to-day basis. Fortunately, most younger disabled individuals have a greater capacity to adjust and adapt to new situations than older individuals. In fact, after a rehabilitation program, these younger people often lead satisfying and productive lives.

All patients experience varying degrees of stress in dealing with the effects of spinal cord injury. However, if preexisting psychosocial problems—chronic drug and alcohol abuse; recognized psychiatric illness; criminal behavior; or severe, unresolved family disruption—exist, the ability to adjust to permanent and dramatic changes in life-style is compounded. Extreme depression, suicide attempts (sometimes the cause of spinal cord injury), or a history of psychiatric illness will be signs of the need for immediate psychiatric referral.

Continuous psychosocial assessment

Psychosocial assessment is a continual, on-going process. The emotional or psychological profiles of patients and families are gradually portrayed to the staff during the weeks of hospitalization. Nurses and others contribute a great deal of information for assessment through direct daily observation and interaction with both patients and families; counseling professionals continue to gather and interpret data; and all team members share their observations of a patient and family's progress through the rehabilitation process.

Throughout the period of adjustment to disability, nurses and others must be able to recognize additional problems that threaten the patient's self-worth. These may include feelings of guilt, helplessness, role confusion, and low self-esteem.

The rehabilitation team must also consider family dynamics. Too often health professionals think of the family as a reliable support structure, somewhat like another health professional, without realizing the full impact of disability on the family unit. Even the strongest families can become exhausted during the process of rehabilitation. Coping with a disabled family member may create a number of internal problems: altered or even reversed roles (for example, the homemaker who must become the bread-winner); altered financial status; added responsibility for physical care tasks, especially bowel and bladder management, which may be awkward or even repulsive for both patient and family; and numerous other practical difficulties, such as caring for the children or the elderly within the home. Children of the disabled seem to get lost in the shuffle, often without recognition or access to the support system they so badly need. Thus, skilled history taking, interviewing, and sensitivity in daily interpersonal interactions are essential to assess current patient and family strengths, problems, and needs.

Goal Setting

Planning and implementing goal-oriented care during rehabilitation must lead the patient and family to take responsibility for managing the effects of disability and maintaining optimal physical and psychological health. Counseling professionals must collaborate with the nurse and other team members in working closely with the patient and family to establish attainable goals that are compatible with assessment data. For example, coping with the effects of disability requires consistent and positive behavioral changes. When an individual's background is unstable and strong support systems are not available, behavioral changes, though not impossible, are slow and difficult to achieve. Unrealistic expectations are both harmful and frustrating to patients, families and staff members. Realistic goal setting must not be equated or confused with reducing standards of care. While patient input and involvement in determining goals increase the likelihood of attainment, in practice it is difficult to know just how and when this participation can be maximized. This difficulty is largely due to the fact that rehabilitation is a dynamic process, which denotes evolvement and change. Patient participation in goal setting must be based on continuous assessment of the psychological and other aspects of disability.

The theoretical framework developed from the concept of the adjustment or grieving process directs planning toward setting objectives and planning interventions that acknowledge a patient's special needs in each phase of grieving. For example, highly anxious patients in the early stages of grieving are unable to set long-term goals for themselves or carry out activities consistently without supervision. Others who are more self-directing need opportunities for greater input and involvement.

Although the goals of care in the acute stage are largely determined by the health care team, the nurse can do much to promote independence and prepare to ease the transition of the patient from the "sick role" to that of a well person by continually setting appropriate expectations, encouraging patient responsibility, and communicating the message, "I am going to care for this now, but in the future you will be responsible for completing or supervising this task yourself." This type of involvement conveys messages of concern and recognition of the patient's abilities and importance.

Well-meaning health professionals often work toward a goal of creating independence for the patient and family while at the same time removing decision making from the patient. A classic example of this is a forced rigid compliance with schedules for rehabilitation activities established without adequate initial input from and involvement with the patient and family. When the rehabilitation process is viewed as a learning process, it is a shared experience in which the health professionals seek and respect the patient and family's opinions and concerns.

Implementation

Having established goals related to assessment data, it is important to collaborate with counseling professionals to implement an approach that will best help patients and families capitalize on strengths and resources.

Good assessment is really good intervention, because empathetic, attentive listening is therapeutic.

> It is important to recognize and respond to patients' and families' need for communication and to capitalize on a warm, trusting relationship with them to encourage expression of feelings and concerns. People feel good when they are listened to and their integrity as human beings is confirmed. This ultimately increases satisfaction with the care provided and cooperation with the recommended program of treatment (Szasz 1980: 8).

Developing a positive relationship between patients and families and health care team

The entire health care team, from the immediate onset of injury, can do much to promote or destroy feelings of trust, self-worth, and hope for the future. A major premise of this book is that *rehabilitation begins the moment of injury*. As such, the critical care team can make a significant contribution toward developing an honest, trusting relationship between patients and families, and health care professionals that will last throughout the entire rehabilitation process.

In reality, the medical priorities surrounding spinal cord injury often overshadow the psychological needs of the patient and family following initial trauma. But psychological support is of the utmost importance regardless of how much physical care is required (Weller and Miller 1977a).

Whether and when to give a prognosis during the early stages is a very delicate issue. Many times physicians do not discuss prognosis unless the patient asks, mostly from fear of "upsetting" everyone too much. However, if the issue is not tackled, the patient, the family, and the medical team are off to a very uncertain start.

One successful approach involves the physician, facilitated by the nurse, arranging to meet with the family soon after admission (within 24 hours after injury). At this time the physician explains what spinal cord injury is and its implications in general; limitations of current medical practice in terms of regenerating the spinal cord; the patient's level and completeness of injury; probable outcomes; and the positive aspects of rehabilitation. The subject is approached gently and with empathy in privacy. Especially when the patient's injury is incomplete, the physician guards against being either too pessimistic or too optimistic. The nurse, who is aware of the contents of the discussion, supports the physician's explanation, corrects any misunderstandings, alerts the physician to any problems, and helps the family to verbalize and begin to cope with their sorrow.

A similar approach is used with the patient, generally within two to three days after injury, depending on the patient's physical and emotional stability. Since patients can be extremely ill at this time, explanations must be very simple and invariably require further explanation. The physician emphasizes that there can be further discussions when the patient is feeling better.

Initially patients and families find it very difficult to believe the prognosis. Both the patient and family need to be able to talk about the actual circumstances of the accident, thereby are helped to grasp the reality of the situation, and to mobilize their coping mechanisms. Families may feel helpless at this time. They may hover over the patient or flee in panic. How quickly and how well family members organize themselves and their daily schedules around the hospitalization are indications of their coping strengths and the amount of support that the family can give the patient. Families should be encouraged to maintain as many routines as possible and should be discouraged from making rash decisions at this time, such as selling a home that may be difficult to renovate for wheelchair accessibility.

Following this straightforward approach, nurses must deal with such questions or statements as: "What do you think?" "What does that doctor know anyway?" "Why didn't they just let me die? I wish I were dead." These times are stressful even for the most skilled and experienced nurses.

In retrospect, many people with spinal cord injuries remember expressing such feelings and say now they mostly appreciated the nurse's just being physically present. It was reassuring to know they could cry and express grief without fear of being abandoned. However, a pessimistic attitude or lack of positive feedback on what the future can hold has the potential of creating even more negativity. Coming from an able-bodied person, responses such as "I understand how you must feel" or "You owe it to your family to live" tend to arouse more anger and frustration. It is more helpful to say something like: "I am trying hard to imagine how you must feel. It must be dreadful, but I do know of people who have a similar injury to yours who are enjoying productive lives" (and then give an example). The latter response conveys messages not only of concern but also of realistic hope.

Promoting self-concept and self-esteem

Following spinal cord injury, the patient's and family's self-concept and self-esteem are very vulnerable. Past experiences and immediate environmental factors influence the way people feel about themselves. Thus the therapeutic environment, of which the nurse is a part, plays a significant role in helping people incorporate vast changes in self-image.

To create a therapeutic environment that will help people adjust to physical disability, the nurse and the interdisciplinary team must be committed to a comprehensive philosophy of care (see Chapter 1) and must demonstrate a positive attitude with a flow of positive feedback toward people in the rehabilitative process.

Counseling professionals focus on helping

patients and families understand how past experiences influence the present situation; explore immediate factors that they consider negative; and choose alternate activities and directions that will help them to live up to their values. These concepts also give direction to nursing interventions, especially regarding those factors in the immediate environment that can be manipulated.

From the moment of injury, implementing general nursing care with a preventive and restorative focus contributes to a sense of independence and helps minimize feelings of helplessness and loss of control. Encouraging self-care promotes self-esteem. Every small thing that patients can do increases their feeling that independence may be possible. Nurses can structure, schedule, and simplify tasks so that the patient will be successful and thereby receive positive reinforcement. For example, instead of trying to eat a full meal, encourage a quadriplegic patient to concentrate on one specific task at any meal, such as managing a sandwich with a sandwich holder at lunch. This task—rather than cutting up food, which is much more difficult, or expecting participation at every meal, which is too fatiguing in the early stages—provides an opportunity for a positive experience. It is important to use specialized knowledge and skills to find practical ways of applying this concept. Throughout the text specific guidelines are given on when and how patients can be expected to participate in their care. For example, participation in the intermittent catheterization program can begin within a few days of injury by self-regulation of fluid intake. Some patients can learn self-catheterization as soon as they are able to sit up 45° in bed.

Thompson and Lott give a good example of the connection between self-care and self-esteem.

A well planned and early developed bowel program, and a reliable bladder training program commenced during the beginning of the rehabilitation phase can initiate a sense of independence: *a sense of autonomy* so that the patient does not have to dwell on shame and doubt. . . . *Success at physical and physiological tasks can blend into success at social reconditioning.* A night out with others—with a consistent control of bodily functions—can lead to the kind of self-certainty which fosters greater interactions in the future. [Emphasis added. Thompson and Lott 1980: 42]

Many times *denial* of injury prevents a patient from engaging in self-care activities or a family from supporting rehabilitative programs. Initially, it is easier for a family to avoid the consequences of injury, since the physical changes are less obvious while the patient is still on bedrest. The realization comes when the patient is first mobilized to a wheelchair and still cannot move. The efforts of staff members as they lift or transfer the paralyzed patient emphasize the reality of the situation. True denial occurs infrequently, but sometimes hope of recovery or such statements as, "I am going to walk out of here," are confused with denial (Treischmann 1980). As long as the patient is participating in the rehabilitation program, these statements are an understandable and natural reaction to sudden disability. Only if the avoidance of the effects of injury is obsessive and interferes with treatment does it become detrimental.

Many patients do not wish to participate in suggested activities and programs because, "I will walk again, so why bother?" Some physical recovery serves to strengthen beliefs that disability is not permanent. In the early stages of the rehabilitation program, patients must be convinced that working with the disability as it is today avoids deterioration of any muscle strength and is the best preparation for any return of function. No time is wasted. This approach does not shatter all hope but does not reinforce unrealistic expectations either. It usually helps both patients and families resolve some inner turmoil. It is an honest way to respond and one in which the nurse can feel comfortable.

It is important to continue to offer realistic responses to patient and family concerns without taking all hope away. For example, one patient asked the nurse, "Are you going to teach me how to walk today?" The nurse responded, "I really wish I could, but today I want to go over your catheterization technique so you can manage better at home this weekend." Another nurse said, "I just can't deal with his statements on a serious level so I joke with him." The latter type of communication can add to patient and family discomfort and decrease the positive effects of a therapeutic relationship.

Behavioral methods to engage a patient in the rehabilitation process are continually receiving greater recognition. Since behavior is sensitive to the influences of the environment, it is believed that if the external consequences can be controlled, behavior can be modified—that is, positive behavioral responses can be increased and undesirable or negative behavioral responses can be reduced. Terms such as *behavior modification*, *operant conditioning*, and *contingency management* refer to this basic principle.

Behavioral methods are designed to enhance traditional care goals and objectives and in no way propose any change in the basic philosophy of helping patients and relating to them in a meaningful way (Berni and Fordyce 1973). Because the rehabilitation process is a learning process, the principles of learning apply. Learning results in a behavioral change. Behavioral change theories are explored further in relation to the educational considerations presented in Chapter 8.

The educational process for the patient and family also facilitates the adjustment process. The rationale for focusing on patient and family education in the acute phase of spinal cord injury is expressed in the following objectives (Fukuyama et al. 1977):

- To increase patient and family knowledge and understanding of the effects of spinal cord injury on physical, vocational, social, and psychological functioning
- To increase the participation of family members in the patient's rehabilitation program and decrease feelings of isolation, hopelessness, and anxiety
- To reestablish communication channels among family members and enhance mutual support in emotionally dealing with disability
- To direct the patient and family toward discharge and realistic planning for the future

Throughout rehabilitation it is crucial that all health care professionals realize that a person's basic personality does not change just because of a spinal cord injury. People adapt psychologically through self-concept and self-esteem. However, the health care team can significantly influence feelings—either positively to promote psychological growth or negatively to restrict it.

Coping with difficult behavior

If the concept of *aggression* can be viewed in a broad context, certain principles of management apply to a variety of difficult behaviors. Ellison describes *overcontrol* of the aggressive drive as equated to inactivity, passivity, and withdrawal; *undercontrol* at its extreme is equated with violent, rageful, destructive behavior (Roy et al. 1976). Naturally there is a wide variety of behavior in between. Therefore a definition of aggressive drive might be "a state of inner tension causing discomfort to individuals and energizing them to take some action against the environment to relieve this unbearable state." Behavioral patterns become dysfunctional when people are unable to develop a satisfying relationship with the environment. For people with spinal cord injuries the disability is the situational crisis that triggers behavioral responses, but their methods of relieving the tension largely depend on previous patterns of handling aggression.

The basic concept of aggression is not a negative one. Aggression is a powerful drive that enables us to grow, achieve, separate from family, and assert our individuality. Quite often a patient who displays great anger during rehabilitation does reasonably well in the long run.

Ellison goes on to explain that there are basic principles that make seemingly dissimilar behaviors more understandable; for example, the same inner feelings that make patients verbally abusive one day may make them hide under the covers the next. Ellison and others advocate the following principles for relief of problems:

- Manipulating the environment to keep the opportunities for expression of independence and individuality as congruent as possible
- Providing outlets to channel or "siphon off" temporary spillover of aggressive behavior that accompanies movement or growth in the adjustment process
- Encouraging patients to develop their own

control system over aggressive impulses, and becoming a helper in this endeavor rather than simply another provider of outside control
- Realizing that overcontrol of the aggressive drive is an emotionally draining state and encouraging patients to channel this energy more effectively

Manipulating the environment In the reality of an institutional setting it may seem impossible to manipulate the environment in any meaningful way, but there are things that one can do. Usually the first rules to be examined are visiting hours in a critical care setting. Many times five minutes per hour is the recommended limit. This type of contact is often inconvenient for the family and does not best meet the patient's needs, particularly if the patient requires a prolonged stay. A mutually agreeable alternative should be worked out; even in a ward setting exceptions can be made. For example, a mother who worked in the afternoon wished to help her son with lunch. Although this time was not within regular visiting hours, the exception helped the mother feel useful and the son was pleased because he understood her need. If a patient cannot sleep during the night, she might be allowed to read in the lounge or watch television. If such requests become habitual, however, the patient may benefit from referral to a counselor or examination of the reasons for such persistent insomnia.

The nurse must remain flexible, but not without caution. Allowing privileges just because of a disability is no service to the patient; it may place unrealistic expectations on the family and eventually deteriorate into an unmanageable situation.

Providing outlets Limited opportunities for both physical and emotional releases of tension are very real problems for patients with spinal cord injuries. Advanced medicosurgical techniques have contributed to earlier mobilization, and socialization opportunities are increasing, but significant difficulties still exist.

Gross motor activities provided by a physical therapy program tend to relieve physical tension. Manipulating heavy medicine balls, using punch bags, or wheeling around outside are some examples.

There must also be opportunities to vent frustration and anxieties verbally. One problem is lack of privacy in an institutional setting, particularly in acute care. Physical space for private discussions and relaxation is needed; simply drawing curtains does not provide a sound barrier. Some of the most meaningful conversations between the nurse and the patient inevitably take place in a bathroom!

Above all, patients should participate in decision making as much as they can, so that they can take an active part in regaining health. When patients are not making good choices in relation to their physical care, it is part of the educational process to try to find ways of making the educational content more meaningful and relevant so that patients will be more committed to it. Nurses can try to help patients realize that making good choices about physical care enhances their health and ensures greater freedom to pursue other activities of which they are still capable.

To reinforce these capabilities, creative collaboration, with counseling professionals in particular, can explore ways in which the patient's authority can be exercised. For example, if a telephone is available, businesspeople can still participate in handling finances, and teenagers can maintain peer contact. Involving teenagers in decision making is infinitely more difficult. Learning to be self-directing or that one's behavior has certain consequences is a normal developmental task for teenagers, so they may not be ready to make decisions about their own care. Many rehabilitation facilities have structured in-house patient groups involved with formal decision making about policies. These opportunities present patients with constructive outlets for their aggression and opportunities to exercise authority. In such settings well-rehabilitated peer counselors can be invaluable in acting as role models to effect needed change; in helping patients see the positive aspects of rehabilitation; and in benefiting from the present opportunities for future productive activities in the community.

Encouraging personal control

A visitor left some alcohol for a quadriplegic patient tucked between his legs and the wheelchair. When the nurse became aware of this, she took the alcohol from the patient without any preliminary discussion. Physically unable to stop her, the patient retaliated by running into her with his electric wheelchair.

This is outside control and its likely result.

In another situation a patient and visitor were drinking alcohol at the patient's bedside. The nurse approached them kindly but firmly, restated the regulations and reasons for alcohol control and requested cooperation. Typically the patient responded "Come on, don't you ever take a drink?" The nurse realized the focus was not on her behavior but on the patient's and proceeded to remove the alcohol. Although presented with a choice, the patient felt embarrassed, belittled, and became very angry and shouted obscenities at the nurse. Later he apologized, and at this point the nurse and the patient were able to discuss more meaningfully how his behavior related to consequences and what other alternatives could be explored to increase his independence.

Here the nurse encouraged the patient to control his own behavior and acted as a helper in his efforts.

The critical point in the latter interaction was when the patient became angry. The nurse felt hurt and was moved to the point of tears, but with support from fellow staff members was able to regain composure. When the patient apologized, the nurse chose to confront the patient and said, "After all we have been through together, how could you talk to me like that? I realize that you are under a lot of stress, but wheelchair or not, you cannot expect to treat people like this without alienating them." In this way the nurse alerted the patient to his responsibility for the consequences of his actions. An honest response from the nurse is wonderful because it makes patients start feeling like "real" rather than "disabled" people. Although seldom mentioned in professional literature, the feeling of forgiveness is also important in a situation like this. Forgiving demonstrates a willingness to carry on and communicates confidence in the patient and hope for the future. If these everyday situations are managed well, the individual will have a better chance with others in the future.

Anger often surfaces as the ability to deny begins to break down. Paralyzed people have the added frustration of having limited physical ways to express pent-up anger. Verbal abuse is a common outlet. Patients may project their anger on the staff who care for them. Families may also be targets, and may in turn displace their anger on staff.

Family and staff can find anger directed at them very hard to handle (Morant 1978). To the staff, the patient's anger may seem ungrateful, unreasonable, hurtful, and sometimes frightening. Some staff members take attacks personally, experiencing feelings of guilt or inadequacy; some return the patient's anger, sometimes inappropriately; some atone for their inner anger by forcing themselves to be especially nice; and some accept the criticisms and complaints at face value and wear themselves out trying to please someone who cannot be pleased. Family members also become confused and hurt by the patient's antagonism. Nurses can help by seeking explanations of these actions and helping patients and families verbalize and deal with their feelings.

Staff members need to recognize their own anger. Such feelings are not shameful in a "professional" person. If team members are assured that their anger is a normal response, feelings of guilt and shame tend to recede. Staff may feel less anxious when they realize that patients' anger is partly their way of turning a festering rage at themselves outward rather than holding it in and aggravating their gloom.

No normal person can bear too much abuse, nor should one try. Patients' destructive hatred must be channeled into learning and labor if they are to achieve their full potential for recovery. All concerned must have appropriate outlets for expression of feelings.

Recognizing overcontrol   Too much control of aggression can lead to withdrawal and aggravate depression. The severity of withdrawal or depression is related to the support of family and staff, previous management or problems, and personal values. It is best to allow patients to withdraw at first if they wish, then gradually to draw them out of the bed or room for short periods. Some patients are "loners," and some withdrawal may be quite normal for them. This should be indicated by their history. For example, a patient may not wish to rely on staff members for personal psychological assistance but prefer to solve problems alone. This prerogative should be respected. Indirect intervention could include assessment of the patient's personal resources outside the hospital if help is needed.

Severe or prolonged withdrawal signals the need for psychiatric consultation.

A middle-aged quadriplegic man, injured in a skiing accident, became increasingly withdrawn approximately four weeks after injury. He began by refusing to get up in the wheelchair. Gradually he refused to eat, had difficulty sleeping, ceased to respond verbally, and finally passively resisted any verbal or physical contact. The psychiatrist began treatment with antidepressant medication in conjunction with psychotherapy. As all attempts to encourage participation in his care were futile, the psychiatrist suggested that the patient be allowed to regress to a fully dependent role to regain his strength before new activities were gradually introduced. The patient began to work through his numerous marital, family, and vocational problems that had existed before the injury. This approach met with relative success and the patient was finally able to participate in a rehabilitation program and return to his rural home. However, one year later family disruption and resultant problems were again evident.

Use of drugs   The routine use of antidepressant or tranquilizing drugs is not generally recommended. Patients are better off facing problems when supportive assistance is readily available, rather than postponing inevitable reactions when resources may not be forthcoming. Moreover, addiction is a major problem, and it can occur within four to six weeks to such commonly used drugs as diazepam (Valium).

Coping with a crisis situation

One problem that is unique to nurses is dealing with uncooperative, depressed, or angry patients while trying to give care that is essential to maintain physical integrity. Interactions can escalate into crisis situations. Typically these situations are most pronounced during the evening or night, when reactions to significant experiences encountered during the day, or on return from passes, seem to surface.

Approaching these situations using a crisis intervention model should make nursing management more successful for the patient and less stressful for the nurse. Techniques emphasize a more straightforward person-to-person approach rather than in-depth psychoanalytical counseling.

Stressful events are part of life, but it is not the events that activate crisis. Crisis occurs when our interpretation of these events leads to stresses so severe that we can find no relief. This interpretation is based on the works of Hoff (1978), who bases crisis theory intervention on a belief that people can develop or mature psychologically throughout life. This does not imply that during the heat of an unpleasant confrontation with a patient, nurses are supposed to be thinking of the significance of the patient's personality development; what they should remember is the opportunity for growth and learning from an unpleasant experience, rather than withdrawal, alienation, and deterioration. Upsetting outbursts can then be viewed as an opportunity for developing and gaining life experiences or perhaps even as a turning point in the patient's life. People who recognize that everyone has potential for vast growth can be most helpful in crisis management.

Hoff explains that people cannot remain in the psychological turmoil of crisis forever, because the accompanying anxiety is too painful. The emotional discomfort stemming from extreme anxiety prompts a person to reduce the anxiety to an endurable level as soon as possible. Possible outcomes are:

- The person returns to the precrisis (usual) state as a result of effective problem solving made possible by internal strengths and social supports.
- The person not only returns to the precrisis state but actually grows from the crisis experience through discovery of new resources and ways of problem solving.
- The person lapses into neurotic or psychotic behavior. Sometimes it is difficult to differentiate between extreme emotional or behavioral responses that are normal and those that are more psychiatric in nature, but most rehabilitation patients are not psychotic.

Several techniques can be applied to coping with a crisis situation. These include listening actively and with concern; encouraging open expression of feelings; helping the patient to gain understanding of events that lead to crisis, to accept reality and to explore new ways of coping; linking the patient with social contacts and activities; and reinforcing the newly learned coping devices after resolution of the crisis. These techniques, some actually preventive, apply in everyday ward situations when caring for patients with spinal cord injuries. Crisis intervention techniques are really a way of assessing and organizing concerns and helping the person do something about them—a model for "putting it all together."

Much of the data collected during assessment determines why people go into crisis. A hospital setting is a better place than most to do some preventive work. As mentioned previously, good assessment provides empathetic and attentive listening, which is therapeutic in itself. The following example indicates how crisis behavior can sometimes be prevented.

Mary, a 47-year-old homemaker, married with four children, was referred to a major neurological center (two weeks after injury) after being diagnosed as experiencing "hysterical" paralysis at a local hospital. Following neurological assessment, her injury was accurately diagnosed as a central cord injury at C_{5-6} cord segment (without bony injury). A comment by the nurse expressing how fortunate Mary was to have escaped a complete injury elicited a hostile response. Mary insulted the nurse's youth and appearance and accused her of being stupid because she had no idea of what life was all about. The nurse was able to look beyond this response and identify several events that culminated in this inappropriate behavior. Although Mary was able to walk and therefore did not "look" that disabled, upper limb and torso weakness rendered her dependent for many activities of daily living and personal hygiene. In addition, she had just experienced a negative relationship with local health professionals who did not believe her complaints, was menopausal, had a daughter who had just left home, and was worried about her husband being left alone with a young woman who was hired to care for the other children. The nurse perceived a severe threat to Mary's self-concept and self-esteem and referred her to a social worker, who initiated marital and family counseling and made alternate child-care arrangements. This enabled the entire interdisciplinary team to proceed with a more empathetic approach. The staff also took immediate steps to resolve some of Mary's hostility toward local health resources, because she would require their supportive services to return home as soon as possible.

When a nurse must deal with an angry outburst and resistance to physical care, it is extremely difficult to control inner feelings or even to begin to understand the underlying cause for the patient's behavior. It is normal to feel hurt and enraged, and nurses should be prepared to give themselves and their patients time to cool off.

Tony, a 17-year-old boy, and youngest of four children, was injured in an alcohol-related diving accident at a high school graduation party. He was diagnosed as having a fracture dislocation of C_5 and C_6 vertebrae with complete quadriplegia at C_7. Several weeks after injury, although still in a Halo brace, he was able to go home on a weekend pass. He returned late on Sunday night, and the nurse was hurrying to get him into bed. Something went wrong and a very unpleasant scene followed. The nurse simply stated she was not prepared to deal with that type of behavior but would return before she went off. It is almost a natural reaction to tell the patient you can't stand this scene one more time but it is far more helpful to focus on the experiences of the day rather than dwelling on previous, similar negative reactions. Tony eventually explained that he had attended a family reunion where his parents insisted on doing everything for him, from pushing his chair around to grinding up his meat! An old auntie had sympathetically patted him on the head. Overwhelmed by these responses, Tony had remained silent only to explode later at the nurse.

These types of experiences point toward the need for assertiveness and social skills training among others. Once the causes of the behavioral outbursts are identified, the nurse can proceed with counseling professionals to encourage the patient to reflect on how to approach the same situation another time; to examine his feelings; and to think about what to do to get other people to react more positively toward him. Many different forms of therapy, including role playing and group interaction, can be employed to facilitate achievement of these new coping techniques.

The patient who consistently experiences extreme difficulties in controlling aggressive behavior may be unable or unwilling to become involved in the rehabilitation process.

Janice, a 17-year-old with C_5 quadriplegia, was from an extremely unstable family background and before injury had serious problems socially and at school. Janice received a number of associated injuries necessitating several surgeries and a prolonged stay in a critical care setting. When admitted to the rehabilitation center, she adamantly refused to get up each morning and resisted treatment. Her obnoxious, unreasonable demands and continual scenes were disruptive to those around her, and professional resources were tapped to exhaustion. At one point when Janice refused to cooperate with any rehabilitation activities, she was discharged to a nursing home. Almost a year later, Janice was able to see more clearly what her goals were and she returned to the rehabilitation center. Although significantly delayed, the course of rehabilitation progressed. Janice is now living independently with a group of disabled people in the community and is completing her high school education in preparation for college entrance.

Drug and alcohol abuse precipitates unmanageable behavior that can pose a threat to patients and to those around them. This problem typically increases as rehabilitation progresses. Reasonable policies with disciplinary action, such as administrative discharge following repeated offenses, only provide temporary solutions. Boyink and Strawn (1980) point out the necessity for clear-cut rules on how many infractions constitute a reason for disciplinary action. The policy must then be supported by all staff members and known to all patients. This encourages the patients to become more responsible for the consequences of their behavior. If policies are not enforced, continued use of alcohol and drugs is condoned and the staff feel angered and unsupported. Liaison with community-based drug and alcohol abuse programs is helpful for specific problems.

Boyink and Strawn explain that illicit use of alcohol and drugs, particularly among the more vulnerable youth population, is influenced by two major factors: *boredom* and the *inability to deal with the reality of disability*. Mind-altering substances provide an escape. In conjunction with the more traditional psychological interventions, management of recreational and leisure time emerges as an important element in achieving productivity. Nurses, particularly on evenings and weekends, have important roles to play in supporting this therapy.

These situations, among others, reflect the importance of goal setting as part of the intake process. If patient and professional goals and expectations are not compatible or harmonious, it may be best to delay admission to a rehabilitation center. Occasionally the risks of physical deterioration in settings where rehabilitation is not an area of expertise can outweigh untimely involvement, although this can arouse moral and ethical dilemmas. These situations also point to the pressing need for development of as many entry, exit, and reentry opportunities as possible to the rehabilitation process to accommodate individual needs.

Evaluation

The outcome of rehabilitation is a result of the patient, the family, and all aspects of the therapeutic environment working together. The rehabilitation milieu must be flexible enough to meet individual needs as patients and families help to define these needs. Comprehensive physical and psychosocial rehabilitation ensures opportunities for achievement of goals that will lead to increased autonomy. Methods of delivering care include interdisciplinary assessment; direct, individual, and family counseling; and varied support services. Such a comprehensive approach has a preventive and restorative focus from the moment of injury and is influenced by the positive attitudes of each health care team member. Each of these aspects must be continually evaluated.

During the rehabilitation process, evaluation of psychological and social adjustment is largely determined by professional judgment. Evaluation encompasses such factors as feedback from the patient and family; ability to set realistic goals and solve problems; and patterns of behavioral change. Achievement of patient and family health education goals also reflects the degree of psychosocial adaptation. In general, the more complete educational goals, the greater the degree of adjustment. The ultimate success or failure of the rehabilitation process will eventually be determined by the ability of the person with a spinal cord injury to live productively in the community at large. Productivity may or may not include financial, vocational, and physical independence, but it must reflect personal satisfaction with one's own life-style.

SELECTED REFERENCES

Berni, R., and Fordyce, W. 1973. *Behavior Modification and the Nursing Process.* St. Louis: C. V. Mosby. *A description of patient management problems that outlines practical techniques to apply behavior modification to accomplish patient care goals and objectives; includes analysis of behavior, reinforcement of behavior, practical management, ethical issues, and future trends.*

Boyink, M. A., and Strawn, S. M. 1980. Spinal cord injury: post acute phase. In *Comprehensive Rehabilitation Nursing.* Eds. N. Martin, N. B. Holt, and D. Hicks. New York: McGraw-Hill. *Overall assessment and planning, and related nursing care in later rehabilitation phase.*

Dunn, M. 1977. Social discomfort in the patient with spinal cord injury. *Archives of Physical Medicine and Rehabilitation* 58 (June): 257–260. *A group of spinal cord injured men rate 20 situations in order of social discomforts.*

Fukuyama, K.; Kelly, J.; and Little, J. 1977. Unpublished material on patient and family education. *A group of staff nurses present rationale for establishing a formal health education program on an acute spinal cord injury unit.*

Gunther, M. S. 1980. The threatened practitioner: work under stress. In *Comprehensive Rehabilitation Nursing.* Eds. N. Martin, N. B. Holt, and D. Hicks. New York: McGraw-Hill. *Skillfully analyzes the nursing service at work, explores factors that cause stress for the nurse, and focuses on management activities that help. Highly recommended.*

Hoff, L. A. 1978. *People in Crisis: Understanding and Helping.* Menlo Park, Calif: Addison-Wesley. *Straightforward approach using everyday language to teach people how to understand, identify, and help other people in crisis; includes information about helping self-destructive people and those whose health and self-image are threatened. Highly recommended.*

Hohmann, G. W. 1975. Psychological aspects of treatment and rehabilitation of the spinal cord injured person. *Clinical Orthopedics and Related Research* 112 (Oct.): 81–88. *Discussion of "normal" reaction to the experienced loss, observations of people with pre-existing psychopathology, and exploration of psychological aspects of pain, sexual adjustment, and the impact on the family. Gives insight into the process of adjustment. Highly recommended.*

Kozier, B., and Erb, G. 1983. *Fundamentals of Nursing.* 2nd ed. Menlo Park, Ca.: Addison-Wesley, Ch. 33. *Review of development of self-concept and self-esteem.*

Leinart, B. K. 1979. Attitudes of nurses toward spinal cord injury patients. *Journal of Association of Rehabilitation Nurses* 4 (Jan./Feb.): 7–9. *A comparison of attitudes of nurses working in acute, intermediate, and rehabilitation areas; stresses the importance of professional attitudes as an integral force determining the degree of success in patient adjustment to disability.*

MacLean, S. 1981. Discharge planning for spinal cord injured patients. Unpublished material, University of British Columbia, Vancouver, B.C. *Examines the rehabilitation process as it applies to three young quadriplegic patients.*

Morant, C. 1978. The role of a psychiatrist on an acute spinal cord injury unit. Unpublished material. Shaughnessy Hospital, Vancouver, BC. *Focuses on the role of the psychiatrist in managing stress encountered by the interdisciplinary team.*

Roglitz, C. 1978. Team approach in the acute phase of spinal cord injury. *Journal of Neurosurgical Nursing* 10 (3): 117–120. *Focuses on the interaction between the nurse and the social worker to enhance staff communication, development, involvement, and understanding of others, which ultimately improves quality of individualized patient care.*

Roy, C., Sr., et al. 1976. *Introduction to Nursing: An Adaptation Model.* Englewood Cliffs, NJ: Prentice-Hall. *Presents a model of nursing focusing on the nurse's role as a helper to patients in adapting to stress rather than a provider in meeting needs. In-depth exploration of self-concept, self-esteem, role function, the physical self and experiencing loss, and related problems in these and other areas.*

Sadlick, M., and Penta, F. B. 1975. Changing nurse attitudes toward quadriplegics through use of television. *Rehabilitation Literature* 36 (9): 274–278. *A technique for promoting more positive attitudes toward potential patient outcomes during rehabilitation.*

Shontz, F. 1975. *The Psychological Aspects of Physical Illness and Disability.* New York: Macmillan. *Superior background reading exploring cyclical adjustment to disability.*

Szasz, G. 1980. A guide to the interpersonal skills of history-taking. *Beta Release* (Journal of the Canadian Diabetes Association) 5 (2): 2–8. *A clear and concise practical overview, especially for the student professional, to enhance the skills of interviewing in clinical situations. Highly recommended.*

Thomas, E. J. 1966. Problems of disability from the perspective of role theory. *Journal of Health and Human Behavior* 7(1) Spring: 2–14. *Examines with insight acquisition of new behaviors and roles.*

Thompson, D. D., and Lott, J. D. 1980. Psychosocial redevelopment of the spinal cord injured person. *Spinal Cord Injury Digest* 2 (Winter): 6–9. *Description of the psychosocial aspects of treatment, rehabilitation, and community environment and how these relate to reprocessing of Erickson's life span development stages.*

Treischmann, R. 1980. *Spinal Cord Injuries, Psychological, Social and Vocational Adjustment.* New York: Pergamon Press. *The only existing work exclusively devoted to the psychosocial impact of spinal cord injuries. Includes an exhaustive critique of the literature with a view to dispelling myths and stimulating research to develop future strategies.*

Virginia Spinal Cord Injury Care and Teaching Manual. 1980. The Virginia Spinal Cord Injury System, University of Virginia Center and Virginia Dept. of Rehabilitation Services, Woodrow Wilson Rehabilitation Center, Box W–279, Fisherville, Va 22939. *Approach directed to patient and family regarding psychosocial and sexual issues.*

Weller, D. J., and Miller, P. M. 1977a. Emotional reactions of patient, family, and staff in acute-care period of spinal cord injury: part 1. *Social Work Health Care* 2 (Summer): 369–377. *Describes and analyzes stages of adjustment in the acute postinjury period with treatment implications and their significance in later rehabilitation. Focuses on introductory material and patient responses.*

———. 1977b. Emotional reactions of patient, family, and staff in acute-care period of spinal cord injury: part 2. *Social Work Health Care* 3 (Fall): 7–17. *Considers emotional reactions of family members and staff with further implications for treatment.*

Wool, R. N., et al. 1980. Task performance in spinal cord injury: effect of helplessness training. *Archives of Physical Medicine and Rehabilitation* 61 (July): 321–325. *Explores possibility of significantly influencing psychological recovery by using rehabilitation strategy aimed at providing success experiences.*

Young, J. S., and Northrup, N. E. 1979. *Statistical Information Pertaining to Some of the Most Commonly Asked Questions About Spinal Cord Injury.* National Spinal Cord Injury Data Research Center, Good Samaritan Hospital, Phoenix, Ariz. *Data collected from 1973 through 1978. Ready reference in question-answer format. Subheadings include demography, etiology, length of hospital stay, cost of hospitalization, use of ongoing services, social and vocational achievements, and life expectancy.*

SUPPLEMENTAL READING

Aadalen, S. P., and Stroebel-Kahn, F. 1981. Coping with quadriplegia. *American Journal of Nursing.* 81 (8): 1471–1478. *Presents a description of coping with the physical and emotional trauma one of the authors experienced after becoming quadriplegic. Good discussion of adaptive mechanisms used by patient and family.*

Alexander, J. L., and Willems, E. P. 1981. Quality of life: some measurement requirements. *Archives of Physical Medicine and Rehabilitation* 62 (June): 261–265. *Explores current views of quality of life issues. Describes quantitative, subjective measurements of "what people do, where they do it, with whom they do it, and how they do it" to assess progress through the rehabilitation process. From these "behavioral vital signs" it is possible to predict life-styles in the postdischarge or community environment.*

Bassler, S. F. 1980. Development of a resource support system for nurses caring for spinal cord injured patients. *Journal of Neurosurgical Nursing* 12 (4): 195–198. *Description of how a planned program of information, guidance, and education was offered to nurses faced with implementing a new Regional Spinal Cord Injury Center.*

Bishop, D. S. 1980. *Behavioral Problems and the Disabled, Assessment and Management.* Baltimore, Md: Williams and Wilkins. *Deals clearly with behavioral problems; addresses the problems of sleep and pain; provides an overview of problems unique to the disabled child; and describes staff interaction in various settings. Specific chapters are devoted to crisis intervention techniques, to spinal cord injury, and to the relationship between alcohol and drug abuse and physical medicine and rehabilitation.*

Buscaglia, L. 1975. *The Disabled and Their Parents.* Thorofare, NJ: Charles B. Slack. *In a very humanistic readable style, describes how disabled persons, their families, and even professionals can suffer more pain than is caused by the disability itself when competent, sound, reality-based guidance is not forthcoming. Chapter 13 deals with becoming disabled later in life. Highly recommended.*

Church, C. S. 1981. Social work involvement with families at the acute stage of spinal cord injury. *Model Systems' Spinal Cord Injury Digest* 3 (Winter): 49–53. *Describes function of the social worker at the acute stage of spinal cord injury: to help families deal with their own feelings and provide support to the patient.*

Harriman, M., and Garfunkel, M. 1981. The value of self-help groups in spinal cord injury rehabilitation. *Model Systems' Spinal Cord Injury Digest* 3 (Fall): 26–33. *Advocates the formation and integration of self-help groups within rehabilitation programs. Four types of self-help groups are proposed. Self-help groups emphasize mutuality and interdependence and provide an opportunity to share feelings and information.*

Hart, G. 1981. Spinal cord injury: impact on clients' significant others. *Rehabilitation Nursing*, January-February, pp. 11–15. *Findings from interviews, beginning within hours after injury, suggest significant others have many needs, including: to feel adequately informed, to feel helpful to the client, and to feel the client is getting good care. To benefit the client, the nurse must listen and react to the concerns and needs of significant others as part of the rehabilitation approach.*

Howell, T., et al. 1981. Depression in spinal cord injured patients. *International Journal of Paraplegia* 19 (5): 284–288. *Evaluation of 22 patients with spinal cord injuries with standardized interview and diagnostic process for depression. Five patients had diagnosable depressions, which is higher than the incidence in the general population but lower than anticipated.*

Jacus, C. M. 1981. Working with families in a rehabilitation setting. *Rehabilitation Nursing* 6 (3): 10–14. *Describes how the health care professional can plan family involvement, highlighting points of entry for professional intervention as families experience various adjustments.*

Kinash, R. G. 1978. Experiences and nursing needs of spinal cord–injured patients. *Journal of Neurosurgical Nursing* 10: 29–32. *Describes some physical and psychosocial needs using numerous direct quotations from paraplegic and quadriplegic patients; includes major needs and concerns, sources of comfort and discomfort, guidelines for intervention, and some conclusions. Meaningful information for those giving direct bedside care.*

Kuenzi, S. H., and Fenton, M. V. 1975. Crisis intervention in acute care areas. *American Journal of Nursing* 75 (5): 830–834. *Describes use of the crisis theory in initial management where physical care is the focus; gives meaningful and practical direction to nurses for interaction with patients and families to prevent crisis behavior (incorporates the grieving process).*

Lamonica, E. L. 1979. *The Nursing Process: A Humanistic Approach.* Menlo Park, Calif: Addison-Wesley. *An examination of the nursing process using humanistic, multimedia techniques. A creative approach to learning that corresponds to current trends.*

Lawson, N. C. 1978. Significant events in the rehabilitation process: the spinal cord patient's point of view. *Archives of Physical Medicine and Rehabilitation* 59 (Dec.): 573–579. *Report of a research study using tape-recorded daily logs, hospital staff ratings, behavioral measure of verbal output, and an endocrine measure to determine significant events during hospitalization. Results suggest that prolonged depression is counterproductive to the rehabilitation process and that important people in the patient's life exert a most significant influence. Discusses programmatic implications.*

Longo, D. C., and Williams, R. A. 1978. *Clinical Practice in Psychosocial Nursing: Assessment and Intervention.* New York: Appelton-Century-Crofts. *Translation of complex and abstract psychosocial concepts into meaningful behavior at the bedside; contains helpful chapters on anxiety, life change, human adaptation and illness, and the therapeutic process with adolescents experiencing psychosocial stress.*

Loomis, M. E., and Horsley, J. 1974. *Interpersonal Change: A Behavioral Approach to Nursing Practice.* New York: McGraw-Hill. *An introductory text on operant conditioning for nurses. Includes treatment approaches for depressed and self-destructive behaviors.*

Marinelli, R. P., and Del Orto, A. E. 1977. *Psychological and Social Impact of Physical Disability.* New York: Springer. *Superior general background reading. Extensive bibliography.*

McHugh, M. L., et al. 1979. Family support group in a burn unit. *American Journal of Nursing,* December, pp. 2148–2150. *Description of nurses beginning a family support group for relatives of those suddenly catastrophically injured; includes the evolvement process of the group, discusses threatening situations and resolutions used by the nurse, and distinguishes between support and psychotherapy. Advantages can readily be related to caring for patients with spinal cord injuries.*

Mitchell, C. J. 1978. Social service innovations. In *National Spinal Cord Injury Model Systems Conference Proceedings.* April 1978. *Discussion of development and role of social service in a specialized spinal cord injury service.*

Pepper, G. 1977. The person with spinal cord injury, psychological care. *American Journal of Nursing,* August, pp. 1330–1342. *In an effort to help nurses understand the disabled person's often perplexing behavior, the author has correlated the adjustments of the severely injured person with the developmental tasks of the infant, child, and adolescent (including those of trust, autonomy, and initiative). Again it should be emphasized that stage theories of disorganization, especially described as regression, are not, and should not be, universally applicable.*

Rogers, J. C., and Figone, J. J. 1979. Psychosocial parameters in treating the person with quadriplegia. *American Journal of Occupational Therapy* 33 (7): 432–439. *The development of a more flexible, comprehensive treatment model that gives priority to developmental status, changing life goals, interpersonal relationships, and social roles. Highly recommended.*

Rohrer, K., et al. 1980. Rehabilitation in spinal cord injury: use of a patient-family group. *Archives of Physical Medicine and Rehabilitation* 61 (5): 225–229. *A report on a program of one-day workshops held for patients with spinal cord injuries and their families. Stresses education, as well as a therapeutic sharing of feelings.*

Romano, M.D. 1976. Social skills training with the newly handicapped. *Archives of Physical Medicine and Rehabilitation* 57 (June): 302–303. *Describes the premise that restoring an individual's social competence maximizes the probability of success of the physical rehabilitation process.*

Tucker, S. J. 1980. The psychology of spinal cord injury: patient–staff interaction. *Rehabilitation Literature* 41 (5–6): 114–121. *Reviews and analyzes current knowledge about the psychology of spinal cord injury; focuses on the emotional reactions of the patient and the less-recognized but vitally important emotional reactions of the staff. The author is a psychotherapist and has a spinal cord injury herself. Extensive selective bibliography. Highly recommended.*

Wiley, L., Ed. 1978. Family centered conferences for better trauma care. *Nursing '78* 8: 71–77. *Nursing grand rounds format reviews a series of interdisciplinary conferences for a quadriplegic patient during acute care, emphasizing and explaining how to enhance independence, help face reality, and prepare for the future. Highly recommended.*

———— 1979. Realistic goals don't mean failure. *Nursing '79* 9 (5): 55–58. *Nurses explore personal feelings when limit setting, consistency, and reality confrontation do not always achieve the optimal outcome for a patient with a self-destructive, sociopathic personality.*

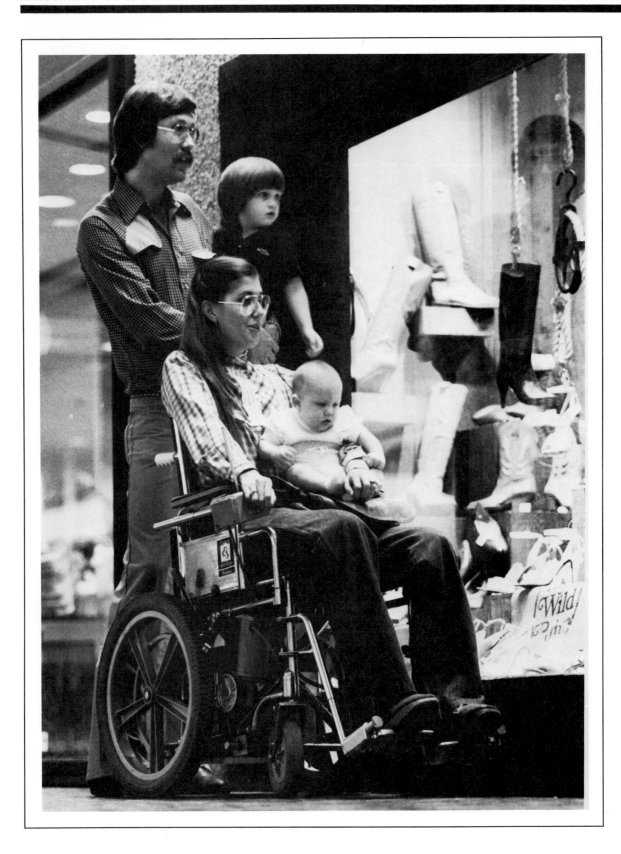

Chapter 7

Sexual Health Care

George Szasz, M.D.

CHAPTER OUTLINE

OBJECTIVES

- To describe sexual consequences dysfunctions in relation to spinal cord injury
- To describe current approaches to sexual problem management
- To describe the nurse's role in sexual health care including sexual care practice methods for the nonspecialist nurse
- To develop communication skills to obtain and give sexual information
- To develop an awareness of personal attitudes, recognize personal limitations, and seek assistance when needed

A 52-year-old woman, married for 28 years and the mother of three sons, suffered an incomplete injury to the C_{6-7} segments in a car accident. Two months after her injury, and just after her husband left at the end of visiting hours, she turned to the nurse: "I think I want to talk to somebody about our sexual life. This was very important to my husband . . . to me too. You know . . . not that we are like kids, but we enjoy each other. I guess I can live without it, but it was so much part of our life."

It is not surprising that this woman turned to her nurse for help, but what did she expect of the nurse? This is how the woman explained it: "I don't know. I didn't know who to talk to. I know that my husband is worried, but he's so shy. I suppose he could go to our family doctor, or the doctors here, but they're all so busy, and there's no privacy here. Actually I feel embarrassed about the whole thing. Talking about sex somehow doesn't fit in with all these sick people. . . . And here I am . . . middle aged, can't move my legs, can't even urinate without help. I guess I should worry about the legs and forget the sex part, and yet, I can't. I thought the nurse might have some answers. How do other women get over this? Is sex over? Or can I do something? Will I satisfy my husband? Will I feel anything? Will my husband ever look at me like he used to?"

This woman's questions are not unusual at all. In the last few years increasing numbers of patients, partners, and family members want intelligent exploration of their sexual dysfunctions and disabilities. Anticipating patients' requests for information, a number of spinal cord injury units and rehabilitation centers have begun programs that consider patients' sexual needs. The specific role of the nurse in this has not been clear. Should the nurse be involved in sexual care? If so, should this involvement be limited to informal and private discussions with the patient, or should it be a formally assigned task? In either case, should the interaction be reported at the team meetings? Should the patient's physicians be informed about the patient's concerns? Should the nurse give advice? If so, what guiding principles should be followed? Who should set these? To whom should the nurse be accountable if something goes wrong, and who should reward the nurse for excellence in the practice of sexual health care? Or should there be a separate "sexual health care service" staffed with specially trained personnel? If so, what would be expected of the nurse, and how could the nurse make the best use of such a service? The answers to these questions are now evolving. The purpose of this chapter is to help this evolution.

GOALS OF HEALTH CARE

Goals of health care for helping patients and families adjust to sexual consequences of spinal cord injury are:

- To provide a comprehensive service, including assessment and treatment of physical, social, and emotional components of patients' sexual functioning
- To make available early consultation services to all patients and families
- To offer continuous assessment, education, and therapeutic features to patients and families as they move through various stages of rehabilitation

SEXUAL CONSEQUENCES OF SPINAL CORD INJURY

Sexual Functioning Status

Nursing histories often include a question about "any problems in your sexual life." If the patient answers "No," it is difficult for the nurse to know whether the patient has no sexual problems or does not even know what areas are covered by the question. Even if a male patient reveals a concern like: "Will I be able to satisfy my partner?" the nurse will still not know whether the patient is worried only about his erection problem or also about, for example, his ability to become a father. Obviously, "any problem in your sexual life" is too general. Many patients will require a list to decide areas that might fall into the "sex" category. Staff members reviewing the nursing history would also find the answers to specific questions valuable, because these would reflect the patient's sexual functioning status at the time of admission to the hospital and at various occasions thereafter.

There are six categories that are useful in establishing the patient's sexual functioning status.

1. *Sexual response status* reflects the physiological ability of the patient to experience genital sensations, erection, ejaculation, vaginal lubrication, orgasm, pelvic thrusting, and other responses to stimulation.
2. *Sexual activity status* indicates the available motor functions that might be used, for example, for embracing, caressing, and intercourse.
3. *Sexual interest status* reveals the degree to which the patient wants to be involved in sex activities.
4. *Sexual behavior status* gives information about availability of partners and the skills in social interaction processes that may lead to sexual activities.
5. *Sex organ status* describes the anatomical integrity of the genitalia and the sexual problems caused by urinary drainage apparatus, genitourinary infections, or surgery.

6. *Fertility status* reveals evidence of the need or ability to procreate or the nature of contraception desired.

The definition of a person's sexual functioning status may be difficult sometimes because meanings of *sexual health* and *sexual losses* vary greatly. For example, what is normal and healthy in sex, and how would one define a patient as sexually healthy? Put another way, at what point would health professionals want to be involved with a patient's sexual life to save that patient from sexual ill health, and at what point would health professionals say: "The treatment is finished; our tests show that you are now sexually healthy"? The consideration of this fundamental question will have to be sidestepped in this chapter. Not enough is known about the biology of sexual behavior to declare that, for example, continuation of various sex practices is a condition of good health and therefore sexual health care is a must for every patient. Also, sexual losses mean different things to different people. For example, a surgeon was overheard to say: "If I had a spinal injury, the last thing I would worry about is sex." A nurse said: "I applied to work on this unit because they have a sex rehabilitation program here." A 24-year-old patient who suffered an incomplete lesion in the lower lumbar and sacral neurological levels said: "You know, it just kills me to think that I might never get it up, you know, hard like it used to be. I just don't feel like being complete. I feel sexless. There's a void . . . as if I wasn't a man anymore." A 42-year-old married man who suffered a complete injury to the T_{10-11} area commented: "We are just thankful to God that I survived. We have three healthy children. Sex was not that important to my wife, and now it's not important to me either." A staff member in an acute spinal cord injury unit was overheard to complain: "If he could get his mind off sex, he might do okay. Doesn't he understand that he has got to do his physical therapy?"

The surgeon who would not worry about sexual losses explained what he meant by saying, "As far as love is concerned, yes, at first intercourse had a lot to do with it, but now our relationship doesn't stand or fall with it. If I were in this situation, and had a choice, I would rather walk than get sexual feelings back. I can't see myself without my work." The nurse explained that to her intimate physical acts were the way to express love and affection. She said, "I was married before. Sex problems were the cause of our deepest distress. Now I wish we could have gone for help." The young man said, "To me sex means pleasure. It's also a way to show how much I like my partner. I also wanted to have a child. It's the difference between being a boy and being a man." The older man said, "We used to enjoy intercourse. Stimulation with the hand? No! That's for kids. I don't think my wife would stand for that anyway! Best to forget it." The staff member who complained about a young man's preoccupation said: "Yes, of course, sex is important, but everything has its time and place. This is time for physical therapy, not for sex. Besides, this is a hospital, not a pleasure dome."

The variety of interpretations of what sex is about or what a sexual loss may represent makes it virtually impossible to organize a sexual health care service with the universality, urgency, and discipline of, for example, a bladder or bowel care program. An added complication is that while some patients are distressed enough to say that "life is not worthwhile" without access to the sexual options (whatever this may mean to the individual), most patients and their partners feel embarrassed about expressing sexual needs at any time, but particularly at the time of a physical crisis. The roots of these feelings are part of our cultural heritage, which still holds that sexual desirability and the right to sexual practices belong to the young, the healthy, the whole, and the beautiful. Even though these ideas have begun to change outside the walls of hospitals and long-term care institutions, the change within is slow. Some professionals unwittingly stifle patients' expressions of sexual problems, because never having received training in this area, they are not sure how to assess or treat patients suffering from these problems. Many patients have a sense of foreboding about their sexual losses, but they have no words to specify their complaints, even if they have the courage to complain. This is why nurses may be approached with mumbled comments, like "I guess I will be a bachelor for life," or "Maybe my wife should get another man," or "I won't be attractive to him now."

This is why the list of sexual status categories is useful in clarifying the patient's problems. In the following pages these categories will be discussed in more detail. Because these categories overlap, they will be grouped under three headings:

1. *Sexual response*
2. *Sexual practice* (including the interest, activity, and behavior status categories and the condition of the genitalia)
3. *Fertility* (including contraceptive issues)

The section on *sexual response* will be the largest, because the physical methods of its assessment will also be included.

Sexual Response

In conceptualizing the sexual physiological damage in a spinal cord injury, it is useful to think of the sexual response as a complex reflex. Like other reflexes, this one requires certain stimuli to initiate reactions, nerve tracks to carry the stimuli to various centers, returning nerve tracks, and organs that react. One characteristic of the sexual response is that the reaction of the genitalia sets off further stimuli, which in turn escalate the intensity of the sexual response. Another characteristic of this response is that eventually the whole body becomes involved in the process so that apart from genital changes there may be changes in muscular tension, blood pressure and heart rate, and perhaps even the level of certain hormones circulating in the body. The stimuli may be "mental"—erotic materials, situations, or thoughts—or "touch"—applied to the genitalia or to other parts of the body. Rhythmic, rubbing action applied to the genitalia is usually the most effective stimulating action in a person with intact neurological pathways. If carried on long enough, such stimulation may lead to a full sexual response. In men the genital aspects of this response include erection of the penis and orgasm. The male orgasm has two parts: an inner tension caused by the secretion of seminal fluid, and the pleasurable release of this tension in the ejaculation of the seminal fluid. In women these two parts of the orgasm are not well identified, but the orgasmic experience starts with a suffusion of warmth in the vaginal area, increase in the lubrication, and strong inner tension, and ends with pleasurable release.

Rhythmic rubbing of the breasts, neck, inner thighs, perineum, or perianal areas may also produce high sexual tension and may lead to orgasmic responses. It is not understood yet how the brain identifies a stimulus as sexual or nonsexual. For example, stimuli arising from washing the genitalia, examining the breast, dressing or undressing, combing hair, or body contact when lifting could be identified as sexual by the brain of the receiver, even though the giver or doer (the nurse or the physician) had no sexual intention at all. The nerve tracks in the brain and the neural reactions necessary to translate a situation or an action into a sexual response are also not well-understood.

Direct touch stimulation of the genitalia is believed to be carried to the S_{2-4} segments by the pudendal nerve. There are probably other autonomic sensory pathways too, but these are not understood. From the sacral area the messages are conducted to the brain through the lateral spinothalamic tracts. Two separate events seem to take place in the brain then:

1. Signals are sent down to the T_{11-12} and S_{2-4} segments to *release* the erection reflex in men and the vaginal lubrication reflex in women. The sequence of events suggests that in an able-bodied person the brain continuously suppresses erection and lubrication *until* the right stimuli arrive. Then the brain seems to let go, and the reflex reaction is released. When the spinal cord is severed at a high level, the brain's suppressing action is removed from the cord segments below the damage, and touch reflex erection and lubrication may occur freely in response to any touch stimulus. If the cord is severed in the sacral segments, the lower reflex center is damaged, and there is no reflex reaction to touch in the genitals. However, as the level of the damage is below the T_{11-12} segments, responses to mental stimuli may find their way through the autonomic nerve pathways leaving the cord at the T_{11-12} levels, and mental reflex erection may occur.

2. Neuromuscular tensions develop. In the able-bodied person the development and the release of this tension can be monitored through

such extragenital changes as elevation in pulse and respiratory rates, increase in the blood pressure, changes in body temperature, appearance of oral and nasal secretions, decrease in auditory and visual acuity, rhythmic musculoskeletal movements, and changes in the mental state of the individual, usually toward a decreased awareness of pain and discomfort. The vaginal changes are characterized by swelling of the outer third of the vagina and a "tenting" or "tubbing" of the inner third of this organ. In the internal portion of the male genitalia the measurable events consist of sperm transportation in the vas deferens, seminal fluid secretion, injection of this fluid into the prostate and the urethra, sequential closing and then opening of the internal and external sphincters of the urethra, and rhythmic contractions of the urethra and pelvic musculature, resulting in ejaculation.

Sexual response with complete lesions

When a spinal cord injury is complete at any level, the brain becomes isolated from signals arising in the genitalia. While erection and vaginal lubrication may still occur in response to either touch or mental stimuli, there can be no orgasmic response arising from or detected in the genitalia. Mental responses will still be processed, and extragenital circulatory and respiratory responses are quite possible. A reported side effect of the circulatory changes is headache, presumably caused by dilation of certain cerebral blood vessels.

The following examples illustrate patients' concerns about losses in genital sensations, ability to have predictable erections, ejaculations, vaginal lubrication, or orgasm. Use Table 7–1 and Figures 7–1 to 7–3, to explain the reasons for the patients' problems. (Some of the explanations are provided in italics.)

A 36-year-old man, married for eight years, suffered a complete injury to the C_{4-5} segments. While still in the intensive care unit, he asked the nurse for a mirror to see his penis while he was being catheterized. "How come I have an erection when I can't feel anything? Will that last?"

(Complete injury to the C_{4-5} cord levels stops incoming signals from the genitalia from reaching the brain. There will be no genital sensation or ejaculation and orgasm arising from genital stimulation. Brain control over erection has been released and touch will cause lasting erection.)

TABLE 7–1 ■ GUIDELINES TO EXPECTED SEXUAL DYSFUNCTIONS FOLLOWING COMPLETE LESION

	T_{10}–L_1 Segments or Above	L_2–S_1 Segments	S_2–S_4 Segments
Genital Sensations	Lost: communication between genitalia and the brain is interrupted	Lost: vague internal feelings possible; some visceral connections to brain still present	Lost: communication between genitalia and the brain interrupted
Erection (Touch)	Still possible: sacral segments intact; genital–sacral reflex connection intact. Called "somatic" or "touch" reflex erection	Possible: sacral reflex connection intact	Not possible: sacral segment destroyed and genital–sacral reflex lost
Erection (Mental)	Not possible: fibers coming to T_{10}–L_1 segments, bringing necessary signals are interrupted	May be possible: sympathetic pathways from brain open to bring necessary signals to T_{10}–L_1	May be possible: T_{10}–L_1 segments intact and still able to mediate signals from brain; called "mental" or "psychogenic" erection
Ejaculation/Orgasm	Not possible: necessary genital–brain–genital contact lost	Cannot occur: necessary genital–brain–genital contact lost. Seminal flow possible because sympathetic fibers coming to T_{10}–L_1 segments may bring necessary signals	Not possible: genital–brain–genital contact lost. In male, seminal flow may be possible because signals originating in brain and coming through sympathetic fibers to T_{10}–L_1 segments can reach genitalia. For reasons not understood these signals may diminish "mental" erection
Erotic Mental Feelings	May be experienced: pulse rate and blood pressure changes possible if mouth, neck, and other intact areas stimulated	May be experienced: pulse and blood pressure changes possible if intact areas of body stimulated	May be experienced: pulse rate and blood pressure changes possible if intact areas of body stimulated

A 28-year-old man, unmarried but living with a female partner, was injured in the sacral area. He was already walking with crutches and braces when he said: "I can't understand it. I get a bit of swelling in my penis when I am in bed with her. Then I get a sticky fluid coming out of my penis—just a few drops—and then all the swelling is gone. It kills me! I feel like . . . I feel worthless. What's the use? I'm not even half a man."

(The sacral area was damaged, and potential for touch reflex erection is gone. Mental stimuli may get through the T_{10}–L_1 segments, causing some erection. The same fibers also carry signals for seminal flow. For reasons not yet understood, when flow occurs erection usually diminishes.)

A 42-year-old married woman with a T_{12} complete cord injury said: "Orgasm was very important to me. Any chance for it now?"

(Not from genital stimulation. Whenever the cord is completely severed, genital signals cannot get to the brain to generate neuromuscular tensions. However, she may become highly responsive to face, neck, and breast stimulation.)

Sexual response with incomplete lesions

The effects of incomplete lesions on the sexual response depend on the damage to the specific pathways and cellular structures. For example, in central cord lesions, the sexual response might not be disturbed. If a partial lesion in-

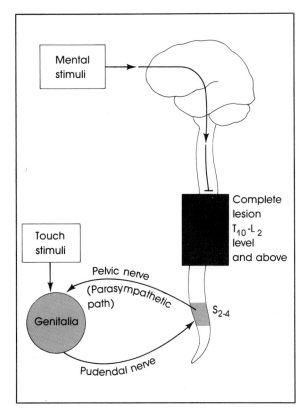

FIGURE 7–1 ■ Complete lesions at $T_{10}-L_2$ segments and above allow touch erection/lubrication. Ejaculation and orgasm in men and orgasm in women not possible from genital stimulation.

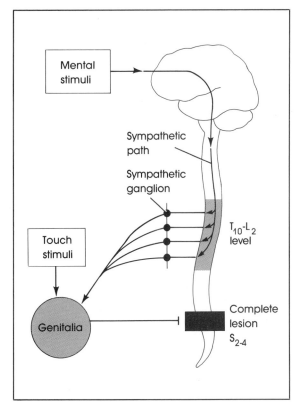

FIGURE 7–2 ■ Complete lesions at the S_2-S_4 cord segment and below allow "mental" erection and seminal flow in men. Orgasm not possible from genital stimulation.

volves the dorsolateral or ventrolateral sides of the cord, sensory or motor sparing may occur and some aspects of the response may be possible. If the lesion is a hemisection of the cord (Brown-Séquard's syndrome), some responses remain, but the eventual outcome is not predictable. (Incomplete lesions are detailed in Chapter 5.)

Diagnostic tests

There are two tests of value to determine if male or female orgasmic reactions might occur in response to genital stimulation.

1. The *pain* or *heat/ cold sensation test* is used to check out the sensory pathways between the genitalia and the brain. A pin is used to cause pain sensation in the genitalia, and hot/cold stimuli are used to find out if the patient can differentiate between various temperature levels in the genital region. These tests give information about the lateral spinothalamic tracts. The tracts are considered intact if a pinprick on the penis or on the women's genital area is immediately perceived as sharp and painful (Figure 7–4), or if hot and cold stimuli are immediately and correctly identified.

2. Another test requires the patient to *contract the anal opening on command.* This test provides information about the motor fibers going to the genitalia from the brain, along the fibers of the pyramidal tract systems. If the patient can correctly perceive pain, heat, or cold and is able to contract the anus voluntarily, the basic tracts are open for genital sensation and for male and female orgasmic reaction. If either one or if both these tests are negative, the patient will not be able to experience orgasm or ejaculation because somewhere along these nerve tracts an injury

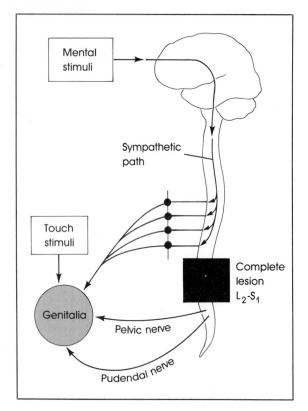

FIGURE 7–3 ■ Complete lesions at L_2–S_1 cord segments result in a dissociated reaction. Both touch and "mental" erections are possible in men, but these are not coordinated. Orgasm in men and women not possible from genital stimulation.

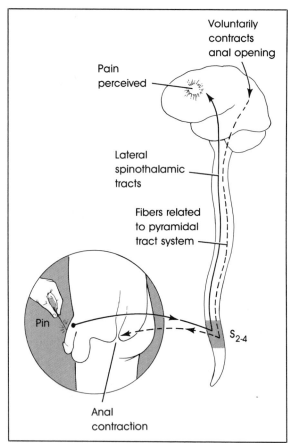

FIGURE 7–4 ■ Testing the lateral spinothalamic tract and descending fibers of the pyramidal tract system. If both are "open," genital sensation and orgasm are likely.

has occurred, blocking signals from reaching the brain. The male patient, however, may still be able to have reflex touch or mental erection, depending on the level at which the injury has occurred. Three reflexes are tested to clarify the situation:

• Squeezing the tip of the penis normally elicits the bulbocavernosus reflex. See Figure 7–5. This indicates that the sacral segments of the spinal cord are open, and reflex "touch" erection is likely to occur.

  The significance of the bulbocavernosus for women is still not understood. The bulbocavernosus reflex can be tested in women by pressing the clitoris to elicit anal contraction.

• The examiner's finger is placed in the patient's anus to test for the anal tone reflex. See Figure 7–6. Contraction of the internal muscles over the examiner's finger indicates that this reflex is intact, which confirms that both the sacral and the lumbar segments of the cord are intact. When both the bulbocavernosus and the anal tone reflexes are present, the reflex touch erection is usually strong, because the level of the injury is higher up in the cord.

  Although the anal tone is tested in the same manner for women as for men, the significance of this reflex is not understood either.

• To find out if the injury is below or above the T_9 level, the examiner squeezes the testicles to elicit pain. See Figure 7–7. The sensory fibers of the testicle enter the spinal cord at the T_9 level. If the patient cannot feel any sensation when the testicles are squeezed, the lesion is above the T_9 level, and there is no possibility

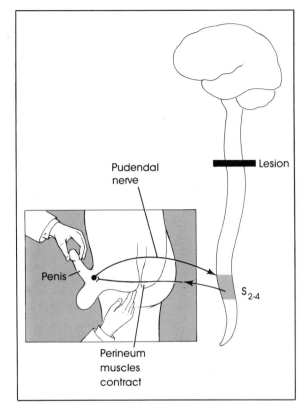

FIGURE 7–5 ■ Testing the bulbocavernosus reflex in men. If present, sacral segment is open. Lesion must be above sacral segments. In men touch erection is likely.

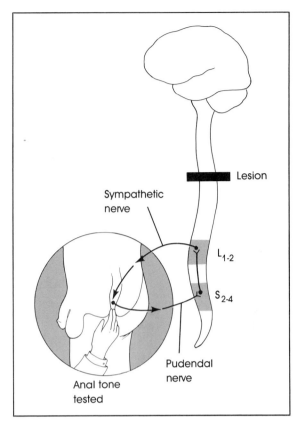

FIGURE 7–6 ■ Testing the anal tone. If present, sacral and low thoracic and high lumbar segments are open. Lesion must be above L_1. In men touch erection is likely to be strong.

for "mental" erections, because the fibers necessary for this type of erection emerge at around T_{11-12}. However, if the patient experiences acute testicular discomfort, the lesion is likely to be below T_{10-12}, and the chances are strong that "mental" erection may occur.

On rare occasions a spinal cord injury occurs at the neurological $L_2–S_1$ level, so that the bulbocavernosus, anal tone, and testicular pain can be elicited, but there is no perception of pain in the genitalia, no anal tone, and no voluntary ability to contract the anus. In such a situation both mental and touch reflex erection may be expected, although of poor quality. Orgasm and ejaculation will still not be possible.

Dysfunctions related to time after injury

When the reflexes begin to return after the initial period of spinal shock, some of the sexual responses may be exaggerated. For example, in

a person with a complete high lesion, strong and lasting erections may occur in response to even the gentlest genital irritation. This response may last for days and must be differentiated from priapism, which is an erection due to clotting of the blood in the penis. If the erect penis becomes even more erect with touch or if erection subsides when touch is removed, the condition is not likely to be priapism.

Erection in response to mental stimulation may not appear for several months after the injury. It is not known why this time delay occurs.

Other factors influencing the sexual response

An interesting feature of erections related to mental stimulation is that they may be accompanied by a flow of prostatic fluid. Often when this secretion appears, the erection weakens.

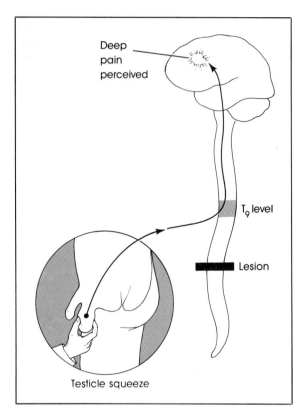

FIGURE 7–7 ■ Testing for testicle-squeeze-induced pain. If present, lesion must be below T$_9$. Possible mental erection in men, sometimes with flow of seminal fluid.

The mental stimulation may be something seen, heard, imagined, or dreamed. Touching on the chest, neck, ears, or throat may also provide mental stimulation. Some women report orgasmic experiences during dreams or when strongly concentrating on erotic fantasy. Spinal cord injured men do not seem to have this facility. Erections resulting from mental stimulation may be subject to interference by concerns over ability to perform sexually, by preoccupations with other worries, by depression and anger, and by centrally acting sedatives or tranquilizers, including alcohol.

The somatic or touch reflex erection may be negatively influenced by some antispasmodic medication. Both somatic and mental reflex erections may be lost by an external sphincterotomy. Although no clear risk figures are available, reports suggest that less than 20% of the patients having the operation suffer this side effect.

Sexual Practices

Three categories of the sexual functioning status will be reviewed under this heading: sexual interest, sexual activities, and sexual behavior.

Interest

Sexual interest and disinterest are poorly understood even in the able-bodied person. *Interest* is often a combination of desire to experience certain sensations arising from caressing or genital play, the wish to be sexually useful to a partner, and the hope that one will be a desirable partner. Without regard to the extent of the injury, motivation to engage in various sex acts may be related to the need for intimacy, feelings of belonging, and pleasure; mutual search for orgasmic experiences; expression of love, affection, and passion; or a need for relief from anxiety and boredom.

A 24-year-old married woman suffered T$_{12}$–L$_1$ complete injury. One year after the injury she said: "You know, I'm really horny, and it's in my head. I never thought how much sex has to do with your head, but sitting in this wheelchair is like being isolated. I used to get a kick out of chasing my husband when he came out of the bathroom. Now I have to close my eyes and think back to the good old days."

Sexual *disinterest* can be caused by chronic pain, discomfort, malaise, and tiredness related to the complications of spinal cord injury. Sedatives, antispasmodic medications, and psychotherapeutic drugs may temporarily depress interest level; and drab living quarters or the physical environment of hospitals or institutional settings may also "turn off" sexual interest.

Four weeks after his injury a 32-year-old unmarried man with an incomplete injury at the C$_{6-7}$ level said, "You know, sex just hasn't been on my mind at all. I'm not surprised, mind you . . . too much else on my mind. Also I haven't slept well for days. It worries one a bit. I used to be pretty active."

Still other negative factors include preoccupation and worry about finances, the job situation, and housing; relationship discord; depression and feelings of hopelessness; and sexual dysfunctions that either existed before the injury or were caused by the neurological damage.

On some occasions the partner's disinterest is more significant than the patient's loss of zest.

A 57-year-old married man, injured at the C_{5-6} level at age 45 and now a complete quadriplegic, said: "Yes, I do get the occasional desire, but my wife just shut down. She says it doesn't bother her—why can't I just forget it too?"

Sex activities may become a chore or a duty, or may turn into oppressing, distressful events.

One woman partner explained it this way: Before his injury he used to grab me while I was in the kitchen. I said "No! Don't do it!" But he knew I wanted it, so he carried on, and finally we just rushed into the bedroom. Now, I wheel him into the bedroom, help him transfer, take his pants off, and wash his penis after I take the condom catheter off. Then I get undressed, sit on top of him, and move till I get bored. I haven't had a climax since he was injured. Yes, I kind of want it, but this is just not my way!

Sexual activities and behavior

Sex acts may be classified as solitary (masturbation) and partner-related acts. The latter might be subdivided into caressing, kissing, genital fondling, oral sex activities, and vaginal and anal intercourse. Most of these activities may be carried out in a heterosexual or homosexual relationship. Homosexually oriented people with spinal cord injuries may be concerned about rejection by "straight" staff members, in addition to their concerns over other aspects of their disability.

Sexual behavior represents courting activities. The focus is on establishing or maintaining a relationship that includes sex activities. The behavior may vary in different cultures and within the cultural context individuals have their own customs. Presenting oneself as a desirable partner may require the ability to dance or drive a car; facility with words; or deeds, such as dressing, walking, and eating in socially approved ways. Strong social norms dictate what is right and wrong. Many people with spinal cord injuries feel that they cannot compete with others under the existing rules; some feel totally unattractive and a burden on a partner.

Able-bodied people enjoying the company of friends with spinal cord injuries may be concerned about points of etiquette. This concern is caused by a feeling of responsibility for the welfare of the person with a spinal cord injury. Again the injured person is perceived as "ill." People who are ill need looking after! Indeed, it is not unusual for an able-bodied partner to approach a nurse and ask for information. "What is it like for a spinal injured person? How do they go to the bathroom? Do they need constant supervision? Is there sex for them?"

The sex partners of persons with spinal cord injury may also be concerned about fulfillment of their own needs:

A 24-year-old woman partner of a 22-year-old man with a complete lesion at C_4 said, "What I really miss is his caresses. Sure I can sit on top of him, but his arms and hands are . . . just useless."

A spinal cord injury causes several types of problems.

1. Technical problems caused by the weakness or loss of function of arms, hands, and legs. Undressing, assuming desirable positions, holding, touching, stimulation with hands, and moving in rhythm with the partner may not be possible.

A 42-year-old woman suffered a partial injury to the T_{4-5} level of her spinal cord. She had only vague sensations in response to hot/cold testing of her genitalia, and she was unable to contract her anal opening on demand. This indicated that it would be unlikely for her to experience orgasm from genital stimulation. This news did not concern her: What worried her most was the weakness in her legs. "I used to hold my lover close to me with my legs around his body. And I used to move. Now I am like a sack of potatoes. I won't be any use to him in sex."

2. Concerns over the appropriateness of acts other than intercourse. To many people the norm is having the erect penis inside the vagina. Manual or oral stimulation is often thought of as a "preliminary act" that leads to the "real thing." To some people anything other than intercourse is "perverse." Among able-bodied people, this focus on intercourse, rather than on enjoyment, is a major cause of erection dysfunction and loss of interest. Among people with spinal cord injuries, this belief may inhibit any experimentation with sex acts other than intercourse.

A 46-year-old man with complete lesion in the sacral area complained: "We've been married for 24 years. The wife never wanted anything but intercourse. I told her I don't have erections. Why can't I rub you with the fingers? But she says that's not normal; she doesn't want to learn anything new like that; and besides, if I can't come, she doesn't want it either."

3. Worries about the possibility of being victimized.

A 20-year-old man suffered a C_{6-7} complete injury. He revealed that in the past he had homosexual as well as heterosexual experiences. "My friends were sitting around the bed, and we talked about my strong erections. Michael said, You're lucky! You can get it from front and back and you wouldn't even know it! I don't like this idea of being used."

Others feel that they are already victims for rape. There are indeed reports of rape committed against women with spinal cord injuries, but there are also stories about quadriplegic men, whose reflex erections were capitalized on without consent by women.

4. Concerns about the genitalia and about bowel and bladder accidents. Both men and women tend to worry about offensive genital odors. Urinary cleanliness and menstrual hygiene care is discussed in Chapters 12 and 15. A recurrent concern among men is that their penis may have become smaller. They notice that when applying the condom drainage device, the shaft of the penis appears to be shorter than before. The reason for this is not clear. Perhaps the weakness of the pelvic floor is responsible for this change. In any case, when pressure is applied to the perineum, the penis becomes longer again.

Bladder and bowel accidents may occur more commonly when sex acts occur spontaneously. If there is time for planning, most people restrict their fluid intake and empty their bladder. Bowel accidents are more difficult to avoid, particularly if the routine calls for bowel care only every second or third day. Women may have more problems with this than men, presumably because the penis inside the vagina activates bowel reflexes. There will be further comments about these problems in the "management" section of this chapter.

While this list has portrayed problems, patients also report new possibilities.

A 29-year-old married man, who had suffered a complete lesion at C_{6-7} level six months before, said, "It was quite surprising! She never could come with me inside. I used my fingers. Now I can't move my hands so we said what the hell, there is that erect penis. So she sat on me and wow! She went over with a bang! It's better for her than before. I get a charge out of it too."

Fertility and Contraception

Many people with spinal cord injuries have urgent concerns about fertility and contraception. "If I can't be a father what else could we do?" "Is there some way to get sperms out of me?" "Can a person with a spinal injury adopt a child?" "My boyfriend is quadriplegic. Should we use a contraceptive?" "I used to be on the pill before my injury. Is this still all right to use?" "Will I fit in my wheelchair if I get pregnant?" "How can the baby come out of me if I cannot push?"

An early concern of women is a missed period. Clinical experience suggests that in many instances menstrual periods are delayed until two to four months after the injuries. Thereafter the periods resume a predictable regularity. Regular menstrual periods are presumptive evidence of female fertility potential.

Women in their childbearing years are able to get pregnant in spite of their injury, although it is not known whether they are as fertile as able-bodied women of comparable age. The fertility of men with spinal injuries is very much subject to dysfunctions. However, even a small volume of seminal fluid, a very low sperm count, and the presence of nonmotile or deformed spermatozoa show some capability for fertilization. Lack of erection ability or inability to experience penile sensations or orgasm is not a reliable indicator of infertility. Physical examination and search for sperms (if there is any mucus flow) must be done before any conclusion can be made about a man's fertility.

If infertility is proven in the man, adoption procedures or artificial insemination by donor are the currently available family planning methods. Internal and external electrical stimulation, the use of vibrators on the penis and of injections of prostigmine into the spinal fluid have been tried but have not yet proven to be reliable methods to stimulate ejaculation or seminal flow.

If a couple's fertility is established, the question is who is going to assume responsibility for birth control. Experience has shown that in a stable couple relationship the person who is most motivated and most able physically should be in charge of the birth control procedures. However, if the person is single or has casual relationships, it is important not to make assumptions about the partner's birth control measures. In such situations it is best for the disabled person to assume the responsibility for protection.

Methods of birth control can be viewed as "you-do-it" or "done-to-you" procedures. The you-do-it methods necessitate some motor and intellectual performance from the person. When these are lacking, the done-to-you methods are useful. Condoms and withdrawal are the you-do-it methods used by men. Both methods require a certain level of motor coordination for correct application. The you-do-it methods used by women include barrier creams and foams, the diaphragm, oral contraceptives, and rhythm methods. Appropriate insertion of anything into the vagina requires specific physical abilities. Few people think that oral contraceptives have complex requirements. Yet appropriate use of oral contraceptives includes a series of motor acts that may be beyond the abilities of some quadriplegic women. The done-to-you methods available to women include intrauterine devices, tubal ligation, hysterectomy, abortion, and depot hormone injection. Vasectomy is the only done-to-you method currently available to men.

Virtually every birth control method is reputed to have some hazards. Some of these side effects are accentuated in the spinal injured because of the nature of the disability. For example, the thromboembolic hazard in the use of oral contraceptives containing estrogen may make this method inappropriate for a woman with a spinal cord injury who spends a large part of the day in a wheelchair. Progesterone-based oral contraceptives may cause weight gain and contribute to depression. Intrauterine devices may be inadvisable when a woman cannot feel discomfort indicating possible uterine perforation or pelvic inflammatory disease, or when increased menstrual flow would be difficult to cope with. Tubal ligation has few if any contraindications specific to physically disabled people. Hysterectomy has the added attraction of reduc-

ing the hygienic problems associated with menstrual flow. Postcoital contraceptive medication and even abortion might be considered for a person who has been sexually assaulted.

APPROACHES TO MANAGEMENT

The principles of one to one management may be stated with some degree of rationality, when a person or couple complains of a sexual dysfunction, disinterest, fertility problem, or other sex-related difficulty. However, institutional approaches to management of these problems are still fairly haphazard.

One-to-One Management

Treatment approaches can be visualized as psychological (talk- and guidance-oriented), medical (involving medications), physical (using external devices, appliances), and surgical (using internal devices). A combination of these approaches may be employed from time to time and the contact with the therapist may be short term, long term, regular or sporadic, open ended or time limited. Some of the treatment approaches may require involvement of the partner and sometimes a group format is used.

Psychological approach: sex therapy

The goals of the psychological approach are to dispel myth, increase freedom of choice, and support the patient's right to feelings and to the expression of feelings. The methods may include *education* to increase biological and self-knowledge; *reassurance* about adequacy; *diminishing* of *hesitation* toward alternative sex activities; and *increasing acceptance* of viewing and touching one's own and the partner's body. These basic methods are often combined into more specific therapy formats. *Marital* and *communication therapies* are used to attend to interpersonal disagreements and to promote direct and intimate discussions between partners; *sex therapy* is applied to treat specific sex dysfunctions.

Sex therapy differs from other psychological treatment methods in two respects:

1. Its goals are essentially limited to the relief of the patient's sexual symptoms.
2. Its methods include prescribed sexual experiences.

These goals shift the couple's attention from intercourse and orgasm to giving and receiving pleasure. The couple learns that apprehensions about any sex act may cause erection, ejaculation, and orgasmic difficulties and may lead to sexual disinterest. An expectation of the therapy outcome is that as various nonintercourse sex acts are gradually accepted by the couple as pleasure-producing, those acts will be approached with less apprehension.

Sex therapy requires a degree of concentration on the sex problem and an exclusion of other problems for a limited period of time. For this reason, it is not often suitable to the life situation of people with acute or recent spinal cord injuries. However, the components of the therapy, namely, education, reassurance, and sexual skills practice, can be used in various combinations and to appropriate levels of intensity just about any time after the injury. The prescribed sexual experiences represent the unique feature of this sexual care approach.

Using this approach in the case of the 46-year-old man with a complete lesion in the sacral area who complained that his wife didn't "want to learn anything new" (see 6 on pp. 127–128), the patient and the partner would be educated about various pleasure-yielding physical activities. They would also be helped to become more comfortable with words expressing their sexual feelings and needs. All of this would help them acquire a wider appreciation of the range of "normal" in sex practices. The wife would become more comfortable with viewing and touching his genitalia and would experience less disappointment with his lack of erection. She would gain more courage to guide her partner with language such as, "I like this. Now a little more pressure. Continue. Now higher," rather than, "That's no good. I don't know what I want. Try something else." The husband would worry less about intercourse being the one and only real sex act. Once relaxed, he might experience erec-

tion from mental stimuli and gain pleasure from stimulation of his breasts, face, neck, or lips.

Obviously, some people are more suitable for this type of an approach than others. To assess suitability, the patient's main complaints have to be clarified first. For example, in the case considered here it would be important to establish whether the main problems are really lack of erection and worries over the wife's refusal to participate in sex acts other than intercourse. Other problems could be the man's disinterest in sex activities or his hidden fear of failure in an intercourse situation; his lack of genital sensation; or his worry over dribbling while being caressed. His wife may have lost sexual interest before the accident; she may or may not have been regularly orgasmic even with the penis inside her; and she may not now enjoy (or may never have enjoyed) the manner in which he stimulates her. On top of all this, hand or oral stimulation may be against her principles. The clarification of the man's problems involves a painstaking review of these possibilities. The therapist's approach is to ask questions in a nonthreatening way. For example, in trying to find out if the wife has been orgasmic before her husband's accident, the therapist might proceed as follows:

THERAPIST: Now I have to ask you a question about orgasms. Would this be all right with you? (This is asking for permission.)

WIFE: Okay.

THERAPIST: Well, I wonder if you have read that many women don't normally experience orgasms? (This is preparation for acceptance in case she does not have orgasms.)

WIFE: Yes.

THERAPIST: I wonder what your own experiences were? (This is an open question, inviting more than a yes or no answer.)

WIFE: Well, I had orgasms but always with intercourse. I don't know why. Maybe my mother told me never to touch myself.

The second step in the assessment is to review the couple's preinjury sexual interest level and sexual practices, including frequency, timing, location, and situations producing "turn on" or "turn off" of interest. Then postinjury sexual practices must be recounted and compared with preinjury experiences.

These two steps yield a rich store of data on the sexual functioning status of this couple, their sexual losses, the meaning of their loss, their beliefs about the right or wrong in various sex acts, their flexibility in this area, their interest in each other, and their willingness to evolve new activities. These are the resources or burdens that they bring to the therapy.

The third step would be a physical examination of the man. This would define the physiological limitations of his erection, ejaculation, and orgasmic process. Of particular interest in this specific case example would be the testicle squeeze test (see Figure 7–7). If he felt acute deep pain in response to the squeeze, the chances for erections produced by mental stimulation would be very good. The physical exam would also review his ability to hold and caress his wife and move in bed and his urinary equipment requirements. The wife would be encouraged to participate in this examination to learn about his remaining potential.

In the fourth step of the assessment, the couple's sexual goals would be explored. A list would have to be developed of their desired acts, the desired frequency of these acts, and safeguards for privacy, birth control, and so on.

The fifth step would be a search for conditions that might contraindicate the use of the psychological sex therapy method. Contraindications include untreated depression, heavy use of tranquilizing medication, obvious evidence of marital strife, and lack of time to engage in the proposed program.

The sixth step would be a review of the other treatment approaches, in case they are applicable in the management of this couple's sexual difficulties in addition to, or instead of, the psychological methods.

Medical approach

The goals of the *medical approach* are limited, because there are no known medications that directly increase sexual interest or restore erection, ejaculation, or orgasmic experiences. Medications used to reduce anxiety, relax spasms, or provide rest or painfree periods may help indirectly, presumably because the patient may feel more zestful. There are many medications, however, that, at certain dosage levels, interfere with interest and function. Drugs that may decrease interest and impair the sexual response include sedatives, analgesics, anticholinergic and antiadrenergic drugs, muscle relaxants, estrogens, and the major tranquilizers.

The medical approach is used for two purposes:

1. To ensure a healthy and painfree existence in the face of a crippling condition
2. To limit the patient to medications that are least likely to interfere with the physiological process of sexual functioning

The therapist must remember the sexual side effects of illness and of the medications used to treat the patient; must inquire systematically about changes in interest, erection, lubrication, and the orgasmic and ejaculation process; and may have to recommend alternate medications if untoward changes do occur.

Physical approach

The goal of the *physical* approach is to give technical assistance to patient and partner in the physical aspects of sex activities. On a general level, promotion of independent movement, dressing and undressing, cleanliness, and secure bowel and bladder management are part of this approach. Occupational and physical therapists may wish to conceptualize a "bedroom scene" and apply principles of the *activities of daily living* training toward the requirements of sexual interaction. On a more specific level, the patient may need technical advice about positions in bed or the use of, for example, a water bed or extra pillows under the hips. Unfortunately, no specific information is available about the relative value of these, but using common sense, and working with the couple, one can identify solutions to problems that may baffle the patient. For example, patients with high cord injuries may not be able to lift their arms to embrace their partner when lying down but might be able to offer a hug when sitting up. Just to call the patient's attention to such a maneuver introduces a whole new set of possibilities for sexual play.

The use of external prosthetic devices to promote erection or replace the penis with a rubber model has not been studied. Common sense must rule: If it is of value to a couple, then it has a place in the management of the sexual problem. Sometimes a rubber band is used at the base of the penis to hold the blood in the penis and prolong an erection. This procedure has little value, and there are some dangers involved, for example, bruising the skin or the spongy tissues of the penis, and possibly causing thrombosis in the damaged blood vessels.

Management of catheters during the act of intercourse is worked out by patients. Women report no technical problems when they tape the catheter to the skin of the lower abdomen or the inguinal region. Men may wish to disconnect their catheter, fold it back over the penis and apply a condom to cover both. Urine on the external female genitalia or in the vagina does not cause significant problems, however.

Surgical approach

The *surgical approach* to the management of sexual problems is limited to insertion of an internal penile prosthesis. This device makes possible a reliable erection of the penis. While long-term outcome studies are not yet available, current experiences suggest that the inflatable prosthesis is more applicable to the needs of people with spinal cord injured than rigid devices. The major concern with both is that pressure sores may develop in the shaft or in the perineum.

A secondary benefit of the inflatable prosthesis is that it makes it easier to use the condom for urinary drainage. The prosthesis does not promote ejaculation and it does not restore sensation to the penis. It seems to be of greatest value to patients with incomplete injuries, many of whom have unreliable and incomplete reflex erections.

Choosing the right approach(es)

In considering the sexual problems of the couple discussed, it appears that the medical and physical approaches may be valuable additions to the psychological approach. However, serious consideration may have to be given to the use of the surgical approach, because that is the only one that might provide the patient with an erection. This, of course, would not help him with orgasm. Now the assessment would have to include the wife's reaction to all this. His comment, "If I can't come, she doesn't want it either," may be a warning of more problems in the future!

Institutional Approaches to Management

Over the last 40 years there have been three administrative approaches to the sexual concerns of patients and partners.

1. To *deny* or repress sexual expressions. The philosophy behind this approach is partly that sex is an inappropriate area for professional exploration; that the patient's whole attention should be focused on return to work; and that it may be a further strain on the patient to learn about the sexual disabilities on top of other problems.

2. To *tolerate* expressions of sexual needs and even to offer some answers or suggestions when this appears to be appropriate or when one or two interested nurses or other health professionals are willing to get involved. This approach is usually haphazard and often undertaken with only token support from the medical staff. It is characterized by a well-meaning surge of interest in the plight of *some* patients; exclusion from consideration of the needs of the *young* and the *old;* dependence on a few interested staff members; and a "wait-and-see" attitude in most of the nursing staff and the medical staff. If an untoward incident occurs, such as a phone call from a wife who is upset that "someone talked sex with my husband," the staff member involved may be reprimanded and memos ("I don't wish to have my patient exposed to sexual counseling" or "there will be no sexual discussion in the intensive care unit") may fly!

3. To *organize a program* of sexual rehabilitation.

The organized approach

An organized program has to have clearly defined goals that are acceptable to the staff members. There must also be a clearly stated outline of the nature of the specific services required, the type of personnel who will be responsible for offering various aspects of this patient–partner care service, and their relationship to the other team members. The relationship has to be spelled out in terms of the referral methods and the role of staff members "before the specialist arrives," the methods of reporting back to staff members, and the inclusion of reports in the agenda of team meetings. A protocol must be drawn up to introduce the service to the patient and the family and to communicate with the staff of the next institution assuming the care of the patient. The plan must provide ongoing staff education and introductory education for new staff members; coordination with other programs; means of supervision, consultations, backup services, and in-service training programs; materials, supplies, and physical space for various required procedures. In addition there may be a need for a protocol to manage conflicting areas for the staff. For example, the staff may have to agree whether this type of service is appropriate for children, or whether to provide a private room for undisturbed experimentation by a couple.

A model of the organized approach

There are few models of the organized approach, but one example is the Sexual Health Care Service in the Acute Spinal Cord Injury Unit of Shaughnessy Hospital, Vancouver, B.C. The service is offered by two sexual health care clinicians (whose background is in one of the health care professions) who work with a physician specializing in sexual medicine. The service includes staff education and research in addition to patient, partner, and family care.

The care services consist of assessment, education, and sexual skill training. These services are extended to the patient's present or intended sexual partner and the patient's family (parents of adolescents, for example). The services can be followed through various steps:

1. *Soon after admission.* The patient's primary care nurse takes a nursing history, and in the course of obtaining data from the patient, inquires about any concerns the patient may have about sexual functioning. The nurse offers reas-

surance that such concerns are common and tells the patient that there is a specialized care service on the ward and that the sexual health clinician will introduce herself later. The existence of the service is brought to the attention of the partner and family as well. This first step legitimizes the early ventilation of sex-related concerns and establishes sexual rehabilitation as a routine part of the unit's medical program.

2. *Introductory visits.* The sexual health clinician visits the patient frequently. During the first few brief meetings with the patient and members of the family, the clinician tries to elicit any sex-related concerns to help the patient organize these concerns; to obtain preliminary evidence of physical dysfunctions; and to outline the future steps in the rehabilitation process. The physical examination, the brief diagnostic procedures, the clear questions, and the direct approach all tend to legitimize the patient's inquiries and give an air of openness and competence to the program.

3. *Assessment.* By the second month, most of the patients are over the acute phase of their injury and are usually ready for a major assessment of their sexual potential.

If a partner is available, first a private assessment is made of the partner's past experiences, present sexual tensions, and methods of resolution. The partner is then invited to participate in the patient's assessment, which includes a physical examination.

This assessment deals with each of the six categories of the patient's sexual functioning status (see the section Sexual Consequences of Spinal Cord Injury). Specific alternatives are then explored and on occasions demonstrated. For example, the partner may want to see how to bring on a reflex erection, or both may want to know what position in intercourse may be most feasible. Some patients may want to know about sexual aids.

A private room is made available to the couple for their unobserved use at their convenience. A record of the assessment is summarized under the various headings of the sexual functioning status list. After review with the patient and partner, the summary is placed in the chart. No final diagnosis is made because the patient's physical and social circumstances may change in the future. Follow-up, therefore, becomes very important.

4. *Follow-up visits.* Follow-up visits are carried out to correct areas of confusion and mis-information, to monitor changes in the patient's sexual functioning pattern and marital and social relationships, and to encourage experimentation with alternative sex activities. The follow-up includes preparation for discharge and periodic progress visits thereafter.

Some patients do not wish to have follow-up visits. Other patients wish to delay experimentation and begin their probings in their home environment. Patients who have no partners may be encouraged to experiment by themselves.

Outcome evaluations of this program are inadequate. In this service the objective of the patient care services is to provide treatment on the basis of assessment. This requires a highly individual approach to each patient and a range of goals that can be very broad, from reassurance and relief gained through accurate information, to a reorientation of the patient's perspectives about the acceptable range of sexual expression.

Immediate and retrospective reviews indicate that in nearly all instances the clinician's interaction with patients and partners leads to a clear definition of the patient's functioning in sex response, sexual activity capabilities, interest level, fertility status, and urinary-bowel hygiene relevant to sex activities. About two-thirds of the patients and partners are able to refocus their sexual expectations on goals consistent with their physical disabilities. This process may take several months or several years. It is not yet possible to assess the relative significance of a number of factors, such as the clinician's input, the behavior of the existing partner (or the appearance of a new partner), the success of vocational reorientation, or the financial status of the family.

One important observation is that the nature and severity of the injury is not the important determinant of the outcome of the sexual rehabilitation. Two factors that seem to help the patient refocus and work toward realistic sex-related goals are (1) active, varied, and satisfying sex relationships before the injury and (2) an interested and adventurous partner. If these factors are missing, or if one or both partners are consumed by anger related to the catastrophic injury, it is more difficult for the clinician to help the couple to achieve significant goals in the short-term treatment.

The following illustrates the complexities of the sexual rehabilitation process and the involvement of a partner:

■ *PERSONAL VIEWPOINT*

At the age of 35, Gus sustained a spinal injury at T_9, resulting in complete paraplegia at that level. His wife, Kate, was 33 years old and their two children were 10 and 7 years old at the time of the injury.

Gus was referred to the sexual health care clinician when he expressed concern that his wife might leave him. The clinician described the service and reassured him that many men worry about their marriages. Gus said he feared that he could not get an erection and that his wife might become sexually frustrated.

Kate admitted that she had many anxieties, including sexual tension. She was embarrassed talking about sex but said that their sexual life had been very important to her.

(Personal Viewpoint continues)

In subsequent visits during the next two weeks, Gus revealed that he and his wife had, in their 12-year-marriage, explored a variety of sexual activities including mutual oral and manual genital stimulation and intercourse in various positions. Physical touch was important to him even though he did not feel it. The findings also indicated that "touch" erections would be possible, but "mental" erections, ejaculation, and orgasm would likely be lost.

With Gus's permission, the clinician interpreted these physical findings to Kate in a separate interview. Kate said she enjoyed and needed physical touching and caressing, but preferred orgasms through intercourse. She admitted that she would like to initiate sexual play, but felt shy and therefore did not. Although their sexual play was varied, she said it was not usual for them to talk to each other about their feelings and desires.

The clinician emphasized to both partners that the initial test results were not final and that the genital assessment would be repeated. It was suggested that they might wish to begin to explore various body sensations that might offer sensual feelings and to monitor changing feelings and responses to genital touching. A private room was made available to them for this intimate experimentation and testing of their remaining sexual abilities.

Two months after admission, Kate said she had touched her husband's penis on one occasion when they were cuddling together. Knowing how an erection would come was comforting to both, and they were interested in attempting intercourse.

Another physical examination at this time, with Kate present, showed no changes in Gus's genital functioning. The exam-

ination also showed that Gus could trigger his bladder to empty, remove his condom, and clean his penis without assistance. Examination of his mobility for sexual activity showed that he could undress and transfer himself to bed, but he needed assistance with his shoes and socks. He could assume a supine or side-lying position and could easily move his arms and body to caress and stimulate his wife. A major problem area was their difficulty in talking openly about their sexual desires. Following another interview together, Kate was able to tell Gus that she would like to initiate some sexual play. He was pleased.

Before his first weekend pass home, Kate and Gus said they hoped to have intercourse. He was worried, however, that she would not be satisfied sexually, because he couldn't move his pelvis and be as physically active in intercourse as he had been in the past. Kate was worried that she might hurt his back if she sat on top of him, and both were uncertain about how they would sleep together for the first time.

After consulting with the orthopedic surgeon, the clinician was able to reassure them that Gus's back was stable and that Kate would cause him no harm. After the weekend, they said that although the experience was different for both, Kate was able to come to orgasm. Gus was pleased that he could satisfy her in this way, and he himself felt physically relaxed after their sexual play.

Soon after, Gus was transferred to the long-term rehabilitation center. The clinician maintained contact with the couple to help them continue reestablishing their sexual relationship in the transition from hospital to home.

PRACTICE METHODS FOR NONSPECIALIST NURSES

Although a sexual rehabilitation program may have to be provided as a specialty service, it cannot function without the interested and knowledgeable support of other staff members. Patients do approach nurses, therapists, psychologists, social workers, brace makers, and even housekeepers with their sex-related concerns. If there is a specialist backup, both patients and team members might feel more at ease discussing sex issues. One nurse said, "The conversation could always be closed by me telling the patient, 'Why don't you go see the sex counselor?' or 'I don't know the answer to this, but I'll ask the sex specialist.'" But even without a specialist around, patients want to explore their sexual situation. The nonspecialist nurse might consider three basic approaches to patient inquiries: detection of concerns; clarification of the complaints, questions, or concerns; and information giving.

Detection of Concerns

A patient's sexual concerns may surface

- Directly in the form of well-formulated questions or statements
- Indirectly through various sex-related comments, innuendos, or behaviors; through non-compliance with the rehabilitation program; or through behaviors that interfere with the nurse's work
- In response to questions in nursing histories or other forms of inquiry by the nurse

The purpose of case finding is to legitimize the patient's sex-related inquiries. It is a way to say that "sex is spoken here," however haltingly. The nurse can explain her limited qualifications for sexual counseling, assist the patient by clarifying the concern, offer information, or help the patient to find out about better sources of information.

Direct inquiries

Mrs. Smith, the 52-year-old woman (discussed at the opening of this chapter), married for 28 years and the mother of three sons suffered an incomplete injury to the C_{6-7} segments of her spinal cord. Two months after her injury she turned to the nurse: "I think I want to talk to somebody about my sex life."

This is direct sexual inquiry. This plea for help gives the nurse an opportunity to acknowledge the appropriateness of this question, to state her own limitations in this area, and to invite further revelations from the patient on a low anxiety level.

NURSE: Oh, I'm glad! You're feeling comfortable enough to talk about sex (*acknowledgment*). I guess you know that I don't have special training in sexual counseling, but I would be glad to listen. Would I do? (*This indicates limitation and invites further information.*)

PATIENT: I'd like that, if you would listen.

NURSE: I might have to ask you a few questions too. (*This is asking for permission to explore when appropriate.*)

PATIENT: I could talk to you.

NURSE: Should we arrange a time then? Like around 2 o'clock, just after your treatment? (*This gives an official seal of approval to the discussion, lowering the anxiety level.*)

Others might approach the nurse with clear-cut questions: "I don't feel my penis. Does this mean that I can't have sex anymore?" or "How long will my reflex erection last?" or "Which position would we use while my brace is on?" or "Could you tell me about artificial insemination?" Again, the response to these inquiries should contain an acceptance of the question and a statement of the nurse's limitations in this area. Then it's up to the patient to continue the conversation. If the nurse is unable to answer the patient's inquiry, a statement like this would be appropriate: "This is a very important question. I just don't know the answers. Would it be all right with you if I check out who could help you with this?" If the question is within the nurse's sphere of knowledge, the nurse may begin to clarify the patient's worries and offer appropriate information. These methods will be discussed later.

Indirect expressions

Examples of indirect expressions of sexual concerns include repetitive references to one's past sexual prowess; repeated compliments about the nurses desirable physical attributes; jokes with sexual connotations; hypothetical questions like, "If you were my wife, would you want to go to bed with me?"; or statements like, "Maybe my husband should find another woman. I will be useless to him," or "I think I'll be a bachelor forever." Patients may make sexual propositions to the nurse or may expose their body, ask for genital care more often than required, hold onto the nurse when it's not appropriate, or attempt to caress the nurse's face or body.

PATIENT: (for the third time in half an hour) Say, you still did not answer me. Would you come to bed with me?

NURSE: Jim, I am not upset with what you are saying, but I want you to know that I don't want to go to bed with you. Is this clear? (This rejects the patient's behavior but not the patient.)

PATIENT: Clear, Shmeer. How am I supposed to know what I can do?

NURSE: You're worried? (This open question invites more information.)

PATIENT: Worried?!

NURSE: Well, you know, some of the other men are worried that they can't get an erection, or that they can't meet women, and so on. What would concern you most? (This is clarification mixed with reassurance that patient's worry is not unique.)

Without making too much fuss, the nurse defused a bothersome situation and gave an opportunity to the patient to express his sexual concern directly. The nurse was now able to respond to the patient's concern and at the same time proceed with other tasks without having to dodge inappropriate requests.

Sometimes what the patient does or says is not an indirect expression of sexual concerns or desires, but behavior representing indirect complaints about the treatment program, or concerns over not making good progress in recovery. The nurse's task here is to find out what these expressions really mean. For this reason, other members of the team should know about the nurse's experiences with the patient. Often other nurses will report similar experiences; by comparing notes they may uncover a pattern of patient behavior that clarifies the problem and indicates the appropriate nursing action.

Doug, a 28-year-old man, married six weeks, suffered a C_{6-7} injury. Two months after his injury he was being prepared for his first weekend home visit. Although usually a cooperative and well-motivated patient, he became abusive to the staff, yelled at his wife, and refused to participate in physiotherapy. When the physiotherapist suggested to him that the exercise would help him to transfer into his bed, he said: "You'd think I'm training for my second honeymoon."

Doug's nurse picked up on this and attempted to clarify.

NURSE: Is that the way you feel?
PATIENT: What way?
NURSE: Like you're going on your honeymoon?
PATIENT: Are you kidding?
NURSE: Well no, but I can imagine that you might feel some pressures. (This is acceptance of feeling.)
PATIENT: What the hell are you talking about?
NURSE: Well, we somehow haven't talked about you and Jane being in the same bed. (This directs the interview toward the sexual area.)
PATIENT: Maybe we didn't talk because it's none of your business.
NURSE: Perhaps not. Have you talked with Jane about this? (This is further directing.)
PATIENT: No. What's there to talk about?
NURSE: Well, this first visit home is kind of an experiment. (This focuses the discussion.)
PATIENT: So?
NURSE: It might be worthwhile to make a plan. What is it that you and Jane want to experience? (This focuses with an open question.)
PATIENT: There you are. Sex raises its ugly head.
NURSE: I did not say sex, or intercourse, or erection, or orgasm. Maybe the two of you want to try something, maybe not. What I am saying is that you and Jane may want to agree before the weekend what your plans are. She might just want to know how the two of you can be side by side. (This gives options and responsibilities to the patient.)

PATIENT: Yeah. Hm . . . Is this written down somewhere?

NURSE: Well, no; but when Jane comes in today, we could make a list together.

PATIENT: I wouldn't mind it.

This brief illustration shows how the nurse disarmed the patient's angry outburst, clarified the main concern, and helped the patient acknowledge his hurt and fear. The patient now could explore alternatives with dignity. The nurse accepted sexual issues as part of the person's daily life, and used common sense and interviewing skills to handle the situation.

Joe, a 39-year-old married man, suffered a C_{6-7} complete injury. An external sphyncterotomy was proposed to assist him with his urinary flow. While at first he seemed pleased with the suggestion, rather abruptly he started to berate the nurse who usually assisted with his catheterizations. Joe also said, "I'm going to sue that doctor if he doesn't do it right." These and similar outbursts were quite uncharacteristic of his previous behavior. Eventually, just a few days before the scheduled operation, his wife told the head nurse that the patient was "petrified with worry because he heard from other men that his erection will be lost after this surgery." When the nurse explained to him that "it would not likely happen," he was still unsatisfied but agreed to the surgery.

His erection failed to materialize for about six weeks after the operation. While this was not unusual following this type of surgery, Joe was depressed, uncooperative, and refused to be treated by the urologist involved. Even after the episode was over, he remained withdrawn and angry. Looking back on this situation, the nurses agreed that the patient was labeled "an angry man" and no concerted attempt was made to investigate the sexual causes for his behavior, even though the nurses knew that many patients are concerned about this operation.

Russ, a 28-year-old unmarried man, suffered a partial lesion at the C_{6-7} level. While still in the intensive care unit he wanted to know about his chances to become a father. When someone suggested to Russ that the answer to this was way down the line, he became angry, asked to see a specialist to find out if the "sperms could be taken out of me and somehow frozen for later use." His request was ignored and his subsequent outbursts were explained at the team meeting as "loss of self-image" or a "struggle to reestablish his image."

Two weeks later his girlfriend arrived from out of town and revealed that she was ten weeks pregnant. She also told the nurse that just before the accident they were planning to have her then seven-week-old pregnancy aborted because of their interpersonal difficulties. Now their dilemma was whether she should go ahead with the abortion or have the baby; and if so, should they separate now or get married and see how things would go?

In the light of this story, the patient's extreme agitation to have his sperm checked was not unreasonable. He had to know whether the baby she carried was his last chance to become a father. In this instance, however, the staff acted in a judgmental way and did not clarify the concerns. The patient lost his trust in the staff members and robbed himself of the opportunity to express his concerns, to hear others' reactions, and to consider the various alternatives for resolving the difficult situation. Parental pressures also forestalled further discussions. The couple got married; she had the baby; two months after that they separated and later divorced.

Barbara, an 18-year-old woman (partial C_{6-7} cord injury), was engaged in a light-hearted conversation with a male nurse about fashions and clothing styles while doing her exercises in the physiotherapy room. Discussion focused on the differences between "sexy" and "sensuous" clothing, and she turned to him for an opinion.

One would not immediately identify this conversation as a cry for help, yet Barbara recalled the incident several months after her discharge from the unit. She said, "I desperately wanted to know, am I attractive enough for a man to have interest in me sitting in a wheelchair, and do I still come across as a sensuous person in a wheelchair? But nobody heard my questions!"

Nursing histories

Nurses can use history taking to inform patients and families that their expressions of sexual concerns are just as welcome as any other relevant concerns or questions about the condition.

NURSE: Now I have a question about sexual functioning. Many persons have some worries about this. Have you or your wife (husband) had any concerns in this area? (This is a form of reassurance, "My questions are routine; you are not the only one who might have some problems.")

PATIENT: I'm not so sure I know what you mean.
NURSE: Can I give you examples of some common concerns? (This is asking for permission.)
PATIENT: Uh-huh.
NURSE: Well, many men (women) wonder if they will be able to satisfy their partners; others worry whether they will be able to get some satisfaction; and others worry whether they can still become fathers or mothers. (This is clarification.)
PATIENT: Yes, to all!
NURSE: You know, these are difficult areas for everybody. I am glad that you don't mind talking about them. We don't have a sex specialist on the ward, but we will get the best information to you over the next few weeks. (This gives reassurance, states limitations, and asks permission to continue.)
PATIENT: You mean everybody will know about my problems?
NURSE: These problems are just as important as your other difficulties. We will respect your privacy. The doctor and two or three of the nurses looking after you will have to know about these concerns so that you can get the best information. (This is explanation, forewarning.)
PATIENT: I guess that's okay.
NURSE: Would you like a pamphlet that mentions sex problems?
PATIENT: No, not now. I will wait till I can talk to you about this again.
NURSE: Okay. But be sure to bring up these questions again if you feel that your questions haven't been dealt with! (This puts some responsibility on the patient.)

The early introduction of the idea that "sex is spoken here" lowers the patient's anxiety that this area might be ignored. It also helps the nurses: the sexual concern will be part of the problem list now, and it will be a relatively easy task to approach the patient again some appropriate moment in the future with: "You may remember, when I took your nursing history, you said that you were worried about some sexual issues. Would this be the right time to talk about it?"

Other ways of letting the patient know about sexual care services would be in a pamphlet de-

scribing the services offered in this treatment unit. Some patients prefer to read about sexual alternatives, rather than discuss them. For example, a 45-year-old wife of a doctor suffered a T_{12}–L_1 fracture with complete paraplegia. She thought sexual health care was a "wonderful idea," but she preferred to "read about it rather than talk." She studied the few pamphlets the nurse gave her, but did not ask any questions. She was seen, however, introducing other female patients to her reading material.

Another way of introducing this topic may come from other staff members (for example, a social worker, physician, or psychologist) who take on the responsibility of describing how these concerns can be looked after on the unit.

Clarification of Concerns

Once a patient's complaint or concern is out in the open, it has to be clarified. To which of the six categories of "sexual concerns" listed earlier in this chapter does the patient's complaint belong? Is it worry about erections and orgasms, loss of interest, loss of the partner's interest, new relationships, active participation in sex acts, or managing urinary or bowel control during a sex act? Is it a concern about becoming a father or mother, or about contraception? Clarification translates the patient's diffuse worries into manageable bits. It also reassures patients that their concerns are not unique. The following example shows how clarification helped the 52-year-old mother of three mentioned earlier (p. 126).

NURSE: Here I am. We have at least 15 minutes now.
PATIENT: I hope I'm not holding you up. I don't even know where I should start! I've never known anybody with my type of injury before. Does it cause any sex problems?
NURSE: Well, you know, just the other day one of the other patients said exactly the same thing and asked the same question. (This reassures the patient.)
PATIENT: You mean other people ask about sex too? That makes me feel better. I thought I might get reprimanded or something.
NURSE: More and more people want to get proper information now. But sex means so many things. How would you feel if I asked you

a few questions to find out what areas concern you?

PATIENT: Well, I only thought about intercourse, but why don't you go ahead. I *am* glad you're here.

NURSE: You did mention intercourse. (This lets the patient set the limits.)

PATIENT: Yes, that's a worry. Could my husband lie on top of me without doing more damage to my spine?

NURSE: You mean when the fracture is healed?

PATIENT: Well, certainly not now! Or do people want this in the hospital? (The patient is now set up to receive information.)

NURSE: Most people want to be hugged and held. That can be done here, certainly. And when your fracture is healed, it would be perfectly safe. Your husband may have to place your legs so that he can position himself.

PATIENT: So you say that we could try intercourse later? I must tell him tonight! You know, I *know* he just did not dare to ask me!

NURSE: There might be other areas that you want to check out, too.

PATIENT: I'm sure, but this is the best news yet. Let's leave it at this; then later I can ask you more.

In this instance this is all that the patient wanted to handle. Now that she had developed a special trust in the nurse, she would later ask for more information.

Information Giving

Information giving is a form of "sexual first aid." It is most appropriate when the patient already has a specific concern about sex. Giving specific information is an organized approach to the patient's distress. Once the main complaint is isolated and the reason for the timing of the question is understood (for example, after a visit by family, a television program, diagnostic comments by a medical attendant, or comments by other patients), the nurse has a good opportunity to clarify misinformation and provide relevant new information. Equally important is a "closure" to the brief discussion. This may consist of a promise for more information, a check

with someone more expert in the situation, or a discussion with the partner.

The nurse will have to accept the patient's statements without cover-up or offering false hope; clarify specific complaints and misinformation; and if it appears to be in the best interest of the patient, arrange for a visit with someone more familiar with the issues.

Megan, a 49-year-old woman, suffered a low thoracic level, incomplete injury. She was divorced but had a partner who entered the picture after her injury. He visited her frequently, but she became depressed after the visits and then gradually lost interest in her bowel training and physiotherapy. Although they had access to a "private room" for sex experimentation, Megan refused to go there after the first visit. Eventually she told him that he should find another partner. He opened up the possibility of a sex problem when he asked the nurse about "another position." In the process of clarification Megan eventually revealed to the nurse that she used to be proud of her ability to "move my seat and satisfy my partner." Unable to do her customary movements she felt useless as a sex partner and as a person. The nurse asked her permission to check with the physiotherapist about alternate positions. The physiotherapist devised a small band that helped keep the patient's ankles together and let her "clasp" him. By the time this was discussed and tried out, the patient's partner was able to convince her that he loved and enjoyed her *as she was*.

The following are a few techniques that may help the nurse in giving "sexual first aid":

1. *Ask for permission.* Whenever a new sexual area is about to be discussed, a good approach is to ask: "Can I ask you a question about your relationship?" or "I would need to know if you have experienced an erection in the last few days. May I ask you about this?" If the patient says "No, I don't want to talk about it," the nurse can safely reply: "I'm glad I asked you first. I wouldn't want to invade your privacy." While the nurse should stop this line of questioning, the reason for the patient's somewhat frightened reply may need to be investigated.

2. *Be specific.* Most patients find it easier to deal with well-stated questions than generalities. For example, "What sort of erection did you notice this morning?" is a question that can be an-

swered with some specificity. "What was going on down below this morning?" is such an unclear way of asking that the answer might not be trustworthy.

3. *Avoid irrelevant questions.* A useful rule is to ask oneself: "Why did I ask this? Could I explain the reason for my question if the patient challenged me?" If the answer is "yes," the question was not irrelevant.

4. *Start with reassurance.* "Many women with spinal injury go through periods of loss of interest, but tell me . . . this loss of sexual interest that's concerning you now . . . have you ever experienced it before your injury?"

5. *Proceed from least sensitive to more sensitive areas.* "I wonder . . . in your conversations with your friends, have you heard about self-stimulation? Have you read about it? What sort of feelings have you had about it? Many young children stimulate themselves—what was your experience as a child? What has your experience been in the last few years?"

6. *Use language that is clear to the patient.* The language can be medical, slangy, or earthy, depending on the patient's needs and the nurse's comfort. Patients sometimes say "organism" meaning orgasm; "pee-nuts" instead of penis; "clidoris" instead of clitoris. In these instances correction may be embarrassing, but letting the patient know that "not that it makes any difference, but here we usually say *orgasm*" may be helpful.

Practicing to Provide Care

Nurses need to practice to fulfill a role in sexual health care. Even if they have a great deal of knowledge about the sexual consequences of spinal cord injury and the best of intentions, they may feel so awkward, vulnerable, and concerned about causing hurt to the patient that a sexual conversation is impossible. One way to acquire the necessary confidence is to practice various conversations. Alternating roles , nurses can rehearse various ways of detecting concerns, or giving "sexual first aid." Audiotape or videotape equipment is useful because it is possible to review style, sound level, points of hesitation, methods of reassurance, clarity, and so on.

In some institutions nurses participate in "desensitization" programs, which include viewing explicit sexual films, discussing reactions to sex-related words, and describing sex acts. The value of these programs is not clear. Perhaps a more fundamental approach to acquiring a facility with sexual conversation is to reflect on the fact that health professionals are motivated in their work by their desire to help people. There is plenty of evidence that sex problems are distressing to most patients. Their desire to talk and enthusiasm about receiving information usually motivates health professionals to help. This motivation leads the nurse to seek more knowledge, better communication skills, and sometimes, a nursing position in an environment where the sexual consequences of the patient's disability are formally considered.

SUPPLEMENTAL READING

Bregman, S. 1975. *Sexuality and the Spinal Cord Injured Woman: Guidelines Concerning Femininity, Social and Sexual Adjustment Designed for Physically Disabled Women and Health Professionals Who Work With Them.* Minneapolis, Minn: Sister Kenny Institute. *Small booklet based on interviews with 31 spinal cord injured women. Purposes of this booklet are to provide a knowledge of sexual possibilities, awaken sexual imagination, and encourage women to be open and honest with their sexual partners.*

Cole, T. M.; Chilgren, R.; and Rosenberg, P. 1973. New programme of sex education and counselling for spinal cord injured adults and health care professionals. *International Journal of Paraplegia* 11:111–124. *Description of a two-day workshop on sex education. Format included exposure to a programmed assortment of explicit slides and films of sexual activity and periodic small-group discussions led by trained group leaders.*

Comarr, A. E., and Vigue, M. 1978. Sexual counseling among male and female patients with spinal cord and/or cauda equina injury, parts 1 and 2. *Ameri-*

can *Journal of Physical Medicine* 57(6): 107–122 and 57(10): 215–227. *Presentation of a model of sexual counseling of disabled persons used over an 18-month period at Rancho Los Amigos Hospital. Also includes results of interviews and neurological examinations of 153 male patients and 21 female patients.*

Comfort, A., Ed. 1978. *Sexual Consequences of Disability.* Philadelphia, Pa: G. F. Stickley. *Textbook for health professionals dealing with several areas of illness in which sexuality may be affected. Some chapters specifically on the disabled person and sexual health.*

Cressey, J. M., and Comarr, A. E. 1981. Sexuality and spinal cord injury. *Spinal Cord Injury Digest* 3(Spring): 23–34. *Describes model of sexual counseling and reeducation with individuals and groups. Summarizes information on the physiology of spinal cord injury sexuality and explores expectations of men and women after injury.*

Crewe, N. M.; Athelstan, G. T.; and Krumberger, J. 1979. Spinal cord injury—pre and post injury marriages. *Archives of Physical Medicine and Rehabilitation* 60(6): 252–256. *A study of the preinjury and postinjury marriages of 55 spinal cord injured persons and their partners. Results show that postinjury marriages tend to be happier than preinjury marriages.*

Cross, L. L., Ed. 1978. *Female Sexuality Following Spinal Cord Injury.* Bloomington, Ill: Cheever Publishing. *Resource book for female patients, spouses, families, and health professionals. Based on interviews and written in question and answer format. Easy to read and follow. Topics include menstruation, birth control, pregnancy, delivery, and breastfeeding.*

Golji, H. 1979 Experience with penile prosthesis in spinal cord injury patients. *Journal of Urology* 121:288–289. *Short report of 30 spinal cord injured patients given penile prosthesis implants. Detailed evaluation of 20 patients 3 to 27 months postoperatively.*

Griffith, E. R., and Treischmann, R. B. 1976. Treatment of sexual dysfunction in patients with physical disorders. In *Clinical Management of Sexual Disorders.* Ed. J. Meyer. Baltimore, Md: Williams and Wilkins, pp. 206–225. *Chapter on problems of sexual dysfunction associated with physical disabilities. Differentiated between primary (organic cause) and secondary (behavioral) dysfunctions. For health professionals.*

Held, J. P.; Cole, T. M.; Held, C. A.; Anderson, C.; and Chilgren, R. A. 1975. Sexual attitude reassessment workshops: effect on spinal cord injured adults, their partners and rehabilitation profes-

sionals. *Archives of Physical Medicine and Rehabilitation* 56: 14–18. *An evaluation of five sexual attitude reassessment workshops offered to spinal cord injured patients and rehabilitation professionals.*

Higgins, G. E. 1979. Sexual response in spinal cord injured adults: a review of the literature. *Archives of Sexual Behavior* 8(2): 173–196. *Critical review of the literature on sexual response in spinal cord injured adults. Pulls together several authors' target behaviors of erection, ejaculation, attempts at intercourse, and male and female orgasm. Suggestion for further research included.*

Hodges, L. C. 1978. Human sexuality and the spinal cord injured: the role of the clinical nurse specialist. *Journal of Neurosurgical Nursing* 10(Sept.): 125–129. *Description of a clinical nurse specialist with expertise in field of human sexuality. Role described as that of a clinician, teacher, and consultant.*

Hohmann, G. W. 1972. Considerations in management of psychosexual readjustment in the cord injured males. *Rehabilitation Psychology* 19: 50–58.

Kaplan, H. S. 1974. *The New Sex Therapy: Active Treatment of Sexual Dysfunctions.* New York: Brunner/Mayel. *Text for professionals. Describes biological and psychological determinants of sexual dysfunction, principles of sex therapy, and common male and female dysfunctions.*

Kinsey, A. C., et al. 1947. *Sexual behavior in the human male.* Philadelphia: W. B. Saunders. *Although text is 20 years old it is still considered an up-to-date resource. Report of male human sex behavior compiled after 9 years of data collection.*

———. 1953. *Sexual behaviour in the human female.* Philadelphia: W. B. Saunders. *Similar to Kinsey's report of males except this text reports female sex behavior based on 15 years of data collection.*

Latimer, A. M. 1981. Accountability for the sexual awareness of the spinal cord injured patient. *Rehabilitation Nursing* 6(4): 8–11. *Article written to increase the rehabilitation nurse's knowledge of the sexual potential of the spinal injured person and assess their own attitudes in dealing with sexual concerns.*

Masters, W. H., and Johnson, V. E. 1966. *Human Sexual Response.* Boston: Little, Brown. *Classic text on normal human sexual response. Directed to health professionals.*

Miller, S.; Szasz, G.; and Anderson, L. 1981. Sexual health care clinician in an acute spinal cord injury unit. *Archives of Physical Medicine and Rehabilitation*

62: 315–320. *Describes role of a sexual health clinician, a nonphysician specialist trained to diagnose and treat sexual dysfunctions of disabled persons.*

Schoenfeld, L.; Carrion, H. M.; and Politano, V. A. 1974. Erectile impotence, complications of external sphincterotomy. *Urology* 4(6): 681–685.

Szasz, G. 1978. Sexuality curriculum for physiatrist, physiotherapist, and occupational therapist. In *Sex Education for the Health Professional: A Curriculum Guide.* Eds. N. Rosenzweig and F. P. Pearsall. New York: Grune and Stratton, pp. 175–185. *Outlines a program in which rehabilitation therapists learn to deal with the sexual rehabilitation of spinal cord injured and other chronically ill patients.*

Szasz, G.; Miller, S.; and Anderson, L. 1979. Guidelines to birth control counselling of physically handicapped. *Canadian Medical Association Journal* 120: 1353–1358. *A series of suggested steps for counseling well-motivated physically handicapped men and women.*

———. 1980. Sexual rehabilitation of the acute spinal injured. In *Medical Sexology, the Third International Congress.* Eds. R. Forleo and W. Pasin. Littleton, Mass: PSG Publishing, pp. 422–426. *Description of a rehabilitation program designed to meet the sexual needs of acute spinal cord injured patients. Describes program offered at the Acute Spinal Cord Injury Unit at Shaughnessy Hospital, Vancouver, B.C., Canada.*

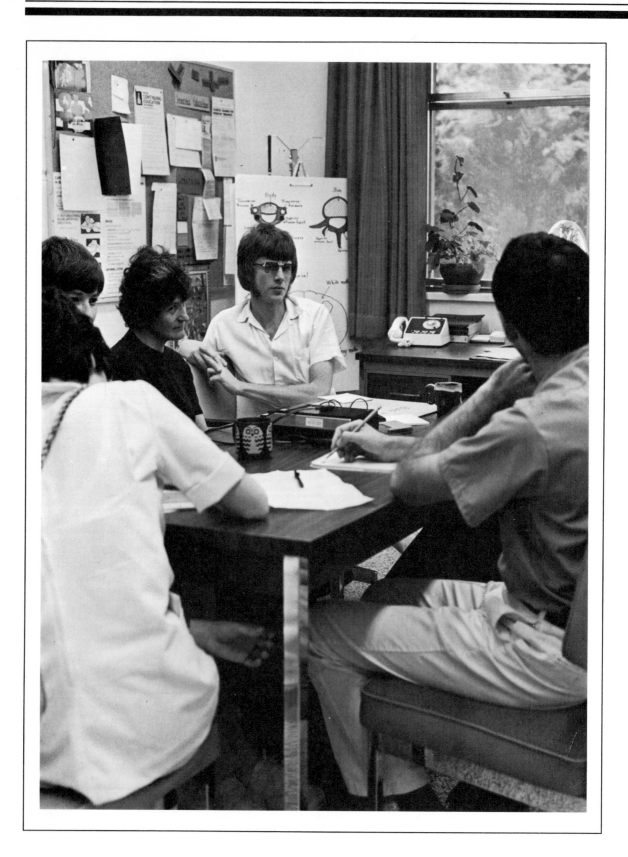

Chapter 8

Patient and Family Health Education*

OBJECTIVES

- To identify patient and family health education goals
- To define learning and describe factors that affect learning
- To identify desirable qualities that enhance the role of the nurse as educator
- To show how to apply the nursing process to health education by assessing learning needs, developing behavioral objectives, implementing educational activities, and evaluating the teaching–learning process

---

* This chapter was developed with the assistance of Jane Andrew, O.T., M. Ed., Patient and
  Family Health Education Coordinator; G. F. Strong Rehabilitation Centre, Vancouver, B.C.

Significant benefits will accrue to patients, families, and staff from a planned coordinated health education program. The following are among the very pertinent reasons for developing a planned patient education program:

- Planned patient education programs offer a means to obtain information that can better equip patients to make decisions and carry out behaviors that safeguard their well-being and permit them to meet their own health care needs.
- Planned patient education programs help ensure that the patient receives correct, non-conflicting information from each staff person involved, that is, the patient experiences continuity and consistency of the educational component of care. [American Hospital Association 1979: 41–42]

The total adjustment of patients and families to a different life-style is the most significant goal of the rehabilitation program. Therefore, patients and families should be given maximum opportunity to explore new health habits, roles, responsibilities, and social functioning. This may require that time be made available from the more traditional rehabilitation program. Learning to cope with leisure time, particularly after discharge, is one such nontraditional area that must be included in the health education process.

The working definition developed for this chapter defines patient and family health education as any information or knowledge, skills or techniques, and attitudes needed by an individual and family to understand and manage the disability and maintain optimal health.

GOALS OF HEALTH CARE

Successful health education of people with spinal cord injuries and their families significantly contributes to the entire rehabilitation process.

We are witnessing a change in the attitude of the health professional and the consumer toward patient education. The consumer rights movement, the requirements of governmental and accred-

iting agencies, and today's emphasis on prevention of health problems attest to this change. With this change comes the challenge of providing accumulated knowledge with a fresh approach. [McCormick and Gilson-Parkevich 1979: preface]

The goals of this chapter are:

- To develop an educational process for those who face serious disability imposed by traumatic injury
- To acquaint the patient and family with the disease process, extent of disability, and the treatment approaches that are being used
- To affect attitudinal/behavioral changes in patients and families so that they will assume an active role in the rehabilitation and in the maintenance of optimal health, including management of the disability throughout life

Implicit in the goals of patient and family education is the principle that the patient and family have a right to be part of the process of determining rehabilitation goals. Health care workers must not allow their dedication and expertise to abridge this fundamental right. In order to make informed decisions about and commitments to their participation in the rehabilitation process, patients and families must be properly informed about the disease process, the extent of residual disability, the services available in the rehabilitation process, and the functional and other outcomes that may depend on the rehabilitation process. The patient and family must then realize they are responsible for the consequences of their decisions and resultant actions.

In order to achieve the goal of patient and family participation in decision making, the "system" and the entire treatment team must not only permit it but also actively encourage it. In practice this means that the patient must be involved in determining the goals of the rehabilitation and discharge plan. The patient, family, and staff must clearly state and mutually understand their expectations and responsibilities very soon after injury. The discussion should include the reasons for admission, services to be provided, effort required, estimated length of stay, and expected outcomes of the various stages of the rehabilitation process. If the participant's expectations and acceptance of responsibilities are not congruent or compatible, possibly participation or timing is inappropriate. If there is agreement, the ensuing process will be meaningful and relevant to the patient and family, and having been involved in making the rehabilitation plan, they will be committed to it.

FACTORS TO CONSIDER WHEN PLANNING AND CONDUCTING EDUCATION

Learning is a process that results in a behavioral change or the acquisition of a skill. To illustrate these definitions let us consider the education necessary to promote optimal urinary function. Activities to attain this goal may include the performance of intermittent catheterizations. Knowledge of the basic anatomy and function of the urinary system, the principles of emptying the bladder at specific regular intervals, and the rationale for using selected techniques will help the patient understand why catheterizations promote optimal urinary function. The information constitutes the knowlege base. The actual physical skill of catheterization is the technique used to meet the goal. It is usually easier to teach the patient and family appropriate knowledge and skills. However, the key question is whether the patient or the family will use the skills; this brings up questions of attitude. The attitudinal component of education is a complex issue involving interest and value judgments supporting the application of acquired knowledge and skills. The behavioral changes made as a consequence of learning help patients and families assume an active role in health care.

Learning is affected by many factors, both positive and negative. Factors that affect learning may be thought of as those directly related to the abilities of the patient and family and those that depend more on the environment, of which the nurse is a part. Some internal factors that affect learning for patients and their families are self-concept and self-esteem, age, educational background and life experience, emotional status, and physical health.

Self-Concept and Self-Esteem

As people mature, self-concept evolves from that of a dependent personality to that of a self-directed adult with the need to be seen by others as self-directing.

> Adults have a need to be treated with respect, to make their own decisions, to be seen as unique human beings. They tend to avoid, resist and resent situations in which they feel they are treated like children—being told what to do and what not to do, being talked down to, embarrassed, punished, judged. Adults tend to resist learning under conditions that are incongruent with their self-concept as autonomous individuals. . . . Once an adult makes the discovery that he can take responsibility for learning, as he does for other facets of his life, he experiences a sense of release and exhilaration. [Knowles 1972:40]

In the aftermath of spinal cord injury, a patient and family's self-concept and self-esteem are particularly vulnerable. The sensitive nurse will be aware of this fact and will take measures to promote feelings of self-worth and minimize feelings of helplessness. To enhance readiness to learn, the nurse should try to strengthen the learner's self-image and promote self-confidence. Implementing the general interventions outlined in Chapters 6 and 7 will help provide psychological support, which in turn promotes learning. For example, the critical care nurse who has skillfully involved the patient and family in nursing care activities communicates recognition of their capabilities and of the importance of their involvement. This preparation develops interest and fosters positive attitudes toward personal health care in the future.

It is important that the nurse continue to involve the patient and family in planning, implementation, and evaluation of health education. This gives the patient an opportunity to see the relevance of learning the activity at hand and thus be more committed to it. If we accept the principle that the patient is the ultimate decision maker and is responsible for the consequences of decisions and actions, in other words is self-directing, we must give the patient as much opportunity for input and involvement as possible during learning (Shaw 1981).

Age

The patient's age provides information about the developmental status of the patient and family. Throughout adulthood, growth encompasses fulfillment of new roles, such as a mate, parent, community member or leader, son or daughter of aging parent, or pensioner.

It is important to understand how normal learning needs to fulfill adult roles must be integrated with health education. For example, a teenager may appear to be exclusively concerned with appearance and attractiveness to the opposite sex. This concern reflects a normal learning need necessary to establish sexual identity and begin the process of exploring what qualities are desirable in a future partner. To proceed with educational aspects of care before personal appearance has been attended to may be devastating and completely block learning. The adult who is dependent on assistance for a bowel procedure may have difficulty accepting help from a family member because it endangers the patient's perceived role as a spouse or independent son or daughter. The elderly are worried about burdening their families. If returning home and remaining there is to become a reality, possible changes in adult roles must be assessed with great care and insight.

The physiological aspects of aging also affect learning. The possibility of diminished visual and auditory faculties, general physical deterioration, and slowed thought processes must be considered.

Educational Background and Life Experience

Knowledge of educational background and life experience will give nurses some idea about a person's interest in maintaining health and the ways in which a person will learn. Generally, the higher the level of education, the greater the working vocabulary and exposure to learning. Depressed socioeconomic status or cultural difference can often hamper the person's understanding of the English language.

Life experience can provide a helpful background conducive to learning; or it may be detrimental if a behavior has to be unlearned. For example, establishing controlled regularity with a neurogenic bowel dysfunction depends largely on dietary intake. The patient who practiced good dietary habits before injury will achieve regulation of bowel movements more easily than a patient whose dietary habits must be unlearned and then corrected. Generally, the older the person is, the greater the tendency to be rigid, which makes behavioral change more difficult.

Emotional Status

Sensitivity to the learner's present emotional status is a key factor affecting learning. Disinterest, increasing agitation, or openly expressed hostility signal underlying concerns that interfere with learning.

> Sensitivity to the patient's anger, fears, and problems is an essential element in a flexible educational program. If, for example, a patient suffers an emotional reverse due to frustration in physical therapy, no teaching is attempted until feelings of inadequacy or rage have beem ameliorated. Or, if a patient seems singularly disinterested in the lesson of the moment, and the nurse perceives concern about a family problem, the lesson is deferred and the more compelling situation is explored. Efforts are then initiated to help with the resolution of the problem before further attempts at teaching are made. [Engstrand 1979: 17]

Psychosocial adjustment following spinal cord injury is another factor to consider, particularly if denial is a problem with either the patient or the family. When hoping for a "miracle cure" negates all else, nurses should encourage the patient to focus on the disability as it is today, and emphasize how important it is to maintain optimal health in case any function should return. This approach usually resolves some of the patient's inner turmoil and helps the patient and family become more open to learning.

Physical Health

When people are ill, the amount of strength and energy they are able to devote to learning is limited. However, Stauffer (1980) injects reality into the situation when she states that whether the patient is "feeling angry, sick, depressed, or just plain miserable, he must absorb an amount of information comparable to a difficult college course, and absorb it well enough to put into immediate daily use once he goes home."

The most stressful times in terms of physical illness for people with spinal cord injuries are the initial recovery period after injury and when infections or setbacks are experienced during the rehabilitation program. During these times, however, the nurse can continue with health education by developing interests and fostering positive attitudes about involvement in health care.

The Therapeutic Environment

One key concept in ensuring successful patient and family health education outcomes is that of helping an adult learn—that is, demonstrating observable attitudes and behaviors that communicate a sense of concern or interest, patience, and a desire to share knowledge, skills, expertise, and points of view acquired through formal training and experience. This emphasizes the role of the nurse as *facilitator* and *resource person*, rather than an authority figure. The total concept of adult education in health care is that professionals have a responsibility to share information and expertise that is vital to maintaining health and to do so in a way that is meaningful for the patient and family.

To create a learning climate the nurse and the patient and family must feel at ease. A relationship that is open to communication and is respecting and constructive will best help the patient and family learn. A positive interpersonal relationship between the nurse and the learner is essential to the process. Primary nursing is also conducive to health education because it fosters a continuous nurse–patient and nurse–family relationship.

THE NURSING PROCESS AND PATIENT AND FAMILY HEALTH EDUCATION

By progressing through each phase of the nursing process—assessment, goal setting, implementation, and evaluation—the nurse uses a systematic method to ensure that the care provided is geared to the individual needs of the patient and family. This method is also applied when providing patient and family health education. Consider how the following basic questions illustrate this process.

1. What does the patient and family need or want to learn? What change in behavior is desired? Why is it important that the patient and family learn? (Assessment)
2. What will the patient and family be able to do and how well at the conclusion of the teaching/learning? (Goal setting or establishing behavioral objectives)
3. On what basis should the education be organized? How should the educational content or material be presented? What teaching aids will facilitate learning? (Implementation)
4. How will the nurse and patient and family determine if learning occurred? (Evaluation)

The nurse must draw on both professional and personal experiences to assess learning needs and determine educational content; to develop behavioral objectives, which can then be evaluated; to find creative ways of communicating, encouraging learner participation, and facilitating feedback; and to apply behavioral change theories.

Assessment

Two major components constitute the broad assessment involved with patient and family health education. To fulfill the responsibility of nurses as educators, nurses must meet learning needs directly related to maintaining health and managing disability, while remaining aware of the psychosocial and other needs of the patient and the family. On an individual basis, nurses must consider factors that affect learning while identifying specific learning needs. Flexibility is an important concept in health education. Integrating awareness of such factors as the person's self-concept, self-esteem, and physical and emotional health enhances learning. For example, if the patient is emotionally upset or physically ill, the nurse should deal with these issues before presenting an educational activity.

The scope and depth of the teaching–learning process involved with severe disability can be overwhelming for both the health professional and the patient and family. The complexity of this situation strongly emphasizes the need for a systematic, coordinated approach to learning on an interdisciplinary level to determine what information is needed; to ensure consistency of content; and to include appropriate team members in determining, implementing, and evaluating educational objectives.

Nurses are concerned with several primary areas, including neurogenic bladder and bowel dysfunction, care of the skin, and respiratory and cardiovascular system management, as well as various aspects of nutrition, physical activity, independent daily living skills, and psychological adjustment. Throughout the book specific educational needs are addressed.

Nurses use professional knowledge and expertise to help patients and family select educational content. This is the information the patient and family will need to know in order to maintain optimal health and manage the disability themselves. In selecting material the nurse must be sure that the content is meaningful and relevant to the patient and family if they are to become involved in the learning process.

Timing is an important factor in attaining relevance. It is significant to remember that adults tend to view education as a process necessary to cope with a present problem (Knowles 1972). If, for example, a patient is preparing for an initial outing, it is more meaningful to learn how to apply a condom and what to do if an "accident" should occur than it is to learn about medications and bladder infections. The latter information is more relevant when the patient is about to go back to work, because bladder infections may cause absenteeism from the job.

Although professionals may be well aware of learning needs, the patient may not be as receptive for a variety of reasons. The initial exploration may appear to be limited in terms of what the patient wants to know, but developing awareness of what the patient needs to know is part of the educational process.

Our real task as nurses is to communicate clearly what behaviors are necessary to meet the desired objectives, to clarify the patient's wants and needs, and to present realistic alternatives (Shaw 1981). For example, when teaching essentials to prevent pressure sores, the nurse must provide a knowledge and skills base that focuses on reasons for skin breakdown and preventive measures necessary to avoid pressure sores. If the patient has difficulty understanding the significance of this education, one reinforcement measure is to demonstrate how unpleasant the alternatives are. The personal cost of ineffective behaviors can sometimes be demonstrated to the learners by confronting them with the consequences of failure (Engstrand 1979). A pressure ulcer is deforming and its appearance grotesque. Yet visual examination of pressure sores and a discussion of how they developed can motivate patients to learn preventive behaviors.

Goal Setting

Throughout the rehabilitation process it is important that the nurse communicate what behaviors are required to meet the goals of planned patient and family health education. A model that clearly conveys the expectations of the health professional allows the patient and family to identify what they know now and what they need to know in the future to maintain optimal health and manage the disability. This type of communication is facilitated by developing specific behavioral objectives.

For the purposes of this chapter, *behavioral objectives* are statements that express, in demonstrable terms, what is to be learned and, when appropriate, how well. Behavioral objectives include the use of action verbs, such as *states, demonstrates,* or *performs,* so that learning can be described precisely and, consequently, evaluated. Words such as *understand* or *appreciate* are too vague and should be avoided. Behavioral objec-

TABLE 8–1 ■ BOWEL MANAGEMENT CHECKLIST

INSTRUCTED (insert signature and date)		OBJECTIVES	Name _____ EVALUATED (insert signature and date)	
Patient	Family Member		Patient	Family Member
		1. States how spinal cord injury affects bowel function		
		2. Explains two reasons for developing a bowel program		
		3. Explains four important factors in developing a bowel program		
		4. Performs or describes how to instruct others with bowel evacuation techniques		
		5. States how to evaluate effectiveness of bowel program		
		6. Describes medications related to bowel management including indications for use, precautions when administering, and side effects		
		7. Describes four potential problems and solutions		

tives specify criteria or standards of acceptable performance that relate directly to identified learning needs.

Table 8–1 is a checklist of the necessary objectives related to management of a bowel program. It can also be used to identify learning needs and as an evaluation tool. To initiate the teaching–learning process the nurse discusses the objectives with the patient and family. To evaluate learning the nurse requires the patient to demonstrate or state the specific objectives. This type of form needs to relate to the entire teaching program and must be supported by a formalized body of information to provide consistency in teaching the content. If such a guideline is unaccompanied by supportive material, it means something different to everyone. For example, the third objective reads: *Explains four important factors in developing a bowel program.* In order to present and evaluate the patient and

family health education necessary to achieve this behavioral objective, the nurse must supply specific information about nutritional and fluid intake, physical activity, planning a consistent evacuation time, and developing a responsible attitude. In other words, the "important factors" should be specifically documented. The seventh objective—*Describes four potential problems and solutions*—requires supportive information including measures to prevent, recognize, and relieve symptoms of constipation, diarrhea, hemorrhoids, and autonomic dysreflexia. If this support information is not available, one staff member may consider only prevention as a potential problem, while another may focus only on relief of abnormal symptoms.

Inconsistency in educational activities causes confusion, discouragement, and incomplete education for the patient and family. As a result, the patient and family may not take their active role in managing the disability and maintaining health. When based on inconsistency, the desired behavior change is not likely to occur.

Implementation

Having established behavioral objectives related to specific learning needs, it is important to review the documented content, specifically, what is to be taught. Implementing the teaching process requires decisions to be made about who will do the teaching and when, how, and where it will occur. Implementation involves organizing learning experiences in a systematic way, selecting resource materials, and supporting desirable changes in behavior.

Patient and family health education should be an integral and scheduled part of the total rehabilitation program, which is offered as routinely and consistently as any other health care service. Staff and patients should schedule educational activities during day hours, rather than relegating education to spontaneous sessions during evenings or on weekends when the patient is more likely to be tired, interested in visiting, or other leisure activities. Scheduled sessions may be planned on both an *individual* one-to-one and a *group* basis. For example, many aspects of patient and family health education require teaching on a one-to-one basis because of the intimate nature of the tasks involved; however, a nurse may establish group sessions to teach the basic essentials of bowel, bladder, or skin care, which are common to everyone.

Generally, health education in nursing is done on a one-to-one basis and often on the spot—that is, during care or assistance with an activity. On-the-spot teaching can be effective for reinforcing learning and providing practical application of knowledge or a skill, but it is not always the most effective method for teaching and learning, because it is not the prime purpose of the activity. Teaching a skill by demonstration and return demonstration can only be effective if the steps and procedures are consistent among the various staff from whom the patient is learning. Without documented procedures, points may be taught somewhat differently by different staff members. This difficulty is compounded by the lack of scheduled time for educational programs. Formalized programs provide consistency, are more efficient in terms of staff time, and therefore make the overall teaching program more effective.

Printed and audiovisual materials enhance the learning process, but do not replace the nurse as educator or facilitator. There are several characteristics to keep in mind when selecting or developing supplemental educational materials.

- The most effective materials are liberally illustrated and speak simply and directly to the problem without medical jargon. This type of material is comprehensible to people with limited reading ability and not offensive or insulting to those with more education.
- Aids should be accessible and easy to use. Videotape and slide–tape presentations are the most likely formats for audiovisual material. To encourage use and minimize risk of breakdown, equipment should be simple to operate.
- Audiovisual materials can be tied in to reference material from the patient library. Flexible library hours will accommodate families as well as patients.
- "Workbook" teaching manuals for the patient and family can be used continuously and extensively following discharge.

Although teaching aids may be planned and produced in-house, an increasing amount of material can be borrowed or purchased, often at a lower cost. There are a number of manuals designed specifically for people with spinal cord injuries and their families currently available. See the Supplemental Reading list at the end of this chapter. The nurse can review the contents of these valuable resources to ensure their timing and relevance and plan comprehensive educational activities.

It is important to give recognition and support when desirable changes in behavior occur. This behavioral approach is described as *operant learning*, or *conditioning*, and is gaining recognition as an effective adjunct in rehabilitative care (Trombly 1966; Sand et al. 1973; Berni and Fordyce 1973; Cheshire and Flack 1978–79; and Norris, Noble, and Strickland 1981). Operant learning is based on the functional principle that behavior can be modified—that is, behavior is sensitive to influence by consequences. When a behavior is met with positive reinforcement, such as praise or encouragement, that behavior is most likely to be repeated in the future. If a behavior elicits a negative consequence, such as criticism or a disinterested response, that behavior is less likely to be repeated in the future. Operant learning does have a place in education to accelerate occurrence of desirable behaviors. Health care professionals use this behavioral approach with varying degrees of intensity and awareness. For example, as a subtle way to reinforce positive peer influence, more and more rehabilitation facilities design group interaction with successfully rehabilitated individuals as role models.

There is a distinct role in operant learning for clinical counseling professionals. Patients may need help with personal problems or concerns to be more open to learning experiences. In addition, those specifically trained in the behavioral sciences are a valuable resource to the nurse engaged in clinical application of behavioral change theories.

The combined expertise of health professionals and innovative educators seems most likely to improve teaching techniques and stimulate learning (Engstrand 1979). The *Spinal Injury Learning Series* (SILS) (Norris, Noble, and Strickland 1981) is such an approach. The theory is presented in a book

> based on award-winning films and seven years of research, [which] describes a new approach to achieving independent living for some 10,000 newly injured persons each year. This book is designed for physicians, nurses, therapists, counselors, educators, and patients. Detailing the hard facts and procedures which a person with a spinal cord injury must acquire to manage one's self-care, the book describes four subjects: Introduction to Spinal Cord Injury, Bowel Care, Bladder Care, and Skin Care. A clear explanation of the communication and psychological theories upon which the series was based is provided. The results of a four-year experimental research project in six model system spinal cord injury centers are stated.

Currently the SILS approach offers 20 one-hour sessions based on a fee-for-service to the patient. The spinal cord injury center will provide equipment and supportive services and will pay the SILS company a participation fee for the educational materials used each session. Such materials include standards, audiovisual materi-

als, testing aids, and a patient notebook. The materials will be continuously updated and improved.

Evaluation

"Basic to all processes of creativity is the ability to evaluate . . . to select, to reject, and to critically determine the value of what has been done" (McCormick and Gilson-Parkevich 1979:153).

Evaluation is an ongoing shared process by which the nurse and the patient and family can determine whether learning has occurred. Evaluation is directly related to the behavioral objectives documented in the planning process. When learning is defined in terms of a behavioral change or a capability, it can be evaluated. Most often the shortcoming in health education is the lack of evaluation. Without criteria or standards supported by specific content, it is difficult to determine when and how adequately an activity has been learned.

There are many ways to evaluate learning. Some methods include open discussions, direct questioning and observation, return demonstrations, and comparison of pretest and posttest results. Written tools should be simply designed and easily tabulated; checklists or rating scales are good formats. The checklist in Table 8–1 is an example of a simple evaluation tool.

The following points should be kept in mind when selecting methods to evaluate learning (Program Planning Guide 1977:67):

- Exactly what is it that you want to find out? Whether the learners "know" something? Whether they "can do" something? How they "feel" about something? [Evaluating attitudes is far more difficult than evaluating knowledge and skills.] Be sure to specify that "something" as clearly as possible.
- What does common sense tell you would be the best way to find out? Have the learners answer questions—written or oral? Have them carry out a procedure? Have them solve a problem of some kind? Have them teach another patient? Have them role play back to the nurse?
- How much time is available? How much help do you have (or do you need)? Interviews and skills demonstrations require a low learner–instructor ratio.
- How important is the element you are considering evaluating? Something the learners *must*

know or be able to do, or just something that would be "nice"?

Evaluation should occur throughout the educational process to measure the extent to which learning has occurred. Patient and family health education is increasingly gaining recognition as an integral process that most significantly influences the ultimate outcome of rehabilitation. Therefore, evaluation data may not only indicate necessary changes in teaching techniques and learner participation, but they may redirect the entire rehabilitation process.

SELECTED REFERENCES

Berni, R., and Fordyce, W. 1973. *Behavior Modification and the Nursing Process.* St. Louis: C. V. Mosby. *A description of patient management problems that outlines practical techniques to apply behavior modification to accomplish traditional patient care goals and objectives; includes analysis of behavior, reinforcement of behavior, practical management, ethical issues, and future trends.*

Cheshire, D. J. C., and Flack, W. J. 1978–79. The use of operant conditioning techniques in the respiratory rehabilitation of the tetraplegic. *International Journal of Paraplegia* 16: 162–174. *Explains how behavioral change theories were applied in the clinical setting to improve pulmonary function using incentive spirometry.*

Engstrand, J. L. 1979. A nursing challenge; effective patient education. *Journal of Association of Rehabilitation Nurses* 4(5): 15–18. *Presents a relevant overview of the educational process in rehabilitation; offers valuable guidelines for nurses involved with spinal cord injured patients and focuses on preventable complications of disability, in this case pressure sores.*

Implementing Patient Education in the Hospital. 1979. American Hospital Association, 840 North Lake Shore Drive, Chicago, Ill. 60611. *Includes definitions and reasons for and guidelines to development of education in health care.*

Joint Committee on Health Education Terminology. 1973. *New definitions.* Health Education Monographs, no. 33. *Clarifies definitions to give clearer future directions.*

Knowles, M. S. 1972. *The Modern Practice of Adult Education.* New York: Association Press. *Classic text on principles and methods involved with adult learning.*

McCormick, R. D., and Gilson-Parkevich, T. 1979. *Patient and Family Education: Tools, Techniques, and Theory.* New York: John Wiley and Sons. *Practical guidelines for designing, presenting, and evaluating educational activities in a pediatric setting.*

Norris, W. C.; Noble, C. E.; and Strickland, S. B. 1981. *Spinal Injury Learning Series.* Jackson, Miss: University Press of Mississippi. *Educational program purchased on a fee-for-service basis; currently offers education on bowel, bladder, and skin care with plans to expand and continually update content.*

Program Planning Guide for Health Professionals. 1977. Vancouver, BC: Department of Adult Education, University of British Columbia. *Presents principles of planning continuing education.*

Sand, P., et al. 1973. Fluid intake behavior in patients with spinal cord injury: predictions and modification. *Archives of Physical Medicine and Rehabilitation* 54:254–262. *Applies behavioral change theories in a clinical setting to enhance nursing care.*

Shaw, L. 1981. The patient as an adult learner. *Association of Operating Room Nurses Journal* 33 (2): 233–239. *Uses a problem-centered approach to adult learning; focuses on preparing the nurse to teach and on assessing the patient's readiness to learn in a hospital environment.*

Stauffer, S. 1980. A master-plan for teaching the patient with spinal cord injury. *Registered Nurse* (July): 56–60. *A brief overview of major educational areas.*

Trombly, C. A. 1966. Principles of operant conditioning: related to orthotic training of quadriplegic patients. *American Journal of Occupational Therapy* 21: 217–220. *Application of behavioral change theories in a rehabilitation setting.*

SUPPLEMENTAL READING

Craig Hospital, 1979. *Nursing Patient Education: A Program to Help the Spinal Injury Patient Manage an Altered Lifestyle.* Craig Hospital, Rocky Mountain Regional Spinal Injury Center, 1–8. *Describes how* the nursing, education, and media departments combined resources to present goal-oriented patient education; includes factors to consider for preparing the nurse-teacher, assessment of the patient and family, and educational content and documentation.

Rohrer, K., et al. 1980. Rehabilitation in spinal cord injury: use of a patient-family group. *Archives of Physical Medicine and Rehabilitation* 61(5): 225–229. *A report on a program of one-day workshops held for people with spinal cord injuries and their families. Education is stressed, as well as a therapeutic sharing of feelings.*

Smith, M. C. 1977. Self-care: a conceptual framework for rehabilitation nursing. *Journal Association of Rehabilitation Nurses* 2 (Mar.–Apr.): 8–10. *Offers guidelines to validate a patient's perspective of abilities, disabilities, and goals as a vital part of comprehensive learning assessment.*

Ulrich, M., and Kelley, K. M. 1972. Patient care includes teaching. *Hospitals* 46: 59–65. *Presents rationale for promoting patient and family education.*

Welnetz, K. 1981. Health teaching for spinal cord injured patients and families during acute hospitalization. *L'axone:* Canadian Association of Neurological and Neurosurgical Nurses 3(2): 5–8. *Project identified learning needs of 52 patients in an acute hospital. Presents guidelines for specific learning content during this phase of care and reinforces importance of learning as a continual process throughout the rehabilitation period.*

The following resources are designed for patient and family health use. See also suggested resources in Chapter 19.

Engstrand, J., and Stuart, B. 1979. *Patient Handbook of Self-Care Procedures.* 2nd ed. Birmingham, Ala. Spinal Rehabilitation Center of the University of Alabama. *Series of pamphlets in three-ring binder, workbook format. Includes orientation to a specific rehabilitation center and numerous step-by-step procedures for people with spinal cord injuries, particularly for use in the home.*

Fallon, B. 1975. *So you're paralysed.* . . . The Spinal Injuries Association, 126 Albert St., London NW17NF, England, pp. 52–62. *A concise handbook with an easy-to-read, humanistic approach to the many facts about spinal cord injury. Addresses the importance of attitude in the adjustment process, which leads into the many aspects of care that must be recognized as important. Also valuable as introductory reading for many staff members.*

Ford, J., and Duckworth, B. 1974. *Physical Management for the Quadriplegic Patient.* Philadelphia, Pa:
F. A. Davis Co. *Detailed photostory accompanied by easy-to-read text; includes managing wheelchairs, transfer activities, personal hygiene, bowel and bladder procedures, and some community living skills. Helpful for patients, families, attendants, and professional staff.*

Garfunkel, M., and Goldfinger, G. 1982. *Living with Spinal Cord Injury Questions and Answers for Patients, Families and Friends.* New York University Medical Center, New York Regional Spinal Cord Injury System (400 E. 34 St., N.Y., N.Y. 10016). *Readable question/answer format guide, for example, Is financial assistance available after spinal cord injury? Can spinal cord injured persons work or go to school? Focuses on life after rehabilitation. Creative photography reinforces positive attitudes communicated in this booklet.*

Goldfinger, G. H., and Hanak, M. A. 1981. *Spinal Cord Injury: A Guide for Care.* New York Regional Spinal Cord Injury System. *A concise handbook directed toward patients, families, and attendants. Creative photography and style reinforces positive attitudes.*

King, R. B.; Boyink, M.; and Keenan, M., eds. 1977. *Rehabilitation Guide.* Chicago: Rehabilitation Institute of Chicago. *In a three-ring binder, workbook format, this rehabilitation guide explains how the body is affected by spinal cord injury and uses a problem-solving format to present management techniques. Strong focus on prevention.*

Meyer, P. R., et al. 1980. *Spinal Cord Injury: A Guide for Patients and Their Families.* Chicago: Midwest Regional Spinal Cord Injury Care System. *Excellent introductory guide for acute care period; includes goals, objectives and medical definitions; describes initial care, physiological changes, psychological adjustments, and surgical interventions; outlines roles of the team members, including the role of family members.*

Virginia Spinal Cord Injury Care and Teaching Manual. 1980. Virginia Spinal Cord Injury System, University of Virginia Center and Virginia Dept. of Rehabilitation Services, Woodrow Wilson Rehabilitation Center, Box W-279, Fisherville, Va. 22939. *Soft-cover workbook designed for personalized patient and family use, for example, What is the level of your injury? What type of bladder do you have, and what are the possible goals for management of your bladder? Also includes numerous opportunities for patients to enter information, such as current medications, dosages, side effects, precautions. A list of questions and a teaching/evaluation checklist are included at the end of each comprehensive section. Includes helpful section on psychosocial-sexual factors. A valuable teaching and resource aid.*

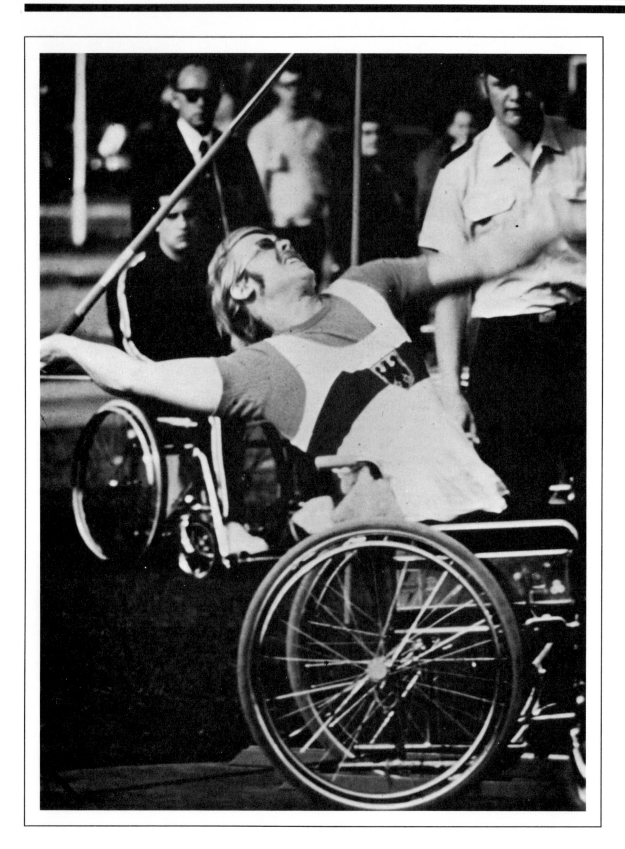

PART IV

MAINTAINING PHYSIOLOGICAL FUNCTIONS

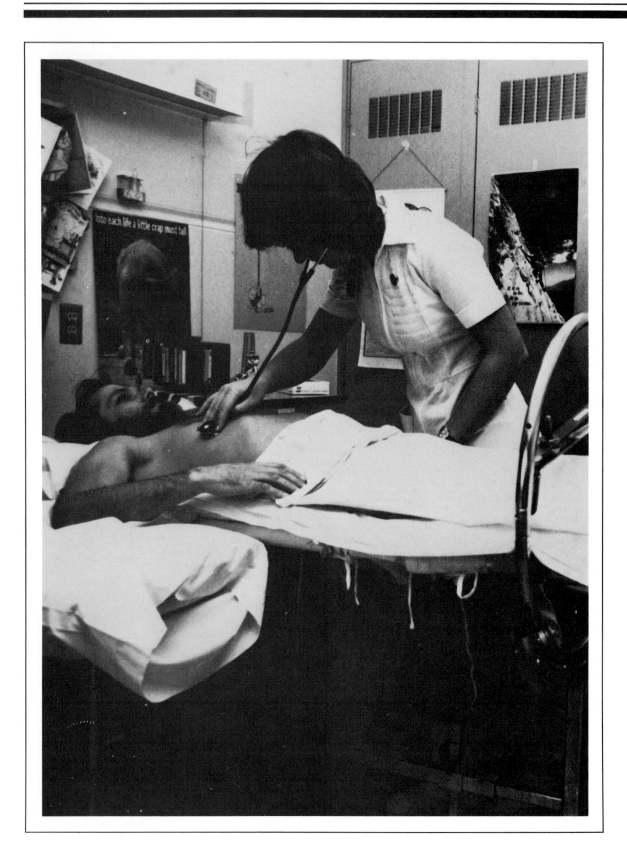

Chapter 9

Promoting Optimal Respiratory Function

CHAPTER OUTLINE

OBJECTIVES

- To explain how respiration is impaired by spinal cord injury
- To correlate expected dysfunctions of the muscles of breathing with the level of injury diagnosed
- To identify spinal cord injured patients who are at additional risk of developing pulmonary complications
- To describe assessment techniques and diagnostic procedures
- To describe innervation, function, and impairment due to spinal cord injury of four major muscles or muscle groups involved in the work of breathing
- To describe preventive measures that promote adequate ventilation and combat retention of secretions
- To describe restorative measures to reestablish adequate ventilation and perfusion
- To describe care for a spinal cord injured patient with hypoxia, atelectasis or pneumonia, pulmonary edema, pulmonary emboli, and pneumothorax
- To explain appropriate self-care skills to patients and families
- To describe long-term implications associated with respiratory function for a quadriplegic person

GOALS OF HEALTH CARE

Repiratory insufficiency is a most serious threat to the patient with a spinal cord injury. In fact, "all quadriplegics and most paraplegics should be considered to have some degree of respiratory insufficiency until proven otherwise" (Carter 1979). The acute management phase requires constant and expert care to prevent life-threatening situations while patients adjust to altered respiratory functioning. For many people with quadriplegia prophylactic chest management is necessary throughout life.

The goals of health care are:

- To ensure adequate gas exchange by:
  —providing sufficient tidal and minute volume
  —maintaining lung elasticity and chest wall flexibility, and strengthening existing muscles of respiration
  —recognizing and managing poor ventilatory stimulus
  —facilitating inspiration and expiration by supportive measures as required
  —preventing, identifying, and promptly treating infections or any other complications
- To promote optimal circulation for oxygen delivery and carbon dioxide removal at a cellular level
- To teach patients and families care to prevent pulmonary complications

Care of the patient with respiratory insufficiency demands a well-defined and well-coordinated program. A number of disciplines may collaborate on chest treatment: the respiratory physician, the nurse, the physiotherapist, and the respiratory technician. Communication of plans to the patient, family, and health team is a most important aspect of respiratory care. The nurse providing 24-hour care plays a key role in this care.

ASSESSMENT OF RESPIRATORY FUNCTION

The initial assessment of respiratory function requires meticulous recording of the history and physical findings to provide an accurate data base. Future assessments can be compared with this information to monitor deterioration or improvement.

Assessment of current respiratory status and knowledge of the diagnosed level of lesion make it possible to predict what muscles will have impaired function, what compensations may occur, and what potential problems can be anticipated. This helps the team prepare for management of complications or emergency situations.

The detail in which a history and physical examination is completed by the nurse will depend on the urgency of the situation and to what extent other team members are involved.

Ability to perform an adequate assessment of respiratory function is vital in any setting since breathing difficulty can develop rapidly at any time during the rehabilitation period.

Respiratory Physiology

Respiration is a process that can be described in three phases: ventilation, alveolar–capillary diffusion, and transport of gases. The following descriptions are based on the works of Kozier and Erb (1983) and Holloway (1979).

Ventilation
Ventilation is the basic act of breathing, that is, inspiration and expiration. Oxygen and carbon dioxide are exchanged between the atmosphere and the alveoli of the lungs. Essential requirements for ventilation are adequate atmospheric oxygen, clear airway passages, and good compliance, or elasticity, of the lungs and thorax.

Depending on the nature and extent of the cord injury, the paralyzed patient has major difficulty maintaining a clear airway and preserving chest movement. Impaired function of the breathing muscles results in poor chest expan-

sion and inability to manage secretions effectively, severely compromising ventilation. The severest consequence occurs with high cervical cord injury that results in total loss of spontaneous respiration. The varying degrees of respiratory involvement related to levels of injury are in the section Physical Examination later in this chapter.

Alveolar–capillary diffusion
Alveolar–capillary diffusion is the exchange of oxygen and carbon dioxide between the alveoli of the lung tissue and the pulmonary capillaries. Factors influencing the movement of gases across the respiratory membrane are the thickness and surface area of the membrane, the coefficient of the gas (determined by its solubility and molecular weight), and the pressure differences on each side of the membrane. The pressure exerted by each gas is called the *partial pressure.* This pressure is measured by diagnostic arterial blood gas analysis to evaluate adequacy of gas exchange. Changes in the pressure gradients are most important clinically and depend on the relationship between ventilation and blood flow (perfusion) in the alveolar–capillary units (Holloway 1979).

As the work of breathing becomes more difficult with paralysis, the physiological dead space tends to increase. *Physiological dead space* is the combination of *anatomical dead space,* which is the air normally in the tracheobronchial tree up to the terminal bronchioles, and *alveolar dead space.* Abnormal alveolar dead space is created when the air in the alveoli cannot participate in gaseous exchange because the alveoli are without capillary blood flow. Alveolar–capillary units are ventilated but not perfused. Following high thoracic or cervical cord injury, lack of chest movement and difficulty managing secretions increase atelectasis, decrease exchange, permit alveolar collapse, and hence increase physiological dead space. This contributes to chronic alveolar hypotension seen with quadriplegic patients. Capillary shunting, referring to these alveolar–capillary units that are perfused but not ventilated, is a common cause of hypoxemia with any critically ill patient, when retained secretions (such as in atelectasis) block alveoli with mucus and prevent ventilation.

Transport of gases

Transport of gases in the blood to and from the body cells occurs for the metabolic process of oxygen use and carbon dioxide excretion. This final phase is also called *cellular respiration*. Oxygen and carbon dioxide transport depends on adequate cardiac output with a normal red blood cell count and hematocrit. Most of the oxygen is carried in the hemoglobin of the red blood cells. Most of the carbon dioxide is carried in the return circulation as bicarbonate (HCO_3) inside the red blood cells. Carbon dioxide is an important factor in the acid-base balance of the body.

In people with spinal cord injuries the volume of the circulating blood may be compromised when blood pools in the extremities. Newly injured patients also tend to develop cardiac arrhythmias; if they have multiple injuries, they may suffer additional hemorrhage or dehydration. These factors severely and adversely affect cardiac output, blood composition, and therefore cellular respiration.

History

Diagnosis of high thoracic or cervical cord injury

The diagnosed level and extent of cord injury are the foundation on which to base an assessment of respiratory function. The most important thing to remember is that *all quadriplegic patients are in potential danger of developing respiratory insufficiency*. Although many quadriplegic patients are not in obvious or severe respiratory distress on admission, the high risk of deterioration requires monitoring for three to seven days after injury. The danger is particularly serious when the onset is gradual and insidious because it is difficult to recognize by the unskilled observer. It is important to consider the post-injury time interval because:

- Buildup of potential *cord edema* and/or *cord hemorrhage* increases neurological deficit that may extend to involve diaphragmatic function, causing threatened respiratory function progressing to loss of spontaneous respirations.

- Paralysis adds extra work to the remaining muscles of breathing (the strain has been estimated as nine times greater than normal). Extreme *fatigue* may progress to exhaustion and respiratory failure.

If onset of respiratory difficulty is solely related to cord edema or fatigue, however, loss of spontaneous respirations is usually temporary.

Associated injuries

Associated chest trauma, most frequently fractured ribs, is common in high-velocity injuries such as occur with motor vehicle accidents or falls. These are most frequently associated with fractures of the thoracic spine. Due to loss of sensation and absence of referred pain, some injuries may not be apparent.

Head injury can also be associated with high-velocity accidents and most frequently is associated with trauma to the cervical spine. Resulting increased intercranial pressure will depress the neural drive controlling respiration rate. It is important to note whether the patient experienced any period of unconsciousness.

Blood loss from internal or external hemorrhage can diminish systemic arterial oxygen pressure (tension) (PaO_2). Neural tissue is most sensitive to continual oxygenation, so cardiopulmonary function must be restored as early as possible to prevent further damage to susceptible neurons in the spinal cord.

Aspiration

Aspiration is suspected with any patient who has been unconscious. If gastric contents contaminate the lung, the patient will have a severe inflammatory response.

Aspiration is also associated with water-related accidents such as diving into shallow water. Near drownings cause fluid to contaminate the lungs, which leads to alveolar collapse and widespread atelectasis.

Preexisting pulmonary and related complications

It is important to note any preexisting pulmonary disease or infections, thoracic surgery, smoking history, cough or sputum, dyspnea, or shortness of breath on exertion. Other complicating factors are low activity tolerance and obesity; allergies, particularly asthma; and anemia, which will significantly affect the oxygen-carrying capacity of the blood. This information may be obtained from relatives or friends if necessary. Any complications may profoundly affect the course of respiratory care.

Systemic fluid overload is another condition that is hazardous to respiratory function, because excess fluid will eventually collect in the lung. The nurse must check the patient's intake and output record carefully, especially after transport, to detect imbalance. Fluid overload, as a result of overcompensation to combat neurogenic hypotension, is a common problem.

Advanced age

Older patients (over 50 years) have problems similar to those of heavy smokers and those with chronic obstructive pulmonary disease. There seems to be increased pulmonary shunting with a lowered PaO$_2$. Reduced compliance with some chest wall rigidity and less lung elasticity also occurs. Finally, cleansing of the respiratory tract is less efficient due to a decrease in phagocytic activity and cilliary action (Spence and Mason 1979). The older paralyzed person is especially susceptible to pooled secretions and numerous related problems.

Physical Examination

The nurse should be familiar with the patient's history and physical assessment as recorded on the medical record and by communication with other health team members. Knowledge of the patient's general response to the treatment plan since admission and the specific response during the preceding 24-hour period is necessary. The physical examination reveals the patient's current respiratory status and includes observation of the airway; inspection of the chest and abdomen for ventilation; palpation, percussion, and auscultation of the chest; and observation of extrathoracic signs and symptoms of distress.

Observation of airway

Airway obstruction is commonly associated with injuries to the cervical spine and loss of consciousness. Eventually, retaining secretions or choking on food may become a problem. When coughing mechanisms are ineffective, the patient's attempted coughs sound very quiet, are nonproductive, and occur in rapid succession. Movement in the throat is not accompanied by chest expansion. The patient is in obvious distress, with a flushed face and frightened appearance until assistance can be obtained.

Inspection for ventilation

Chest assessment requires knowledge of external chest landmarks in relation to underlying respiratory structures. See Figure 9–1. Inspection of ventilation includes assessment of thoracic size and shape, respiratory rate and rhythm, chest expansion, and abdominal movement. (Chest assessment techniques are summarized in Procedure 9–1.)

Thoracic size and shape The normal chest is symmetrical, with the anteroposterior dimension smaller than the lateral dimension. When the chest is unusually shaped or has a bony pro-

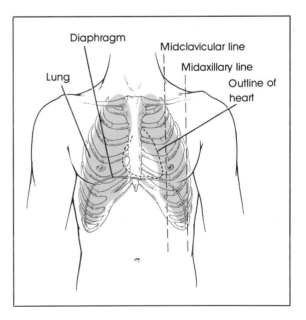

FIGURE 9–1 ■ External chest landmarks in relation to underlying respiratory structures.

PROCEDURE 9–1 ■ CHEST ASSESSMENT

Purpose

The purpose of chest assessment is to determine the patient's respiratory status, especially to detect retained secretions and to evaluate the effectiveness of the therapy. The techniques of inspection, palpation, percussion, and auscultation are included.

Action	Rationale
1. Place the patient supine and remove clothing or bed covers below the waist.	To observe all the muscles used in breathing, especially the diaphragm, a good view of the chest *and* abdomen is necessary.
2. Inspect chest for abnormal shape or asymmetry.*	
3. Count respiratory rate.	An increased rate of shallow respirations is an early sign of respiratory insufficiency.
4. Observe pattern of respiratory rhythm.	Be alert for periods of sleep-induced apnea in quadriplegic patients.
5. Observe chest expansion and abdominal movement. Describe chest expansion as normal, increased, or decreased. (Further assessment requires spirometry.)*	Signs of abnormal or increased work of breathing include: • Exaggerated use of accessory muscles in the neck and shoulders • Paradoxical or abdominal breathing • Inability to breathe deeply • Inability to cough
6. Palpate the chest with fingers on each side of the rib cage, thumbs pointing toward the sternum. Observe movement of your hands as the patient breathes.*	As the patient breathes, thumbs should move apart equally. Asymmetry of chest expansion exists if they do not. A condition such as fractured ribs may cause asymmetry of chest expansion. Tactile fremitis or vibratory tremors may also be felt on palpation of the chest wall.
7. Percuss the chest systematically by tapping the chest from the apices to the bases of the lungs. Compare from side to side and at each level. It is also possible to percuss diaphragmatic excursion on the posterior chest.*	Abnormal dullness on percussion is indicative of retained secretions.
8. Use a stethoscope to auscultate all lobes of the lungs. Proceed systematically as for percussion.*	Retained secretions cause: • Bronchial sounds • Diminished breath sounds • Increased or decreased fremitus • Adventitious sounds (rales and rhonchi)
9. If possible, place patient prone and repeat techniques.	The prone position can aggravate breathing by limiting impaired chest expansion and abdominal movement.

* The Halo-thoracic brace limits the use of these techniques.

(*Procedure continues*)

PROCEDURE 9–1 ■ (continued)

Action	Rationale
10. Observe the posterior chest for spinal curvatures.	Spinal curvatures may also limit chest expansion and may have predisposed the patient to initial injury. For example, a patient with kyphosis, a humpback deformity of the posterior spine, is more prone to injuring the cord from a relatively minor fall.
11. Observe amount and nature of secretions.	
12. Check vital capacity and compare with baseline data.	A reduced vital capacity indicates deterioration in pulmonary function.
13. Interpret serial comparison of arterial blood gas analysis.	Early deterioration in respiratory function is detected by a decrease in Pao_2 and/or an increase in $Paco_2$ values.
14. Collaborate with physician to determine significance of chest X-ray findings.	Chest X rays are of limited value in early detection of retained secretions because microatelectasis, which causes small airway closure, cannot easily be seen.

tuberance, it will be necessary to modify procedures for turning, positioning, and fitting to allow for adequate chest expansion.

Respiratory rate and rhythm Normal respiration in the adult occurs at a regular, rhythmic rate of 14 to 20 breaths per minute, inspiration being shorter than expiration. A number of complex interactions involving the central and peripheral nervous system and the musculature of the chest wall control the rate and rhythm of breathing. Intimately tied to the neural drive regulating respiration are feedback mechanisms made possible by chemoreceptors, mainly sensitive to carbon dioxide levels in the blood.

The central nervous system provides both *voluntary control* (*cortical*) and *involuntary control* (*autonomic*) to regulate respiration. An example of voluntary control is the breath control used in singing. Autonomic control regulates breathing during sleep.

Complete apnea results from cord damage at or above segments C_4 when diaphragmatic action is lost. This is due to interruption of the pathway from the brain to the spinal cord and peripheral nerves (in this case the phrenic nerve). Both voluntary and involuntary control are absent.

However, even if the patient has phrenic nerve control, autonomic control can be altered by spinal cord injury in the cervical area. Damage to these fibers in the spinal cord may interrupt the delicate feedback communication pattern to the medulla. The respiratory center then becomes less responsive to increases in blood carbon dioxide levels, which normally stimulate respiration (Bergkofsky 1964).

This predisposes the quadriplegic patient to the unusual syndrome of *central alveolar hypotension,* more commonly referred to as *sleep-induced apnea* or *Ondine's curse.* (In ancient folklore, Ondine, a sea nymph, placed a fatal curse on her unfaithful mortal husband that when he next fell asleep he would stop breathing. In other words, he would lose autonomic control of respiration.) The body's insensitivity to hypercarbia is characterized by periods of apnea. The patient may be able to breathe normally when awake but "forgets" to breathe during sleep. Lethargy and headaches may occur in the morning. If the condition is severe, hypoxemia can build to fatal levels.

Nurses must carefully observe resting quadriplegic patients, especially during the night. Recovery from sleep-induced apnea should occur in three to five months (Zeluff et al. 1977).

Chest expansion and abdominal movement *Chest expansion* depends on adequate neural drive from the respiratory center in the medulla

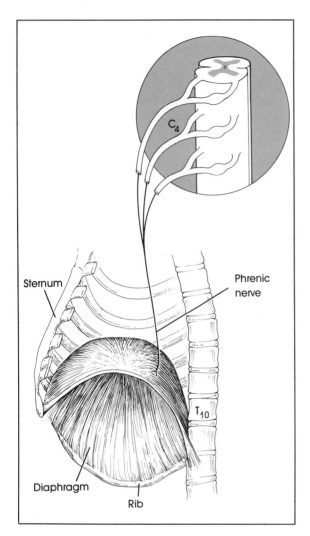

FIGURE 9–2 ■ The diaphragm, the most powerful muscle for breathing, receives innervation from the C_4 cord segment with lesser contributions from C_3 and C_5 cord segments.

and stable musculature and skeletal structures of the thorax. The lungs are suspended in the flexible thoracic cage, which is bound by the sternum in front, the spinal column in back, the rib cage encircling, and the diaphragm below. Each lung has a covering of visceral pleura, which is closely related to the parietal pleura lining the thoracic cavity. The lung has no muscle tissue itself and does not actively contract but responds directly to the muscular expansion and contraction of the thorax. *Inspiration* occurs when muscular expansion of the chest creates a nega-

tive (subatmospheric) pressure in the lung, and air is pulled into the alveoli. Normal *expiration*, a much more passive phase, occurs when intrapulmonary pressure becomes greater than atmospheric pressure; the chest muscles relax; and the lungs recoil, returning the thoracic cage to its resting position.

The *work of breathing* or *mechanics of breathing* are the movements required to achieve inspiration and expiration. The active phase of inspiration requires more effort, because it expands the thorax in three directions to increase the anteroposterior, lateral, and vertical dimensions. The major muscles involved in breathing are the diaphragm, intercostal muscles, and to a lesser extent the accessory and abdominal muscles.

The *diaphragm* is a strong sheet of muscle separating the thoracic and abdominal cavities. See Figure 9–2. It is convex above and concave below. The diaphragm is attached to the lower border of the rib cage and inserts into a common central tendon. As this tendon contracts, the diaphragm flattens, lowering the upper dome shape to pull downward and enlarge the thoracic cage. It also moves abdominal viscera downward. This "plunger" effect creates negative pressure in the lung. Diaphragmatic action is the dominant force involved in normal quiet breathing and adds power to coughing and sneezing.

The diaphragm is innervated by the phrenic nerve arising primarily from the fourth cervical cord segment but receiving small contributions from the third and fifth cord segments. Lesions at or above this level cause diaphragmatic paralysis and loss of spontaneous respiration. This creates a need for lifelong artificial respiratory support. Lesions occurring below the cervical plexus (C_{1-4}) may allow partial or full diaphragmatic function, but respiratory function will be subnormal due to involvement of the remaining muscles of breathing. Diaphragmatic movement may be described as strong or weak. One side may be functioning but the other not.

The *intercostal muscles* are a large number of small muscles located between each pair of ribs. See Figure 9–3. Contraction of the *external intercostal muscles* elevates the rib cage, leading to expansion of the anteroposterior and lateral dimensions of the chest wall. These muscles may be responsible for 30% to 35% of effective ventilation (Cheshire and Flack 1978–79).

The intercostal muscles are innervated by the upper thoracic cord (T_{1-7}). Lesions above T_6 or T_7 paralyze intercostal function, which destroys the ability to cough and breathe deeply.

Coughing requires strong respiratory muscle contractions to build up the high pressures that force air out of the lungs. This cleansing mechanism is vital to remove foreign particles or mucus from the bronchial tree. Both quadriplegics and high paraplegic patients have difficulty producing an effective cough. Assessment of this problem in high paraplegic patients may be deceiving because they appear to be breathing normally. Close observation, however, shows that they have difficulty taking a deep breath.

When intercostal muscles are not moving, *paradoxical respiration* is evident. Paradoxical respiration, also referred to as *abdominal breathing,* is a familiar condition in quadriplegia when the diaphragm is the sole remaining muscle of breathing. The paralyzed muscles of the thoracic cage passively collapse with inspiration (as the diaphragm descends) and expand with expiration (as the diaphragm ascends) (Tyson et al. 1978). As this is the reversal of normal ventilatory movements, the condition is easily recognized. In the unconscious patient paradoxical breathing is the most important diagnostic sign of cervical injury.

The *accessory muscles of breathing* are the sternocleidomastoid and scalenus muscles located in the neck and upper chest. The accessory muscles help elevate the upper rib cage during inspiration (Figure 9–4).

These muscles are also innervated by the cervical cord (C_{2-7}). Only very high injuries totally impair the function of the accessory muscles. Quadriplegic patients tend to overwork these muscles. It is possible to observe patients heaving deeply, with excessive shoulder movements, to compensate for the loss of other chest muscles.

The major muscles of expiration are the *abdominal muscles* (Figure 9–5). The internal intercostal muscles also aid in expiratory movements. The muscles of the anterior abdominal wall decrease the size of the thoracic cage by pulling

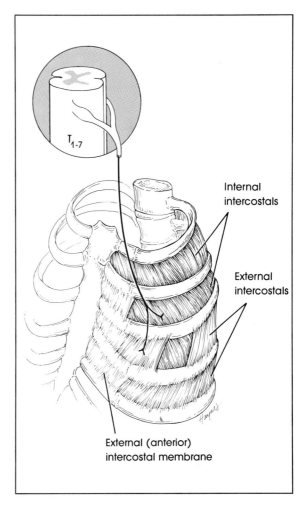

FIGURE 9–3 ■ The intercostal muscles aid in chest expansion and are innervated by the T_{1-7} cord segments.

downward and inward on the rib cage and forcing the abdominal viscera upward against the diaphragm. These muscles provide resistance to a working diaphragm and thus help return the thoracic cage to its resting position. The most recent literature suggests that 60% to 65% of breathing capacity is generated from the combined actions of the diaphragm and accessory muscles (Cheshire and Flack 1978–1979).

The abdominal muscles are innervated by the lower thoracic cord (T_{6-12}). Lesions occurring at this level paralyze abdominal muscle function and particularly interfere with forceful expiration (such as in coughing).

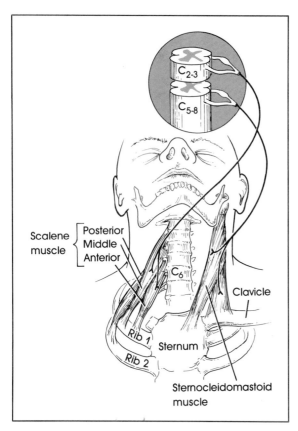

FIGURE 9–4 ■ The accessory muscles are most often preserved following a cord injury, and therefore they become overworked. They elevate the upper rib cage during inspiration and are innervated by the C_{2-8} cord segments.

Palpation, percussion, and auscultation

The techniques of palpation, percussion, and auscultation are used to assess vibrations transmitted throughout the respiratory system. Procedure 9–1 further details these techniques.

In *palpation* the hands are placed on the patient's chest to help determine the symmetry of chest expansion. The initial assessment is usually limited to the anterior chest while the patient is supine due to necessary immobilization.

Percussion involves tapping the chest to assess the position, size, and density of underlying structures. When percussed, normal lung tissue has a resonant sound. Diminished vibrations occur when structures are more solid. This dullness may be heard normally, as over the heart and liver, or abnormally when large amounts of retained secretions clog lung tissue.

Auscultation of the chest using a stethoscope is used to determine breath sounds, voice sounds, and adventitious or abnormal sounds.

Breath sounds are described as *vesicular* — soft, quiet sounds heard over much of the lung as air passes into the alveoli (particularly on inspiration); *bronchial* — loud, tubular sounds heard over the major bronchi and trachea (mainly on expiration); and *bronchovesicular* — a combination of the two. Bronchovesicular sounds occur when the bronchi come close to the lung surface, which is mainly at the apices and between the scapulae posteriorly. Diminished or absent sounds indicate abnormality. Location is also important. Bronchial sounds should not occur where vesicular sounds should be, and so on.

Voice sounds are transmitted through the respiratory system and can be detected as vibrations on the chest wall. These vibrations are termed *fremitus*. An increase in fremitus, as occurs with consolidation of a lung, or decrease or absence of fremitus, as occurs with obstruction of a bronchus, indicates abnormality.

Listening for *adventitious sounds* superimposed on breath sounds is probably the technique used most frequently by nurses. As with assessment of vital signs, it is not the isolated assessment, but the comparison of data to indicate deterioration or improvement, that is most helpful. For example, it is important to listen to the patient's chest before and after a session of chest physiotherapy to determine the effectiveness of the treatment. The chest should be auscultated in a systematic fashion similar to that used in percussion.

Describing adventitious sounds can be confusing, as a wide variety of terms are used in the literature. For clarification it is better to describe the characteristics of abnormal sounds rather than simply to label them. The most common descriptions are of rales and rhonchi. *Rales* are continuous, moist, crackling, or bubbling sounds that are more evident on inspiration as air passes through alveoli that are partially collapsed or filled with fluid. *Rhonchi* are discontinuous, drier sounds—sometimes described as musical, whistling, or wheezing sounds—that are more evident on expiration as air passes through a tracheobronchial tree that has been narrowed, by lung secretion, for example. Occasionally, a pleural rub or grating sound of breathing may be heard.

Extrathoracic signs and symptoms of distress

Extrathoracic signs and symptoms of distress may include sternal indrawing, trachea tug, nasal flaring, facial tension, and shortness of breath.

Other signs and symptoms of respiratory insufficiency are reflected in the cardiovascular and central nervous systems. These systems are most sensitive to hypoxia and CO_2 retention in the blood. Observe for compensatory tachycardia; poor color ranging from peripheral cyanosis involving the extremities to central cyanosis (which can be detected by a bluish tinge of the lips, tongue, and mucosa of the mouth); and subtle changes in level of consciousness such as restlessness, irritability, or confusion (progressing to coma if unarrested).

Nurses should never underestimate the negative effects of severe pain, anxiety, or agitation on respiratory function. It is important to listen to the patient. If a patient claims difficulty in breathing, the nurse should assess the total respiratory picture, including an assessment of the chest and related systems and of the artificial airway and mechanical ventilator if in use. If the patient is still not comfortable, it is best to check the arterial blood gases.

Diagnostic Procedures

Pulmonary function tests

Pulmonary function tests, especially those performed at the bedside, are becoming increasingly useful to assess pulmonary volumes and pressures in prevention, recognition, and treatment of pulmonary complications in patients with spinal cord injuries.

The following normal values are based on findings for the young adult male (Kozier and Erb 1983). The values are about 20% to 25% less in the female. Other variables depend on age, build, physical condition, and position, so a reading within 20% of the predicted normal value

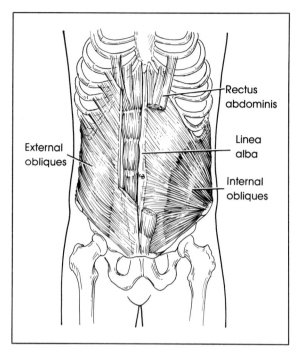

FIGURE 9–5 ■ The abdominal muscles, innervated by the T_{6-12} cord segments, must be intact to produce a forceful cough. Ineffective coughing is a major cause of respiratory insufficiency for persons with spinal cord injury.

may be acceptable, with an even wider range for the quadriplegic patient. Abnormal values seen with quadriplegia are based on Cheshire and Coats (1966), Carter (1979), McMichan et al. (1980), and Ledsome and Sharp (1981). It should be noted that as research and management techniques improve, abnormal values once considered acceptable will likely not remain so.

The amount of air in the lungs can be divided into *pulmonary (lung) volumes*. Two or more pulmonary volumes combine to form a *pulmonary (lung) capacity*.

Lung volumes

1. *Tidal volume* (TV). The tidal volume is the amount of air inspired and expired in normal quiet breathing. Its normal value is 500 mL. Eventually a stable, uncomplicated quadriplegic patient under basal conditions requires a tidal volume of 350 mL.

2. *Inspiratory reserve volume* (IRV). The inspiratory reserve volume refers to the amount of air forcefully inspired in addition to the tidal volume. Its normal value is 3000 mL. Especially at the onset of injury, the inspiratory reserve volume is somewhat decreased. This is due mostly to the flaccid paralysis of the intercostal and abdominal muscles occurring with spinal shock, creating an unstable chest. Eventually the inspiratory reserve volume should improve, although it will always be slightly subnormal.

3. *Expiratory reserve volume* (ERV). The expiratory reserve volume refers to the amount of air forcefully exhaled below the tidal volume. Its normal value is 1100 mL, and it measures a person's ability to cough. It has been estimated that with quadriplegia the expiratory reserve volume is decreased to from one third of normal to virtually nothing. This decrease is expected to be permanent.

4. *Residual volume* (RV). The residual volume is the amount of air, approximately 1200 mL, left in the lungs after exhalation of the tidal volume and expiratory reserve volume. This residual volume of air is involved with the gaseous exchange between the alveoli and pulmonary capillaries. Because of difficulties with forceful exhalation of air, this value is at least 10% higher than normal with quadriplegia. If the ERV is nonexistent, the RV is totally elevated and mechanical ventilation is needed. (It is not possible to measure this at the bedside.)

Lung capacities

1. *Total lung capacity* (TLC). Total lung capacity is the total of all the volumes and is the maximum volume to which the lungs can be expanded. Its average value is 5800 mL. An overall decrease is common in patients with spinal cord injuries.

2. *Inspiratory capacity* (IC). The inspiratory capacity is the tidal volume and the inspiratory reserve volume combined (about 3500 mL). Again a slight decrease is anticipated with cord injury.

3. *Vital capacity* (VC). The vital capacity is the most important value to consider in patients with spinal cord injuries. It can be measured quickly and easily at the bedside with a spirometer. The patient is instructed to take a deep breath and expel as much air as possible.

The vital capacity consists of the tidal volume, the inspiratory reserve volume, and the expiratory reserve volume (4600 mL). This combines all the lung volumes except the residual volume and indicates the patient's ability to take a deep breath. The normal value is approximately 4600 mL. Initial readings average from 1150 mL to 1600 mL (approximately 25% to 35% of the predicted normal value). With the passage of time and appropriate treatment, such as chest physiotherapy, deep breathing with assisted coughing, and/or mechanical ventilation for an interim period, values significantly improve (Figures 9–6 and 9–7).

> Patients with spinal cord injury at C_5 and below have a forced vital capacity (FVC) that may be expected to be about 30% of predicted normal in the acute stage. Patients with injury at C_4 usually have smaller FVC. A significant increase of the FVC can be expected within five weeks of injury with an approximate doubling at three months. Patients in whom the FVD decreases to less than 25% of predicted normal are likely to develop respiratory failure requiring ventilator support. [Ledsome and Sharp 1981: 44]

Cheshire and Flack (1978–79: 163) explain:

> It is in the context of the ability of the patient to handle a respiratory infection that the vital capacity becomes of critical importance. In the patient with respiratory infection, the greater the vital capacity, the greater the ability to move secretions from the alveoli to the airways, hence minimizing the chances of consolidation and the complications of inadequate gas exchange in the alveoli. The majority of quadriplegic patients are unable to bring secretions to the mouth, but with an adequate vital capacity they are able to bring secretions to the airways, and with assisted coughing, can bring secretions from the airways to the mouth.

4. *Functional residual capacity* (FRC). The functional residual capacity consists of the expiratory reserve volume and the residual volume (2300 mL). It is the amount of air left in the lungs after normal expiration and generally remains within normal limits with spinal cord injury.

Summary There are several important factors to remember about pulmonary function tests:

- Evaluation made on a trend developed in consecutive readings is more valuable than an isolated reading.
- Anxiety, sedation, and other injuries significantly affect pulmonary function during the acute stage.
- The time factor after injury is critical. As spinal shock passes and flaccid paralysis converts to spasticity, improvement should occur. Increased intercostal and abdominal muscle tone tends to stabilize the chest and cause more effective contractions to aid respiration.
- Breathing exercises help strengthen inspiratory muscles, but the major problems lie with impaired expiratory flow, which hampers the patient's ability to produce an effective cough.
- The VC is the single most important pulmonary function test to assess coughing ability.

Arterial blood gas analysis

Adequate or insufficient gaseous exchange in the lungs is reflected by arterial blood gas analysis, which is an essential component of assessment for all spinal cord injured patients.

A blood gas sample should be included in the admission workup. Serial evaluations provide a consistent picture of results and are most valuable for assessment thereafter. For example, a blood gas sample obtained before chest physiotherapy one day and after the treatment the next will not accurately reflect the patient's status.

Analysis includes PaO_2, $PaCO_2$, and a measurement of the acid-base balance (expressed in mEq/L or base excess). The normal values are as follows:

PaO_2	80 to 100 mmHg
$PaCO_2$	36 to 44 mmHg (plus or minus 4 mmHg)
pH	7.36 to 7.44
HCO_3	23 to 28 mEq/L or
Base excess	+2.5 to −2.5

When considering the desired PaO_2, the time interval after injury is important. Initially, maintaining a PaO_2 at or above 80 mmHg is recom-

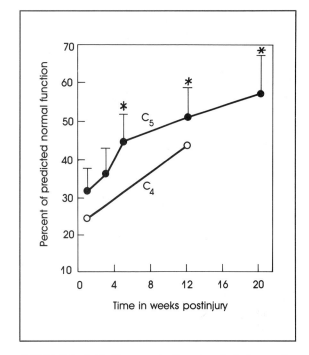

FIGURE 9–6 ■ Changes in functional vital capacity (FVC) at intervals following spinal cord injury in five patients with lesions at C_4 and in eleven patients with lesions at C_5. Vertical bars indicate the standard error of mean. The asterisks indicate that the values are significantly different from the values measured at one week after injury. (From J. R. Ledsome and J. Sharpe, unpublished material.)

mended because "spinal cord oxygen tension in experimental paraplegia quickly falls below normal tissue requirements, even in the absence of systemic hypoxemia. Systemic hypoxemia may therefore increase the severity of spinal cord injury" (Tyson et al. 1978). Damage is greatest to neurons close to the injury site for an estimated 72 hours following the event.

Gradual adjustment to maintaining a minimal PaO_2 of 60 mmHg may be generally considered acceptable by some for an uncomplicated, stable quadriplegic patient under basal conditions. However, with advancements in respiratory management and rehabilitative techniques, more recent literature suggests that the PaO_2 and $PaCO_2$ are nearer normal following the acute period.

The $PaCO_2$ is generally considered a more accurate reflection of alveolar ventilation. The

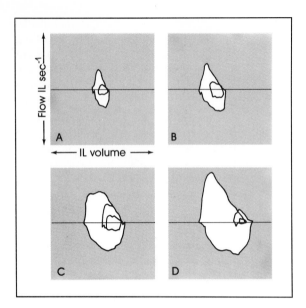

FIGURE 9–7 ■ Changes in the maximum expiratory flow volume curves in one patient with complete C_5 quadriplegia at intervals following spinal cord injury. (A) On admission 24 hours after injury. (B) One week after injury. (C) Three weeks after injury. (D) Six months after injury. Note the significant increase in function as time progresses. (From J. R. Ledsome and J. Sharpe, 1981.)

quadriplegic patient has a tendency toward hypercarbia, a buildup of CO_2 the blood. Hypercarbia is most often associated with inadequate chest movement and hence inadequate ventilation. The chest needs to move; therefore with quadriplegia, diminished potency and decreased coughing ability are particular problems. A $PaCO_2$ of 45 to 50 mmHg can be anticipated, especially during the acute period.

Measurements of acid-base balance should generally be within normal limits. The nurse should be alert for development of respiratory acidosis caused by hypoventilation. When CO_2 is retained in the body, excessive production of carbonic acid causes the pH to fall below 7.35. The $PaCO_2$ rises. Respiratory arrest is imminent if the $PaCO_2$ is elevated above 60 mmHg. The quadriplegic patient may tolerate slightly higher levels due to the chronic elevation of $PaCO_2$. The HCO_3 may remain normal or increase. The patient may attempt to blow off CO_2 by increasing the rate and depth of respirations. It is most important to note any change in the level of con-

sciousness ranging from confusion to coma. Renal compensation does not reach a maximum level for five to seven days to stabilize acid-base imbalances. Therefore, immediate treatment may include mechanical ventilation to control carbon dioxide blood levels, administration of bicarbonate to neutralize acidosis, and treatment of associated electrolyte imbalances.

The analysis of blood gas results may reveal another complication, metabolic alkalosis. Loss of metabolic acids through vomiting and nasogastric tube drainage associated with paralytic ileus will cause a rise in pH and HCO_3 while the $PaCO_2$ remains within normal limits. Metabolic alkalosis is discussed further in Chapter 12.

Chest X ray

A chest X ray must be taken on admission to assess the patient's current pulmonary status, detect associated trauma, rule out preexisting pulmonary complications, and establish baseline data. Serial chest X rays are valuable in evaluating treatment of such complications as pneumonia.

It is important to remember and to remind others that while it is customary for chest X rays to be taken with the patient in a semi-Fowler's or upright position, in cases of spinal injury the initial chest X rays are taken with the patient supine due to immobilization. A pneumothorax, for example, which would be clearly visible in a standing patient because the air would rise to the lung apices, would be more difficult to see in a supine patient because the air would diffuse over the entire space between the lung and the chest wall.

NURSING INTERVENTIONS

Preventive Measures

Prophylactic chest treatment focuses on promoting adequate ventilation and preventing retention of secretions. To be effective, the techniques used must be practiced diligently. It should be mentioned that early mobilization, made possible by advanced medicosurgical techniques, has dramatically reduced problems associated with stasis of secretions.

To promote adequate ventilation

Upper airway obstruction The first priority of respiratory care is to ensure a clear airway. Nasopharyngeal and oral suction, placement of an oral airway, side positioning (which may involve emergency logrolling the patient when an unstable spinal fracture is not yet protected with traction), bag ventilation, intubation, and ventilatory support may be needed. Life-saving techniques must be oriented to cervical spine injury to reduce the risk of further neurological damage. For a review of these emergency procedures see Chapter 3.

Aspiration of vomitus blocking the airway is another potentially fatal complication for the patient with quadriplegia. Burke and Murray (1975) emphasize that unrecognized paralytic ileus is probably the most common cause of sudden death in the quadriplegic patient during the first 48 hours when decreased coughing ability leads to aspiration of stomach contents, resulting in respiratory arrest. Associated abdominal distension also inhibits diaphragmatic movement. To ensure a patent airway prophylactic use of nasogastric drainage to evacuate stomach contents is recommended.

Severe nasal congestion is common and troublesome for people with quadriplegia and is aggravated by the supine and prone positions. This may be partly due to the interruption of the cervical sympathetic fibers supplying the face and nose (Carter 1979). Anticongestant nose drops are of little value in alleviating the difficulty; turning the patient from side to side is more helpful.

Patients may tend to gag or choke on food particles as they gradually resume a full diet. During mealtime, staff must provide adequate supervision and a communication system so patients can indicate that help is needed. The assisted coughing technique and/or oral suctioning will help clear the airway. See Procedure 9–4. It's a good idea to have a portable suction machine handy in a communal dining setting.

Stasis of secretions Regular turning plays an important role in preventing secretion stasis in dependent areas of the lung. Even a minor adjustment to the patient's position promotes comfort and prevents accumulation of secretions. In one study (Hoffman 1977), continuous reading of PaO_2 and $PaCO_2$ were monitored in a patient on a respirator. There was remarkable improvement in arterial blood gas values within fifteen minutes after a position change. The patient should be turned every two hours or more frequently if desired.

To prevent cramping or restricting diaphragmatic movement, it is necessary to position the patient in correct body alignment when recumbent and support good body posture when sitting. If an abdominal binder is applied, it should not extend over any portion of the rib cage. If the patient's chest is abnormally shaped, a Halo vest may inhibit chest expansion.

The prone position aids drainage of secretions and allows full percussion of the posterior chest. However, in the newly injured patient, the position may be difficult to tolerate or contraindicated, as with chest trauma or when mechanical ventilation is used. An undesired autonomic *vagovagal* response triggering cardiopulmonary arrest is sometimes linked with sudden and profound changes in position immediately after injury. Most quadriplegic patients nursed on a Stryker frame with cervical traction experience neck pain when turning or have problems with chest expansion.

To combat retention of secretions

Manual techniques used to clear the chest Manual techniques used to clear the chest are often referred to as *chest physiotherapy* and include breathing exercises, assisted coughing, vibration and percussion, and postural drainage.

The need for and evaluation of treatments is determined by the chest assessment. (To review chest assessment techniques see Procedure 9–1.) A *moist, unproductive cough* is the first sign of retained secretions and requires vigorous treatment. Other symptoms are increased rate of shallow breathing, dyspnea, or repeated ineffective attempts to cough. Treatments are generally given every 2 to 4 hours. Most seriously ill patients will not tolerate more than 15 minutes per session. The patient's tolerance and general condition must be taken into account to avoid fatigue. Exhausting the patient defeats the purpose. Procedure 9–2 outlines some helpful planning techniques to minimize this problem.

PROCEDURE 9–2 ■ PLANNING CHEST CLEARING TECHNIQUE SESSIONS

Purpose

The purpose of planning chest clearing technique sessions is to improve effectiveness of the sessions and conserve patient energy.

Action	Rationale
1. Coordinate interdisciplinary team members to plan treatments that coincide with regular turning times.	To promote rest and sleep periods for the patient.
2. Capitalize on peak periods when medications such as analgesics or bronchiodilators will be most effective.	To promote patient comfort and maximize action of medications.
3. Avoid mealtimes or oral feedings by 30 minutes.	To prevent aspiration.
4. Maintain adequate systemic hydration; avoid over-hydration.	Adequate hydration liquefies secretions sufficiently for expectoration; overhydration leads to fluid accumulation in the lungs.
5. Carefully explain each session to patient (and family when necessary).	To maximize patient cooperation. Vigorous chest therapy can be initially frightening to both patients and families.
6. Check to see that the airway is clear before proceeding. Preoxygenation with a higher percentage of oxygen before oral or tracheal suctioning may be used with all chest clearing techniques.	

Breathing exercises will build strength of existing muscles of respiration and promote adequate ventilation. See Procedure 9–3.

Assisted or diaphragmatic coughing will help clear the airway of secretions or trapped food particles. This technique is of lifelong value to all quadriplegic and many high paraplegic patients. Even though high paraplegic patients may seem to be breathing normally, their ability to cough may be severely impaired. See Procedure 9–4.

Vibration and percussion (or clapping) are usually used in conjunction with *postural drainage* to prevent retention of secretions. See Procedures 9–5 and 9–6. These techniques are used, for example, when the patient is on initial bedrest or has had a relapse caused by infection.

As the chest clears, treatments are reduced. Manual techniques are considered effective when respirations are unlabored, lungs are clear on auscultation with air entry to all lobes and vital capacity, and arterial blood gases are within normal limits for the patient. If the patient's condition deteriorates, restorative measures must be considered.

Incentive spirometry Incentive spirometry is based on the fundamental principles of neuromuscular exercise and behavioral psychology (Cheshire and Flack 1978–79). The objective is to provide a practical means to increase the patient's vital capacity and thus increase coughing ability to combat intercurrent respiratory infection. Neuromuscular exercise is based on repetitive and increasingly difficult movements, in this case to strengthen the diaphragm and other muscles of breathing. Gradually, the patient is able to take deeper breaths and exhale more forcefully. Operant conditioning techniques use positive reinforcement to encourage desirable behavior. When the patient's efforts to breathe deeply are acknowledged by positive consequences, such as praise from a nurse or other patients, this behavior is more likely to be repeated again in the future. Thus the nurse's enthusiasm is a key influence on the success or failure of this technique.

The Spirocare Incentive Breathing Exerciser (distributed by Marion Laboratories, Kansas City, Mo.) is a device that provides positive

PROCEDURE 9–3 ■ BREATHING EXERCISES

Purpose

The purpose of breathing exercises is to ensure air entry to all parts of the lung by encouraging slow, relaxed, and deliberate deep breathing. This procedure can be used with incentive spirometry, which helps motivate the patient when vital capacity can be measured to monitor progress.

Action	Rationale
1. Instruct patient to take deep breath in through nose and exhale through mouth (rate: 6 to 10 breaths per minute).	
2. Place hands on diaphragm to help patient focus attention (even though patient may not be able to feel your hand).	
3. If cervical traction is in place, provide prism glasses.	Restriction of head movements limits field of vision.

feedback through its system of brightly colored lights and digital display to encourage the patient to perform sustained maximum inspiratory movements. The system is goal oriented. The desired volume range is selected and displayed on one panel. The measurements of the patient's efforts are displayed on the adjacent panel so that results can be compared directly.

Carbon dioxide rebreathing therapy The technique of rebreathing CO_2 may be used for selected patients to improve deep breathing ability and combat formation of atelectasis. The desired effects are initially to increase the respiratory rate and then to increase the depth of respirations and stimulate coughing. See Procedure 9–7.

Intermittent positive pressure breathing treatments (IPPB) IPPB is given to aerate and humidify underventilated areas of the lung created by the quadriplegic patient's inability to sigh and deep breathe regularly. Promoting alveolar distension in this manner may actually stretch the lungs and thorax. When IPPB is used as a strictly prophylactic measure, the desired effects must be weighed carefully against the possibility of intrathoracic pressure creating cardiovascular embarrassment by interfering with venous return to the heart. In patients with spinal cord injuries and circulation that is already compromised, nurses must be alert for delirium, lowered blood pressure, reflex tachycardia, and impaired peripheral circulation (Rau and Rau 1977).

At the first signs of chest congestion, aerosol medications such as bronchodilators and mucolytic agents may be administered to enhance the effects of this deep breathing technique. A typical treatment may consist of 2 mL Mucomyst, 2 mL 1/4% Neosynephrine, and 0.5 mL Bronkosol added to the nebulizer (Carter 1979). Humidification is increased when sterile water is added to the nebulizer. The IPPB ventilators may be used with a mouthpiece or tracheostomy adapter.

Treatments are usually ordered every four to six hours. Each treatment must be followed with manual techniques sufficient to clear the chest of mobilized secretions. Suctioning may be necessary. As the chest clears, treatments are gradually discontinued.

Ultrasonic nebulization The ultrasonic (electronic) nebulizer produces a fine nonheated mist from distilled water. It is used in conjunction with manual methods to clear the chest; to loosen thick, tenacious bronchial secretions; and to stimulate a cough reflex. This combats consolidation and atelectasis in the alveoli.

The mist created by the nebulizer is delivered to the patient by an oxygen flow system. Treatment sessions must not exceed ten minutes and *must* be followed immediately by clapping, vibrating, and assisted coughing with postural

PROCEDURE 9–4 ■ ASSISTED COUGHING

Purpose

The purpose of assisted coughing is to help the patient expectorate secretions when partial or complete paralysis of the abdominal muscles and inability to take deep breath reduce effective coughing and to prevent accumulation of secretions extending down the bronchial tree.

Action	Rationale
1. Instruct patient to breathe in deeply and "double cough," that is, cough twice in succession without inspiration between.	This adds more expulsion force for a more efficient cough.

2. Place forearm over upper abdomen and diaphragm. Place other hand over chest wall. Move hand around until most effective spot is found.

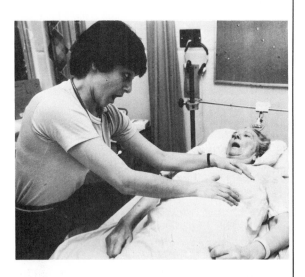

3. Maintain an even and firm pressure directed inward and upward and a "bounce" pressure as patient attempts to cough. Timing is crucial. Apply pressure *only* after inspiration is complete.

4. If patient is in chair, from behind place clasped hands over diaphragm and assist with a sharp pull inward and upward on cough or after inspiration. Paraplegic patients may fold arms over upper abdomen to assist own efforts, but quadriplegic patients need strong support.

Strength requires weight of assistant's body but not sufficient to cause the patient pain.

---

drainage to clear the chest. Otherwise, a dangerous excess of fluid will remain in the lung, which defeats the purpose of the treatment. Treatments are contraindicated if the patient has fluid retention or pulmonary edema. Bronchospasm resulting from inhalation of the mist can be a problem for some patients. Medications are not compatible with this system; ultrasound may degrade the drug, and calculation of the dosage inhaled is unreliable.

Restorative Measures

Serious insult to respiratory function often requires nursing the patient in a critical care setting. It is not within the scope of this text to provide a comprehensive guide for the care of the critically ill patient, but rather, how to build on existing knowledge and skills to meet the additional needs of patients with spinal cord injuries. To benefit most from the information about restorative measures, nurses should be familiar with in-depth physical assessment of the chest and should be comfortable caring for the patient requiring supplemental oxygen, an artificial airway (including deep tracheal suctioning), and mechanical ventilation. Recommended reading for review of these topics is included at the end of this chapter.

Oxygen therapy

Supplemental oxygen is usually necessary on admission and may be required at intervals

PROCEDURE 9–5 ■ VIBRATION AND PERCUSSION (CLAPPING)

Purpose

The purpose of vibration and percussion (clapping) is to dislodge and mobilize secretions in the bronchial tree. Secretions can then be expectorated or suctioned out. These techniques are used in conjunction with postural drainage.

Action

1. Auscultate the patient's chest before each treatment.

2. Place whole hands in contact with affected area of the chest wall. To vibrate chest, apply vigorous, rhythmical, intermittent pressure during expiration.

Rationale

To establish baseline data for comparison at end of treatment. This technique may be modified to fine tremor in presence of rib fractures.

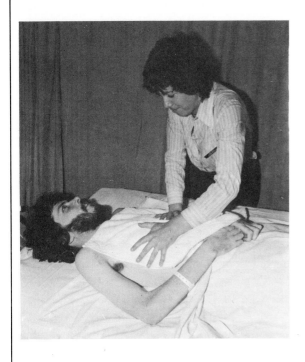
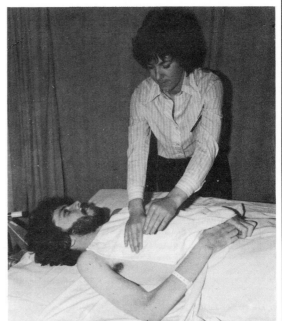

3. Place relaxed, cupped hands over affected area of chest and perform rhythmical percussion. This is called clapping.

4. Work from more dependent to less dependent areas of the lung.

5. If necessary, assist the patient to expectorate (as in Procedure 9–4) or suction out the secretions.

6. Auscultate the patient's chest after treatment.

This technique is contraindicated in the presence of rib fractures, pneumothorax, or acute cardiac disease, for example.

You may wish to hand ventilate the intubated patient on a mechanical ventilator; coordinate your efforts with the co-worker suctioning.

This will determine the treatment's effectiveness.

PROCEDURE 9–6 ■ POSTURAL DRAINAGE (TRENDELENBURG POSITION)

Purpose

The purpose of postural drainage is to promote gravity-assisted drainage of secretions. This position enhances effectiveness of vibration and percussion techniques. Unless contraindicated by associated injury, such as head injury, it is desirable to proceed with postural drainage with all spinal injured patients (within limitations of orthopedic alignment, tolerance, and type of immobilization bed in use).

Action	Rationale
1. Tip or tilt entire bed to lower head of bed approximately 18 inches.	This is possible on immobilization beds (Stoke-Eggerton tilting bed, the Wedge Stryker turning frame, and the ICU stretcher bed). Regular beds require placement of solid blocks under the foot.

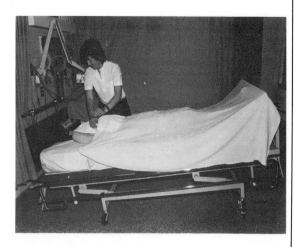

2. Place patient in side-lying (alternate) supine or prone position.

3. To treat complications in specific lung segments, collaborate with physiotherapist to choose appropriate position.

When a patient is not allowed to sit up, the most difficult area to drain is the apices of the lungs. Sometimes tilt table therapy is possible.

---

throughout the rehabilitation period should pulmonary complications arise. Nurses must recognize the need for supplemental oxygen. Symptoms include rapid, shallow respiration or dyspnea; a pale or dusky color eventually leading to peripheral or central cyanosis; possible coolness of the extremities; and tachycardia. Restlessness or subtle altered changes in judgment or behavior may be the first sign of a change in the level of consciousness. Irritability, confusion, and drowsiness progressing to coma may follow. In addition, a decrease in the vital capacity or a lowered PaO_2 on a blood gas analysis may occur.

In an effort to compensate for limited chest expansion, paralyzed patients will breathe through both nose and mouth; therefore, oxygen is generally delivered via face mask and *must* be humidified to prevent drying of mucosa and secretions. A regular mask is used to deliver an oxygen concentration of 40% to 60%; a mask with an attached rebreathing bag yields a higher concentration; and a Venturi mask is needed to deliver lower concentrations of 24% to 40%. This mask is designed with increased exhalation ports to prevent rebreathing carbon dioxide. To achieve the necessary high air flow, narrow tubing, which is not compatible with humidification, must be used. As the use of dry oxygen is undesirable, humidified compressed air with an atmospheric concentration of 21% oxygen may be the best alternative.

PROCEDURE 9–7 ■ CARBON DIOXIDE REBREATHING THERAPY

Purpose

The purpose of carbon dioxide rebreathing therapy is to improve deep breathing and to stimulate coughing. This therapy is a preventive measure to combat atelectasis formation.

Action	Rationale
1. Fill a reservoir bag with a mixture of 10% CO_2 and 90% O_2 (from a prepared tank).	
2. Have the patient hold the mouthpiece securely in mouth (or use a securely fitted mask) and wear nose clips.	There must be a complete seal between the patient's mouth and the reservoir bag.
3. Ask the patient to breathe in and out through the mouth until more and deeper breaths are taken and coughing is stimulated.	
4. Discontinue treatment if the patient complains of dizziness or headache.	This indicates too much CO_2 in the blood.

Artificial airways

An artificial airway is necessary when a patient develops an upper airway obstruction, copious amounts of secretions interfering with airway patency, or the need for mechanical ventilation.

When dealing with spinal injuries, upper airway obstruction may be a problem at the scene of the accident or on admission to the emergency room. Accumulation of secretions and the need for mechanical ventilation tend to have a more gradual onset; hence elective intubation is more likely. Anticipated dysfunction and length of time the patient is expected to be intubated will influence the type of airway selected.

Psychological preparation for elective intubation can help relieve the fear and anxiety associated with the discomfort, total dependency, and inability to talk. Reassurance that this is a temporary measure offers some relief, but it is more important to establish a system of making the patient's needs known. As this problem is most severe when the patient is on a mechanical ventilator, it will be discussed in that section.

Endotracheal intubation Endotracheal intubation is useful for emergency or for short-term intubation (approximately 72 hours). This airway is most often selected for the paraplegic patient with associated chest problems and may occasionally be used for postoperative management.

Endotracheal tubes extend from the nose or mouth to the trachea. The nasotracheal route is preferred for cervical injuries as less manipulation of the head and neck is required during insertion. Endotracheal tubes are not recommended and are poorly tolerated by quadriplegic patients (particularly conscious patients) as they tend to induce retching, vomiting, and excess salivation, which are extremely hazardous.

Tracheotomy A *tracheotomy* is selected for long-term management (longer than 72 hours). It is useful for the quadriplegic patient or the paraplegic patient with preexisting lung conditions or severe chest injury. This airway is essential for the quadriplegic patient requiring permanent mechanical ventilation and is used when a patient is intolerant of an endotracheal tube.

Tracheostomy tubes are inserted during an operative procedure. The surgeon makes a horizontal incision between the second and third tracheal rings just large enough to admit the tracheostomy tube. A tracheotomy is ideally an elective procedure, but may be undertaken as an extreme emergency measure. Advantages include ease of removal of secretions, reduction of anatomical dead space to reduce the work of breathing, less chance of tube displacement, and increased patient comfort. Complications include that of the procedure itself, hemorrhage, tracheal trauma, and airway obstruction.

Whenever a tracheostomy tube is in place, a major safety precaution is to place a tube of the same size at the patient's bedside. In addition, a sterile tracheostomy dressing tray, with retractors or tracheal dilator forceps, should be placed in a central position to facilitate emergency tube replacement.

There are two main types of tracheostomy tubes:

1. The *disposable Portex-plastic cuffed tube.* Most patients requiring a tracheostomy will also require initial mechanical ventilation, so Portex-plastic cuffed tubes are used to provide a good seal for the respirator. The inflated cuff occludes the space between the tracheostomy tube and the trachea to prevent air from escaping. The wide-bore tube with a soft cuff (high residual volume) is recommended to facilitate suctioning and minimize pressure on the trachea. The cuff must be deflated periodically to relieve all pressure on the wall of the trachea. The patient can also speak when the cuff is deflated.

2. The *reusable metal tube (uncuffed).* Metal tracheostomy tubes are more suitable for long-term or permanent use mainly because the small size minimizes tracheal damage and the design facilitates easier cleaning. They are generally used when mechanical ventilation is no longer required to ease removal of secretions and decrease the effort involved in breathing by reducing physiological dead space. With advancements in preventive and restorative measures in respiratory care, the need for a permanent tracheostomy is no longer as great. The stabilized ventilator-dependent quadriplegic person uses this uncuffed tube to "talk around" when air escapes through the mouth and nose on expiration. Metal tubes are available in narrow diameter and short lengths to provide the smallest functional artificial airway possible. There are no cuff problems to cause necrosis. The metal tubes have two parts: the outer cannula and a removable inner cannula. To clean, the nurse simply removes the inner cannula, cleans it with normal saline or hydrogen peroxide to remove crusting, and returns and locks it into place.

Mechanical ventilation

Patients with very high cord injuries suffering instant diaphragmatic paralysis will require immediate resuscitation and lifelong ventilatory support. Occasionally patients with severe chest trauma may also need immediate artificial respiration. For the most part, as previously mentioned, intubation and mechanical ventilation is an elective measure undertaken when a number of factors have been considered.

Deterioration of respiration is mainly caused by extreme fatigue as the work of breathing is increased and/or neurological edema expands to impair phrenic nerve function. Nurses can assist physicians to identify and minimize such general problems as poor cardiovascular status, pain, sleep deprivation, or abdominal distension, which may be interfering with respiratory function. Nurses will observe the nature and rate of respirations, particularly watching for ineffective, rapid, shallow breathing; increasingly noisy respirations; and approaching periods of apnea (or near apnea) leading to eventual signs of severe distress. They must recognize the onset of such pulmonary complications as hypoxia, atelectasis, pneumonia, and pulmonary edema. Certainly associated chest injuries or preexisting disease can profoundly affect the patient's course of treatment.

The physician will consider the diagnostic findings in light of values acceptable for the stabilized quadriplegic person to determine to what extent the present illness will alter these values. When it becomes obvious that the patient will not be able to maintain adequate respiratory function if the present course continues, mechanical ventilation is necessary and used to avoid complete respiratory failure.

Nurses can capitalize on the observation time to prepare the patient and family psychologically for mechanical ventilation. It is important to minimize apprehension so the patient does not fight the machine and increase breathing difficulties.

Types of mechanical ventilators The most commonly used ventilators are described as pressure-controlled or volume-controlled machines (see Fuchs 1979 and Holloway 1979).

1. The *positive pressure–cycled ventilator,* such as the Bird Mark 7 or the Bennett PRII, ends the inspiratory phase when a preset pressure has been reached. In other words, providing the airway is clear, the predetermined pressure will deliver the desired volume of gas. If the airway is obstructed or restricted in any way, however, the predetermined pressure will be attained earlier and only part of the volume of gas will be delivered.

2. The *volume-cycled machine* ends the inspiratory phase when a predetermined amount of gas has been delivered. Certain safety mechanisms abort the inspiratory phase if extreme pressures are reached while the ventilator is attempting to deliver the preset volume of gas. Volume-cycled machines include the Bennett MA–1 and MA–2, Ohio 560, Emerson, and Ergstrom ventilators.

For several reasons, the volume-cycled ventilator is more desirable for patients with spinal cord injuries. Poor lung compliance and secretion retention problems make it difficult for the quadriplegic to maintain a clear airway; thus, the use of a pressure-cycled ventilator is limited. Airway closure causes the preset pressure to be attained rapidly, ending the inspiratory phase before the desired volume of gas is delivered. It is difficult to estimate from the preset pressure the actual volume of gas the patient is receiving. The pressure-cycled machine also increases intrathoracic pressure and thus can aggravate the already impaired venous circulation to the heart.

Each type of respirator can be used in a variety of modes to ensure inspiration:

- The *assist/control mode* assists patients to take a breath if they trigger the machine or delivers a breath if they fail to do so. This mode is desirable for patients with weak chest musculature or weak neural drive resulting in irregular respirations and is suitable for initial mechanical ventilation for most patients with spinal cord injuries.
- *Assisted ventilation* is used when patients can initiate a respiration by triggering the ventilator to deliver the preset volume or pressure. This

mode is used for patients with spinal cord injuries when they are recovering from initial fatigue or neurological edema involving diaphragmatic function. At this stage, weaning should be considered.

- *Controlled ventilation* delivers a preset volume or pressure at the desired rate regardless of patient effort or lack of effort. This mode is needed for apneic patients, most notably ventilator-dependent quadriplegic patients with high cord injuries.
- It is also possible to change either the timing or pressure settings that influence the expiratory phase. The most frequently used expiratory maneuver for patients prone to secretion retention leading to alveolar collapse because of small airway closure is *Positive End Expiratory Pressure* (PEEP). PEEP is based on the fundamental principle of airway expansion on inspiration and airway collapse on expiration. PEEP maintains a positive pressure of 1 to 15 cm H_2O at the end of each expiration. To demonstrate this, take a deep breath, exhale part of it, and breathe in again. The pressure in the lungs is not allowed to return to normal atmospheric pressure and you have increased the resting volume of the lungs or the functional residual capacity (FRC). The application of PEEP causes alveoli to stay open longer maintaining oxygenation of pulmonary capillary blood. By combating small airway closure, it is possible to maintain or increase FRC and lung compliance and help prevent hypoxia and increased work of breathing.

Physiological problems of prolonged mechanical ventilation

Prolonged mechanical ventilation, so often encountered with quadriplegia, aggravates a number of the complications common to any patient requiring mechanical ventilation. Major potential problems include insufficient or excessive ventilation or oxygenation, water imbalances, infection, atelectasis, gastrointestinal complications, and a pneumothorax (Holloway 1979). Patients with spinal cord injuries are particularly subject to infection, gastrointestinal complications, and a pneumothorax. The major potential problems associated with long-term management of the artificial airways required are infection, excessive secretions, and necrotic changes associated with pressure caused by the tracheostomy tube.

Infection and excessive secretions Measures to prevent or treat infection and measures to manage excessive secretions go hand in hand. Astute chest assessment will reveal early signs of congestion. Infection may be detected by the presence of a moist cough or an increased amount of purulent secretions, often accompanied by an elevated temperature.

Nursing care measures are directed toward liquefaction and removal of secretions and avoidance of introducing infection. Measures include providing constant airway humidification and ensuring adequate systemic hydration to liquefy secretions and to promote bronchial drainage. Measures with a preventive and restorative focus have been previously described. Problems of caring for patients with atelectasis and pneumonia are addressed later in this chapter.

Meticulous sterile technique while suctioning the trachea is probably the single most important factor to prevent introducing infection. It is best to avoid excessive suctioning by choosing the most effective times to clear mobilized secretions—that is, right after turning and promptly following chest physiotherapy or chest treatments. Rigid cleaning schedules for equipment must also be followed. Most institutions have a policy of changing the ventilator tubing every twenty-four hours and replacing the sterile water in the humidification system every eight hours. The nurse will also provide good mouth care and care to the tracheostomy site every four to eight hours as needed and will consult with the physician about changing the tracheostomy tube weekly, because mucus tends to crust outside the airway on the tracheal mucosa.

Tracheal necrosis To minimize the risk of tracheal necrosis, Portex-plastic tubes with high residual volume soft cuffs are recommended for use with mechanical ventilation. As previously mentioned, this type of airway ensures minimal pressure on the trachea at the cuff site. Tubing should be supported so that the tube itself is not malaligned and causing undue pressure on the trachea. Secure all tubing before and after turns. A rare but serious complication that may develop even after extubation is a *tracheoesophageal*

fistula. This complication is caused by necrotic changes in the trachea and is more likely to develop if a large nasogastric tube has also been used. The nurse should observe for oral or tube feeding in tracheal aspirate. During the early stages this is more commonly caused by difficulty in swallowing while the tracheostomy tube is in place. If tracheal aspirate is not contaminated until four to six weeks after intubation, it is more likely that a fistula has formed. The patient may complain of a severe burning sensation during or after meals; this is caused by food contamination of the fistula. Diagnosis is confirmed by X ray or endoscopy, and surgical repair is usually necessary.

Gastrointestinal problems Patients with spinal cord injuries often develop gastrointestinal problems. Air swallowing can cause severe gastric dilatation, which complicates an already existing paralytic ileus, which in turn hampers respirations. The severe emotional and physical stresses of trauma, plus side effects of frequently used steroid therapy, increase the risk of gastric ulceration and hemorrhage. (An antacid regime and nasogastric decompression are recommended for promoting optimal nutrition and are presented in Chapter 11.)

Pneumothorax The longer the patient is mechanically ventilated, the greater the number of risk factors involved, and the greater the tendency to develop a pneumothorax. Early recognition and nursing interventions are discussed in detail later in this chapter.

Communication problems encountered during prolonged mechanical ventilation

Communication is a major concern for patients requiring mechanical ventilation. The longer the patient is mechanically ventilated, the more complex the situation becomes as the need for communication becomes greater and greater. To compound the situation, awareness of prognosis may have progressed to severe depression manifested in anger, rage, or complete withdrawal. In a desperate attempt to maintain some control over the environment, the patient usually becomes extremely rigid and develops definite staff preferences, which cannot always be met. It is difficult to provide really helpful information and to ease the obstacles that are blocking communication. The nurse who is able to care effectively for a patient in this situation possesses wonderful skills much to be admired and is a valuable resource person. Such a nurse will treat the patient with respect, appreciating what respiratory failure and spinal cord injury implies to the individual; will manage the respirator and related equipment comfortably; will minimize the stressful effects of an intensive care setting; and will establish a basic communication system. The following measures will help nurses handle difficult situations when the patient becomes severely agitated:

• Consider the patient's preinjury personality to help anticipate responses during illness. Often the social worker can obtain this information from family members.
• Consider internal sources of anxiety. The person dependent on a respirator is in constant fear of disconnection from the machine or possible mechanical failure that could lead to suffocation and death. Hypoxia may cause secondary confusion, and the physical and emotional trauma surrounding the sudden onset of paralysis will contribute to a severe anxiety state.
• Consider and try to eliminate environmental factors contributing to stress. "We situate critically ill people in an alien, often crowded, and highly stressful environment—one over which they have little or no territorial or spatial rights and one in which they are generally helpless and totally dependent upon the interventions of nursing and medical personnel" (Gowan 1979: 342). These adverse effects are often described as sensory deprivation or overload and sleep deprivation. Some measures used to reduce these effects are: allowing a few personal belongings at the bedside, providing clocks and marking off days on a calendar to maintain orientation, dimming lights at night and during rest periods, and organizing care to allow for much-needed sleep. It is generally valuable to create as "homey" an atmosphere as possible with colored linens, window drapes, and even posters on the ceiling.

When delivering nursing care, it is important to establish a trusting rapport to make the patient feel secure. If this is achieved, communication becomes much easier. Simple measures, such as protecting the patient's modesty or avoiding conversations "over" patients that do not include them are of utmost importance. *Gentle* moving of patients will convey messages of caring and concern. Patients may see the ventilator as a projection of themselves. Nurses should address the patient before making any ventilator adjustments. It is also helpful for nurses to introduce themselves, discuss the activities planned during the shift, and explain each procedure carefully. Much verbal support is needed.

Devices To facilitate communication a fenestrated, low-pressure, cuffed tracheostomy tube may be introduced (see Figure 9–8). This device has a removable inner cannula that exposes an opening on the upper surface of the outer cannula, which allows the patient to talk during expiration. Unfortunately, suctioning

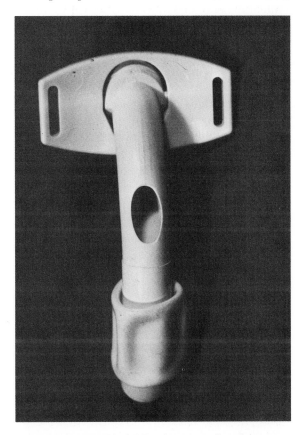

FIGURE 9–8 ■ The Shiley fenestrated tracheostomy tube. (Distributed by Shiley Sales Corp., Irvine, Ca 92714.)

may be difficult with this device. During insertion, the suction catheter tends to catch on the window opening of the outer cannula. Reinsertion of the inner cannula at this point may push secretions back down into the lung. To accommodate the inner cannula, it is necessary to use a small catheter (French size 12), which is not large enough to remove tenacious or copious amounts of secretions.

An innovative technique, still in the experimental stages, is the use of an *electrolarynx**. This is an artificial, electrically stimulated larynx that enables the patient to communicate quickly and effectively. Successful use depends on the patient's overall articulation ability and availability of a good placement site.

Eventually, patients with high cervical cord injuries who will remain ventilator-dependent, will be able to talk. A portable ventilator system is compatible with the metal, uncuffed tracheostomy tube and, on expiration, allows for vocalization around the tube. See Chapter 17 for care of patients requiring a permanent artificial airway and portable mechanical ventilation.

Nonverbal communication systems   Most often some type of nonverbal system is needed to establish effective communication. The most suitable approaches for patients without use of their upper limbs are scanning and encoding techniques.

In the *scanning technique*, a person presents various symbols or words to the patient, who remains passive until the correct item is chosen. Simple examples are:

- Yes/no guessing or questioning. Present the patient with choices, one at a time, or pose questions in such a way that only a "yes" or "no" answer is needed. This may require a system, such as one blink for "yes" and two blinks for "no." The questions include requests for information about pain, nausea, air hunger, or the need for suctioning. As sensation is diminished elsewhere, increasing awareness of discomfort over the head, neck, and shoulders is common, particularly headache or itchiness on

the face. Nurses should include these questions and others about preferences and preexisting conditions.
- Scanning of a poster board. A poster board, or a set of cards on a ring, can contain a list of questions, commands, pictures, or symbols individualized to patient needs. The nurse can point to the choices individually and ask the patient to respond using the "yes" or "no" blink system.

Encoding techniques are techniques where the message items to be communicated are indicated by multiple signals from the patient. A simple example of this technique uses a vocabulary matrix like the one illustrated in Figure 9–9A. The patient specifies the word(s) of the message by indicating the two appropriate numbers; one in the horizontal column and the corresponding number in the vertical column. For example, if the desired word was *juice,* the patient would indicate number 5 from the horizontal line A and number 2 from the vertical line 0. The numbers can be indicated by using the blink method. An example of a more complex system is shown in Figure 9–9B. The nurse must be the direct selector pointing to individual words and letters (note the letters are set up like a typewriter keyboard to prepare the patient for future skills that will require the use of a mouth stick). The patient again uses a blink system for indicating desired words.

The scanning techniques are simple to operate and require little effort on the part of the patient. Unfortunately such communication is slow. The encoding techniques provide a faster means of communication and an access to a larger vocabulary. They require, however, greater physical control and higher cognitive abilities than the scanning technique. For the spinal cord patient who requires a nonvocal communication aid for a short period only, a simple scanning device is suggested. Whatever system is used, the nurse must *initiate* and *encourage* its use for the patient to become comfortable with it. For longer periods more sophisticated electronic environmental aids should be investigated by the occupational therapist.

Liaison activities   To combat feelings of isolation and loneliness, the nurse can provide a

---

* For more information on this largely experimental device, contact the Department of Speech Pathology, Northwestern Memorial Hospital (Wesley Pavilion), Chicago, Illinois.

LINE "A" FIRST	A 1	A 2	A 3	A 4	A 5	A 6	A 7	A 8
O 1	WHO	LEG	FOOT	PAIN	WATER	DOCTOR	P.T.	S.P.
O 2	WHAT	ARM	HAND	SCRATCH	JUICE	NURSE	O.T.	S.W.
O 3	WHEN	BACK	NECK	SUCTION	FOOD	BED		
O 4	WHERE	HEAD	EYES	TURN	HOT	WHEEL CHAIR		
O 5	WHY	NOSE	MOUTH	WASH	TISSUES	LIGHT	I	YOU
O 6	HOW	BOWEL	BLADDER	TIME	COLD	FAN	YES	NO

A

SUCTION	SCRATCH	FOOD	WATER	PAIN	YES	NO				
TIME	HOT	COLD	JUICE	TURN	I	YOU				
WASH	1	2	3	4	5	6	7	8	9	0
BED	Q	W	E	R	T	Y	U	I	O	P
LIGHT	A	S	D	F	G	H	J	K	L	;
FAN	Z	X	C	V	B	N	M	,	.	?
TISSUES	BOWEL	BLADDER	LEG	ARM	WHO	WHAT				
DOCTOR	EYES	HEAD	BACK	NECK	WHY	WHEN				
NURSE	P.T.	O.T.	S.P.	S.W.	WHERE	HOW				

B

FIGURE 9–9 ■ (A) A vocabulary matrix as shown here is a simple example of an encoding system. (B) This matrix can become more complex with the addition of numbers and letters. Actual charts measure approximately 9 × 12 inches.

key liaison role between the patient and other team members or the family and visitors. For example, staying at the bedside to support the physician or visitor in their initial attempts to communicate can ease the situation and make the visit more meaningful. Also, patients frequently have questions about their treatments, such as "When can I eat?" or "How long will I be on this machine?" Nurses can try to clarify some of these concerns before the physician's visit, perhaps by talking to previously intubated patients for more ideas.

When verbal communication is not possible, the patient becomes increasingly aware of nonverbal communication. Facial expression, for example, can quickly communicate cheerfulness, anxiety, or frustration. In addition, touching patients, especially where their sensation is still intact, will enhance communication of feelings and concerns.

Gradual withdrawal from mechanical ventilation and artificial airway support

Most patients with spinal cord injuries require a gradual withdrawal or *weaning process* from ventilator support. Generally, the longer the period of time on the respirator, the longer the process. The entire concept of *gradual* withdrawal from ventilator support is based on increasing the tolerance and strength of existing respiratory muscles and facilitating the return of strength in weaker muscles. This concept is basic to beginning any exercise program, such as building up stamina to jog for increasingly longer periods.

Criteria to begin the weaning process These criteria will be met as the patient's general condition stabilizes and as neurological edema and spinal shock subside. Diaphragmatic function strengthens, and, with reflex contractions of the chest musculature breathing improves.

Criteria to begin the weaning process include:

- Tolerance of a reduced concentration of inspired oxygen (FIO_2), ideally to that of room air

- Acceptable pulmonary function studies and arterial blood gas values (as compared to standards for a stabililzed quadriplegic person)

- Freedom from infected secretions, water imbalances, or other pulmonary complications that are not under control

- Stable blood pressure and pulse

When criteria are met, the process to be used is explained to the patient. The two methods of ventilatory support are:

1. Gradually increasing periods of time off the ventilator
2. Use of intermittent mandatory ventilation (IMV) while the patient is still on the respirator

The latter is a newer, more successful approach to freeing patients from ventilator support.

Monitoring techniques To monitor patient progress before, during, and after initial weaning periods spent off the ventilator or when ventilator IMV settings are adjusted, *serial arterial blood gas analysis* can be used. Recently *ear oximetry* has been introduced to the weaning process to reflect arterial oxygen saturation (PaO_2) more accurately. It is a reliable and practical technique useful for continuously monitoring patients at risk of rapidly changing states of oxygenation. After cleaning and application of a va-sodilator cream, a small device (ear piece) is fitted to the patient's ear lobe. In a recent study, Saunders, Powles, and Rebuck (1976) concluded that the Hewlett-Packard 47201 A model offered several added advantages for use in a clinical situation. It is described as a simple robust instrument; easy to apply and comfortable to wear; insensitive to position on the ear and to differences in skin pigmentation; and simple to operate with stability of characteristics. The noninvasive technique of ear oximetry can also replace the use of an arterial line or repeated puncture for blood gas samples and the patient is free to move about in the wheelchair.

Time periods off the ventilator If the plan is to wean the patient by gradually increasing time periods off the respirator, planning and timing are essential. The best time to initiate the weaning process is when the patient is most rested and the greatest number of people are around. This reassures the patient in case of possible breathing difficulties. For example, the nurse might complete morning care, allow a rest period, and take advantage of peak periods of pain medication. The airway must be clear before beginning the weaning process and the patient should be in the most comfortable position to ease breathing, perhaps a side-lying position with the head of the bed elevated. Constant evaluation of physical and psychological tolerances is essential. See Procedure 9–8.

Intermittent mandatory ventilation (IMV) IMV is physically and psychologically less traumatic for the patient then increasing time periods off the respirator. The patient is encouraged to breathe spontaneously while a controlled number of mandatory breaths are delivered by the ventilator. That is, breaths from the ventilator are interspersed at timed intervals while patients are breathing on their own. For details of this method see Procedure 9–9.

Gradual withdrawal from ventilatory support is usually successful; however, there are rare problems associated with psychological dependence on the respirator. Some interesting work is being done with biofeedback techniques to help patients with this problem (Corson et al. 1979).

Discontinuing the artificial airway The quadriplegic patient in particular can rarely tolerate the removal of a tracheostomy tube in one step. A gradual process of discontinuing the artificial airway must take place. This process can start when the patient is able to maintain spontaneous respiration, maintain acceptable blood gas values on room air, and manage secretions effectively. An intact gag and swallow reflex should also be present.

Most often, a metal tracheostomy tube is used to replace a larger Portex tube. Every few days the tube is changed to a smaller size to reduce the stoma size (a number 6 is the minimal tube size recommended before starting to close the airway for short periods). Steps to reduce the stoma size can begin while the patient is on a ventilator. Convenient and safe techniques for changing tracheostomy tubes during mechanical ventilation are presented in Procedure 9–10.

To facilitate gradual accommodation to closing the artificial airway, a small *plug* can be used to occlude the tracheostomy tube and allow intermittent periods of natural breathing and communication. The airway must be clear before inserting the plug into the tracheostomy tube. The patient may only tolerate this a few minutes each hour to start, but the time can gradually be increased. Observation is needed for a 72-hour period, while the tracheostomy is continuously plugged. Final extubation can be performed if the patient is breathing easily, vital signs are stable, and the vital capacity and arterial blood gases are maintained at an acceptable level.

Another method uses the *Kistner tracheal button*. The tracheostomy tube is removed and replaced by the Kistner button, which allows minimal inspiration of air while it occludes the stoma on expiration so the patient can talk (Adams 1979). Most of the air is warmed and humidified as it is inspired through the nose and mouth. If a constant open airway is needed, a *fenestrated* tube (with an opening that also allows air to pass in and out of the nose and mouth) will make communication possible. Techniques used for extubation are described in Procedure 9–11. Hoarseness and sore throat can occur on extubation. No treatment is usually necessary. The patient should be monitored for excessive fatigue, ease of respirations, maintenance of adequate vital capacity and stable vital signs. Should distress occur, reintubation may be necessary.

SPECIFIC NURSING INTERVENTIONS FOR PULMONARY COMPLICATIONS

Hypoxia

Hypoxia is a diminished availability of oxygen to the body cells and can be caused by internal or external environmental factors. With spinal cord injury the causes of hypoxia are usually related to *impaired neural impulses to breathing muscles.* This results in ventilation problems as airway resistance increases and lung compliance decreases. The other major cause of hypoxia is *hemorrhagic or neurogenic shock,* which leads to low cardiac output and decreasing volumes of circulating blood to transport gases.

Goals of care

- To identify patients at risk of developing hypoxia
- To recognize the patient in need of supplemental oxygen
- To maintain, on admission, a desired PaO_2 of 80 mmHg. As mentioned previously, early avoidance of systemic hypoxia will lessen the chance of lower oxygen tension in the spinal cord and thereby prevent further neurological damage. Later in the rehabilitation phase a PaO_2 of 60 mmHg is acceptable for a quadriplegic under basal conditions

Nursing interventions

1. Practice preventive measures to control risk factors. To keep chest clear, avoid airway obstruction, maintain a regular schedule (every two hours), perform chest physiotherapy, and give IPPB treatments as ordered by physician. Also initiate treatment to control predisposing factors to hypoxia, such as hemorrhage.
2. Observe for early signs and symptoms of hypoxia: increased rapid, shallow breathing; noisy respirations; dyspnea; pale color; tachycardia; and restlessness or irritability. Extrathoracic signs and symptoms will develop eventually if hypoxia is severe.

PROCEDURE 9–8 ■ INCREASING TIME PERIODS OFF THE VENTILATOR

Purpose

The purpose of this procedure is to gradually withdraw the patient from dependence on the mechanical ventilator by slowly increasing the time periods off the ventilator and, thereby, increasing the strength of the respiration muscles. Respiratory insufficiency must also be prevented.

Action	Rationale
1. Plan to initiate periods off ventilator when patient is most rested and comfortable.	To maximize patient tolerance to procedure.
2. Stay with patient, offer reassurance, and give constant feedback on progress.	To maximize patient cooperation and minimize fear. Psychological support is a key factor to ensure success.
3. Assess current respiratory status. Perform chest assessment and ensure that the airway is clear. Obtain arterial blood gases for baseline data or use ear oximeter.	To prevent respiratory insufficiency, weaning criteria must be met.
4. Detach the ventilator source and attach a T-piece to the airway from a humidified oxygen source.	This is usually set 10% higher than the FlO$_2$ on the ventilator to compensate for less accurate control of inspired air.
5. Ask the patient to watch you breathe and to breathe with you.	This, in itself, will help to regulate breathing and minimize feelings of panic. Panic can lead to hypoxia and respiratory arrest.
6. Observe diaphragmatic movement and look for movement of accessory muscles in neck, shoulders, and abdominal muscles.	The objective of gradual removal of patients from mechanical ventilation is to activate these muscles.
7. Monitor pulse and respiratory rate every 5 minutes.	Respiratory distress is indicated by: • Tachycardia or an increase in the heart rate greater than 20 beats per minute • Tachypnea or an increase of respiratory rate greater than 30 beats per minute

(Procedure continues)

3. Give oxygen supplement as ordered by physician. If high concentrations of oxygen by mask are ineffective, intubation and mechanical ventilation needs to be considered.
4. Confirm cause with physician and initiate treatment as ordered for underlying condition.
5. Evaluate effectiveness of treatment according to level of outcome criteria reached:

   • Normal, unlabored respirations at a rate of 12 to 20 breaths per minute
   • Blood pressure and pulse within normal limits for patient
   • Alert and oriented
   • Good color, free from cyanosis
   • Arterial blood gases within acceptable range of PaO$_2$ 60 to 100 mmHg and PaCO$_2$ 35 to 50 mmHg

Atelectasis and Pneumonia

Atelectasis is a partial or complete collapse of the lung. Alveoli and blood vessels may be involved, leading to diminished blood flow and decreased gaseous exchange to the affected area. *Microatelectasis* or early small airway closure is

PROCEDURE 9–8 ■ (continued)

Action	Rationale
8. Continually observe general tolerance to procedure.	Be alert for additional signs and symptoms indicating respiratory distress: • Excessive apprehension • Extreme fatigue • Excessive sweating above the level of lesion
9. If the patient is not too distressed, arterial blood gases should be drawn before returning to the ventilator to monitor patient's progress or monitor constant ear oximetry readings (preferred method). Clarify with physician what fluctuations are acceptable for individual patients and adjust timing accordingly.	Poor tolerance and therefore general indications to reduce time spent off the ventilator include: • A fall of Pao_2 to below 60 mmHg • A rise in $Paco_2$ of more than 10 mmHg • A decrease in pH to below 7.25 (Adams 1979) Oxygen saturation indicated by oximetry should not fall below 60 mmHg.
10. Plan weaning periods to start "on the hour."	For ease in scheduling subsequent time periods off the ventilator.
11. Increase time spent off the ventilator gradually from 15 minutes each hour to a whole hour, then 2 hours, and so on as tolerated.	
12. Progress to full days off the ventilator and resume use only at night, then discontinue mechanical ventilation.	As quadriplegic patients are prone to sleep-induced apnea, careful evaluation should be made for *several nights* before mechanical ventilation is discontinued.

scattered and not detectable on chest X ray. This subtle problem is a danger to any postoperative or immobilized patient.

Pneumonia results in inflamed, edematous alveoli, blocked with fluid. The lungs become saturated, heavy, and solid, thereby inhibiting gaseous exchange and creating an environment prone to infection. Pneumococcus bacteria, viruses, or aspirate of foreign material are prime causes of infection.

Due to immobilization, poor chest expansion, and inability to cough effectively, patients with spinal cord injuries are predisposed to *hypostatic pneumonia*. The mechanism by which this develops is described by Larabee (1977). Because the patient is lying down, the pressure of abdominal contents forces the diaphragm to rise higher in the chest, and the great vessels of the chest tend to fill with blood. The bronchioles are crowded, which increases their tendency to be obstructed by mucus. In addition, gravity pulls the mucus to the dependent side of the bronchioles. The upper surface of the bronchioles tends to dry out and crack, providing a site for infection, while the lower surfaces allow mucus to pool and become more easily obstructed.

These two conditions, related to secretion retention, are discussed together, as the nursing goals and interventions are similar.

Goals of care

• To identify patients at risk of developing atelectasis or pneumonia
• To recognize early signs of congestion and initiate early treatment
• To assist patient with removal of secretions by clearing dependent areas of lung
• To provide adequate lung expansion
• To prevent or control infection

PROCEDURE 9–9 ■ INTERMITTENT MANDATORY VENTILATION (IMV)

Purpose

The purpose of this procedure is to gradually withdraw the patient from dependence on the mechanical ventilator, thereby increasing the strength of the respiration muscles. Repiratory insufficiency must also be prevented.

Action	Rationale
1. Plan to initiate IMV when patient is most rested and comfortable.	This maximizes patient's tolerance to procedure.
2. Collaborate with physician to reduce the FIo_2, ideally to room air, and discontinue PEEP.	The use of PEEP makes it more difficult to inspire air.
3. Assess current respiratory status. Perform chest assessment and ensure that the airway is clear. Obtain arterial blood gases for baseline data or use ear oximeter.	To prevent respiratory insufficiency weaning criteria must be met.
4. Collaborate with physician to *select* the IMV rate.	It is important to remember the concept of IMV, that is to stimulate muscles which have become weakened through disuse. The diaphragm gets lazy because the ventilator is doing the work of breathing. Therefore, if the patient has been maintained on ten breaths per minute, cutting the IMV rate to eight breaths per minute is not effective. Setting the IMV rate at four breaths per minute, with a volume of 800 to 1000 mL aids in CO_2 retention, which will stimulate breathing.
5. Set the IMV rate as ordered by the physician.	The ventilator will deliver this number of mandatory breaths per minute: • The Bennett MA–1 can be adapted to allow patient to breathe spontaneously from an attached separate source of humidified oxygen or compressed air (this may be an additional wall outlet or tank). Simultaneously, the ventilator is set to deliver a predetermined number of breaths per minute. The MA–1 system will deliver a breath despite patient's effort or lack of it. • The newer MA–2 is sensitive to patient's next inspiratory effort. In this synchronous intermittent mandatory ventilation (SIMV) mode on the MA–2, the ventilator delivers demand breaths in response to patient's breathing efforts.
6. Encourage patient to breathe spontaneously. In the beginning ask patient to watch you breathe and breathe with you.	This, in itself, will help stimulate and regulate breathing.
7. Observe diaphragmatic movement and look for movement of accessory muscles in neck, shoulders, and abdominal muscles.	The objective of gradual removal of patients from mechanical ventilation is to activate these muscles.

(Procedure continues)

PROCEDURE 9–9 ■ (continued)

Action	Rationale
8. Initially, monitor pulse and respirations every 5 minutes. Gradually reduce monitoring but observe patient closely following future adjustments to ventilator settings.	Respiratory distress is indicated by: • Tachycardia or an increase in the heart rate greater than 20 beats per minute • Tachypnea or an increase of respiratory rate greater than 30 beats per minute
9. Continually observe general tolerance to procedure.	Be alert for additional signs and symptoms indicating respiratory distress: • Excessive apprehension • Extreme fatigue • Excessive sweating above the level of lesion
10. Monitor serial blood gas analysis or use ear oximetry (preferred method) and adjust ventilator accordingly. Clarify with physician what fluctuations are acceptable for individual patients.	Poor tolerance and therefore general indications that IMV rate is set too low include: • A fall of Pao_2 to below 60 mmHg • A rise in Pao_2 of more than 10 mmHg • A decrease in pH to below 7.25 (Adams 1979) Oxygen saturation indicated by oximetry should not fall below 60 mmHg.
11. Progress to full days when IMV is not required at all. Resume IMV only at night, then discontinue mechanical ventilation altogether.	As quadriplegic patients are prone to sleep-induced apnea, careful evaluation should be made for several nights before mechanical ventilation is discontinued altogether.
12. Provide humidified oxygen or air via a T-piece or trach mask.	This protects artificial airway.

Nursing interventions

1. Practice preventive measures to mobilize secretions. Patients at risk will require a regular change of position at least every two hours, a vigorous chest physiotherapy program with emphasis on vibration and clapping with postural drainage, and IPPB treatments given as ordered. To promote lung expansion, high pressures, gradually increased to 40 cm H_2O, may be indicated.

2. Observe for signs and symptoms of retained secretions, the earliest of which is a *moist cough*. Note the amount and nature of any sputum. Perform a routine chest assessment, and be alert for dullness on percussion, tactile fremitus, and presence of rales and rhonchi. Examine diagnostic findings for abnormal arterial blood gases, a lowered Pao_2 and/or elevated $Paco_2$, decreased vital capacity, and signs of consolidation on chest X ray.

3. Give oxygen supplement as ordered. The physician may increase the FIo_2 or flow rate. If mechanical ventilation is in use, the physician may increase the sigh mechanism in frequency and/or volume to ensure adequate deep inflation of the lungs. Positive end expiratory pressure (PEEP) may be applied to keep small airways open longer.

4. Liquefy secretions for ease of removal. Ensure that adequate humidification is available on all supplemental oxygen. The ultrasonic nebulizer may also be used.

PROCEDURE 9–10 ■ CHANGING TRACHEOSTOMY TUBE

Purpose

The purpose of this procedure is to change the tracheostomy tube either for cleaning or to reduce size of stoma and to perform the procedure without causing respiratory insufficiency or patient discomfort.

Equipment

- Metal tracheostomy tube set including an obturator, inner and outer cannula, and tie tapes
- Rigid plastic adapter for connection between the tracheostomy tube and the respirator fitting
- Oxygen source
- Sterile gloves and masks
- Scissors
- Tracheal dilators (Trousseau)
- Spare Portex-tube within easy reach
- Sterile dressing tray; tracheostomy dressing
- Hand resuscitation bag
- Suction equipment and catheter

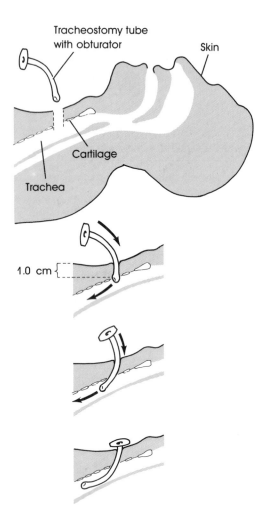

Action	Rationale
1. Explain the procedure to the patient. Point out that the procedure is not painful but may stimulate coughing.	This helps relieve fear and gain the cooperation of the patient. If the patient is apprehensive or panics during the procedure, breathing difficulty will be aggravated.
2. Check suction equipment for working order. Connect catheter (correct size for tracheostomy tube) to suction tubing. Leave suction turned on.	In an emergency, equipment must be immediately available.
3. Have hand resuscitation bag with tracheostomy adapters and an oxygen source at hand.	Emergency equipment is useless unless connecting adapters fit correctly.

(Procedure continues)

PROCEDURE 9–10 ■ (continued)

Action	Rationale
4. Have a set of tracheal dilator forceps on hand.	Should the tube become accidentally dislodged, these special forceps will open the stoma and allow air entry.
5. Open dressing tray and tracheostomy set and prepare sterile field.	
6. Rinse tracheostomy adapters with sterile water and place at edge of sterile field.	Adapters are often soaked in antiseptic solutions.
7. Place sterile lubricant on sterile field.	
8. Don sterile gloves and check to see that the inner cannula fits easily into the outer cannula. Also check to see that the tracheostomy adapter attaches securely to the *inner* cannula.	Technically the sterilized components of metal tracheostomy sets are interchangeable, but with use this is not always so.
9. Place the obturator inside the outer cannula and apply a small amount of sterile lubricant to the tip of the obturator. The tracheostomy dressing may be placed around the tube at this time.	
10. Suction patient to clear airway if needed and preventilate with a couple of 'sigh' breaths before disconnecting the ventilator.	This increases patient tolerance to procedure.
11. Snip the tie tapes and deflate the cuff before removal. Use your dominant hand for maneuvering the metal tracheostomy tube.	
12. Using one hand (nondominant hand), quickly but gently remove the Portex-tube; with the other hand insert the metal tracheostomy tube. Advance the tip of the obturator approximately 1.0 cm (about 3/8 to 1/2 inch) to allow entry into the trachea; continue advancement using a continuous circular motion.	Attention must be directed toward the curvature of the metal tracheostomy tube, which necessitates the movements described. Slight hyperextension of the neck also eases insertion.
13. Immediately remove the obturator; insert the inner cannula (which has the adapter already attached); and connect the respirator tubing.	
14. Allow the patient several respirations, then proceed to suction through the new tracheostomy tube.	This ensures the patency of the new artificial airway.
15. Auscultate the chest and observe for chest wall expansion.	This is necessary to check for adequate air entry.
16. Secure tube with the tapes. Knot tapes rather than tying in a bow.	This prevents accidental extubation.
17. Place a piece of elastic over the respirator tubing at the tracheostomy connection site and anchor to each side of the outer cannula.	This prevents accidental dislodging of respirator tubing.
18. Assess respiratory status.	

PROCEDURE 9–11 ■ REMOVAL OF TRACHEOSTOMY TUBE

Purpose

The purpose of this procedure is to remove the tracheostomy tube without causing respiratory distress and to minimize patient discomfort.

Equipment

- Suction apparatus
- Scissors
- Sterile glove
- Light gauze dressing (sterile)
- Micropore tape

Action	Rationale
1. Explain procedure to the patient. Point out that the procedure is not painful but may stimulate coughing.	To promote patient cooperation. Apprehension and panic aggravate breathing difficulties.
2. Have suction equipment close at hand.	
3. Auscultate the patient's chest and clear airway, if necessary, before proceeding.	
4. Snip the tie tapes.	
5. Don sterile gloves.	
6. Use a circular motion to quickly, but gently, remove the tube.	The curvature of the metal tracheostomy tube necessitates the movements described. Slight hyperextension of the neck also eases removal.
7. Cover the tracheostomy site with a light gauze dressing and micropore tape.	To avoid skin breakdown, do not use waterproof tape which will completely occlude the area and trap secretions.
8. Change the dressing every 8 hours or when soiled. Wipe area with saline or sterile water and dry.	Mucus can wet the dressing from the inside. Watch for food and liquids contaminating the dressing on the outside. Allow tracheostomy site to dry and heal naturally. Avoid repeated cleansings and harsh solutions.
9. Assess respiratory status.	

5. Assist physician to remove severe, massive mucus plugs during bronchoscopy.

6. Observe carefully for signs and symptoms of infection. Monitor temperature rectally every four hours [or more frequently if elevated over 40°C (104°F)] and observe sputum for increased amounts or purulence. Take daily specimens for culture and sensitivity. Prevent or control infection by using meticulous suctioning techniques and take measures to avoid any other systemic infections, such as a bladder infection, that will decrease the patient's general resistance.

7. Administer therapeutic courses of antibiotic drugs as ordered. Report culture and sensitivity results before antibiotic courses are commenced to prevent development of resistance. Since there is a high risk of this complication in long-term care, prophylactic drugs must be used cautiously.

8. Evaluate effectiveness of treatment according to level of outcome criteria reached:

- Unlabored respirations at a rate of 12 to 20 breaths per minute

- Normal body temperature
- Unproductive cough or sputum, free from infective organisms
- Lungs clear on auscultation
- Chest X ray clear without evidence of consolidation
- PaO_2 60 to 100 mmHg and $PaCO_2$ 35 to 50 mmHg
- Vital capacity within normal limits for patient

Pulmonary Edema

Pulmonary edema causes the lungs to swell and become heavier with fluid, which increases the work of breathing and makes gaseous exchange more difficult. Pooling of blood in the pulmonary system is most often associated with failure of the left side of the heart. A buildup in pulmonary capillary pressure ultimately causes rapid transudation of fluid into the alveoli and interstitial spaces of the lung. Some conditions that threaten patients with spinal cord injuries are fluid overload, shock, cardiac arrhythmias, and pulmonary complications, such as pneumonia or pulmonary emboli.

Goals of care

- To identify patients at risk of developing pulmonary edema
- To recognize the onset of pulmonary edema
- To decrease venous return to the heart to assist movement of fluid out of the alveoli into the venous circulation
- To maintain adequate ventilation and perfusion

Nursing interventions

1. Practice preventive measures to minimize risk. For example, minimize physical and emotional stress to decrease work of the heart and take measures to alleviate shock and avoid pulmonary complications.

2. Prevent a positive pressure fluid balance in the body. Maintain a detailed intake and output record. Be sure to include amount and type of fluids administered during transport. Vigorous attempts to combat neurogenic shock with massive IV fluid intake are ineffective and cause a major fluid overload problem.

3. Observe for signs of dyspnea, cough, and hypoxia. Note any amounts of pink, frothy sputum; or chest congestion such as rales, which indicates fluid-filled alveoli.

4. Take measures to decrease venous return to the heart and help move fluid from alveoli into the systemic circulation. Elevate the head of the bed if possible. Administer intravenously rapidly acting diuretics and cardiotonics as ordered by the physician. Measures such as application of rotating tourniquets to decrease circulating blood volume are contraindicated due to the decreased peripheral circulation associated with paralysis. Observe for unstable autonomic nervous system control causing sudden onset of shock or respiratory distress.

5. Cautiously administer small doses of IV morphine as ordered to decrease respiratory rate, alleviate pain, and control apprehension. Stay with patient.

6. Insert Foley catheter for accurate output record. (Intermittent catheterizations are not practical when hourly output should be monitored.)

7. Give supplemental oxygen as ordered. Use of IPPB may be contraindicated because the positive pressure created in the chest tends to slow venous return to the heart. Also, if the patient is mechanically ventilated, therapeutic use of PEEP may be desirable to minimize collapse of, or help reopen, alveoli.

8. Evaluate effectiveness of treatment according to level of outcome criteria reached:

- Unlabored respirations at a rate of 12 to 20 breaths per minute
- Blood pressure and pulse within normal limits for patient
- Lungs clear on auscultation
- Pulmonary function tests and arterial blood gas values within normal limits for patient
- No evidence of sputum
- No evidence of fluid imbalance

Pulmonary Emboli

Occlusion of a pulmonary vessel by an undissolved mass circulating in the bloodstream is known as *pulmonary embolism*. This condition is a major complication during the acute stage. The great majority of pulmonary emboli arise from deep vein thrombosis (DVT) in the legs (Casas et al. 1977–78). The danger from pulmonary emboli varies greatly depending on the location and extent of resultant lung ischemia. Small emboli may subside undetected, while a massive embolus may cause respiratory arrest. Three factors predispose any patient to formation of thrombi: (1) stasis of venous circulation, (2) changes in the vein wall, and (3) hypercoagulability of the blood. The main causative factor in the spinal injured patient is sluggish venous return. Paralysis reduces compression and release of pressure or the "milking action" on the veins normally associated with muscular activity. During the most critical period, that is, for approximately three to five weeks after injury, spinal shock compromises the situation even further when flaccid paralysis virtually eliminates muscle tone.

Patients with spinal cord injuries are subject to a number of factors that place any patient at risk: prolonged bedrest, recent surgery, hip or extremity fractures, possible deterioration of nutritional status, obesity, advancing age, preexisting heart disease or lung complications, and, of course, thrombophlebitis with subsequent deep vein thrombosis.

Early detection is the biggest defense against pulmonary embolism. Nurses must be constantly alert to subtle or nonspecific changes in the patient's clinical posture, especially during the first six weeks after surgery, when incidence is greatest. For example, a low-grade fever without evidence of infection may be the only indication that the patient is in potential danger.

Goals of care

- To identify patients at risk of developing DVT and subsequent pulmonary emboli
- To inhibit formation of thrombi by preventing venous stasis, avoiding trauma to or pressure on venous walls, and minimizing effects of hypercoagulability of the blood
- To provide early detection of pulmonary emboli and initiate treatment to prevent recurrent embolization that may cause life-threatening complications

Nursing interventions

1. Practice preventive measures to decrease risk. Take measures to promote venous return to the heart and to protect venous walls from undue pressure or trauma. Avoiding dehydration will help maintain normal blood viscosity and clotting time. Detect thrombophlebitis promptly to enable initiation of early treatment. These nursing care measures, including the detection and treatment of deep vein thrombosis, are described fully in Chapter 10. Remember prevention and early detection are the best defense against pulmonary embolism.

2. Observe for sudden onset of hypoxia, rapid respirations, or dyspnea. The patient may complain of difficulty "catching my breath." Tachycardia and pyrexia are usually present, and the patient is apprehensive. Chest pain may be absent, decreased, or referred due to sensory loss. On chest auscultation, a pleural friction rub or signs of atelectasis or consolidation may be evident. Symptoms may vary from mild to severe.

3. Recognize the possibility of fat emboli when petechiae are seen, particularly on the chest and neck.

4. Stay to calm patient and provide psychological support.

5. Provide complete bedrest. Return the patient to bed if up. To help ease breathing, it may be possible to elevate the head of the bed or change patient to side-lying position and remove restrictive braces or clothing. Be sure to communicate the plan to other team members, since occupational therapy and physiotherapy activities will need to be modified or stopped.

6. Give supplemental oxygen as ordered.

7. Initiate emergency measures to combat shock or institute cardiopulmonary resuscitation if indicated. Massive emboli that often occur bilaterally are a major cause of death in the early stages. Many times there is no evidence of pre-

existing DVT. Some patients have a feeling of impending doom and complain of difficulty in breathing or light-headedness before a sudden arrest situation occurs.

8. Prepare patient for a battery of tests to confirm diagnosis and assess extent of lung involvement. A diagnostic workup will include complete blood work; arterial blood gases, which may show a drop in PaO_2; chest X ray, which may show evidence of infarctions; and an ECG, which may reveal right-sided heart strain. Nonspecific results are frequently valuable to rule out other conditions. Recently *lung scanning* has proven most helpful. A radioactive substance (administered intravenously) travels with the blood to outline flow to the lung tissue. Where blood flow is decreased or absent due to ischemic changes (caused by pulmonary emboli or other lung disorders), uptake of the radioisotope will not be possible. A photograph of the results is placed on the medical record. Areas of normal perfusion will be dark; ischemic areas will be light. All these tests may be repeated on a serial basis to evaluate treatment.

9. Administer anticoagulant therapy as prescribed by the physician to prevent further embolization. Heparin is the drug of choice. Anticoagulant therapy is discussed in conjunction with the management of deep vein thrombosis in Chapter 10.

10. Evaluate effectiveness of treatment by level of expected outcome criteria reached:

- Effortless respiration at a rate of 12 to 20 breaths per minute
- Stable vital signs and normal body temperature
- Chest clear on auscultation, free from pleural friction or signs of consolidation
- Blood work, arterial blood gases within normal limits for patient
- ECG within normal limits (free from signs of right-sided heart strain)
- Chest X ray clear
- Lung scan normal or without signs of further deterioration
- No blood in sputum, nasogastric aspirate, urine, or stool and patient free from other signs of internal bleeding
- No evidence of thrombophlebitis

Pneumothorax

A *pneumothorax* is defined as air in the pleural cavity, that is, air between the parietal pleura of the lungs and the visceral pleura of the chest wall. An *open pneumothorax* occurs with a perforation of the visceral pleura and chest wall providing a continuous opening to the outside air. A *closed or spontaneous pneumothorax* occurs with a rupture of the parietal pleura or underlying lung tissue. When the lung collapses the pleural tear closes. A *tension pneumothorax* is very dangerous, because a valvelike tear allows air to pass in but not out. Risks may vary depending on size; a small, spontaneous pneumothorax may respond to oxygen therapy and bedrest while the air is slowly reabsorbed, but larger ones will create a medical emergency. Patients with spinal cord injuries are most subject to the development of a closed pneumothorax as a complication of mechanical ventilation. There are several risk factors: copious secretions leading to complications such as airway obstruction, bronchitis, or pneumonia; and invasive procedures done in the chest region such as thoracentesis or cardiopulmonary resuscitation (CPR). A patient fighting the respirator can raise intrathoracic pressures to dangerously high levels, as will application of high pressures of PEEP. A patient with fractured ribs may also develop a pneumothorax. The greater the number of risk factors involved, the greater the incidence of pneumothorax. Discussion in this section will focus on spontaneous pneumothorax developing as a major complication of mechanical ventilation.

Goals of care

- To identify patients at risk of developing a pneumothorax
- To recognize pneumothorax promptly to prevent life-threatening situations
- To evacuate air from the pleural cavity and reexpand the lung
- To prevent infection

Nursing interventions

1. Practice preventive measures to minimize risk factors. For example, mobilize and assist patient to remove secretions, stabilize rib fractures, and avoid liberal use of high pressures with PEEP.

2. Recognize onset of pneumothorax immediately. A sudden onset of persistent, stabbing chest pain is the usual symptom. The spinal injured patient may not be able to feel this due to sensory loss or may not be able to communicate discomfort when on the ventilator. The first sign may well come from the ventilator itself when a *sudden increased and sustained pressure is required to ventilate the patient* (peak inspiratory pressure) (Fuchs 1979). Look for signs of hypoxia (tachycardia, tachypnea) and increased dyspnea progressing to distress. Sometimes subcutaneous emphysema on the chest and neck is apparent. The affected side of the chest may be enlarged and fixed (without movement with respiration). On auscultation, breath sounds will be diminished or absent. Look for signs of mediastinal shift (such as a tracheal tug) toward the unaffected side. A chest X ray may show signs of lung collapse and mediastinal shift.

3. While the physician is notified, immediately hand ventilate the patient to help prevent high pressures of air from entering the pleural cavity and causing progression to a tension pneumothorax. If possible, elevate the head of the bed.

4. Assist physician with thoracentesis and establishment of continuous chest tube drainage.

5. Monitor serial chest X rays daily to evaluate improvement or deterioration.

6. Administer analgesics, bronchodilators, and antibiotics or steroid preparations (to avoid secondary infection) as ordered by the physician.

7. Evaluate effectiveness of treatment according to level of expected outcome criteria:

- Alert and oriented
- No chest or referred pain
- Normal respirations at a rate of 12 to 20 breaths per minute
- Symmetrical chest size and expansion
- Normal air entry throughout lungs
- No evidence of subcutaneous emphysema
- Trachea midline
- Blood pressure, pulse, and temperature within normal limits for patient; normal color
- Chest X ray clear without signs of lung collapse or mediastinal shift

SELF-CARE SKILLS

Patients need to know how the level of injury affects their breathing or coughing and how to prevent and treat upper respiratory tract infection. Self-care programs for quadriplegic and high paraplegic patients focus on hazardous complications associated with retained secretions, primarily pneumonia. Patients should learn preventive measures to protect themselves from predisposing environmental factors.

Probably the single most dangerous factor hampering respiratory health is *smoking,* but despite its obvious evils, many patients are unable to give it up. Gadgetry has even been developed to promote independence with this activity! At least such devices promote safety by avoiding burns to the skin or surrounding environment. As skills with arm movements develop, splints can be adapted to hold a cigarette. After prolonged stays in critical care areas where smoking is obviously not allowed, some patients are able to quit outright. Restricting smoking to common areas on ward settings does wonders to curtail the habit. However, especially outside the hospital setting, motivation for change must come from the patient. Successful community programs to stop smoking are generally based on behavior modification techniques.

Avoiding people with a cold or flu, dressing appropriately for the weather to avoid extreme changes in body temperature, and eating a well-balanced diet keep up general resistance and minimize risk of infection. Annual flu shots are recommended.

Should chest congestion or cold occur, patients and families should understand the importance of a high fluid intake (2500 to 3000 mL per day), deep breathing exercises, assisted coughing, postural drainage and clapping, and use of a humidifier. Appropriate team members, such as the community health nurse, should assess the home setting to ensure that these measures are feasible. Patients should take their temperature and call the family physician at the first sign of congestion.

A few patients may require a permanent tracheostomy. This and other techniques of caring for the ventilator-dependent quadriplegic person will be discussed in Chapter 17.

For a review of general information on assessment and implementation of education programs for patients and families, see Chapter 8.

LONG-TERM IMPLICATIONS

When assessing people with quadriplegia or high paraplegia who have been paralyzed for some time, nurses should keep in mind changes in respiratory function that are considered acceptable in light of permanent disability and should adjust baseline data as follows:

- Thoracic size and shape. A decreased anterior/posterior diameter caused by intercostal atrophy or contractures may lead to a rigid rib cage (Thomas, 1977: 251).

- Chest movement. Anticipate permanent paradoxical breathing. The respiratory rate and rhythm should remain normal at a rate of 12 to 20 breaths per minute.

- Pulmonary function tests. Generally speaking, the overall total lung capacity decreases. A tidal volume of 350 mL and a minimal vital capacity of 800 mL is considered acceptable under normal conditions, but a vital capacity of 2000 mL is needed to handle a respiratory infection. The expiratory reserve volume, which measures ability to cough, is virtually absent.

- Arterial blood gas analysis. A PaO_2 of 60 mmHg and a $PaCO_2$ of 45 to 50 mmHg is considered acceptable. Acid-base balance should be within normal limits.

Quadriplegic patients will frequently require assisted coughing and may find postural drainage and clapping necessary to keep the chest clear. However, secretions should be free from infection at all times.

Based on assessment, nurses help patients continue with preventive measures or refer them to appropriate resources such as family physician or physiotherapist. They remain alert for recurrent respiratory tract infections, keeping in mind that there may be underlying causes such as depression or poor nutrition.

SELECTED REFERENCES

Adams, N. R. 1979. The nurse's role in systematic weaning from a ventilator. *Nursing* 9 (8): 35–41. *A comprehensive, well-illustrated guide describing weaning with a T-piece or with intermittent mandatory ventilation (IMV) and weaning from a tracheostomy. Includes criteria for beginning the process, related nursing care, and a sample weaning flow sheet.*

Bergofsky, E. H. 1964. Mechanism for respiratory insufficiency after cervical cord injury. *Annals of Internal Medicine* 61 (3): 435–447. *A technical study investigating the mechanisms underlying chronic respiratory insufficiency (alveolar hypoventilation); explains how and why acute and chronic respiratory failure occurs following onset of quadriplegia.*

Burke, D. C., and Murray, D. D. 1975. *Handbook of Spinal Cord Medicine.* London and Basingstoke: MacMillan Press, Chapter 6. *Brief focus on acute respiratory and metabolic management of the quadriplegic patient.*

Carter, E. R. 1979. Medical management of pulmonary complications of spinal cord injury. *Advances in Neurology* 22: 261–269. *Presents major principles of respiratory insufficiency; summarizes problems common to the typical, the older, and the high-level quadriplegic patient; and focuses on several unique problems such as pleural effusion and cardiac arrest.*

Casas, R., et al. 1977–78. Prophylaxis of venous thrombosis and pulmonary embolism in patients with acute traumatic spinal cord lesions. *International Journal of Paraplegia* 15: 209–214. *A review of incidence and prevalence of deep vein thrombosis, its complications, and the prophylactic use of calcium heparin (a European perspective).*

Cheshire, D. J. E., and Coats, D. A. 1966. Respiratory and metabolic management in acute tetraplegia. *International Journal of Paraplegia* 4: 1–23. *Detailed correlations between the respiratory and metabolic aspects of acute management. Describes concepts and principles of maintaining adequate alveolar ventilation while promoting optimal nutrition and fluid and electrolyte balance.*

Cheshire, D. J. E., and Flack, W. J. 1978–79. The use of operant conditioning techniques in the respiratory rehabilitation of the tetraplegic. *International Journal of Paraplegia* 16: 162–174. *Based on the principles of neuromuscular exercise and behaviorist psychology, incentive spirometry is described as a way to improve respiratory function. Respiratory rehabilitation is designed to help the quadriplegic patient clear secretions and combat respiratory infection. Interprets conflicts in existing literature about mechanisms of breathing after spinal cord injury. Highly recommended.*

Corson, J. A., et al. 1979. Use of biofeedback in weaning paralyzed patients from respirators. *Chest* 76 (5): 543–545. *Reports on a study of two quadriplegic patients who failed to be weaned from a mechanical ventilator until biofeedback techniques were used. Biofeedback supplied information that the patient could use repeatedly to reach the criteria measured the previous day, thereby strengthening the existing muscles of respiration. Techniques described in detail.*

Fuchs, P. L. 1979. Understanding continuous mechanical ventilation. *Nursing* 9 (12): 26–33. *Concise overview of continuous mechanical ventilation with clinically relevant suggestions for recognizing and solving common problems.*

Gowan, N. J. 1979. The perceptual world of the intensive care unit: an overview of some environmental considerations in the helping relationship. *Heart Lung* 8 (2): 340–344. *Describes factors and helpful recommendations to help the patient cope with the psychological (emotional) and physical (sensory) environments that add to the existing stress of critical illness. Extensive bibliography.*

Hoffman, J. 1977. Arterial blood gas analysis as a basic criterion for the management of the neurosurgical patient. *Journal of Neurosurgical Nursing* 9 (1): 29–33. *Integrates pulmonary assessment and intervention techniques for patients with head and spinal cord injuries; includes chart of blood gas analysis for a patient with quadriplegia during the first 14 days after injury. Illustrates anticipated decreased pulmonary function before recovery.*

Holloway, N. M. 1979. *Nursing the Critically Ill Adult.* Menlo Park, Calif: Addison-Wesley. *Superb, clinically relevant reference. Integrates meaningful concepts of anatomy and physiology with the nursing process throughout text. Chapters 9 and 10 on aeration assessment and acute disorders are particularly helpful. Highly recommended.*

Kozier, B., and Erb, G. 1983. *Fundamentals of Nursing: Concepts and Procedures,* 2d ed. Menlo Park, Calif:

Addison-Wesley. *Presents introductory information on physiology of respiration, pulmonary function, assessment, and interventions. Chapter 18 includes step-by-step procedure for intermittent positive pressure breathing therapy.*

Larabee, J. H. 1977. The person with spinal cord injury: physical care during early recovery. *American Journal of Nursing* 77: 1320–1329. *Self-study format presenting overall care of actual and anticipated problems including those affecting respiratory function.*

Ledsome, J. R., and Sharpe, J. 1981. Pulmonary function in acute cervical cord injury. *American Review of Respiratory Disease* 124 (1): 41–44. *Research has implications to improve management of pulmonary function.*

McMichan, J. C., et al. 1980. Pulmonary dysfunction following traumatic quadriplegia. *Journal of the American Medical Association* 243 (6): 528–531. *A current study of pulmonary complications in 22 quadriplegic patients as compared to a retrospective survey of 22 comparable patients. Concludes that vigorous pulmonary therapy is associated with increased survival, fewer pulmonary complications, and less need for mechanical ventilation. Documentation of serial pulmonary function tests demonstrating marked decrease in repiratory function immediately after injury with significant improvement over time. Helpful information for nursing assessment and intervention. Highly recommended.*

Rau, J., and Rau, M. 1977. To breath or be breathed: understanding IPPB. *American Journal of Nursing,* April, pp. 613–617. *Description of treatment goals and nursing care; includes tables of information on hazards and symptoms; procedure for intermittent positive pressure breathing treatment; and comparison of Bird and Bennett respirators.*

Saunders, N. A.; Powles, A.; and Rebuck, A. 1976. Ear oximetry: accuracy and practicability in the assessment of arterial oxygenation. *American Review of Respiratory Disease* 113: 745–749. *A comparative study of three ear oximeters; concludes that ear oximetry is an accurate method of assessing changes in oxygenation and describes the added practical advantages of the Hewlett-Packard 47201A ear oximeter.*

Spence, A., and Mason, E. 1979. *Human Anatomy and Physiology.* Menlo Park, Calif: Addison-Wesley. *Presents foundations in anatomy and physiology, which include the effects of aging.*

Thomas, E. L. 1977. Nursing care of the patient with spinal cord injury. In *The Total Care of Spinal Cord Injuries,* D. S. Pierce and V. H. Nickel, Eds. Boston: Little, Brown, pp. 249–297. *Focus on long-term assessment and optimal maintenance management of respiratory function.*

Tyson, George W., et al. 1978. *Acute Care of the Head and Spinal Cord Injured Patient in the Emergency Department.* Charlottesville, Va: Department of Neurosurgery, University of Virginia. *Includes recognition of impending or manifest respiratory insufficiency in emergency care. Concise overview of emergency care, including neurological assessment and preparation of the patient for transport. Highly recommended.*

Zeluff, G. W., et al. 1977. Ondine's curse. *Heart Lung* 6 (6): 1057–1063. *Discussion of pathophysiology and differential diagnosis of apnea or near apnea in the high cervical cord injured patient; includes descriptions of phrenic nerve testing and surgical considerations to resolve the problem.*

SUPPLEMENTAL READING

General

Fugl-Meyer, A. R. 1971. A model for treatment of impaired ventilatory function in tetraplegic patients. *Scandinavian Journal of Medicine* 3: 168–177. *A rehabilitative focus on respiratory care.*

Guttman, L. 1973. *Spinal Cord Injuries Comprehensive Management and Research.* Oxford, England: Blackwell Scientific Publication. *Classic text on all aspects of spinal cord injury. Includes historical background information; general statistics; legal aspects; detailed anatomy and neuropathology of cord trauma and its effects on all body systems; regeneration; fractures, dislocations, gunshot injuries, and stab wounds; and neurophysiological and clinical management aspects. Extensive bibliography.*

Hudelson, E. I. 1977. Mechanical ventilation from the patient's point of view. *Respiratory Care* 22 (6): 654–656. *Gives insight into patients' perception and offers suggestions to ease some of the difficulties experienced.*

Linn, L. 1979. Psychosocial needs of patients with acute rspiratory failure. *Critical Care Quarterly* 1 (Mar.): 65–73. *Increases awareness of the patient's emotional and individual needs while on a respirator; considers environmental sources of anxiety and offers suggestions to minimize the effect of negative factors.*

Assessment

Carol, M., et al. 1979. Acute care of spinal cord injury, *Critical Care Quarterly* 2: 7–21. *Includes cardiopulmonary assessment and management in critical care. Excellent overview.*

Guyton, A. 1976. *Textbook of Medical Physiology.* 5th ed. Philadelphia: W. B. Saunders. *Detailed presentation of respiratory physiology and abnormalities.*

Pulmonary Function Tests in Patient Care. 1980. American Journal of Nursing Co. *Programmed instruction on assessment and interpretation.*

Tinker, J. 1976. Understanding chest X rays. *American Journal of Nursing* 76: 54–58. *A brief review of gross pathology on chest films, with illustrations of common disorders.*

Vanderheiden, G. C., and Grilley, K., Eds. 1975. *Nonvocal Communication Techniques and Aids for the Severely Physically Handicapped.* Baltimore, Md: University Park Press. *Based on transcriptions of the 1975 Trace Center national workshop series on nonvocal communication techniques and aids, provides detailed descriptions of the problems, tools, applications, and results. Advanced reference book.*

Waldron, M. W. 1979. Oxygen transport. *American Journal of Nursing* 9 (2): 272–275. *Clear explanation of oxygen delivery in relation to body homeostasis; illustrated graphs of the hemoglobin–oxygen dissociation curve helpful for arterial blood gas interpretation. Includes problem-solving section for self-evaluation.*

Intervention

Bromley, I. 1976. *Tetraplegia and Paraplegia: A Guide for Physiotherapists.* Edinburgh: Churchill Livingston. *A clear and detailed guide to physical therapy required by patients with spinal cord injuries.*

Craig Rehabilitation Center, Nursing Care Procedures. 1974. Denver, Colo: Craig Rehabilitation Hospital. *Basic step-by-step procedures, many of which relate to patients with spinal cord injuries.*

Kurihara, M. 1965. Postural drainage, clapping, and vibrating. *American Journal of Nursing* 65 (11): 76–79. *Good explanation of diaphragmatic breathing; chart correlating lung segments to be drained with postural drainage positions and with chest area to be clapped or vibrated. More suitable positions for long-term care.*

Sandham, G., and Reid, B. 1977. Some Q's and A's about suctioning. *Nursing* 7 (10): 60–65. *Photo story of nasopharyngeal and artificial airway suctioning; addresses problems of suctioning the left bronchus and difficulties encountered while on a mechanical ventilator. Includes step-by-step suctioning procedure.*

Tecklin, J. S. 1979. Positioning, percussing, and vibrating patients for effective bronchial drainage. *Nursing* 9 (3): 64–67. *Photo story of manual techniques for bronchial drainage of acutely ill children and adults.*

Trout, C. 1975. *Respiratory Management of the Acutely Injured Patient.* Continuing Education in the Treatment of Spinal Cord Injuries, No. 5. Chicago: National Spinal Cord Injury Foundation. *Excellent presentation of airway management and chest ventilation from the accident scene into the emergency room and the critical care area. Focuses on quadriplegia.*

Potential Problems

Fitzmaurice, J., and Sasahara, A. 1974. Current concept of pulmonary embolism: implications for nursing practice. *Heart Lung* 3 (2): 209–218. *A comprehensive review of risk factors, prevention, recognition, and treatment.*

Molyneux-Luick, M. 1978. Water-sports injuries, the old and the new. *Nursing* 8 (8): 50–55. *Explains physiological effects of fresh and salt water aspiration; presents information on nursing actions to promote optimal blood gases, pH, cardiac output, and central nervous system function; and presents tables of information on assessment and treatment of associated injuries. Especially helpful for nursing the patient with quadriplegia from a diving accident.*

Patient and Family Health Education

Engstrand, J. L., and Stuart, B. J. 1979. *Patient Handbook of Self-Care Procedures.* 2d ed. Birmingham, Ala: Spain Rehabilitation Center of the University of Alabama. *Section on respiratory home care focuses on prevention, postural drainage, and chest percussion and vibration; emphasizes precautions necessary for the quadriplegic individual. Well written in lay language.*

Fisher, M. L. 1979. Helping acutely ill patients put out the fire. *American Journal of Nursing* 79 (6): 1104–1105. *Description of nurses using behavior modification techniques to help the motivated post-surgical patient stop smoking.*

King, R. B.; Boyink, M.; and Keenan, M., Eds. 1977. *Rehabilitation Guide,* Medical Rehabilitation Research and Training Center No. 20. Chicago: Northwestern University and Rehabilitation Institute of Chicago. *Major principles of respiratory management and related home care; includes general respiratory care and tracheostomy equipment and pro-* *cedures. Uses a problem-solving approach for presentation, pp. 81–88.*

Virginia Spinal Cord Injury Care and Teaching Manual. 1980. The Virginia Spinal Cord Injury System, University of Virginia Center and Virginia Dept. of Rehabilitation Services, Woodrow Wilson Rehabilitation Center, Box W–279, Fisherville, Va. 22939. *Section on pulmonary complications (pp. 88–94) includes preventive measures, care during colds, assisted "quad" coughing, and a well-illustrated guide to postural drainage.*

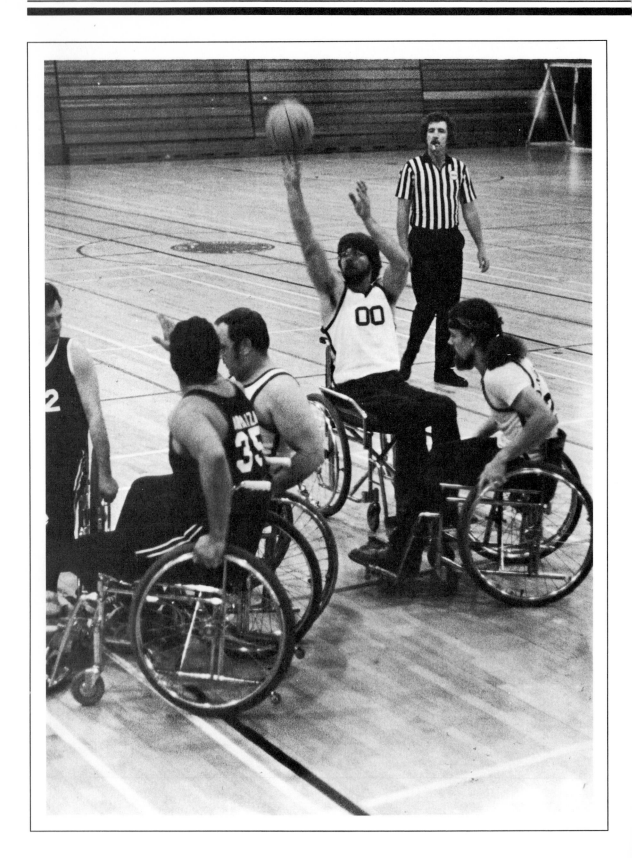

Chapter 10

Maintaining Cardiovascular Function and Body Temperature Control

CHAPTER OUTLINE

OBJECTIVES

- To explain how neural control of heart rate and peripheral vascular resistance and body temperature control are impaired by spinal cord injury
- To describe patients who are at additional risk of developing circulatory and temperature regulation problems and present methods of assessing the condition of those patients
- To discuss preventive measures to preserve cardiac function
- To describe appropriate activities and positioning techniques used to promote circulation to paralyzed limbs
- To explain significance of an elevated temperature as a diagnostic sign

- To present measures used to assist the patient conserve or dissipate body heat to regulate body temperature
- To discuss care of a patient with cardiac arrhythmias, edema, postural hypotension, autonomic dysreflexia (hyperreflexia), and deep vein thrombosis
- To present appropriate self-care skills to teach to patient and family
- To describe long-term implications associated with cardiovascular function and regulation of body temperature for the quadriplegic and high paraplegic patient

GOALS OF HEALTH CARE

Maintaining a desirable environment within the body is largely a function of the autonomic nervous system. This nervous system's influence on actions of the heart and blood vessels provides regulatory control of heart rate and blood pressure and pulse. Autonomic control of sweat glands helps regulate body temperature.

The stability of this internal environment is threatened when intricate communications with the central nervous system are interrupted. The higher the level of lesion, the more complicated the effects become, as greater body area is involved.

Immediately following injury, reactions in response to loss of autonomic nervous system control are extreme. The acute management phase focuses on prevention of complications while gradual adjustment to compensatory functioning occurs. "Local homeostasis" is usually achieved within a year. During that year, the goals of health care are:

- To preserve normal heart rate, blood pressure, and body temperature by preventing:

— abnormal heart action and inadequate tissue perfusion
— abnormal stimuli from triggering an exaggerated autonomic nervous system response
- To minimize negative effects of immobility and a passive vasodilation of the peripheral vascular system on blood flow
- To prevent complications caused by poor circulation and loss of body temperature control
- To be constantly aware of the risks involved and identify developing problems promptly to initiate effective early treatment

ASSESSMENT OF CARDIOVASCULAR FUNCTION AND BODY TEMPERATURE

Assessment of current cardiovascular status and body temperature and knowledge of the diagnosed level of lesion make it possible to predict the extent of autonomic nervous system dysfunction. Anticipation of compensatory function and potential problems helps the team prepare for emergencies and develop long-term care plans. The detail in which a history and physical examination are completed by the nurse will depend on the urgency of the situation and to what extent other team members are involved.

Dysfunction Following Spinal Cord Injury

The explanation of altered functioning of the circulatory or cardiovascular system following a spinal cord injury is not abnormality in the heart itself, but mainly changes in autonomic nervous system control of the influential vascular network. Similarly, this autonomic deficit affects mechanisms regulating body temperature. As maintaining a stable blood pressure, pulse, and temperature are so closely related, they will be discussed together in this chapter. To review the general characteristics of the autonomic nervous system, see Chapter 5.

Circulatory disturbances

Circulation depends on the heart's effectiveness as a pump, peripheral vascular resistance, and the volume and nature of circulating blood. In patients with spinal cord injuries, a threat to circulation is associated with a decrease in peripheral vascular resistance. Problems may also arise from the tendency of newly injured patients to develop cardiac arrhythmias or from complications associated with other injuries or preexisting conditions.

General factors influencing circulation
Blood pressure is a complex mechanism reflecting functional integration of the neurological and cardiovascular systems, and its measurement is a basic indicator of adequate tissue perfusion. Blood pressure is directly related to *cardiac output* and, most importantly, to *peripheral vascular resistance*. Similarly, the *pulse* reflects adequacy of circulation in general and can also be used to assess specific blood flow to the periphery.

Cardiac output is defined as the total amount of circulating blood in the body—approximately 5 liters per minute (at rest). The *minute volume* is computed by multiplying the *heart rate* by the *stroke volume* or amount of blood ejected into the systemic circulation with each ventricular contraction. The cardiac output is determined by the amount of venous blood returned to the

heart and autonomic nervous system stimulation or inhibition of the heart rate.

The heart derives innervation from both the sympathetic and the parasympathetic divisions of the autonomic nervous system. By far the more powerful is the sympathetic stimulation, which increases the heart rate and strengthens cardiac contractions. This is a vital response involved with the body's "fright and flight" mechanism. In a normal resting state there is little sympathetic influence on the heart. The major determinant of the heart rate at rest is the parasympathetic tone. Parasympathetic fibers reach the heart via the *vagus* nerve.

Peripheral vascular resistance is determined by the length and radius of the blood vessels and to a lesser extent blood viscosity. The vascular network responds to local tissue needs and to the central nervous control system.

Local control of blood flow is very important and functions independently to a great extent. Local blood vessel activity is based primarily on oxygen need and levels of carbon dioxide accumulation in the tissues themselves. Decreased oxygen levels in the tissues draw blood flow; increased levels of carbon dioxide shunt blood away from the affected area. The heart is also capable, to a certain extent, of adjusting pump action according to the amount of venous blood returned, and there is a direct relationship between arterial pressure and urinary or fluid excretion.

Central control of blood flow and vessel resistance is accomplished by the combined actions of the vasomotor center in the brain stem and the sympathetic division of the autonomic nervous system. Numerous other intricate factors are involved including the actions of higher brain centers on the vasomotor center and sensitive "feedback" mechanisms located throughout the body. The simplified explanations that follow focus mainly on the integrating function of the sympathetic nervous system, because injury to the spinal cord has the most profound effect on this component.

Sympathetic stimulation alters the radius of blood vessels, thus directly changing the resistance of these vessels and regulating blood flow through the tissues (Guyton 1976). Changing the rate of flow in these numerous and widespread blood vessels ultimately alters the total amount of circulating blood, which plays a major role in cardiovascular function.

Neural control of circulation By far the most important influence on peripheral vascular resistance is the *sympathetic vasoconstrictor system,* which is responsible for maintaining vasomotor tone. It is capable of rapidly shunting blood from the peripheral circulation to more vital organs when preparing the body for stress defense.

Vasoconstrictor fibers are distributed, with rare exception, to all the blood vessels of the body, but most abundantly to the arterial vessels. The supply is especially rich in the kidney, spleen, and skin of the limbs. Vasoconstriction can be accomplished by direct *neural stimulation* of the blood vessels. Secretion of epinephrine and norepinephrine from the adrenal medulla is described as *humoral stimulation* and also causes vasoconstriction. Neural stimulation provides rapid action, while humoral control produces long-lasting chemical effects throughout the body. The sympathetic nervous system also carries vasodilator fibers for innervation of specific secretory sites, but these are of less significance in circulatory control. The blood vessels do not receive parasympathetic innervation.

The *vasomotor center* is located in the reticular formation of the pons and medulla and is greatly influenced by the hypothalamus and other higher brain centers. "Nerve impulses from this center are ultimately transmitted by vasoconstrictor nerves to blood vessels, and the vasomotor center itself is continuously (tonically) active in promoting some degree of vasoconstriction (called *vasomotor tone*)" (Spence and Mason 1983: 526). With spinal cord injury, vasomotor tone is lost mainly due to interference with neural, rather than humoral, control of vasoconstrictor fibers.

Disturbances of circulation after injury For the sympathetic portion of the autonomic nervous system to function correctly, communication pathways between the vasomotor center in the brain stem and vasomotor fibers of the spinal cord and peripheral nervous system must be intact. The sympathetic fibers compose the thoracolumbar outflow of the autonomic nervous system. Injury to the spinal cord at the T_6 segmental level or above will interfere with the sympathetic nervous functions of preparing the body for stress and maintaining vasomotor tone. Injury below the T_6 level allows at least partial sympathetic function to continue. With lower lumbar or sacral cord injuries, the sympathetic nervous system remains intact but loss of reflex activity below the level of the lesion impairs vasomotor control to the lower limbs.

High paraplegic and quadriplegic patients are in the most danger of circulatory disturbance as evidenced by hypotension and bradycardia. The fall in the blood pressure and pulse rate is explained by the loss of vasoconstrictor tone and lack of sympathetic tone to the heart. Both capillary exchange and venous return to the heart are slowed. When circulation is slowed blood tends to pool in the abdomen and lower limbs.

Severe instability of the cardiovascular system is encountered immediately after injury and lasts for several days. A rare but most dangerous phenomenon may occur during this time. Stimulation, such as rapid changes of body position when turning or deep tracheal suctioning, is believed to trigger a vagovagal response. Massive activation of the parasympathetic system, made possible by the intact cranial outflow portion, is unchecked by the usual sympathetic antagonism; therefore stimulation to the heart is strong enough not only to slow, but also to stop, the heartbeat.

Further aggravating an injury to any level of the spinal cord is the superimposed postinjury state of *spinal shock.* As explained in Chapter 5, this neurogenic shock is characterized by loss of reflex activity below the level of lesion with subsequent low blood pressure and pulse rate.

With the passing of spinal shock and general recovery from traumatic injury, segmental sympathetic reflex activity provides some degree of compensatory function. Although a lower blood pressure and pulse rate may persist, cardiovascular function will eventually stabilize.

Abnormal thermoregulatory control

Regulation of temperature depends on the body's ability to maintain a balance between heat production and heat loss. Disturbances in the *thermoregulatory mechanisms* of patients with spinal cord injuries are caused by loss of autonomic control over vasomotor activity and the most important sweat mechanism. Quadriplegic patients, in particular, are unable to maintain a desirable central temperature if they are not protected from changes in environmental temperature. Assuming the temperature of the environment is a condition known as *poikilothermy*.

General factors influencing body temperature
The *heat regulation center* or "thermostat" of the body is located in the hypothalamus at the base of the brain. Input is received from thermosensitive receptors in the skin; the abdominal viscera and spinal cord (to a lesser extent); and central thermoreceptors in the hypothalamus itself that respond to actual changes in the temperature of the circulating blood. Thermoregulatory activity is further influenced by conditions resulting in fever and by environmental temperature changes. The following descriptions of heat production and heat loss are based on the works of Guyton (1976) and Castle and Watkins (1979). Explanations of abnormal control of these mechanisms associated with cord injury are based on the works of Guttman (1973) and Johnson (1971).

Production of heat in the body is actually the amount of energy released when food is metabolized. The rate at which this process occurs is called the metabolic rate and is usually measured under basal conditions. Factors that mainly affect the basal metabolic rate, and therefore directly alter body temperature, are exercise or activity, actions of the sympathetic nervous system, and production of the thyroid hormone. The actual temperature of the circulating blood is also able to accelerate or decrease metabolism.

Again, as in control of circulation, the sympathetic nervous system is most powerful in maintaining immediate physiological control of body temperature. People can also adjust clothing and indoor temperatures to protect themselves from changes in the environmental temperature. Fluctuating levels of thyroid hormone production respond, but only gradually. For example, prolonged exposure to the cold, such as in the beginning of winter, will stimulate production of the thyroid hormone to increase the basal metabolic rate, but the response takes several weeks.

Neural control of body temperature *Thermogenesis*, or conservation of body heat when the circulating blood becomes abnormally cool, re-lies on the anterior hypothalamus to raise body temperature by stimulating mechanisms to vasoconstrict peripheral blood vessels and increase metabolism and muscular activity, including "shivering."

Sympathetic vasoconstriction of the blood vessels of the skin diminishes blood flow to the periphery, thus decreasing the amount of heat loss to the atmosphere. Heat is thereby conserved by circulation of the warmed blood within the internal structures.

Sympathetic stimulation to increase body metabolism produces additional heat. Release of epinephrine into the tissues immediately increases the need for oxygen; this requires acceleration of cell metabolism and thus increases heat production.

Increased muscular activity also produces additional body heat. This may be voluntary, as with vigorous exercise, or an autonomic response to increase muscle tone. Progression to the reflex action of shivering, characterized by rapid muscle relaxation and contraction, is a most powerful mechanism and can almost double heat production in the body. Piloerection, or goose bumps, also occurs as small muscle contractions erect hair follicles. (This is of benefit to lower mammals with thick fur as a means of trapping air to increase thermal insulation.)

Thermolysis, or reduction of body heat, is stimulated when circulating blood becomes abnormally warm and relies on the posterior hypothalamus to stimulate mechanisms to lower body temperature. The thermoregulatory mechanisms act primarily to dilate skin blood vessels.

Disturbances of temperature regulation after injury Injury to the spinal cord above the thoracolumbar outflow of the sympathetic nervous system leaves loss of function in the hypothalamic thermoregulatory mechanisms.

Interruption of the sympathetic nervous system communication with the temperature control center in the brain causes lack of internal control below the level of lesion, mainly from absence of vasoconstriction, loss of the ability to shiver to conserve body heat, and loss of thermoregulatory sweating to dissipate heat. Chronic loss of vasomotor tone and passive vasodilation tends to cause continual loss of body heat.

The ability to control body temperature is directly related to the amount of musculature still normally innervated. People with quadriplegia will be the most severely affected. People with injury to the upper thoracic cord will have only partial function of these thermoregulatory mechanisms. Those with lower injuries may lose certain control of mechanisms below the level of lesion, but enough normal body function is usually preserved to control temperature.

History

Factors negatively influencing the maintenance of adequate circulation and temperature control include diagnosis of high thoracic or cervical cord injury, preexisting cardiovascular complications, associated injuries, and advanced age.

Diagnosis of high thoracic or cervical cord injury

The level and extent of cord injury diagnosed will indicate the severity of symptoms associated with interruption of sympathetic nervous control. Remember that the most critical time to observe for unstable blood pressure, pulse, and temperature is immediately after injury during spinal shock. The long-term problems associated with hypotension and poikilothermy tend to decrease as time passes.

Preexisting cardiovascular disease

It is important to note any preexisting cardiovascular disease. The patient may be well aware of a previous cardiac condition or may only describe subtle changes, such as fatigue on exertion or swelling of extremities, indicating circulatory problems. Complaints of dyspnea, palpitations, and especially chest pain should be investigated thoroughly. Pain can also be associated with vascular occlusion problems, as with intermittent claudication in the lower limbs. Preexisting cardiac disease is not prevalent with spinal cord injury, since the majority of patients are young.

Associated injuries

Patients with multiple injuries may develop internal or external hemorrhage from a variety of sources, which will deplete circulatory blood volume and thus diminish cardiac output. Spinal or neurogenic shock and hemorrhagic shock both cause low cardiac output. When they occur together the situation is more difficult. This problem is discussed further in Chapter 4 on emergency care.

Advanced age

Older patients (those over 50), particularly the elderly, have diminished cardiac reserve and cannot withstand the excessive demands placed on the heart with increases in physical and emotional stress as well as younger people can. The heart becomes a less effective pump as valves thicken and become more rigid, which causes incomplete filling and emptying of the heart with each contraction. Similar loss of arterial elasticity diminishes blood flow mainly to the extremities and the brain. The aging process, then, makes patients more susceptible to congestive heart failure, hypertension, and ischemic heart diseases. This places the older paralyzed person in double jeopardy of developing cardiac and circulatory problems.

Body temperature also tends to decrease with age. Adaptation to changes in the environment is slower due to sluggish action of thermoregulatory mechanisms. For example, older patients find it difficult to keep warm and cannot tolerate as much increased activity at high temperatures.

Physical Examination

Examination of the heart and circulation usually follows assessment of respiratory function. The physical examination reveals the patient's current cardiovascular status and includes cardiac assessment, vascular assessment, and assessment of other related body systems. Observation of body temperature will also be described in this section.

Cardiovascular status

Cardiac assessment   The following is summarized information of techniques used in evaluation of cardiac function. Purely cardiac problems are not particularly common in patients with spinal cord injuries and are not emphasized

PROCEDURE 10-1 ■ INSPECTION, PALPATION, AND AUSCULTATION OF THE HEART

Purpose

The purpose of these techniques is to assess the current cardiac status.

Action	Rationale
1. Inspect and palpate the chest wall. Locate the heart and determine size by describing cardiac borders in relation to external landmarks of ribs, intercostal spaces, and imaginary reference lines, e.g., mid-clavicular or midsternal lines. Palpate the *point of maximal impulse* (PMI)	The *precordium* is the chest area overlying the heart. Note any lifts, heaves, or abnormal pulsations or vibrations of the precordial area.
2. Auscultate heart sounds and describe in terms of intensity, frequency, quality, and duration.	Auscultation techniques allow assessment of heart sounds created by blood flow inside the heart during each cardiac cycle. Heart sounds are low and may be hard to hear, making auscultation difficult. The first sound corresponds to the beginning of ventricular systole (*lubb* sound) and the second sound corresponds to the end (*dupp* sound). Normally a longer pause (the *lubb-dupp pause*) occurs after the second sound. This relationship remains throughout the normal cardiac cycle, and these two sounds may be heard throughout the precordial area.
3. Auscultate heart sounds in a systematic fashion from the aortic area, to the pulmonic area, to the tricuspid area, and finally to the mitral or apical area.	To assess specific valve action, it is best to auscultate in a systematic fashion. *Murmurs* are heard when blood flow within the heart becomes turbulent. These usually result from obstruction, valvular defects, or abnormal vascular communication between compartments of the heart. Abnormal sounds may reveal specific problems, such as valvular insufficiency or stenotic changes.

here. The techniques of *inspection, palpation,* and *auscultation* are used to obtain precise information about the heart. See Procedure 10-1.

Consideration of diagnostic findings will also add to assessment data. Numerous invasive and noninvasive diagnostic aids are available to provide sophisticated information about cardiac function. The following measures are most likely to be encountered in the immediate post-injury period, especially when the patient is suffering from multiple injuries.

• *Hemodynamic monitoring,* through direct placement of catheters in the atria (for obtaining central venous pressure) or pulmonary or systemic arteries, measures cardiovascular pres-

sures and allows arterial or venous blood samples to be obtained without repeated vascular punctures. This method of assessment is usually designated for use only in critical care areas, because obtaining and analyzing pressure measurements and prevention of complications require specialized nursing skills. The advantage of hemodynamic monitoring, that is, the ability to obtain exact blood pressures, must be carefully weighed against the increased possibility of infection, thrombosis, and possibly emboli formation. Certainly gentle range of motion exercises—with careful support of the limb and continuous assessment of circulation to the distal portion of the limb—are mandatory. One source recommends insertion of a femoral arterial line on admission to the emergency room in cases of abnormal initial blood gases, deterioration of respiratory status, or apparent hemodynamic abnormalities (Carol et al. 1979).

- The *electrocardiogram* (*ECG*) is a most valuable and frequently used diagnostic test to aid in the identification and treatment of cardiac arrhythmias. Many physicians believe an ECG is an essential part of the admission workup for any patient over 40 years of age. The demand on cardiac reserve is increased in patients with spinal cord injuries due to the severity of physical and emotional stress associated with the injury. Continuous monitoring is not always practical due to position demands restricting exposure of the chest, such as proning on a Stryker frame. Moreover, meticulous skin care and changing of lead sites are essential to prevent skin breakdown when leads are placed on an area of the chest that is without sensation.

- A *chest X ray* must be included in the admission workup to provide information about heart size, signs of enlargement, calcification of cardiac structures, and alterations in blood flow in relation to the pulmonary circulation. However, many times the patient cannot tolerate being moved to the X-ray department, and initial portable films, which present a more distorted view, may not provide the detailed information desired.

- *Blood work analysis* to examine serum enzyme levels may be useful to detect ischemic heart problems. Certain enzymes are released from damaged tissues, and the enzyme levels peak between 24 and 72 hours after a myocardial infarction. Spinal cord injury itself is not associated with increases in serum enzyme levels unless there is significant damage to skeletal muscles.

Skill at cardiac assessment, particularly auscultation, and interpretation of diagnostic findings requires considerable practice under the direction of a knowledgeable practitioner (Holloway 1979). Although nurses may be unable to diagnose abnormalities, their ability to detect and describe unusual findings may alert a physician to the need of further assessment.

Vascular assessment Impairment of vasomotor control as a result of cord injury may cause short- or long-term changes in the peripheral vascular system. This system is intimately tied to cardiovascular function as a whole. Techniques involved in vascular assessment are *inspection and palpation of the extremities, and measurement of the blood pressure and pulse.* See Procedures 10–2 and 10–3.

Critical observation of circulatory status is required during the immediate postinjury period. Nurses should watch for evidence of a deep vein thrombosis, especially while the patient is immobilized. Edema and postural hypotension can cause problems when mobilization is started. Specific nursing care measures are discussed in detail later in this chapter.

Vascular assessment would be incomplete without consideration of blood work results to indicate abnormal blood composition, inadequate oxygenation, hemorrhage, and fluid or electrolyte imbalances. One source suggests that a CBC with differential, SMA–6, SMA–12, coagulation studies, type and crossmatch, and arterial blood gases be drawn to establish baseline data for all patients on admission (Carol et al. 1979).

Assessment of other body systems Inadequate circulation can be reflected by altered function of other body systems, and examination of pulmonary and renal function and the central nervous system, in particular, should be included in general assessment of the cardiovascular system. Respiratory function depends on cardiac function; left-sided heart failure, for example, causes blood to pool in the pulmonary system, which leads to pulmonary edema. Renal and cardiac functions are also associated. Urine output will decrease to conserve blood volume when compensating for an abnormally low blood pressure. Observation of the level of consciousness is most important as increased restlessness, irritability, or subtle behavioral changes may well be the first signs from the central nervous system of poor oxygenation from inadequate blood flow.

Body temperature

Methods used to determine body temperature include palpating the skin and, of course, measuring by thermometer. For techniques used see Procedure 10–4. Because of extreme lability, determine body temperature regularly, every two to four hours on admission and there-

PROCEDURE 10–2 ■ INSPECTION AND PALPATION OF THE EXTREMITIES

Purpose

The purpose of these techniques is to assess vascular status, especially to detect impairment or obstruction of venous blood flow.

Action	Rationale
1. Inspect and palpate both upper and lower extremities.	Good circulation to the extremities ensures that the skin is warm and dry, pink (if the patient is Caucasian), and free from any swelling. The skin will reflect inadequate circulation by abnormal pallor, a mottled appearance, or a cyanotic tinge. Coolness of extremities and presence of edema also indicate poor circulation.
2. Watch carefully for developing edema in the hands and arms of quadriplegic patients, as well as in the feet and ankles of all paralyzed patients. Always compare limbs bilaterally.	Vasomotor inactivity associated with paralysis causes blood to pool in the extremities. Gravitational forces, especially when a sitting position is assumed, further complicate the situation by overcoming the abnormally low pressure of venous blood returning to the heart.
3. Constantly examine the skin for local lesions.	Initially, lacerations, hematomas, bruises, or even burns may be sustained at the time of injury. During the course of rehabilitation, pressure areas or accidental trauma may occur. Observe these surface areas closely, because stasis of circulation slows the healing process, and the underlying venous structures may be damaged.
4. Examine the involved extremity *distal* to the lesion for increased warmth, redness, and swelling.	These signs indicate an obstruction to venous return. The greatest potential danger is the development of a deep vein thrombosis, predisposing the patient to pulmonary embolism. For more detailed information on general skin assessment and care, see Chapter 15.

after on a daily basis for an eight- to twelve-week period.

Disturbances of temperature regulation due to interruption of autonomic nervous system communication with the temperature control center in the brain causes lack of internal control below the level of the lesion.

Nurses should closely observe the high paraplegic and quadriplegic patient. The higher the level of injury, the greater the body area affected and the more severe the symptoms.

The spinal cord injured patient will always have some degree of difficulty in controlling body temperature, but the severity of this problem subsides as local reflex activity resumes, and the body adapts to the injury. Low body temperature is a particular problem during the state of spinal shock.

GENERAL NURSING INTERVENTIONS

Maintaining Adequate Circulation

To ensure adequate cardiovascular function, nursing care focuses on preserving adequate pumping action of the heart, maintaining desirable blood volume and composition, and pro-

PROCEDURE 10–3 ■ MEASUREMENT OF BLOOD PRESSURE AND PULSE

Purpose

The purpose of measuring the blood pressure is to assess systemic circulation, which reflects the general cardiovascular status. The pulse is also measured to assess systemic circulation. More specifically, it is used to evaluate blood flow to selected body parts [e.g., the pedal pulse (*dorsalis pedis*) is included in assessing circulation to a lower limb].

Action	Rationale
1. Obtain the blood pressure.	The blood pressure indicates the pressure at which blood is forced through the arteries; the systolic pressure is produced when the ventricles contract and the diastolic when the ventricles are at rest. The normal blood pressure range for an adult is generally 110 to 140 mmHg systolic and 60 to 80 mmHg diastolic.
2. Observe for *hypotension* immediately after injury.	Systolic pressures less than 100 mmHg are considered hypotensive. Due to spinal shock, and sometimes hypovolemic shock caused by multiple injuries, all patients may experience an initial fall in blood pressure. High paraplegic and quadriplegic patients will eventually develop a constant low blood pressure. Experience has shown that quadriplegic patients have a blood pressure of about 100/60 mmHg when resting and an even lower pressure when sitting up.
3. Observe for episodes of *hypertension*.	A pressure of greater than 160 mmHg systolic or 100 mmHg diastolic is described as hypertensive. Episodes of hypertension, reaching extremely dangerous levels, can be associated with the autonomic crisis called autonomic hyperreflexia.
4. Take the pulse and describe in terms of rhythm and volume.	The pulse rate is generally between 60 and 100 beats per minute in the adult and of a regular rhythm and normal force.
5. Observe for *bradycardia* immediately after injury.	Bradycardia describes a pulse rate less than 60 beats per minute and tachycardia a pulse rate greater than 100 beats per minute. Bradycardia after injury is due to spinal shock. Tachycardia at this time is a symptom of internal or external bleeding associated with the initial trauma.

moting blood flow in the peripheral vascular system. Measures discussed in this general section are largely preventive. As seen with respiratory function, *early mobilization* has greatly reduced complications, and *vigorous physiotherapy to unaffected limbs* has done much to enhance cardiopulmonary reserve.

Preserving cardiac function

1. *Prevent hypoxia.* A diminished flow of oxygen in the systemic circulation may progress to myocardial hypoxia in the heart. The most common causes of simple systemic hypoxia in patients with spinal cord injuries are impaired neural im-

PROCEDURE 10–4 ■ ASSESSING BODY TEMPERATURE

Purpose

The purpose of assessing body temperature is to determine which nursing care measures are required to help the patient maintain a desirable body temperature. The body temperature is a vital diagnostic sign.

Action	Rationale
1. Palpate the skin surface of the body with the back of the hand, rather than the fingertips.	The back of the hand is more sensitive to temperature changes.
2. Note areas of warmth or coolness and also moisture content.	The body surface may be the same throughout; or cooler in areas of poor circulation; or warmer in localized areas, indicating a problem such as soft tissue pressure or thrombophlebitis. The skin may be dry (as in spinal shock) or moist and clammy (as in hemorrhagic shock).
3. Obtain an oral temperature.	The normal range of an oral temperature is 36° to 37°C (96.8° to 99.6°F).
4. Obtain a rectal temperature. Gently insert a *well-lubricated* thermometer and *hold* in place for 5 minutes.	A rectal temperature is considered most accurate in measuring core body temperature and will measure 0.4°C (0.7°F) more than an oral measurement. Rectal temperatures are recommended for patients in shock or coma, restless or uncooperative patients, or patients receiving oxygen or mouth-breathing (most quadriplegic patients mouth-breathe). Extra care must be taken to avoid rectal trauma when the patient is without rectal sensation and is subject to sudden position change from involuntary leg spasms.
5. Be alert for *hypothermia* early after injury, and in the postoperative and elderly patient.	Most patients with spinal cord injuries suffer from subnormal temperatures due to spinal shock, hypovolemic shock, exposure to the elements at an accident scene, and the air-conditioned surroundings of emergency rooms.

pulses to the breathing muscles, which leads to ventilation problems, and hemorrhagic or neurogenic shock, which lowers cardiac output.

It is important, then, to determine the cause of hypoxia and initiate early treatment. To review identification of patients at risk and treatment of pulmonary complications resulting in hypoxia, see specific nursing interventions in Chapter 9.

2. *Minimize workload of the heart.* Physical and psychological insult, which both occur readily with paralysis, easily increase the workload of the heart. In reaction to this stress, the heart receives increased levels of adrenalin and becomes more irritable; this may cause electrical instability. This leads to less effective circulation, and in turn, decreases oxygenation of vital organs including the heart itself.

To avoid excess cardiac stimulation, take measures to promote adequate rest and psychological comfort and reduce the effects of physical and emotional stress. Stress induces epinephrine production, which in turn causes an increase in oxygen consumption by the heart. Especially during the early stages when intensive care is required, the nurse is responsible for coordinating interdisciplinary care at a tolerable rate for the patient. General measures to protect the patient from the physical and emotional trauma associated with the invasive atmosphere of a critical care unit have been described in Chapter 9. As the rehabilitation process progresses, monitor the patient closely for signs of fatigue associated with increases in physical activity. Carefully observe those with a history of poor tolerance for exercise before injury, such as the obese or the elderly. Be sure to communicate your observations effectively, so therapy programs can be modified if necessary.

Another important nursing measure is to ensure regular evacuation of the neurogenic bowel to avoid any added strain on the heart. (Maintaining bowel function is discussed in Chapter 13.)

3. *Maintain desirable blood volume and composition.* Prevent or promptly treat fluid and electrolyte imbalances. Intravenous fluid administration and electrolyte replacement therapy, as well as adequate nutrition and hydration, are described in Chapter 11. A decrease in the volume of circulating blood may result from hypovolemic or neurogenic shock.

4. *Help the physician control blood pressure with medication.* Hypotension due to neurogenic shock can be treated by medications such as dopamine hydrochloride (Intropin), a sympathomimetic amine. This powerful drug increases cardiac output directly by stimulating the heart muscle and indirectly by stimulating the release of norepinephrine. Dopamine hydrochloride must be carefully titrated, using an infusion pump, to maintain the target blood pressure. Onset of the effect is rapid, within five minutes, and duration of action is about ten minutes. Be alert for adverse reactions of arrhythmias and watch insertion site for signs of infiltration, which will cause necrotic changes.

Promoting blood flow in paralyzed limbs

1. Assist venous return to the heart. As all patients with spinal cord injuries suffer from some loss of strength and ability to move in addition to initial total immobilization, an appropriate activity level must be provided immediately to prevent circulatory complications. Certainly the philosophy of early mobilization with postural changes and wheelchair activity greatly decreases the hazards of immobilization caused by venous stasis.

- Encourage as much activity as possible within limits of orthopedic stability. Active or passive range of motion exercises are essential for patients on bedrest. A physiotherapy program based on the level of lesion and patient tolerance should be initiated soon after admission.
- Introduce mobilization from bedrest to wheelchair activities gradually by a *graded* activity program to avoid circulatory collapse. This is evidenced by the frequently encountered and closely related problems of *gravitational edema* and *postural* (orthostatic) *hypotension.* Ways to prevent or forestall these complications, which are particularly severe with quadriplegia, are described in the section on specific nursing interventions later in this chapter.
- Elevate paralyzed limbs while in bed or in the wheelchair. The following measures may need to be maintained continuously during bedrest if the problem is severe. Otherwise they may be used during rest periods or at night only.
  —Elevate and support limbs with pillows and select arm and foot boards for immobilization beds.
  —Elevate foot of bed 10 to 15 degrees only (to avoid inguinal congestion), unless contraindicated when countertraction is required for cervical injuries.
  The following technique may be used while the patient is in the wheelchair rather than returning the patient to bed.
  —Tip the chair backward and elevate legs to rest or recline on bed or couch. See Figure 10–1. Elevated leg rests for special problems may be required.
  —Practice tipping chair every two to three hours during waking hours. After meals, in between therapy, or when watching television may be convenient times.
- Provide compression forces to muscle bellies and joints. Antiembolitic (elasticized) stockings and ace or tensor bandages are used to exert a supplemental force on the veins. These measures are specifically indicated with edema,

postural hypotension, or thrombophlebitis. Correct application and care is essential to avoid blocking circulation. Antiembolitic stockings are generally preferred for convenience and ease of application. Tensor bandages are required when the patient has an arterial line, when there are associated leg injuries or open areas on the skin, or when elasticized stockings are not large enough to fit.

2. Avoid local trauma to blood vessels. Regular turning to relieve pressure and positioning the patient correctly to reduce pressure on bony prominences help ensure adequate circulation to the skin. Positioning, support, and protection of the extremities, including the arms of quadriplegic patients, are important whether the patient is on bedrest or sitting up in a wheelchair. (Chapter 14 describes specific positioning methods on various immobilization beds.)

Generally, nursing care measures to prevent, recognize, and treat skin breakdown will in turn prevent undue pressure on internal vein structures. Avoid venous punctures in the legs at all costs. Be sure to alert lab technicians to avoid this hazard when obtaining blood specimens. An IV site in the leg should be selected only under extraordinary circumstances. Also, attend promptly minor cuts, blisters, or skin abrasions on the legs and feet. Due to paralysis, the healing process is slow and extra care is needed to prevent infection.

Maintaining Desirable Body Temperature

To maintain desirable body temperature, nursing care focuses on protecting the patient from the environment. Measures to help patients conserve and dissipate body heat are needed.

Helping patients conserve body heat

1. Prevent undesirable cooling of the body. Maintain a desirable environmental temperature of 21°C (70°F) whenever possible. The quadriplegic patient (nursed without blankets) in a constant environmental temperature of 21°C (70°F) will stabilize at a body temperature of 35°C (94° to 95°F) (Cheshire and Coates 1966). Some physicians believe this slight degree of hy-

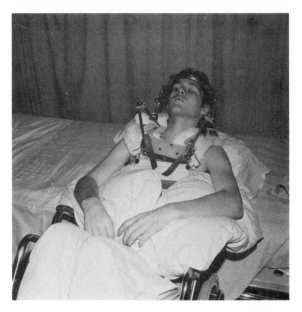

FIGURE 10–1 ■ A convenient rest position.

pothermia is beneficial during the initial post-injury period when hypoxia is most likely to occur. The lowered body temperature decreases the basal metabolic rate, thereby reducing oxygen requirements and reducing the work of breathing. Although there may be immediate therapeutic advantages to this spontaneous cooling, the patient is generally kept covered until complications are ruled out. If patients are going to be outside for activities, or even for a short period during transport, provide warm clothing or covering to protect them from the climate. Carefully observe inactive, poorly nourished, or elderly patients who have difficulty keeping warm at the best of times.

2. Take measures to warm the patient. A hot beverage, a warm bath, or an extra cover, for example, may make the patient comfortable. Keep the patient dry at all times to prevent rapid heat loss. Never use hot water bottles and electric heating devices that may burn desensitized skin.

The postoperative patient with a spinal cord injury can readily develop hypothermia. Immediate placement of warmed blankets on the patient in the recovery room usually prevents further problems.

3. Care for the quadriplegic patient with excessive diaphoresis of the upper body. Sometimes periods of *profuse* sweating above the level of lesion is thought to be a mechanism triggered to compensate for loss of thermoregulatory sweating below the level of lesion. This is most uncomfortable and distressing for the patient although the condition tends to stabilize eventually. The patient must be kept dry to *prevent chilling.* Changes of bed linen or clothing may be necessary every few hours. "Drenching" of bed linen is not uncommon. Flannel sheets or towels used to wrap the patient's torso are most absorbent. Dehydration may occur.

When the problem is prolonged or interferes with daily activities, oral anticholinergic drug therapy can be used to suppress the overactive sweat glands. However, anticholinergic effects may also produce undesirable actions, such as urinary retention.

Periods of excessive sweating may be induced by reflex action of the sympathetic nervous system. Underlying conditions, such as increased bladder pressure from infection or straining with a constipated stool, may cause reflex sweating. Unlike the desired diaphoresis associated with temperature control, the cause of these diaphoretic episodes must be identified and treated.

Helping patients dissipate body heat

1. Prevent undesirable warming of the body. During the summer avoid the outdoors if temperatures are extremely high, especially if high humidity is a factor, or remove extra clothing during exercise or therapy periods to allow heat loss. The patient's oral temperature may well average 38°C (100° to 101°F) at this time (Thomas 1977).

A fan can be used to cool a warm patient (constant air flow aids heat loss by convection). Adjust air conditioning if possible. Another idea, often used by wheelchair athletes, is to carry a water spray bottle. The water vapor sprayed on the skin acts like perspiration to promote heat loss through evaporation.

2. Recognize and treat fever promptly. An elevated temperature is a particularly valuable di-

agnostic sign, as sensory loss frequently renders the patient unable to localize or describe pain associated with infection or other underlying disease processes.

- Detect onset of fever. Frequently the patient will feel chilled, complain of general malaise, fatigue, headache, loss of appetite, and the skin will be warm and dry to the touch. Monitor temperature rectally every two to four hours, or more frequently, to reveal fever pattern. Observe pulse and respirations. Tachycardia and hyperventilation may occur as oxygen requirements increase approximately 18% with each 1°C rise in body temperature. Anticipate some temperature elevation as a reaction to dehydration, hemorrhage, or even surgery in the early postinjury period.

- A constant fever pattern, of sudden onset, is usually associated with infection. Urinary or respiratory tract infections are common culprits in patients with spinal cord injuries. Immediately check for concentrated, foul-smelling, or sedimented urine. Perform a chest inspection and note any signs of congestion. Check for a moist, productive cough that may indicate early secretion retention. A persistent low-grade fever can be associated with thrombophlebitis. Check the lower extremities for any signs.

- An intermittent fever pattern, in which the temperature is elevated for periods and then returns to normal during a 24-hour time span, may indicate an allergic drug reaction, gram-negative bacteremia, or septicemia. This can be very difficult to diagnose. Check the patient's drug profile. Note any penicillins or barbiturates in particular that may cause an allergic reaction. Often a blood culture, obtained when the temperature is next elevated, will be ordered.

- Alert the physician to an elevated temperature. Before specifically treating the source of the suspected infection, obtain urine, sputum, throat, and wound specimens for culture and sensitivity to indicate specific antibiotic therapy. As paralyzed patients are prone to a number of infections over a long-term period, cautious use of antibiotics in the early stages is important to avoid building up drug resistance. Prophylactic use of antibiotics is not recommended.

- Administer antipyretic drugs as ordered to act directly on the vasomotor temperature control center and take measures to promote heat loss from the body surface. Fanning and tepid sponging are usually sufficient to maintain the body temperature around 37.8°C (100°F). Alcohol sponges have a tendency to dry the skin. The use of ice packs or an electric cooling blanket introduces the added risk of "burning" the patient's insensitive skin and is rarely necessary. Should the patient begin to shiver above the level of the lesion, stop the cooling measures in use. The shivering mechanism actually generates heat. The patient may even need to be warmed temporarily to alleviate shivering.
- Replace fluid loss and maintain adequate nutrition. Increase fluid intake to 3000 mL daily unless contraindicated by other conditions. As the basal metabolic rate increases with fever, there is a dramatic increase in the amount of calories needed. Nourishing liquids, such as milk shakes or eggnogs, are usually most acceptable to the anorexic patient. Soup or broth is good, too. Intravenous therapy for fluid and electrolyte replacement may also be necessary.

SPECIFIC NURSING INTERVENTIONS FOR POTENTIAL COMPLICATIONS

Cardiac Arrhythmias

Serious insult of cardiac function may occasionally require nursing the patient in a cardiac care unit. It is not within the scope of this text to provide a comprehensive guide to this type of care, but to point out prevention, assessment, and interventions for some problem areas common to spinal cord injuries. Nurses should, of course, be familiar with cardiac assessment and ECG interpretation.

Cardiac arrhythmias, or irregularities in the rhythm of heart contractions, may be harmless or may progress to fatal complications. Due to

their general high risk of developing hypoxia, hypotension, and fluid, electrolyte, and metabolic imbalances and a high degree of physical and emotional stress, patients with spinal cord injuries are notably predisposed to cardiac disturbances. Accompanied interruption to the autonomic nervous system is thought to release high levels of catecholamines in the blood, increasing sympathetic stimulus to the heart. Abnormal vagal, parasympathetic reactions can slow or stop the heartbeat. The patient with a spinal cord injury is most likely to develop bradycardia or tachycardia and premature ventricular contractions. The most critical time is the 12 weeks immediately following the injury (Comarr 1977).

Goals of care

- To identify patients at risk of developing cardiac arrhythmias
- To identify and control preexisting heart disease
- To preserve adequate cardiac output by maintaining optimum heart action and sufficient core and peripheral perfusion
- To diagnose and initiate treatment early to prevent progression of symptoms causing fatal complications

Nursing interventions

1. Minimize risk conditions. Provide general measures, as discussed previously in this chapter, to prevent systemic hypoxia and therefore myocardial hypoxia, minimize workload of the heart to decrease oxygen requirements, and maintain desirable blood volume and composition. Promote peripheral vascular circulation to avoid complications of edema, postural hypotension, and autonomic dysreflexia. These are all associated with undesirable blood pressure changes. In addition, several other specific measures should be observed:

- Maintain normal fluid and electrolyte balances. Surprisingly severe fluid and metabolic imbalances can and usually do accompany spinal cord injury. It is postulated that increased mineralocorticoid activity leads to sodium retention and potassium depletion (Burke and

Murray 1975). A positive sodium balance causing overhydration adds to circulatory overload. More important is the severe loss of potassium. Hypokalemia delays restoration of smooth muscle function, particularly in the cardiac muscle, so irregularities can develop. The body's buffer systems are severely taxed by pulmonary and renal involvement, which further aggravate the situation. Monitor detailed intake and ouput. Administer fluid and electrolyte replacement therapy as ordered.

- Minimize stimulating effects of increased catecholamines circulating in the blood, characterized by tachycardia and premature contractions. Alleviate pain and promote physical and emotional rest.

- Avoid vagal stimulation leading to uncontrolled bradycardia or cardiac arrest. To decrease catecholamine release and minimize the risk of hypoxemia-induced arrhythmias, suction patients cautiously, particularly those with an artificial airway. Preoxygenate the patient on 100% oxygen before suctioning and postoxygenate for a few breaths too. Observe a time limit of 15 seconds when applying suction to avoid blocking the patient's air supply. Instruct patients not to hold their breath and strain with early bowel evacuations. Also avoid turning patients quickly for the first few days after injury. Although poorly understood, cardiac arrest has occurred following a sudden change of position. Turning may create an undesirable respiratory stimulus. Without time to develop a local homeostasis, the passively dilated venous network may simply be unable to shunt blood adequately to accommodate the position change. For this reason, some physicians do not recommend early use of turning frames. *Severe* vagal instability lasts only a few days after injury.

2.   Constantly observe patients with preexisting heart disease or those at risk of developing cardiac involvement. Some factors to be alert for are advanced age, severe emotional strain, severe pulmonary or renal involvement, a history of smoking, and diabetes. Consult with the physician about continuous monitoring, need for pain relief, and need for oxygen for high-risk individuals. Confirm preexisting diagnosis with physician and initiate treatment measures to alleviate effects of primary disease.

3.   Observe for deterioration in current cardiac function associated with arrhythmias. Look for signs of decreased cardiac output, mainly reflected by depressed level of consciousness, failing cardiac signs, and poor renal function as follows:

- Note subtle changes in the level of consciousness, such as dizziness or slow mentation, which can indicate hypoxia.

- Note falling blood pressure and pulse rate and rhythm irregularities. Compare apical pulse with peripheral pulses to detect any pulse deficit.

- Be alert for signs of heart failure. Increased central venous pressure, jugular vein distension, venous engorgement of abdominal vessels, liver tenderness, anorexia, nausea and vomiting, and generalized dependent edema suggest right-sided heart failure, which causes backup of blood in the systemic circulation. Left-sided heart failure causes backup of blood in the lungs and creates pulmonary signs such as dyspnea, rales, and wheezing cyanosis; pulmonary edema; and hyperventilation leading to respiratory alkalosis. Finally, more generalized symptoms, such as severe apprehension with accompanying chest pain, poor color, and clammy skin with diaphoresis, may well indicate a myocardial infarction.

- Be alert for decreased urinary output with an increased specific gravity and loss of electrolytes or catecholamines in the urine.

4.   Detect arrhythmias by continuous monitoring. See Figure 10–2. The ability to identify a normal sinus rhythm and detect abnormalities is important. Obtain an electrocardiogram rhythm strip and attach to nursing notes every eight hours for routine recording on each shift and when abnormal rhythm occurs. Note and record time of onset, duration, and frequency of arrhythmia. Collaborate with the physician to determine acceptable parameters for the pulse rate and number and pattern of premature ventricular beats allowed. If the patient is hemodynamically stable, intervention may not be warranted. If arrhythmias worsen, however, cardiac output can fall to dangerous levels, causing shock. For example, a sudden onset of bradycardia is dangerous, whereas a gradual onset is a compensatory method to improve stroke volume and maintain cardiac output that is commonly seen with quadriplegia. On the other hand, tachycardia may temporarily increase cardiac output, but eventually filling time to the heart will be so limited that cardiac output falls. Uncontrolled premature contractions indicate cellular irritability and predispose the patient to flutter and fibrillation problems.

Continuous cardiac monitoring may be hampered by the prone position required for traction, limited chest exposure with orthopedic braces, and the equipment needed to maintain pulmonary support, gastric decompression, and so on. Therefore astute history taking, physical examination, and interpretation of diagnostic findings are heavily relied on to monitor hemodynamic status. The greatest emphasis is, of course, on prevention.

5. Administer cardiac suppressants and stimulants, diuretics, and oxygen therapy as ordered by the physician. Also administer analgesics as ordered. Assess pain and anxiety levels frequently. (Often small intravenous doses of analgesics every two hours are most effective.)

6. Detect abnormal laboratory findings (primarily blood hematology, chemistry, electrolytes, and urine and serum osmolality) and respond appropriately.

7. Evaluate effectiveness of treatment by level of outcome criteria reached:

- Pulse 60 to 100 beats per minute of regular rate and rhythm, no pulse deficit, peripheral pulses of equal rhythm and volume bilaterally
- Blood pressure within normal limits for patient (100/60 mmHg is acceptable for a recumbent quadriplegic person)
- ECG in regular sinus rhythm without evidence of premature beats (or within acceptable rate and pattern as decided by physician)
- Heart action able to maintain adequate core and peripheral perfusion as evidenced by alert and oriented mental state, absence of elevated

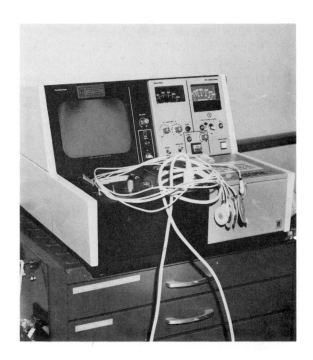

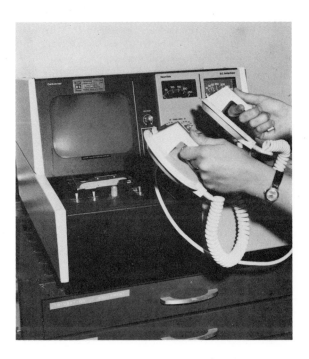

FIGURE 10–2 ■ A compact, portable monitor-defibrillator combination system is well suited to the acute rehabilitative setting. (A) Continuous monitoring mode with patient cable and leads attached. (B) Electrical paddles for emergency care.

venous systemic or pulmonary pressure, no chest pain (angina), and urinary output within normal limits, usually 2 to 3 liters per day

Edema

Edema is the swelling of body tissues from excessive fluid accumulating in the interstitial spaces. The source of edematous fluid is the blood plasma (Kozier and Erb 1983). During circulation the blood plasma enters the capillary from the arterioles and filters into the interstitial space. Fluid, electrolytes, and nutrients are delivered and waste products are removed in this space between the capillaries and the tissue cells. Normally, approximately 90% of the fluid reenters the capillary at the venule end and is reabsorbed into the systemic circulation. The remaining 10% is reabsorbed by the lymphatic system.

Several factors may interfere with this fluid exchange at the capillary level to result in edema. For example, an inflammatory response may cause localized swelling, by increasing the permeability of the capillary wall, or shock will diminish urinary output, which causes fluid retention and generalized swelling. The most common cause, however, is an increase in venous pressure at the reabsorption end of the capillary. When reabsorption is not possible, fluid is trapped in the interstitial spaces and nourishment and removal of waste products at the cellular level is decreased. This is also true of patients with spinal cord injuries. Due to disturbed vasomotor control and decreased tone in paralyzed muscles, circulatory return to the heart is poor, which increases venous pressure. Sluggish venous return is overcome by gravitational forces and *dependent* or *orthostatic edema* occurs. Orthostatic edema is characterized by bilateral, pitting edema in dependent body parts and is relieved by position changes.

Goals of care

- To identify patients at risk of developing orthostatic edema
- To inhibit formation of orthostatic edema by promoting venous return to the heart
- To control orthostatic edema by assisting movement of edematous fluid back into the systemic circulation
- To prevent complications until compensatory function develops

Nursing interventions

1. Assist venous return to the heart. Encourage as much activity as possible within limits of orthopedic stability while on bedrest and during periods when up in the wheelchair. Avoid extended periods of time without a position change or incorrect positioning of limbs that will block circulation. Protect the patient from skin breakdown or other local trauma to blood vessels. Take measures to relieve prolonged or severe hypotension, such as administering blood replacement therapy as ordered by the physician to combat hypovolemic shock or relieving episodes of postural hypotension.

2. Carefully monitor patients with predisposing conditions leading to impaired circulation. Observe all patients closely during the stage of spinal shock when diminished reflex activity causes complete loss of muscle tone and a greater degree of hypotension. The quadriplegic patient will have early problems. The patient with a lower motor neuron lesion that causes flaccid paralysis is prone to chronic problems. Monitor elderly patients closely, as valvular insufficiency and a degree of cardiac failure can occur. Finally, any patient with local trauma to blood vessels from associated fractured extremities to pressure areas will need special attention.

3. Inspect extremities carefully for evidence of any swelling, especially during early mobilization, as most problems occur at this time. Check the patient's lower extremities every few minutes during initial tilt table mobilization and again on return to bed following early wheelchair activity. Edema can also occur in dependent areas while the patient is in bed. Check the sacral area, the hands and arms of quadriplegic patients, and the lower extremities, especially if countertraction is being used. Be sure to support upper and lower extremities securely on arm boards, footboards, or pillows. When up in the wheelchair, paralyzed limbs must always be supported. Elevated wheelchair leg rests are available. Techniques used to position patients on a variety of immobilization beds are described in Chapter 14. Positioning the patient in a wheelchair is discussed further in Chapter 16.

4. Consult physician if edema does not subside with overnight bedrest or if unilateral or sudden edema occurs. Although orthostatic edema is most common, other complications, such as cardiac failure or thrombophlebitis, must be ruled out. The physician may wish to have the involved extremities X-rayed to determine undetected or pathological fractures or heterotopic ossification. Heterotopic ossification is an abnormal excessive bone formation associated with paralysis and characterized by swelling and stiffness of the joints involved and an elevated temperature. Kozier and Erb suggest monitoring the following signs to detect systemic overhydration: weight gain, generalized edema, and puffy eyelids; low output of concentrated urine with elevated specific gravity; apathy, confusion, weakness, or anorexia; and eventual decreases in hematocrit, hemoglobin, and red blood cell count in the blood plasma due to cellular malnutrition.

5. Apply elasticized stockings, which aid venous circulation by compressing muscle bellies and joints. A variety of sizes and strengths of stockings are available on the commercial market. Some come in small, medium, and large sizes. Others must be individually measured to fit the foot, calves, and thighs. To ensure a correct fit, obtain measurements following a rest period, when edema has subsided.

Tensor bandages may also be used, but are not as convenient and tend to slip when a patient sits up in the wheelchair. To promote circulatory return, use spiral turns, wrapping upward from the foot; wrap the entire leg, as far up the thigh as possible; and use circular turns only to anchor and terminate bandaging (using circular turns on the entire leg would impede rather than promote circulatory return). To avoid abrasions to skin without sensation, secure the tensor with one-inch adhesive tape rather than metal clips.

Whatever method is used, success depends on a good fit and correct application. Be sure to apply *before* the patient is mobilized. Continuous monitoring of circulation to the toes and heels is necessary and stockings or bandages must be removed every four to eight hours for inspection and care of the skin.

6. Perform range of motion exercises according to an individualized program. Collaborate with the physician and physiotherapist to plan passive exercise programs. Forced movement of edematous joints may cause additional trauma. With intensive physiotherapy, additional treatment by the nurse may not be required.

7. Evaluate effectiveness of treatment according to level of outcome reached:

- No evidence of sacral or extremity swelling; if minimal orthostatic edema is present, it should be pitting in nature and relieved with rest or position change

- Skin extremities warm and dry to touch without evidence of breakdown
- Full range of motion possible in all extremities without evidence of contractures or pain
- Blood pressure and pulse within normal limits for patient without evidence of severe and prolonged hypotension
- Urine output balanced with fluid intake without evidence of urinary retention
- Hematocrit, hemoglobin, and red blood cell count of blood plasma within normal range

Postural Hypotension

Postural or orthostatic hypotension is a dramatic fall in the blood pressure when the upright position is assumed. The pathology involved is similar to that causing gravitational edema in people with spinal cord injuries, that is, disturbed vasomotor control decreasing the blood supply returning to the heart. Again, lesions sustained at or above the T_{4-6} segmental levels interfere with sympathetic stimulation to the abdominal viscera and lower extremities. Blood tends to pool in these structures, and the sluggish circulation is overcome by gravitational forces when the patient attempts to sit up in bed or transfers to the wheelchair. Blood literally rushes to the patient's feet and the body is unable to make the necessary blood pressure adjustments to preserve circulation to the head, neck, and chest areas. The higher the level of injury, the greater the effects become. Prolonged bedrest is an aggravating factor with any patient, but quadriplegic patients have the most difficulty.

General adaptation to this problem does occur, usually within a year after injury. The critical time is during early mobilization from bed to the wheelchair. This process must be undertaken very gradually.

Goals of care

- To identify patients at risk of developing postural hypotension
- To forestall blood from accumulating in the abdomen and lower extremities when the upright position is assumed
- To prevent complications, such as blackouts or fainting spells, until compensatory function develops

Nursing interventions

1. Assist the patient to adjust to position changes. The physician will outline the activity permitted within the limits of orthopedic stability but the mobilization process must be undertaken gradually according to the patient's tolerance. Thomas (1977) recommends progressions in elevating the head of the bed for increasing periods of time before the patient sits at 90 degrees. When the patient can tolerate one-half hour at 30 degrees, increase elevations in stages until 80 to 90 degrees can be tolerated for one hour. Although a reclining back chair may be needed initially, sitting in a wheelchair can then be attempted. A *tilt table* can be used in a similar fashion. The physiotherapist usually supervises the use of this equipment, but it is a good idea to know how to lower the table should a hypotensive episode occur. Monitor the patient's blood pressure before and after each significant position change and compare with baseline data. The systolic pressure should not drop below 80 mmHg.

Other measures used to prevent hypotensive episodes are the application of long-leg antiembolitic elastic stockings, tensor bandaging of the legs, and abdominal binders. The classic many-tailed scultetus binder may be used, but the straight cotton or elastic abdominal binders are more convenient, especially for repeated use. See Figure 10–3. Do not allow any abdominal binder to extend over the rib cage, making chest expansion more difficult. It should reach from the gluteal fold to the waist. Be sure to apply all supports before getting the patient up.

For extreme or prolonged bouts of postural hypotension, medication such as ephedrine may be given 20 to 30 minutes before mobilization.

2. Carefully observe the quadriplegic patient during early mobilization for signs and symptoms of hypotension. Often the patient can alert you to its onset. Due to cerebral anoxia and sympathetic response above the level of lesion (attempting to raise the blood pressure), the following may occur:

- Weakness, dizziness, pale color, and blurred vision deteriorating to blackouts, or fainting
- Excessive sweating above the level of lesion and tachycardia

3. Promote venous return to increase the blood pressure should a hypotensive episode occur. Immediately lower the tilt table or head of bed. If the patient is up, quickly tilt the wheelchair backward and lower the chair back (Figure 10–4). Instruct the patient to breathe deeply and assist expiration by placing hand on diaphragm. Some physicians believe this movement elicits a vasoconstriction reflex in the chest. Within a few minutes the blackout will usually disappear, and the wheelchair can be slowly returned to its normal position. If these measures are not successful, return the patient to bed, elevate the foot of the bed, and notify the physician.

4. If an episode should occur when the patient is alone, the patient can bend forward to relieve symptoms. To avoid injury from falling out of the wheelchair, secure a safety strap around the lower chest of quadriplegic patients. Provide close supervision and restrict off-ward activities during the early stages.

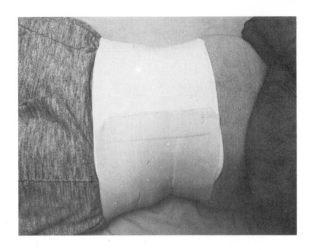

FIGURE 10–3 ■ An elastic abdominal binder with velcro closures; note correct position to allow for free expansion of rib cage for ease with breathing.

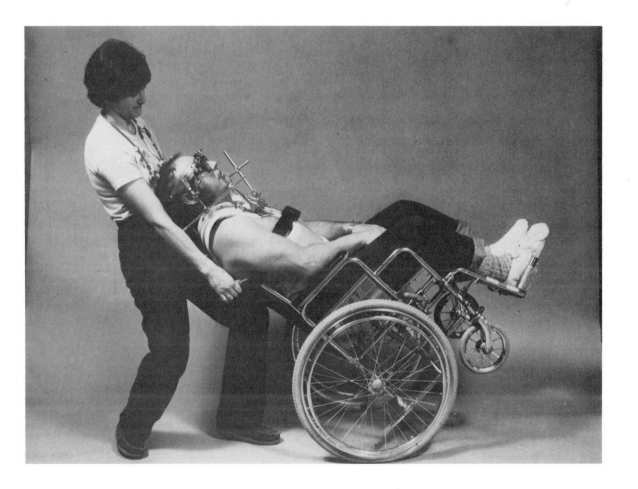

FIGURE 10–4 ■ Promptly tilting the wheelchair back to a reclining position usually prevents or alleviates a fainting spell.

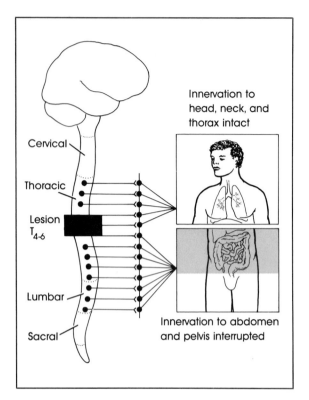

Cervical

Thoracic

Lesion
T$_{4-6}$

Lumbar

Sacral

Innervation to
head, neck, and
thorax intact

Innervation to abdomen
and pelvis interrupted

FIGURE 10–5 ■ Significant interruption of the sympathetic nervous system is evident with an injury at the T$_{4-6}$ cord segments or above.

5. Prepare patient and family to alleviate anxiety should problems occur. Often the patient can alert you verbally of a blackout coming on. Tell the family to notify a staff member and teach them how to alleviate the problem.

6. Evaluate effectiveness of treatment according to level of outcome reached:

- Alert and oriented
- Blood pressure maintained within normal limits for patient, usually 90/60 mmHg for the stabilized quadriplegic person
- Pulse within normal limits for patient without evidence of tachycardia
- Physical strength within normal limits for level of injury sustained
- Patient able to state signs and symptoms of possible onset of hypotensive episodes to alert staff member

Autonomic Dysreflexia

Every RN, nursing assistant, and orderly should be familiar with the onset of *autonomic dysreflexia* or *hyperreflexia* as signs and symptoms may be precipitated by routine bladder and bowel procedures and can quickly progress to dangerous or even fatal levels, creating a medical emergency.

Autonomic dysreflexia is mainly characterized by a sudden, severe headache secondary to an uncontrolled elevation of blood pressure. If untreated, the hypertension may progress to fatal complications, such as cerebral hemorrhage or an acute myocardial infarction.

It is estimated that most quadriplegic people experience autonomic dysreflexia at some time after the spinal shock period has subsided. Although this autonomic response is most frequent and unpredictable during the first year or so after injury, it can occur spontaneously many years later (Comarr 1977).

Autonomic dysreflexia or hyperreflexia is caused by a variety of abnormal stimuli, creating an exaggerated response of the sympathetic nervous system (comprising the thoracolumbar outflow of the autonomic nervous system) due to lack of control from higher centers. This condition occurs mainly when the level of lesion is at the T$_{4-6}$ segmental levels or higher (see Figure 10–5). When lesion is sustained below this level, enough of the sympathetic nervous system is usually preserved to avoid this abnormal functional response.

The condition of autonomic dysreflexia is precipitated by afferent stimuli from localized areas below the level of lesion, mostly from the abdominopelvic region (Taylor 1974). The most frequent source of stimuli is an overdistended bladder. Rectal stimulation, bowel impaction, urinary infection, calculi, or instrumentation (particularly when associated with internal bleeding to some degree) are also common offenders. Later in the rehabilitation process, deep pressure sores, operative incisions, and so on, may also cause problems. Even pregnancy, but most especially labor, can elicit this undesirable response. The mechanisms involved in this unusual condition are (see Figure 10–6):

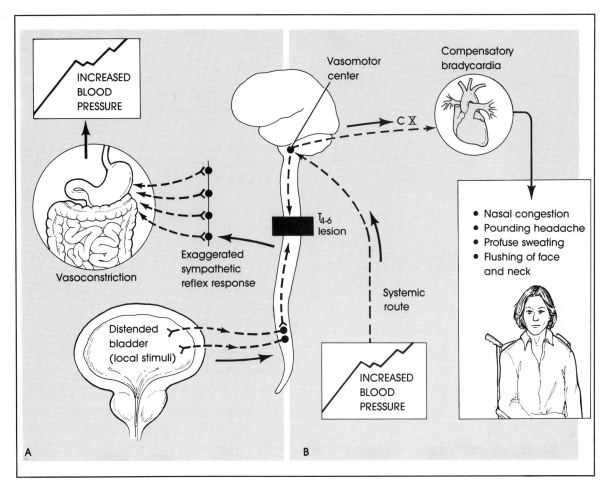

FIGURE 10–6 ■ (A) Local stimuli enter the spinal cord; upgoing communication is blocked by a lesion at T$_{4-6}$ segmental levels (or above); an exaggerated sympathetic reflex response is activated. (B) Communication via systemic routes activates the parasympathetic nervous system, but inhibitive downgoing messages are blocked by the T$_{4-6}$ lesion; parasympathetic response in the cranial outflow overcompensates, causing a number of symptoms experienced above the level of the lesion.

1. Local stimuli (for example, from a distended bladder) enter the spinal cord and ascend to the level of the lesion where communication to the brain is interrupted. An enormous sympathetic reflex response is activated.

2. The result: blood vessel spasm in the abdominal and pelvic organs and vasculature of the skin. This spasm causes vasoconstriction to an area so rich in blood supply that the body's blood pressure rises quickly.

3. Messages indicating this sudden hypertension travel by *systemic routes* other than the spinal cord (communication from distended receptors in the aortic arch and carotid sinuses) to the vasomotor center in the brain. To compensate, the parasympathetic division of the autonomic nervous system lowers the blood pressure by slowing the heart rate and attempting to dilate all blood vessels. Some impulses may be effective, as normal parasympathetic outflow in the cranial and upper thoracic regions may be preserved, but other impulses are blocked by the spinal cord lesion, thus preventing communication with the lower thoracic and sacral autonomic outflow.

4. *The result:*

- Overactive sympathetic vasodilation above the level of lesion causing flushing of the face, neck, and chest; nasal stuffiness or congestion; profuse sweating of the upper body; possible engorged temporal and neck blood vessels; and headache
- Parasympathetic stimulation (through the cranial outflow to the intact vagus nerve) causing bradycardia

Goals of care

- To identify patients at risk of developing autonomic dysreflexia
- To avoid abnormal stimuli from triggering exaggerated sympathetic nervous system response
- To recognize immediately the onset of this condition and initiate measures to lower the blood pressure
- To remove or control abnormal stimuli and prevent dangerous or fatal complications such as cerebral hemorrhage

Nursing interventions

1. Avoid abnormal autonomic response from strong local stimuli. For example, during the intermittent catheterization program, ensure a desirable balance between intake and output. Monitor IV fluids carefully to prevent overhydration or warn patients against drinking several glasses of fluid at one time. Urinary output for each catheterization (including the preceding manual expression measurement) should not exceed 600 mL. Avoid complications such as a urinary infection or calculi formation, which can also stimulate autonomic dysreflexia. Regular evacuation of the bowels should be maintained and constipation avoided if possible. Follow nursing care outlined in Chapters 12 and 13.

2. Closely observe quadriplegic and high paraplegic patients. As previously mentioned this syndrome occurs when the sympathetic outflow to the abdominal organs is not intact, caused by lesions to the T_{4-6} levels and above. Autonomic dysreflexia is more likely to occur when the patient is lying down; the sitting position lowers the blood pressure, as in postural hypotension. Check the history to see if the patient is prone to develop signs of autonomic dysreflexia following any specific procedure.

3. Be alert for the following signs and symptoms, indicating the onset of autonomic dysreflexia:

- Headache (due to elevated blood pressure) of a pounding, severe, and sudden onset. Thoroughly investigate complaints of *any* headache.
- Elevated blood pressure. (Compare with baseline data. Blood pressure of 140/90 may be considered high for some; others may experience obvious extremes of blood pressure of 300/160.)
- Bradycardia, which is most common, or tachycardia may be experienced by extremely high quadriplegic persons.
- Profuse sweating, flushed face, blotchiness of skin above the level of lesion, and goose bumps
- Nasal stuffiness or obstruction
- Apprehension

4. If up in the wheelchair, return the patient to bed and elevate the head of the bed or hold the patient in the sitting position to lower the blood pressure. Postural hypotension is induced in the sitting position. Avoid placing the patient in a chair as it is more difficult to check the possible source of stimuli. During a crisis situation, care will require two or three staff members simultaneously to monitor the blood pressure every few minutes and check for a possible cause. See Figure 10–7.

5. Remove the source of causative stimuli if possible.

- Check the bladder for overdistension, the most frequent cause. If the patient is on an intermittent catheterization program, catheterize immediately regardless of how recently the last procedure was performed. If there is an indwelling catheter, look for kinks in the tubing, plugged connections, or a full leg bag—anything that may obstruct the urinary flow (Taylor 1974). Immediately irrigate or change the foley catheter if obstruction persists.
- Check the lower bowel for stool. Bowel problems often cause onset of autonomic dys-

reflexia during routine evacuation measures. Gently and gradually try to remove stool manually. If symptoms persist, stop procedure. Resume if symptoms subside.

6. Consult the physician promptly if "first aid" treatments are not successful. Although the techniques mentioned are usually effective, miscellaneous problems need to be identified and treated. For example, if profuse bleeding and clotting occur following a urological procedure, the patient will probably have to return to the operating room for surgical intervention.

7. Administer ganglionic blocking agents as ordered by the physician.

During a crisis situation, intravenous medication is required. Comarr (1977) recommends hydralazine hydrochloride (Apresoline) (20 mg per mL) cautiously given 0.5 mL at a time. Should extreme hypotension occur, an antidote to the ganglionic blocking agents, such as metaraminol bitartrate (Aramine), should be kept on hand. If the hydralazine hydrochloride fails to lower the blood pressure, a low spinal anesthetic is given to calm local reflex activity in the abdomen or the lower extremities. These medications should be located in a prominent place for convenience. Some centers use the emergency cart. A lumbar puncture tray to administer the spinal anesthetic should also be easily accessible.

Once the entire episode has passed, an elevated blood pressure and other symptoms may persist. Comarr suggests less potent, oral, antihypertensive medication. The dosage may be titrated as indicated by the blood pressure.

8. Monitor the patient's blood pressure and pulse every four hours for 24 hours following a crisis. The autonomic nervous system tends to remain unstable when the body's reaction has been severe.

9. Provide psychological support. The exaggerated sympathetic response is accompanied by an increased circulation of catecholamines, which increase anxiety. The patient may feel apprehensive and agitated and find it difficult to rest. Explain the body's reaction and make the patient comfortable to promote sleep.

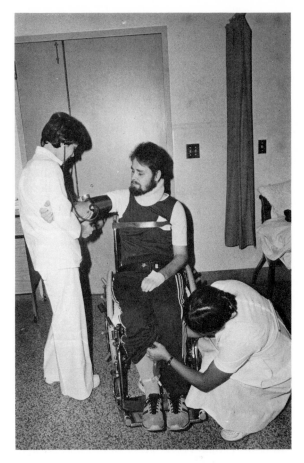

FIGURE 10–7 ■ Two nurses immediately assess a patient who complains of a sudden headache indicating the complication of dysreflexia.

At an appropriate time, the patient must be adequately prepared to cope with this emergency situation outside the hospital setting. Patient education on this subject is discussed later under the heading Self-Care Skills.

10. Reconsider the causes of autonomic dysreflexia for each patient, and initiate nursing actions to prevent further episodes if possible. For example, if rectal stimulation during bowel procedures precipitates an attack, insert a local anesthetic, such as Nupercaine ointment 1% ten minutes before evacuation. Again, it must be stressed, prevention is the best treatment.

11. Evaluate effectiveness of treatment according to level of outcome criteria reached:

- Blood pressure within normal limits for patient (usually 90/60 mmHg for a quadriplegic person in the sitting position)
- Pulse rate within normal limits for patient without evidence of bradycardia
- Patient comfortable without signs of hypertension (no headache, signs of increased intercranial pressure, or signs of heart failure indicating hemorrhage)
- Nasal passages clear
- Skin warm, dry, pink (if the patient is Caucasian), and without blotchiness or excessive sweating above the level of lesion
- Patient calm or able to sleep
- Patient able to state signs and symptoms and causes of onset of autonomic crisis to alert staff member

Deep Vein Thrombosis

Deep vein thrombosis (DVT) is the development of a blood clot in the venous structures. It is particularly common in the abdominopelvic region and lower extremities. Sometimes *thrombophlebitis,* or inflammation of a venous pathway, can be identified before the clot or *thrombus* matures.

A clot—consisting of intact and ruptured platelets that adhere to the blood vessel wall—protrudes slightly. The platelets cause the precipitation of fibrin and other blood elements, which then form the mature thrombus. Once formed, a thrombus can grow in size as more platelets and blood elements stick to it. A thrombus can partially or completely occlude a blood vessel or break free from the blood vessel wall and travel in the bloodstream, at which point it becomes an *embolus.* The embolus is most dangerous when it enters the pulmonary circulation and obstructs blood flow to lung tissue.

The clinical incidence of DVT following injury to the spinal cord is about 15% (Casas et al. 1977–78). This is similar to the average incidence in the general postoperative patient population. Diagnosis by venography and other methods, however, reveals a much higher incidence (Burke and Murray 1975:36). A triad of

factors predisposes any patient to formation of thrombi: stasis of venous circulation, changes or trauma to the vein wall, and hypercoagulability of the blood.

Following spinal cord injury a significant precipitating factor is sluggish venous return to the heart. Impairment of vasomotor control, initial loss of muscle tone, inability to move extremities, and prolonged immobilization contribute to poor circulatory return. Bedrest can cause localized trauma of delicate vein structures by the continuous contact or pressure exerted, particularly on the lower extremities. Patients with spinal cord injuries are also thought to be in a state of hypercoagulability similar to that of the postoperative patient. An increase in the platelet count, in platelet stickiness, and in prothrombin time is often evident following trauma. Blood viscosity also increases if the patient is dehydrated.

Factors that place any patient at risk are advancing age, possible deterioration of nutritional status, obesity, smoking, preexisting heart disease, lung complications, associated hip or long bone fractures, and recent surgery, especially in the abdominal area.

Goals of care

- To identify and observe patients at risk of developing DVT
- To inhibit formation of thrombi
- To detect thrombophlebitis early and initiate prompt treatment to prevent or control DVT
- To prevent embolization that may cause severe complications, primarily a pulmonary embolus

Nursing interventions

1. Discourage clot formation by promoting venous return to the heart, increasing the rate of blood flow in the peripheral vascular system, and preventing blood pooling in the extremities:

- Encourage as much activity as possible within limits of orthopedic stability. If the patient is on bedrest, active and passive range of motion exercises are essential. Be sure to include a full range of passive exercises to the lower limbs during morning and evening care. Also perform ankle-pumping exercises, about five times on each foot after every turn. A physiotherapy program designed according to level of lesion and patient tolerance should be initiated soon after admission. Certainly practicing the philosophy of early mobilization with postural changes and wheelchair activity greatly decreases the risk factors.

• Apply elastic stockings or tensor bandages correctly to exert a compression force on the veins.

• Position limbs carefully to avoid gravitational edema.

• Encourage smokers to quit or at least cut down. Nicotine in cigarettes is believed to constrict the veins, thus slowing blood flow.

Protect venous walls from trauma or pressure as follows:

• Turn and correctly position the patient every two hours. Generally, measures taken to prevent skin breakdown will prevent undue pressure on internal vein structures. Take care to prevent pressure on the susceptible popliteal space behind the knee, a point at which lower limb circulation can be easily obstructed, especially in the supine position. *Never* put pillows under the knees or use a knee gatch when a patient is sitting in bed. Also avoid elevating the legs on pillows because they compress the calf and may press on the popliteal space. Instead elevate the entire foot of the bed (on blocks if necessary). When a patient is in the side-lying position, be sure to place a pillow between the legs. Without a pillow, the legs pressing against each other will compress the veins.

• Avoid venous punctures in the legs at all costs. Be sure to alert lab technicians when obtaining blood specimens to avoid this hazard. An intravenous site in the leg would be selected only under extraordinary circumstances. If such a site is unavoidable, exercise great care when inserting needles and when administering medications intravenously. Techniques must be as nontraumatizing as possible. Vessel injuries commonly occur at intravenous insertion sites.

• Promptly attend to minor cuts, blisters, or skin abrasions on the legs and feet. The healing process is slowed due to already compromised circulation, and extra care is needed to prevent infection and subsequent blood vessel irritation.

Minimize effects of hypercoagulability and promote normal clotting as follows:

• Prevent or alleviate dehydration, thus avoiding an increase in blood viscosity.

• Question women of childbearing age who may be taking birth control pills. Research shows this pseudopregnancy state, accompanied by a slight increase in blood coagulability, may also be a predisposing factor in increasing the tendency for clot formation. The physician will likely order discontinuance of birth control pills, at least temporarily.

• Administer *prophylactic* anticoagulant therapy as prescribed by physician. The desired effects of preventing thrombosis must be carefully weighed against complications of uncontrolled bleeding. Anticoagulation is the subject of worldwide controversy. Some centers in Europe routinely anticoagulate patients on admission until wheelchair activity is possible. In North America this practice is usually reserved for patients with evidence of deep thrombosis or other high-risk conditions.

2. Monitor the high-risk patient closely for thrombophlebitis, especially during the three to five weeks immediately after injury when the incidence of thrombus formation is greatest.

3. Monitor body temperature every morning for at least six weeks after injury. A low-grade fever, unaccompanied by apparent infection, often indicates thrombus formation. The time it takes to get a quick temperature before the daily activities start is always well spent; it can provide valuable baseline data for detecting a host of problems.

4. Observe lower extremities of all patients daily. During morning care is a convenient time. Thrombophlebitis is often discovered by astute nurses and therapists during routine activities. Expose the legs from the groin to the feet. Compare legs bilaterally. Look for any combination of the following signs or symptoms:

- Skin warm to the touch in a localized area. An increased temperature in the affected leg often occurs several days before other signs. If the patient has had a heavy blanket on, expose the legs for 10 minutes to assume room temperature. To increase sensitivity to temperature variation, place your hands in cold water for a few minutes before examination and then use the backs of your hands. Compare various parts of each leg at the same time to detect any variations.
- Asymmetric enlargement in comparison of thighs, calves, or ankles. Obtain leg measurements immediately on admission and compare daily if swelling is suspected. See Procedure 10–5 for further information on technique.
- Swelling and/or redness following the course of a vein. Inspect the calves and popliteal areas closely.
- Possible increase in spasms of affected limb.
- Low-grade fever without other apparent cause. Remember that due to sensory loss the classic Homan's sign or induction of pain on movement will not be present.

5. If thrombophlebitis is suspected, maintain bedrest and minimize limb movement until the diagnosis is confirmed by the physician and further activity orders are obtained.

6. Prepare the patient for diagnostic tests. Ultrasonic recordings or a venogram are used to detect thrombi. If thrombi are present, a lung scan will follow to detect any embolization to pulmonary vessels. Coagulation studies are also included. If thrombophlebitis or DVT occurs, a number of measures can be taken to discourage embolization.

7. Administer anticoagulant therapy as ordered by physician. Low-dose heparin (such as 5000 to 7500 IU every 12 hours) is the drug of choice for several reasons: rapid action, lack of interaction with other drugs, relative ease of neutralization, and low incidence of side effects (Watson 1974). Administration would be contraindicated for patients with brain injuries or with gastric, genitourinary, or other signs of internal bleeding. Heparin is most effectively absorbed intravenously and is generally given via a heparin lock by slow infusion over a five-minute period. Observe the site for signs of infection or infiltration.

To protect the patient against excessive anticoagulation, clotting and prothrombin times and/or platelet counts are frequently monitored (usually 30 minutes before the next dose of medication is due) so that the physician can adjust dosages accordingly. Observe closely for any signs of frank bleeding in sputum, nasogastric returns, urine, or stool. Obtain periodic specimens for occult blood. Minimize intramuscular injections, as bleeding from injection site may persist. The patient is usually anticoagulated until the clinical picture has stabilized and gradual mobilization is resumed. To prevent a state of hypercoagulation, the dosage of heparin is reduced *gradually* as oral anticoagulants are initiated over a five- to seven-day period. Sometimes aspirin is used for its antiplatelet property in preventing thrombus formation. Oral anticoagulants especially tend to be incompatible with many drugs. Check with the hospital pharmacist about interaction with other medications the patient is receiving.

8. If not already done, apply elastic stockings or tensor bandages to exert a compression force on the veins. *Never* use heat treatments on insensitive skin to promote circulation.

9. Carefully elevate the affected limb to promote circulation. Specific activity will be ordered by the physician. Prolonged immobilization is thought by some to aggravate venous stasis. Most agree some form of inactivity is warranted to minimize the chances of dislodging clots.

A conservative approach includes bedrest for five to ten days with the foot of the bed elevated 10 to 15 degrees (with the hip and knee extended). Range of motion exercises are restricted to the upper extremities.

A more liberal approach includes bedrest for a few days only; legs elevated when up in the wheelchair; and maintenance of a full physiotherapy program without exercises to the affected limb.

PROCEDURE 10–5 ■ OBTAINING LEG MEASUREMENTS

Purpose

The purpose of obtaining leg measurements to compile serial data is a method used to detect early swelling that may indicate onset of thrombophlebitis, which may lead to pulmonary embolism. Strict accuracy must be obtained for measurements to be of any value.

Action	Rationale
1. Measure ankle, calf, and thigh circumferences on admission.	To provide baseline data.
2. Obtain measurements at the widest point of the ankle, calf, and thigh.	To provide continuity, some settings prefer calf and thigh measurements to be obtained at a mandatory distance from the kneecap—say 6 or 8 inches (20 cm).
3. Mark the leg with a black felt pen to indicate area to be measured. Apply the tape so it is centered on the line before measuring.	To facilitate accuracy of serial measurements.
4. Obtain serial measurements in the morning before any activity.	If the patient is up before measuring, gravitational edema may give a false reading.
5. As a preventive measure, repeat measurements on a weekly basis.	To detect swelling early that may be indicative of thrombophlebitis.
6. Repeat measurements daily if swelling is present.	To monitor swelling and response to treatment.
7. Record measurements.	Measurements can be conveniently recorded on a flow sheet as shown below.

Leg Measurements

	Left		Right	
Thigh	_____	inches/cm	_____	inches/cm
Calf	_____	inches/cm	_____	inches/cm
Ankle	_____	inches/cm	_____	inches/cm

Action	Rationale
8. Compare measurements of one leg with the other and with baseline data. Look for any discrepancies.	Swelling of one leg may be an early sign of thrombophlebitis. Findings of 1.5 cm increase in size (as compared with baseline or admission measurements) or a 1.5 cm discrepancy (when compared with the unaffected leg) is considered significant for males; a 1.2 cm measurement is considered significant for females.

10. Take measures to avoid postural hypotension and autonomic dysreflexia. Sudden changes in blood pressure could dislodge thrombi.

11. Be constantly alert for signs of embolization to the pulmonary circulation, characterized by sudden onset of hypoxia; rapid, shallow respirations or dyspnea; and severe apprehension. Chest pain may be absent, decreased, or referred due to sensory impairment. Symptoms may vary from mild to severe, depending on the extent of lung involvement. For assessment and interventions, see Chapter 9.

12. Evaluate effectiveness of treatment by level of outcome criteria reached:

- Lower extremities free from signs of swelling, redness, or localized warmth along the course of a vein
- Leg circumference measurements symmetrical and within normal limits as compared with baseline admission data
- No evidence of increased leg spasms
- Body temperature normal
- Anticoagulation studies (clotting and prothrombin times and platelet counts) within acceptable limits for patient
- No signs of blood in sputum, nasogastric aspirate, urine, or stool, and patient free from other signs of internal bleeding
- Ultrasonic recordings and venogram normal without signs of thrombus formation
- Effortless respirations at 12 to 20 breaths per minute without signs of hypoxia or chest discomfort

SELF-CARE SKILLS

Patients will need to know how their level of injury affects their circulation and body temperature. They must learn measures to promote circulation and avoid hazardous complications associated with blood pooling in the extremities, primarily edema, postural hypotension, and thrombophlebitis. The ever-present danger of autonomic dysreflexia and environmental factors predisposing the patient to extreme changes in body temperature should also be included. The program is directed toward the quadriplegic and high paraplegic person, but circulatory difficulties can also be a problem for the patient with a lower motor neuron or flaccid paralysis from a lumbosacral injury.

Instruct the patient in general methods to promote circulation, such as keeping active, elevating legs periodically during the day on a chair or resting in bed, and taking general measures to relieve pressure on skin and bony prominences. Also teach the application and care of support devices, such as elastic stockings and abdominal binders, if recommended for individual use to combat postural hypotension or gravitational edema. Teach the patient how to observe for venous drainage problems. Swelling in the feet, lower legs, and hands of quadriplegic people tends to be a long-term problem. If swelling is not controlled by general measures or does not disappear with overnight rest, a physician should be notified. Any signs of localized redness, swelling, or warmth of one leg only may indicate thrombophlebitis. Instruct patients to take their temperature and notify the physician immediately.

Once mobility is established, postural hypotension is not generally a long-term problem, but it may cause dizziness or blackouts in the early stages when patients are out on day or weekend passes. To prepare the patient and family, include instructions on elastic stocking and abdominal binder application and how to tilt the wheelchair backward to prevent fainting. If the problem occurs when the patient is getting out of bed, instruct them to prop the patient on pillows for 15 to 20 minutes beforehand.

Prepare the patient for an autonomic dysreflexia crisis, emphasizing prevention and early recognition. Teach patients how to check bladder and bowel; instruct them to go immediately to the nearest emergency facility if symptoms do not subside. Recommend that quadriplegics carry some type of medical alert bracelet or information.

Teach patients how to prevent overheating by avoiding direct sunlight in hot weather; staying indoors during extreme summer heat and humidity; being alert for symptoms of heat stroke (light-headedness, headache, fainting, nausea, and vomiting); and drinking 8 to 10 glasses of fluid per day. Emphasize that body temperature should never be over 37.8°C (100°F). Teach patients and families that sponging, water spray, fanning, and air conditioning are all effective cooling measures.

Teach patients to avoid chilling in cold weather by wearing extra protective clothing. Stress never to use hot water bottles or electric heating devices because loss of sensory warning systems makes it difficult to prevent burns to the skin, which are difficult to heal.

For general information on education programs for patients and families, see Chapter 8.

LONG-TERM IMPLICATIONS

When assessing a quadriplegic or high paraplegic person who has been paralyzed for some time, keep in mind changes in cardiovascular function and control of body temperature that are considered acceptable in light of permanent disability. Adjust baseline data as follows:

1. A chronic, passive degree of vasodilation below the level of lesion. However, within a year or so, local reflex activity will resume to provide some compensatory function in vasoconstriction.

2. An average blood pressure of 100/60 mmHg for an uncomplicated stabilized quadriplegic patient. A slightly lower pressure of 90/60 mmHg is common in the sitting position.

3. A lowered pulse rate of 60 beats per minute.

4. A PaO_2 of 60 mmHg and a $PaCO_2$ of 40 to 50 mmHg in quadriplegic people with reduced pulmonary function. Acid-base balance and all other blood work should be within normal limits.

The quadriplegic person may always require elastic stockings and occasionally an abdominal binder to control gravitational edema. If edema does not subside overnight, is of sudden onset, or occurs only on one side, further investigation is needed. Prolonged postural hypotension is also abnormal.

Signs of autonomic dysreflexia can usually be avoided as the patient becomes more familiar with bladder and bowel management. However, severe, sudden episodes can occur spontaneously at any time after injury. Autonomic dysreflexia is a constant complication to anticipate. Take several precautions and collaborate with a physician if a woman becomes pregnant. To avoid an autonomic crisis during delivery, anticholinergic drugs may be given during the third trimester. Certainly special precautions should be taken to alert obstetrical staff on the patient's admission.

Based on your assessment, help the patient continue with preventive measures or refer to family physician or follow-up rehabilitation center if a problem is suspected. Be alert for skin breakdown in all patients with poor circulation. Sometimes underlying problems, such as cardiac failure or inability to provide self-care, will arise.

SELECTED REFERENCES

Burke, D., and Murray, D. 1975. *Handbook of Spinal Cord Medicine.* London and Basingstoke: Macmillan Press, Chapters 4 and 6. *Brief overview of temperature control and venous drainage complications.*

Carol, M., et al. 1979. Acute care of spinal cord injury. *Critical Care Quarterly* 2: 7–21. *Includes cardiopulmonary assessment and management in critical care. Excellent overview.*

Casas, R., et al. 1977–78. Prophylaxis of venous thrombosis and pulmonary embolism in patients with acute traumatic spinal cord lesions. *International Journal of Paraplegia* 15: 209–214. *A review of incidence and prevalence of deep vein thrombosis and its complications and the prophylactic use of calcium heparin (a European perspective).*

Castle, M., and Watkins, J. 1979. Fever: understanding a sinister sign. *Nursing* 9 (2): 27–33. *A review of normal body temperature control, fever patterns, pyretic agents, and related nursing care.*

Cheshire, D., and Coates, D. 1966. Respiratory and metabolic management in acute tetraplegia. *International Journal of Paraplegia* 4: 1–23. *Includes literature review and summarizes causes of hypothermia following spinal cord injury; explores possible clinical advantages of permitting spontaneous cooling (p. 8).*

Comarr, A. 1977. Autonomic dysreflexia. In *The Total Care of Spinal Cord Injuries.* Eds. D. Pierce and V. Nickel. Boston: Little, Brown, pp. 181–185. *Summarizes etiology and characteristics and focuses on medical management of crisis situations; includes preventive aspects and patient and family education.*

Guttman, L. 1973. *Spinal Cord Injuries Comprehensive Management and Research.* Oxford: Blackwell Scientific Publications. *Classic text on all aspects of spinal cord injury. Includes historical background information; general statistics; legal aspects; detailed anatomy and neuropathology of cord trauma and effects on all body systems; regeneration; fractures and dislocations, gunshot injuries, and stab wounds; and neurophysiological and clinical management aspects. Extensive bibliography.*

Guyton, A. 1976. *Textbook of Medical Physiology.* 5th ed. Philadelphia: W. B. Saunders. *Detailed presentation of local (neural) control of blood flow to tissues and body temperature regulation.*

Holloway, N. 1979. *Nursing the Critically Ill Adult.* Menlo Park, Calif: Addison-Wesley, Chapters 2–6. *Clinically superb reference on cardiac assessment, acute disorders, and related nursing care. Includes presentation of arrhythmias and conduction defects, cardiac failure and tamponade, vascular assessment, shock, and fluid and electrolyte imbalances. Describes risk factors, preventive measures, signs and symptoms, and nursing actions. Highly recommended.*

Johnson, R. 1971. Temperature regulation in paraplegia. *International Journal of Paraplegia* 9: 137–143. *Technical descriptions of heat production, heat loss, and the local effect of ambient temperature following spinal cord injury.*

Kozier, B., and Erb, G. 1983. *Fundamentals of Nursing: Concepts and Procedures.* 2d ed. Menlo Park, Calif: Addison-Wesley, pp. 376–380. *Review of tensor bandaging procedures and application of binders.*

Spence, A., and Mason, E. 1979. *Human Anatomy and Physiology.* Menlo Park, Calif: Addison-Wesley. *Includes perspectives on aging throughout text.*

Taylor, A. 1974. Autonomic dysreflexia in spinal cord injury. *Nursing Clinics of North America* 9 (4): 717–725. *Detailed but concise review of pathophysiology, signs and symptoms, nursing and medical management, and patient and family education.*

Thomas, E. 1977. Nursing care of the patient with spinal cord injury. In *The Total Care of Spinal Cord Injuries.* Eds. D. Pierce and V. Nickel. Boston: Little, Brown, pp. 249–297. *Implications for nursing management in long-term care to maintain optimal body temperatures.*

Watson, N. 1974. Anticoagulant therapy in the treatment of venous thrombosis and pulmonary embolism in acute spinal injury. *International Journal of Paraplegia* 12: 197–201. *Detailed article favoring selected use of anticoagulants with early recognition of deep vein thrombosis as opposed to routine prophylactic treatment (a British perspective).*

SUPPLEMENTAL READING

General

Bates, B. 1974. *A Guide to Physical Examination.* Philadelphia: J. B. Lippincott. *Step-by-step graphic guide to physical assessment.*

Claus-Walker, J., and Halstead, L. 1978. Autonomic drugs in spinal cord injury: temporal prescription profile. *Archives of Physical Medicine and Rehabilitation* 59 (Aug.): 363–367. *Examines drugs used to modify the effects of acute hyperactive gastrointestinal irritability (related to peptic ulceration), bradycardia, orthostatic hypotension, neurogenic bladder dysfunction, and autonomic dysreflexia and derives a clearer understanding of the progressive recovery and adaptation process of the autonomic nervous system following spinal shock.*

Evans, D.; Kobrine, A.; and Rizzoli, H. 1980. Cardiac arrhythmias accompanying acute compression of the spinal cord. *Journal of Neurosurgery* 52: 52–59. *Report of a research study with monkeys demonstrated cardiovascular dysfunction associated with autonomic nervous system hyperactivity following spinal cord injury. Clinical application is then discussed.*

Sommers, D. 1979. Reactivity of the cardiovascular system in the tetraplegic. *Clinical Pharmacology and Therapeutics* 26 (3): 344–353. *Suggests rationale for improved cardiovascular responses that occur over time.*

Autonomic Dysreflexia

Erickson, R. 1980. Autonomic hyperreflexia. *Archives of Physical Medicine and Rehabilitation* 61 (Oct.): 435–440. *An in-depth review of autonomic hyperreflexia including causes, definitive medical management, and pharmacalogic prevention. Extensive bibliography.*

Kavchak-Keyes, M. 1977. Autonomic hyperreflexia. *Association of Rehabilitation Nurses* 2 (5): 17–22. *Comprehensive review of pathogenesis and treatment measures with emphasis on planning nursing interventions. Extensive bibliography.*

Nath, M., et al. 1979. Autonomic hyperreflexia in pregnancy and labor. *American Journal of Obstetrics and Gynecology* 134: 390–392. *Clinical description of managing a 36-year-old quadriplegic primipara with the complication of autonomic dysreflexia during labor. Extensive bibliography.*

Deep Vein Thrombosis

Chamberlain, S. 1980. Low-dose heparin therapy. *American Journal of Nursing:* 1115–1117. *Review of low-dose heparin as a prophylactic agent against deep vein thrombosis in high-risk postoperative patients; includes information on subcutaneous abdominal injection as preferred site.*

Cudkowicz, L., and Sherry, S. 1978. The venous system and the lung. *Heart Lung* 7 (1): 91–96. *Comprehensive review of normal venous system and structure, prevention and early signs and symptoms of deep vein thrombosis, with descriptions of Doppler ultrasonic flow probe and impedance phlebography used in diagnosis.*

Hachen, H. 1974. Anticoagulant therapy in patients with spinal cord injury. *International Journal of Paraplegia* 12: 176–187. *A European perspective.*

McConnell, E. 1978. Fitting antiembolism stockings. *Nursing '78,* September, pp. 67–71. *Photostory guide to measurement, application, and patient teaching.*

Perkash, A., et al. 1978–79. Experience with the management of thromboembolism in patients with spinal cord injury: Part I. Incidence, diagnosis, and role of some risk factors. *International Journal of Paraplegia* 16: 322–331. *A review of 50 spinal cord injury patients focusing on problems with diagnosis and consequent implications of anticoagulant therapy (an American perspective).*

Patient and Family Health Education

Engstrand, J., and Stuart, B. 1979. *Patient Handbook of Self-Care Procedures.* 2d ed. Birmingham, Ala: Spain Rehabilitation Center of the University of Alabama in Birmingham. *Patient instruction regarding autonomic dysreflexia.*

Goldfinger, G., and Hanak, M. 1981. *Spinal Cord Injury, a Guide for Care.* New York: Regional Spinal Cord Injury System, New York University Medical Center, Institute of Rehabilitation Medicine, pp. 26–27. *Brief section of this revised primer presents the cardiovascular complications phlebitis and hypotension; includes recognition of signs and symptoms and prevention.*

King, R. B.; Boyink, M.; and Keenan, M. 1977. *Rehabilitation Guide.* Medical Rehabilitation Research and Training Center No. 20. Chicago: Northwest University and Rehabilitation Training Institute of Chicago. *Includes various care procedures related to cardiopulmonary function, such as caring for antiembolitic stockings; also presents autonomic dysreflexia care throughout.*

Scalley, R., et al. 1979. Interdisciplinary inpatient warfarin education program. *American Journal of Hospital Pharmacy* 36: 219–220. *Documentation of an educational program using audiovisual and written material and counseling; includes learning objectives that may be helpful as a pattern for other educational programs.*

Virginia Spinal Cord Care and Teaching Manual. 1980. The Virginia Spinal Cord System, University of Virginia Center and Virginia Dept. of Rehabilitation Services, Woodrow Wilson Rehabilitation Center, Box W-279, Fisherville, Va. 22939, pp. 79–95. *Section on medical complications include autonomic dysreflexia, thrombus, and dependent edema.*

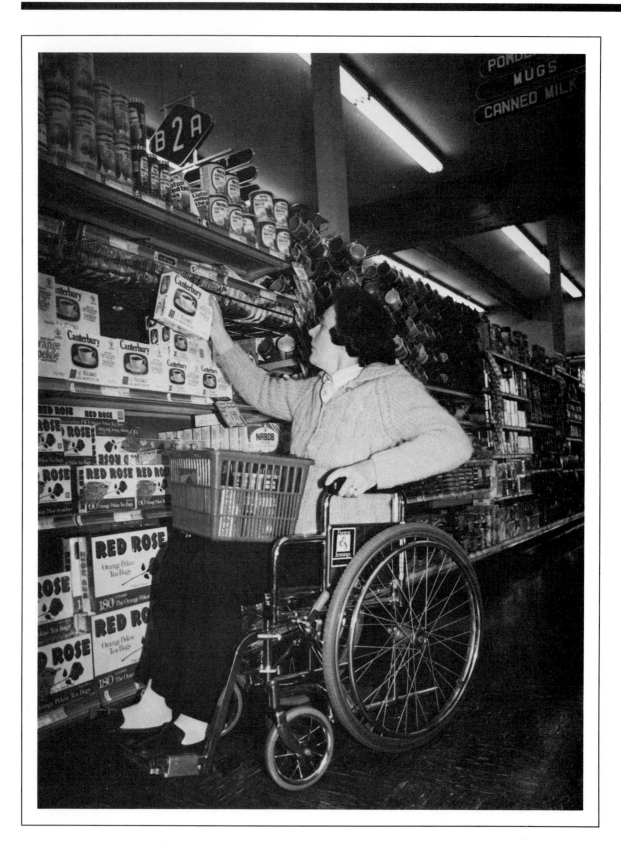

Chapter 11

Promoting Optimal Nutrition

CHAPTER OUTLINE

OBJECTIVES

- To identify health care goals for maintaining adequate nutrition
- To describe the impact of less-than-optimal nutrition on recovery period
- To describe the neural control of the digestive system and dysfunction following spinal cord injury
- To describe the symptoms of patients who risk developing malnutrition
- To give a method of determining current nutritional status by assessing general appearance, examining the gastrointestinal tract, and obtaining specific body measurements
- To specify abnormal laboratory results indicative of threatened nutritional status
- To discuss the significance of negative nitrogen balance
- To help nurses assess ability of patients to feed themselves and provide appropriate assistance
- To describe a well-balanced diet obtained from the four major food groups
- To identify foods that provide roughage to help regulate bowel elimination
- To describe how to care for the patient with paralytic ileus, gastric ulceration and bleeding, malnutrition during the critically ill period, and difficulty in controlling body weight
- To describe the application and care of adaptive feeding aids for the patient with quadriplegia
- To describe appropriate self-care skills to teach patient and family
- To describe long-term implications of maintaining good nutrition for the disabled person

GOALS OF HEALTH CARE

Nutrition contributes to our physical and mental health as well as to our resistance to infection and disease. No one knows how many conditions have roots in faulty nutrition, but we do know that maintaining optimal dietary intake directly influences the success of most aspects of the rehabilitation process. Providing adequate nutrition for patients with spinal cord injuries frequently presents unique problems. This chapter will help nurses recognize potentially fatal complications of the gastrointestinal system, identify the subtle onset of malnutrition, and participate in appropriate interventions. The goals of such interventions are:

- To prevent morbidity from gastrointestinal complications
- To prevent malnourishment by providing adequate nutrients to build, repair, and maintain body systems
- To provide special diets for preexisting or acquired conditions
- To help patients reach and maintain ideal body weight
- To help patients establish regular bowel and bladder patterns
- To increase resistance to infection, promote wound healing, and to prevent the breakdown of skin
- To maintain patients' strength, energy level, and physical ability to take part in rehabilitation programs
- To teach patients the good eating habits essential for health and well-being
- To help disabled people (and families when appropriate) with menu planning, food shopping, and meal preparation

ASSESSMENT OF NUTRITIONAL STATUS

The detail of a history and physical examination completed by the nurse depends on the urgency of the situation and to what extent other team members are involved. Assessing current nutritional status, identifying patients at risk, and recognizing potential and actual problems early are fundamental concepts.

Changes in Status Following Spinal Cord Injury

The digestive system, neural control, and dysfunctions

The gastrointestinal system, or alimentary canal, is a long tubular structure extending from the mouth to the anus and is composed largely of varying layers of smooth muscle. The digestive system is largely controlled by the autonomic nervous system, with the exception of such voluntary acts as chewing, swallowing, and controlling defecation. Generally, with the exception of the distal colon and rectum, innervation to the digestive apparatus is affected only temporarily by cord injury.

The gastrointestinal system readies food for absorption and metabolism and eliminates the largest volume of waste products from the body. Digestion requires a number of motor, secretory, and sensory functions. Although the digestive tract receives innervation from both the parasympathetic and sympathetic divisions of the autonomic nervous system, the parasympathetic division is by far the more essential. The sympathetic nervous system contributes antagonistic control to balance activities of motion and secretion, but it is generally less significant in daily functions. For a review of the general characteristics of the autonomic nervous system, see Chapter 5. In general, unchecked parasympathetic activity results in enhanced glandular secretion (that is, pancreatic and gastric) and relaxed junctional sphincters, such as the pylorus and ileocecal valve. Autonomic nervous system imbalance and release of the external anal sphincter from central control are responsible for the majority of the gastrointestinal complications of spinal cord injury.

Motor functions Motor functions are necessary to propel food through the digestive tract. Parasympathetic stimulation, which is transmitted almost entirely by the vagus nerve from the cranial outflow, maintains tonic contractions (tone) and produces stronger rhythmic contractions when ingestion of food distends the gut. These propulsive movements are referred to as *peristalsis*. With the exception of the immediate postinjury period, when reflex activity is suppressed by spinal shock, motor functions of the gastrointestinal tract largely remain within normal limits following cord injury.

Secretory functions Secretory functions are associated with the chemical digestion of food. The parasympathetic nervous system stimulates production of saliva and other gastric juices to aid in this function. Patients with quadriplegia or high paraplegia may experience *hyperchlorhydria*, a highly acidic condition that occurs most frequently with cervical cord injuries, because the vagus nerve (parasympathetic) is preserved and the thoracolumbar innervation (sympathetic) is interrupted. Stimulation of the vagus nerve causes the secretion of a strong acidic gastric juice, while sympathetic stimulation causes the secretion of a weak, alkaline mucoid juice. When quadriplegia causes interference with sympathetic stimulation, neutralization is diminished and hyperacidity can occur (Pollock and Finkelman 1954).

Sensory functions Sensory functions are closely associated with regulation of dietary intake. Some local element of preserved sensation is believed to occur, since the sensations of hunger and satisfaction remain unchanged following cord injury. The most significant factor is diminished or lost sensory warning mechanisms in the abdominal area. Although referred pain sometimes ascends to the upper body, this loss of pain can disguise or make acute abdominal distress difficult to recognize. Diagnosis relies heavily on radiographic findings.

Other problems

Metabolism takes place following absorption, that is, passage of nutrients through the intestinal wall into blood and lymph systems. This is the body's way of using chemical compounds at the cellular level. Many factors common to critically ill patients—for example, unfavorable pH, elevated body temperature, or concentrated drug therapy including antibiotics—negatively influence this process. Mobilization of skeletal calcium as a result of paralysis and immobilization is also a major problem. Later in the rehabilitation process anorexia, dehydration, or repeated infections may negatively influence metabolism, leading to malnutrition.

Knowing all the facts about proper nutrition is not enough. Disabled persons must be able to overcome obstacles encountered in shopping for food, preparing meals, and often even feeding themselves.

History

Nutritional assessment begins with a review of the patient's history for conditions that change nutrient needs or interfere with nutrient intake, absorption, and digestion.

Patients with spinal cord injuries can develop malnutrition very quickly during the acute stage. At a time when the body needs it most, food intake may be restricted, as with paralytic ileus, or decreased, as with anorexia. Meanwhile accelerated breakdown of nutrients occurs to meet the additional demands imposed on the body by trauma, surgery, infection, or preexisting depletion.

Another major factor to consider is the effect of immobilization on various metabolic and physiological functions. Immobilized patients experience an increase in excretion of nitrogen, calcium, and many electrolytes and a decline in the basal metabolic rate. Patients with spinal injuries may have even more pronounced problems as bedrest may be prolonged to gain orthopedic stability, and restrictive braces or the actual paralysis prevents physical activity. Activity stimulates physiological recovery.

Because muscle mass begins to decrease early and dramatic weight loss is not uncommon

during the initial postinjury period, extensive nutritional assessment and intervention are required. Referral to a nutritional team or dietitian should occur without delay on admission.

Although others may complete a more thorough history, the following information should be added to the general nursing history. As the patient's condition stabilizes, the nurse will interview the patient or family if indicated with regard to weight and height, dietary intake, and elimination patterns. This information can help predict future problems.

Dietary habits

Be alert for the tendency toward greater fluctuations in weight following spinal cord injury. To determine the patient's knowledge, interest, and previous eating habits, the nurse can discuss a typical breakfast, lunch, dinner, and snacks. During this discussion the nurse will note special diets, food allergies, likes and dislikes, fluid intake, and any sociocultural factors that may influence the diet. For example, certain ethnic groups prefer diets excessively high in carbohydrates and fats or low in fruits and vegetables; certain foods may be prohibited for religious reasons; and lack of money often restricts food selection.

Elimination patterns

Although the patient may not have experienced any difficulties with bowel and bladder control before injury, major problems emerge swiftly following injury. Maintaining regular bowel elimination and, to a lesser extent, preventing bladder distension are essential to maintaining a good appetite. Feelings of nausea, diaphoresis, and general discomfort frequently signal problems with elimination and contribute to anorexia.

Physical Examination

The physical examination reveals the patient's current nutritional status rather than identifying risk factors and should include observation of general appearance and vitality; anthropometric data; examination of the gastrointestinal system; consideration of laboratory findings; and assessment of upper body strength, which determines patients' ability to feed themselves.

General appearance and vitality

A well-nourished person appears alert and responsive, has healthy looking hair and skin, and is not overweight or underweight. Some early signs of poor nutritional status include easy fatigability, listlessness, inattentive or even irritable behavior, and anorexia. The mucous membranes of the eyes may look dry or "glassy," and conjunctiva may be too pale or too red. The skin may be dry, or there may be evidence of skin breakdown.

Anthropometric data

The nursing profession as a whole is being encouraged to collect more objective data on a person's nutritional status to assist in prompt intervention and ongoing accuracy in evaluation of nutritional management. Anthropometric data include height, weight, ideal body weight, weight before injury, and measurement of muscle mass and body fat.

It is generally sufficient to record an estimated weight because during the initial stages movement to a bed scale is not worth the added risk of spinal malalignment. Moreover, the weights of orthopedic appliances vary considerably and bias any actual weights that are taken. For example, a Halo-ring device may weigh anywhere from 22 to 26 pounds. The nurse should also record the maximum and minimum weight the patient can remember. A wide discrepancy may indicate that weight control is a problem. Comparing data with a standard weight-for-height table will indicate the general nature of nutritional adjustments that will be necessary.

Recommended weights for the stabilized person with a spinal cord injury are slightly less than those recommended for the general population. The East Orange Veteran's Administration Center has established that for the patient with a paraplegic injury, the recommended weight is 10 to 15 pounds below the Metropolitan Life Insurance ideal body weight for a given height and frame size (Peiffer et al. 1981: 501). For the patient with a quadriplegic injury, the recommended weight is 15 to 20 pounds below that in the Metropolitan Life Insurance table.

Muscle mass and body fat are important factors for the nutritional specialist to consider when assessing nutritional status. Measuring the mid-upper-arm circumference is a good indicator of muscle mass, and obtaining triceps skin fold measurements with special calipers is an indicator of body fat tissue. Findings are compared with standard charts and expressed as a percentage of normal. These simple clinical measurements are becoming more common and are of particular value during the acute stage; however, their validity in the quadriplegic patient is questionable due to impaired muscular activity and associated muscular atrophy in the upper extremities.

The gastrointestinal system

A well-nourished person normally maintains good dental hygiene and is free from bouts of indigestion, constipation, or diarrhea. Procedures 11–1 and 11–2 can be used to assess the function of the patient's gastrointestinal system.

Swallowing problems may arise as a complication for the patient with a tracheotomy. The nearness of the artificial airway to the esophagus interferes with relaxation of the upper esophageal sphincter, necessary to allow food to pass.

Laboratory findings

Certain laboratory findings reveal abnormalities suggestive of nutritional deficiencies. Routine urine and blood analysis may reveal: protein, glucose, and acetone in the urine; low hemoglobin and hematocrit; reduced serum albumen and total protein; abnormal cholesterol levels; and abnormally low serum electrolyte concentrations. Other miscellaneous blood and urine tests may be indicated to measure the end products of metabolism, namely, nitrogen balance and creatinine levels to indicate the catabolism of protein.

Following spinal cord injury, anemia and hypoproteinemia are common manifestations. Also, a high elimination rate of serum albumen, an indicator of visceral protein status, is not uncommon. The creatinine-height index, which is determined by lean body mass or muscle and expressed as a percentage of normal, is a con-

PROCEDURE 11–1 ■ ASSESSING CHEWING AND SWALLOWING ABILITY

Purpose

The purpose of assessing chewing and swallowing ability is to identify problems associated with malnutrition and to promote safety by preventing choking and aspiration.

Action	Rationale
1. First examine the mouth.	Dental caries, absent teeth, and gum disease may be painful and hamper chewing ability. Periodontal problems with reddened, swollen, or spongy gums that bleed easily are most common in patients over 40. A major problem in the elderly is ill-fitting dentures due to shrinking gums.
2. Check for any swallowing difficulties.	Although not associated with spinal cord injuries per se, a patient with a very high cervical cord injury may experience ascending edema, affecting the lower brain stem and subduing the swallowing reflex.
3. To check for gag reflex, brush the eyelash lightly with a piece of soft tissue.	Usually if the blink reflex is present so is an intact gag reflex.
4. Observe the tracheal aspirate for evidence of oral or tube feedings.	
5. Perform a methyline blue test, adding dye to the feedings and observing the tracheal aspirate.	A positive result will confirm the connection between the trachea and the esophagus. It may also suggest a rare but more serious complication, tracheoesophageal fistula. Differentiating the two requires radiology or endoscopy, but a fistula takes two to four weeks to develop, so a positive dye test before then probably indicates swallowing dysfunction (Holloway 1979). Although this problem will usually disappear after the airway is removed, the patient requiring prolonged use may have difficulty meeting nutritional requirements.
6. Closely observe the patient who has just had a Halo-thoracic brace applied.	Maintaining the neck in the desired degree of hyperextension may cause swallowing difficulties. However, with very slight adjustment of the bars by the physician this problem can usually be solved.

stant value regardless of dietary intake. Severe depletion is a significant complication, especially among patients with quadriplegia.

The following factors are positive indicators of nutritional risk (Peiffer et al. 1981: 503–504):

- Body weight—more than 10% below the recommended ideal body weight
- Serum albumin—less than 3.0 gm/dL
- Caloric intake—less than calculated maintenance or anabolic requirement
- Protein intake—less than calculated maintenance or anabolic requirement
- Hemoglobin—less than 12 gm/dL
- Hematocrit—less than 37%
- Creatinine-height index—less than 60% of standard

PROCEDURE 11–2 ■ ASSESSING THE FUNCTION OF THE LOWER GASTROINTESTINAL TRACT

Purpose

The purpose of this procedure is to determine function of the lower gastrointestinal system. The nurse performs an abdominal assessment, observes the consistency and frequency of stool, and looks for systemic signs and symptoms of gastric upset.

Action	Rationale
1. Check the abdomen.	
• First, listen for bowel sounds by auscultating the abdomen in all four quadrants.	Normal bowel sounds are intermittent and vary in intensity. Be alert for absent, occasional, or weak sounds immediately following injury.
• Next percuss and palpate the abdomen.	The techniques of percussion and palpation should follow auscultation as manual pressure applied to the abdomen may change peristaltic activity. (Abdominal assessment is discussed further in Chapter 13.) The abdomen should be soft and flat without evidence of distension, swelling, or rigidity.
2. Recognize physical discomfort.	When large portions of the body trunk are without sensation, appreciation of localized pain or cramping is not possible.
• In addition to the obvious signs of nausea and vomiting, be alert for generalized tension, malaise, anorexia, shoulder tip pain (the most common referred pain); and, in quadriplegic patients, headache, perspiring, or chills.	These signs and symptoms are indicative of abdominal abnormality.
• Above all, be alert for an increased pulse rate or an elevated systemic temperature and/or white blood count without other apparent cause.	This may signal acute abdominal distress or peritonitis, which may cause death if unrecognized or unchecked.
3. Examine bowel elimination patterns in detail.	Lack of control and bouts of constipation or diarrhea greatly affect the patient's nutritional status (see Chapter 13).

Upper body strength

Patients with quadriplegia have difficulty feeding themselves because of weakness of the upper extremities. Nurses will collaborate with occupational therapists to complete a detailed assessment of upper extremity muscle function and provide individualized aids to assist with feeding. In addition to the care and application of these devices, the nurse must also be aware of psychological stresses to patients using them. Patients easily become frustrated when relearning eating skills. Eating is a very social activity and mealtime can sometimes trigger stressful behavior. Refusing to eat or overeating can signal a deeper existing depression. In general it can be a time when physical limitations are most pronounced.

GENERAL NURSING INTERVENTIONS

Physical fatigue and psychological adjustment can directly affect a patient's appetite, and relearning feeding skills practiced since early childhood or being fed is almost unbearable for many patients. Dietitians, nurses, and occupational therapists must work closely together to prevent malnourishment.

General nursing interventions include:

1. Provide appropriate fluid intake. Routine intravenous solutions provide little nutrition. For example, a liter of 5% dextrose in water contains only 200 calories. Vitamin supplements are needed very early and fluids by mouth should be given as ordered as soon as active bowel sounds return. Fluid intake should be maintained at a minimum of 2000 mL every 24 hours unless contraindicated. A patient with an indwelling catheter needs 2500 to 3000 mL; a patient on an intermittent catheterization regime needs a *regulated* pattern of fluid intake to avoid bladder distension. For more information on fluid intake see Chapter 12.

2. Encourage oral intake of food. Following the critical period, a high-protein and often high-calorie diet is needed to improve nutritional status. A high-protein diet must be defined by a percentage of total caloric intake. If the day's protein intake is beyond 22% to 25% of the total caloric intake, the protein will be used for energy and not for the desired building and restorative purposes. Measures to encourage eating include:

- Small, frequent feedings of preferred foods with as pleasant an atmosphere as possible.
- Calm, friendly assistance with feeding. Be patient, but firm, and do not rush. The quadriplegic patient will often develop hiccoughs if forced to eat too quickly.
- Social interaction. Bringing the patient to the dining table, or even in a bed to a communal dining area, encourages socialization and promotes the feeling of health rather than sickness and isolation.

Often families can be most helpful with this aspect of care.

3. Take measures to prevent aspiration:

- If the patient is in cervical traction or must maintain the recumbent position on bedrest, use the *side-lying* position and tilt the entire bed up 20 degrees. Most specialized immobilization beds have a "tilt control."

- If the patient is on a turning frame, position *prone*, not only for safety reasons but also to promote independence as it is easier for patients to feed themselves in this position. See Figure 11–1.

4. Ensure an adequate airway. Use manual techniques to clear the chest at least $\frac{1}{2}$ hour before mealtimes. This allows the patient sufficient time to expectorate secretions and rest. To prevent aspiration, avoid chest physiotherapy for 30 minutes following oral intake. If the patient is being mechanically ventilated, be sure to inflate the cuff on the tracheostomy tube before feeding. Be sure suction equipment is readily available for high-risk patients. Test the equipment before each meal, particularly when mobile suction units are used in communal dining settings. Choking can be a particular problem, especially during the early stages, because of decreased coughing ability. Performing an assisted coughing maneuver (see Procedure 9–4, Assisted Coughing, in Chapter 9) will usually dislodge food particles in the throat, but suctioning may be necessary to clear the airway. A soft diet is easier to tolerate should choking be a recurring problem.

5. Encourage good nutritional habits, including three regular meals and a well-balanced diet. An adequate diet includes recommended amounts of all major food groups: milk and milk products; meat and alternates; breads and cereals; and fruits and vegetables. The body requires proteins, carbohydrates, fats, vitamins, minerals, and water. Table 11–1 outlines nutrients, major food groups, sources, functions, and any changes in requirements of each following injury.

6. Encourage as much activity as orthopedic stability allows. Maintain range of motion and other specific exercises of unaffected limbs to promote digestion, aid in elimination, and minimize protein breakdown, thus ensuring that weight is gained as lean muscle rather than adipose tissue (Holloway 1979).

7. Initiate and maintain regular bowel habits to avoid constipation and diarrhea. For specific nursing interventions, see Chapter 13. A well-balanced diet high in fiber aids regularity. Fiber is a carbohydrate that is not broken down by mechanical or chemical digestion so that it provides roughage needed to regulate elimination of solid wastes. Fiber absorbs many times its weight in water and thus helps soften stools and eliminate toxins and waste products more rapidly. Avoid refined foods such as white bread. High fiber intake is discussed further in relation to bowel management (see Chapter 13).

8. Provide patient and family education. Nutritional counseling should develop or reinforce good eating habits. Although the dietitian is mainly responsible for this teaching program, the nurse has many opportunities to help put recommendations into practice. For example, the nurse may assist the patient with menu selection or encourage visitors to bring nourishing snacks, such as fruit or nuts, rather than candy or sweets. The other major aspect of education involves self-care skills and encouragement of independence with eating, which will be discussed later in this chapter.

SPECIFIC NURSING INTERVENTIONS FOR POTENTIAL COMPLICATIONS

Paralytic Ileus

Paralytic ileus is the absence of normal peristalsis in the small bowel, which allows fluid and gas to accumulate. It is common with all levels of injury to the spinal cord. Its exact cause is unknown, but it is probably related to temporary autonomic nervous system interruption. Onset and severity differ although patients with complete quadriplegia are likely to suffer the most.

Goals of care

- To recognize onset of paralytic ileus
- To prevent aspiration of vomitus
- To provide adequate hydration and nutrition

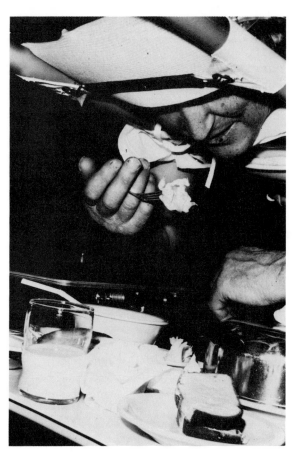

FIGURE 11–1 ■ A quadriplegic man eating in the prone position on a Stryker frame.

Nursing interventions

1. Give nothing by mouth from the moment of injury until the physician has ruled out all paralytic ileus 48 to 72 hours later.

2. Observe all patients with spinal cord injuries for the onset of paralytic ileus throughout the 72-hour postinjury period. Loss of bowel sounds may occur immediately following injury or may be delayed up to 48 hours. Carefully check the patient with quadriplegia for delayed onset. Unrecognized ileus is probably the most common cause of sudden death in the quadriplegic patient during the first 48 hours when decreased coughing ability leads to aspiration of stomach

TABLE 11-1 ■ NUTRITIONAL NEEDS OF THE SPINAL CORD INJURED PATIENT

Nutrient	Food Groups; Best Food Sources	Function	Requirements Following Spinal Cord Injury
Protein	MILK and MILK PRODUCTS MEAT and ALTERNATES, e.g., meat, fish, poultry, eggs, milk, and cheese. Lower quality: soybeans, nuts, breads, cereals, dried beans and peas, and other legumes.	1. To build, repair, and maintain muscle, nerve, connective, and epithelial tissue. Protein accounts for tough fibrous nature of hair, nails, ligaments, and muscular structures. 2. To constitute essential components of enzymes, hormones, antibodies, and other blood proteins. These affect internal environment, stability, and metabolism.	1. Increased supply is needed to: • Repair severe bone and ligamentous injuries • Heal associated wounds • Tolerate postoperative period • Prevent skin breakdown • Fight infections such as those of the respiratory and urinary systems
Carbohydrates (Fiber)	BREADS and CEREALS FRUITS and VEGETABLES, e.g., whole grain breads and cereals, fresh fruit, raw vegetables, rice, pasta, and potatoes.	1. To supply readily available energy. 2. To provide roughage needed to regulate elimination of solid wastes. Fiber is a complex carbohydrate not broken down by mechanical or chemical digestion. Fiber absorbs many times its weight in water to soften stools and eliminates toxins and waste products more rapidly.	1. Increased supply is often needed to provide energy for basic functions in response to illness, e.g., increased respiratory effort of quadriplegic patients during acute phase. Intake should be adjusted as activity increases. 2. Increased fiber in the diet is generally needed to promote bowel control. Fiber must be increased gradually to avoid cramping and discomfort.
Fats	MEAT and ALTERNATES MILK and DAIRY PRODUCTS, e.g., whole or 2% milk, cheese, meat, fish, poultry, nuts, oils, butter, and margarine.	1. To provide a concentrated form of reserve energy, which is stored in adipose tissue and has high calorie value. 2. To protect and insulate body. 3. To promote normal growth and development.	1. Normal supply is required. 2. Reduced supply is required for overweight patients. In addition to the general health hazards of obesity, mobility problems and susceptibility to skin breakdown increase.
Vitamins A B Complex	ALL FOOD GROUPS dark green or yellow-orange fruits and vegetables, e.g., carrots, squash, apricots, and spinach; milk and dairy products; and liver. whole grain cereals and breads, organ meats, and eggs	1. To play dynamic role in metabolism. Absence of vitamins results in malnutrition and specific deficiency diseases. 2. To promote normal energy growth and development and resistance to infection.	1. Supplements almost always required in early stages. 2. Vitamin C in high doses is given to provide acidic environment in bladder to reduce infection.

(Table continues)

TABLE 11–1 ■ (continued)

Nutrient	Food Groups; Best Food Sources	Function	Requirements Following Spinal Cord Injury
Vitamins C	citrus fruits, juices, tomatoes, strawberries, broccoli, and canteloupe		
D	fortified milk and margarine		
E	vegetable oils, wheat germ, whole grain breads and cereals, and margarine		
K	green and yellow vegetables		
Minerals Calcium Phosphorus	ALL FOOD GROUPS milk, cheese, and yogurt	1. To control many chemical mechanisms in the body such as fluid balance, blood volume, and acid-base balance.	1. Specific deficits measured by blood chemistry in early stages and replaced accordingly.
Iron	liver, red meats, whole grain breads and cereals, and green leafy vegetables	2. To provide rigidity to bones and teeth. 3. To regulate excitability of muscular and nervous systems.	2. Calcium and phosphorus deficits occur with paralysis and immobility.
Potassium	fruits and vegetables		
Sodium	salt and high-protein foods		
Water	MILK and MILK PRODUCTS FRUITS and VEGETABLES, e.g., beverages, soups, milk, and juices.	1. To provide a medium for all body fluids (secretions and excretions). In fact, the body requirements for water exceed food. 2. To aid digestion and elimination. 3. To regulate body temperature. 4. To make possible all body functions.	1. Measures to correct dehydration or fluid overload must be initiated according to fluid profile. 2. Water requirements generally increase. Bladder and bowel program largely depend on regulated intake of 2000 to 3000 mL daily.

contents, which results in respiratory arrest (Burke and Murray 1975).

3. Auscultate the abdomen to detect presence or absence of *bowel (peristaltic) sounds.* Place the diaphragm of the stethoscope lightly against the abdominal wall and listen to all four quadrants. Normally, peristaltic bowel sounds are heard as gurgling sounds (at least 5 sounds per minute). Bowel sounds may be described as present, fleeting (occasional), faint, or absent. Bowel sounds are absent during ileus.

4. Be alert for developing abdominal distension. Measure abdominal girth at level of um-

bilicus every eight hours. Progressive abdominal distension may contribute to respiratory difficulties by restricting the movement of the diaphragm and, if untreated, may lead to nausea and vomiting. When ordered, insert a nasogastric tube to decompress the stomach and reduce the risk of vomiting. To minimize gastric irritation, select an air-vented tube and attach to gravity drainage or low intermittent suction. Observe nature of aspirate, and record volume.

5. Check lower bowel for presence of stool. Any stool should be gently removed manually with a well-lubricated, gloved finger. Do not give enemas as fluid will only accumulate and aggravate the situation. A well-lubricated rectal tube in place for 30 minutes at a time, to avoid pressure on desensitized bowel lining, may help relieve flatus.

6. Maintain nothing by mouth and administer intravenous replacement therapy. If untreated, dehydration and electrolyte imbalance are dangers as large volumes of fluid are trapped in the gut and unavailable to the general circulation.

7. Monitor intake and output, including gastric returns, and vital signs as ordered or more frequently according to nursing judgment.

8. Monitor blood hematology and chemistry daily.

9. Detect passing of paralytic ileus by reduced nasogastric returns, return of bowel sounds, and passing of flatus or stool.

10. Be alert for prolonged paralytic ileus, again especially in patients with complete quadriplegia. If ileus persists for longer than 5 to 7 days, hyperalimentation may be considered to supply adequate nutrition. Be alert for any signs or symptoms of gastric ulceration and bleeding.

11. Evaluate effectiveness of treatment according to level of outcome reached:

- Gastric aspiration of less than 50 mL in 24 hours
- Active bowel sounds with passing of flatus or stool
- Abdomen flat without evidence of distension
- Blood hematology and chemistry within normal limits without evidence of bleeding or electrolyte imbalances
- Adequate urine output without signs of dehydration
- Minimal weight loss without evidence of malnutrition

Gastric Ulceration and Bleeding

Neurogenic gastroduodenal ulceration and bleeding is a severe complication of spinal cord injury but may pass unrecognized because the paralyzed person cannot feel the classic symptom of severe or burning abdominal pain. The literature suggests that early detection and management could avoid a number of fatalities (Kewalramani 1979). The terms *stress ulcer* and *acute peptic ulceration* are used to describe gastrointestinal hemorrhage that occurs following spinal cord injury or other physical trauma. Patients with severe cervical cord injury, often with respiratory insufficiency and/or multiple injuries, and those who have undergone early operative procedures are most likely to develop gastric ulceration. The incidence of acute ulceration is probably close to 5% (Burke and Murray 1975 and Kewalramani 1979).

Insult to the autonomic nervous system may cause local circulatory disturbances in the gastric mucosa, which are of paramount importance in initiating the process of ulceration and hemorrhage. Abnormal vasodilation or vasoconstriction may cause ischemic changes, which become a focus for ulceration. Excessive production of acidic gastric juices may further erode existing necrotic areas, particularly in quadriplegic patients, in whom parasympathetic irritation is unchecked because of damage to the sympathetic system.

Preexisting gastrointestinal problems, severe psychological reaction to injury, steroid therapy, parasympathomimetic (cholinergic) drugs, and/or local irritation from a nasogastric tube further predispose the patient to gastric ulceration.

Goals of care

- To identify patients at risk of developing gastric ulceration
- To provide early detection and understand significance of slightly abnormal clinical findings
- To recognize the onset of gastric ulceration
- To control hemorrhage
- To promote healing of gastric mucosa

Nursing interventions

1. Take preventive measures to minimize risk. For example, prevent or recognize and treat systemic *hypoxia* early. (For specific nursing care measures, see Chapter 9.) Take precautions to decrease local gastric irritation when a nasogastric tube is in place; always use an air-vented tube attached to gravity drainage or low intermittent suction.

2. To combat gastric hyperacidity, administer antacids as ordered. This is essential for a patient receiving steroid drugs or a patient with a nasogastric tube used for decompression.

3. Be alert for evidence of bleeding in the gastrointestinal tract; nausea and vomiting; frank hematemesis; abdominal distension; nasogastric returns that look like "coffee grounds," are blood tinged, or show frank fresh blood; and stools that are loose and tarry (melena) or show occult blood on laboratory examination. The onset of acute gastrointestinal hemorrhage usually occurs within 7 to 14 days after injury. It may present as a slow perforation, which is difficult to diagnose because lack of sensation eliminates the classic signs of abdominal pain, tenderness, and muscle guarding. *Shoulder tip pain,* which is referred pain, is a classic sign but not always present.

4. Be constantly alert for signs of hemorrhagic shock; an increased pulse rate (greater than 100 per minute); a drop in blood pressure (systolic pressure 85 mmHg or below); and an acute drop in hematocrit (less than 30%) or hemoglobin (less than 10 gm %).

To differentiate the fatal complication from the relatively common problem of paralytic ileus, Wilmot and Walsh (1973) emphasized:

- *Hemorrhagic shock* is not evident in paralytic ileus unless the ileus has been untreated and the patient has been allowed to progress to a much more serious state of acute gastric dilatation.
- *The pulse rate may be increased.* The blood pressure may already be low from neurogenic shock so it is not as helpful. (Hypotension mechanisms are discussed in Chapter 10.)
- *Shoulder tip pain* is never present in paralytic ileus; if it is present, immediately think of perforation.
- *Vomiting* is not present in paralytic ileus (unless it is untreated) but is present in early perforation.

5. Prepare the patient and assist the physician with diagnostic tests. An abdominal flat plate will reveal air in the peritoneum caused by gastric dilatation. The patient may be too sick to undergo an upper GI series with a contrast media or a gastroscopy. The physician may wish to use peritoneal lavage to rule out peritonitis. Washings should be free from blood, gastric contents, or infection.

6. Institute the following measures as ordered to control gastric bleeding:

- Insert nasogastric tube and attach to low-pressure, intermittent suction.
- Give continuous iced saline lavage.
- Administer antacids.
- Administer blood transfusions and IV replacement therapy.

Surgical intervention may be indicated in rare or unusual cases.

7. Discontinue corticosteroid therapy as ordered, to avoid the associated side effect of gastric irritation.

8. Control pain with analgesics and/or muscle relaxants as ordered.

9. Monitor vital signs and intake and output to assess tissue perfusion.

10. Monitor patient's response to treatment by obtaining daily specimens for blood hematology and chemistry and stool specimens for occult blood. Daily measurements of abdominal girth may also be needed to check amount of distension.

11. Evaluate effectiveness of treatment according to level of outcome criteria reached:

- Regular pulse at rate of 60 to 100 beats per minute.
- Blood pressure within normal limits for patient (90/60 mmHg is considered acceptable for the patient with quadriplegia).
- Urinary output approximately 60 mL per hour.
- Blood hematology and chemistry within normal limits for patient.
- Nasogastric returns free from occult or frank blood with a pH above 3.
- Stools free from occult or frank blood.
- Patient comfortable without feelings of nausea, referred pain, or abdominal distension.

Malnutrition During Critical Period

Immediate life-threatening problems in the critically ill often overshadow nutritional needs, yet metabolic support is a meaningful adjunct to hemodynamic and pulmonary life-saving measures. Malnutrition can cause weakness, fatigue, and poor wound healing; contribute to skin breakdown; and prolong convalescence and rehabilitation.

Trauma causes stress, which dramatically increases energy requirements. An average adult requires 1200 to 2000 calories per day to maintain biochemical functions. Major trauma or surgery may increase this requirement by as much as 50% (Wieman 1978).

The body stores potential energy in carbohydrates, proteins, and fat. *Catabolism* is the process by which these stores are broken down and converted into usable energy. When it is impossible to eat following injury, energy requirements are initially met by catabolism of carbohydrates in the form of glycogen. These stores are depleted within a few hours, and the body then draws on stored protein and fat for energy. Protein breakdown to meet energy requirements (as opposed to its usual function of building and repairing tissue) causes an additional urinary nitrogen loss of 10 to 15 gm per day. Trauma or infection accelerates protein catabolism and produces a negative nitrogen balance. Patients with severe spinal cord injuries have been known to excrete 40 to 50 gm per day, indicating a negative nitrogen balance, which can lead to massive tissue wasting, severe weight loss, dehydration, electrolyte imbalances, and possibly death.

If the patient is unable to eat but has a functional gastrointestinal tract, tube feedings may be considered. If the gastrointestinal tract is not functioning, usually due to prolonged paralytic ileus or associated abdominal trauma, total parenteral nutrition (TPN), or hyperalimentation, may be an alternative. When the patient has not taken anything orally for 5 days, and is not likely to for another week, TPN should be considered (Holloway 1979).

Goals of care

- To recognize patients at risk of developing malnutrition
- To recognize signs and symptoms of inadequate nutrition
- To administer complex nutritional supplements safely and prevent complications
- To ensure positive nitrogen balance

Nursing interventions

1. Complete a nutritional assessment within 24 hours of injury by estimating height and weight and obtaining mid-upper-arm circumference and skin fold measurements. The underweight patient with preexisting depletion is at greater risk.

2. Recognize conditions that increase nutritional needs. Carefully observe patients with quadriplegia who develop respiratory insufficiency; patients with multiple injuries; patients who require early surgical intervention; and patients with infection and elevated temperature.

3. Be alert for conditions that limit oral intake or absorption. Carefully observe patients with quadriplegia who are most likely to develop prolonged paralytic ileus; mechanically ventilated or high quadriplegic patients who may develop gastric distension from air swallowing or swallowing difficulties; patients with anorexia, persistent nausea, or diarrhea; and patients with associated abdominal injuries, which occur most frequently in motor vehicle accidents or falls from a considerable height.

4. Administer nasogastric feedings as ordered. Advanced techniques, tubes, and formulas have made tube feedings safer, more nutritionally sound, and more comfortable for the patient. However, tube feedings are an extreme measure and should be used only when diligent and patient nursing care is unable to overcome anorexia due to physical fatigue or emotional depression. Newer feeding tubes are smaller, softer, and more pliable, and feeding mixtures flow more freely than milk. These improvements reduce the risks of aspiration, tube irritation to the throat and gastric mucosa, and pressure necrosis of the esophageal and tracheal wall. Insertion can be difficult if the patient is uncooperative or if cervical traction or a Halo is in place. It is easier and safer to *place the patient in a side-lying position* during insertion. When the patient has a neurogenic bowel, *diarrhea* and *absorption* may become a problem. Continuous drip feeding over 24 hours is recommended, and Griggs and Hoppe (1979) suggest the following techniques to establish feeds, promote absorption, and control diarrhea:

- To minimize the risk of aspiration, tilt the entire bed or elevate the head of the bed 20 to 30 degrees. If intermittent feedings are ordered, position patient on the right side to promote gravity-assisted emptying of the stomach.
- Begin the feeding at half strength at 50 mL per hour.
- Observe the patient for glucosuria and diarrhea. If this does not occur for 12 to 24 hours, increase the fusion rate by 25 mL per hour each day.
- Once the desired rate is achieved, advance to a full-strength formula.
- If diarrhea, a symptom of osmolar overload, should occur, resume half-strength feedings at 50 mL per hour and gradually increase. Antidiarrheal agents such as paregoric or Lomotil may help and are usually well tolerated. If diarrhea persists, feedings may have to be stopped altogether and resumed in 24 to 48 hours or when diarrhea is controlled. Contact the dietitian to check lactose content of the feeding mixture.
- Nausea may indicate delayed gastric emptying. Stop the feed immediately and attempt to determine cause. Measure abdominal girth to detect gastric dilatation.

5. Administer total parenteral nutrition (TPN) as ordered by the physician. Hyperalimentation, or TPN, is "the intravenous solution infusion of protein as amino acids (nitrogen), hypertonic glucose, and additives (including vitamins, electrolytes, minerals, and trace elements) into a central vein, ideally the superior vena cava" (Colley and Wilson 1979). It is a major advancement in critical care medicine, but to avoid complications it must be implemented by a highly skilled nutritional team, in which nursing has a major role. Nursing the patient receiving TPN is a complex task involving preparing the patient and possibly the solutions, assisting the physician with central venous catheter insertion, administering the solution, maintaining the catheter site, and monitoring the patient for complications. Very strict aseptic technique must be used to prevent infection, which may easily progress to septicemia, and astute observation is required to detect metabolic imbalances. The care of patients with spinal injuries is essentially the same as for any critically ill patient, although the physician may encounter greater difficulty in placing the catheter because neck immobilization restricts access to the paraclavicular region. Observe the patient for signs of respiratory or cardiovascular distress.

6. Evaluate progress toward good nutritional status by level of outcome criteria reached:

- Positive nitrogen balance to signal catabolism is under control
- Condition necessitating use of supplements is improved or alleviated
- Able to take adequate daily nutrients orally
- Increased muscle mass (as measured by upper-arm circumference) and body fat (skin fold measurement)
- Increased body weight (approximately $2\frac{1}{2}$ pounds per week)
- Alert with higher energy levels
- Improved wound healing
- Improved skin tolerance
- Blood chemistry and hematology within normal range

Weight Control

Weight control is singled out as a specific problem, because great fluctuations in body weight are apt to occur during the first year after injury. Excessive weight loss in the immediate postinjury period has already been described. A poor appetite may persist for weeks. However, as mobility and strength return, undesirable weight gain is just as likely to occur. Dietary intake needs to be adjusted to altered activity levels. Overeating can also be linked to depression and perceived changes of body image.

Goals of care

- To maintain acceptable weight for body height and build
- To provide a well-balanced diet including a variety of foods from each of the four main food groups

• To encourage maintenance of recommended dietary intake

Nursing interventions

1. Complete a nutritional assessment to identify potential problems with eating habits and determine the patient's current status. Consult with the dietitian and the patient to determine ideal body weight and develop realistic goals. Although the dietitian is primarily responsible for nutritional counseling, the nurse has a major responsibility in observing dietary intake and identifying any physical or emotional problems that may need referral to other team members. Involvement of the patient, and often the family, is essential.

2. Care for the underweight patient. A poor appetite may be associated with physical or emotional stress. When major physical problems are ruled out, simple fatigue and low energy levels will naturally suppress the appetite. There is a delicate balance between conserving strength and energy and promoting independence. For example, patients may be fed breakfast and dinner but attempt lunch on their own. Encourage as much participation as possible and praise the patient when successful. Encourage friends or relatives to assist with meals. Often they can bring in appetizing snacks. Also offer high-protein, high-calorie drinks every few hours.

Be constantly aware that the underweight, malnourished patient is much more susceptible to pressure and other factors that cause skin breakdown. Frequent turning, correct positioning, and meticulous attention to general cleanliness habits are required. Any number of specialized beds or equipment may be used to minimize risk and prevent skin problems.

Emotional stress may contribute to anorexia. Be sensitive to patients who are embarrassed when they cannot feed themselves; are easily frustrated when trying to achieve feeding skills; and express feelings of hopelessness and depression or act out. Nurses should collaborate with counseling professionals to develop an approach to these deep-rooted problems. Sometimes patients are better left to their own devices; others prefer the peer support and positive social interaction of communal dining. Occasionally a patient may withdraw and completely refuse to eat. Not eating and feeling their "bodies are dead" are signs of severe depression, rather than a normal reaction to an abnormal situation, and a psychiatrist should be consulted. The patient may need antidepressant medication in conjunction with other therapy.

3. Care for the patient who overeats. Some patients feel eating is the only pleasure left in life and tend to consume large meals, frequent high-calorie snacks, and too many soft drinks. When activity is decreased this combination leads to rapid weight gain that is difficult to reverse. Be sure patients are aware of the high-calorie foods in their diet. The hospitalized patient's eating habits can be curtailed to a certain extent, but when the patient goes home, self-motivation is the key. Physical appearance tells you something about the patient's general attitude toward rehabilitation. Ongoing counseling may be needed to promote feelings of self-worth. Obesity in patients confined to wheelchairs makes transfers more difficult, hampers ability to shift weight to avoid skin breakdown, and generally makes such things as dressing or attendant care far more tiring and complicated.

4. *Evaluate progress* toward weight control by levels of outcome reached:

• Body weight acceptable for height and body build
• Normal muscle mass and body fat distribution
• Caloric intake regulated to amount of energy expended
• Adequate nutrients from all four basic food groups included in daily intake

SELF-CARE SKILLS

The Patient with Paraplegia

The patient with paraplegia has little problem eating independently. During the initial stages, when the recumbent position must be

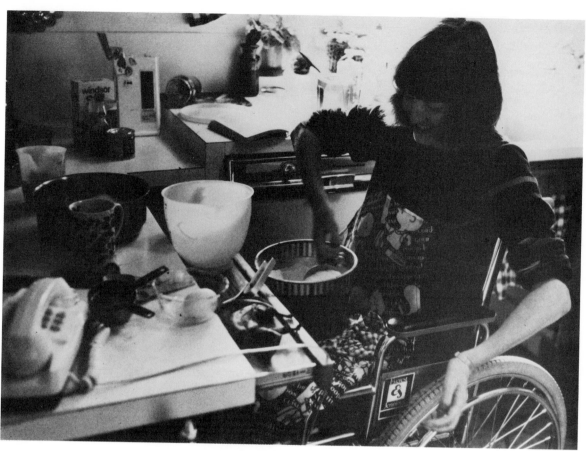

FIGURE 11–2 ■ A quadriplegic woman cooks independently.

maintained, it is much easier and safer to eat in the prone position on a turning frame or in the side-lying position on a regular bed.

When the patient is ready to return home, thought must be given to redesign of the kitchen for wheelchair accessibility, especially if the patient is a homemaker. Many rehabilitation centers, under the direction of an occupational therapist, have preparation classes for home-living skills and offer advice on design following home assessment. Problems such as reaching over sinks, counters, stoves, and shelves must be considered. Managing to grocery shop is another important area of education. See Figure 11–2.

The Patient with Quadriplegia

For the patient with quadriplegia the simple task of eating may be very complex. Close collab-

oration with the occupational therapist is needed to help the patient achieve as much independence with eating as possible. The therapist will complete a detailed assessment of muscle power in the upper extremities to determine the patient's ability to use arms and hands. Appropriate aids and/or splints may then be selected or designed and fabricated for individual use. Nurses should be familiar with the care and application of these individualized aids and must be aware of the exact amount of assistance each patient requires.

Developing self-care skills is a very creative process, and much depends on each patient's interest, motivation, and cooperation, as well as physical capabilities. It is also a changing process. The amount of assistance required during the beginning stages of rehabilitation is not necessarily the degree of assistance that will be required throughout the person's life. With on-

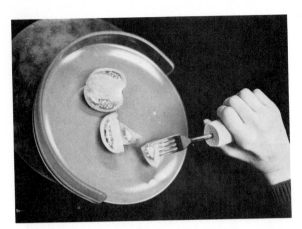

FIGURE 11–3 ■ A quadriplegic woman using a pad-ded handle on a fork. The nonskid plate mat and plate guard shown here are also commonly used aids.

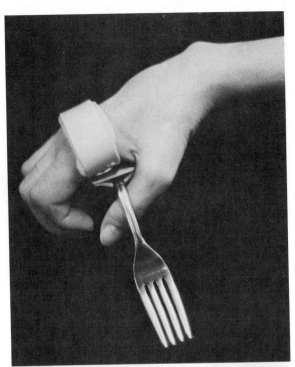

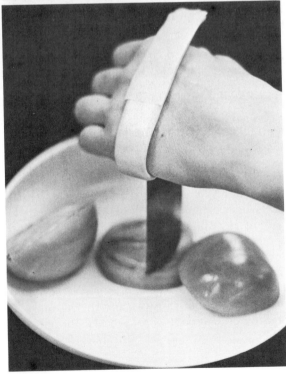

FIGURE 11–4 ■ (A) A fork is inserted into the uni-versal Palmer cuff. (B) Using a special knife attached to a cuffed device, a patient cuts food with a rocking motion.

going therapy and practice, existing muscles do strengthen, and coordination can improve.

There are increasing numbers and varieties of self-care aids currently available. Particularly sophisticated are the bioengineering aids being developed to help individual patients eat inde-pendently. The ability to feed oneself depends on three basic movements: movement of the fingers, including ability to stabilize a utensil; ability to flex (drop) and extend the wrist; and ability to move the arm sufficiently to bring food to the mouth. Adaptive aids capitalize on exist-ing abilities to support these basic movements.

Patients who can move their fingers may in-terlace utensils between their fingers and man-age with minimal assistance to set up a tray, reach a straw, cut meat, and so on. Others may need padded utensils, which are easier to ma-neuver. See Figure 11–3. (This can be accom-plished by wrapping IV tubing around a fork even when the patient is in the intensive care unit!) If the finger function is very weak the uni-versal Palmer cuff may be used. See Figure 11–4. Utensils are inserted into a pocket on the cuff. A splint may be added to help stabilize a weak wrist and enable the patient to take advan-tage of any arm movement. See Figure 11–5. Dynamic splints may be used to convert wrist power for a pincher grasp. See Figure 11–6. When arm movement is impaired, sling supports can be added to help the patient overcome grav-

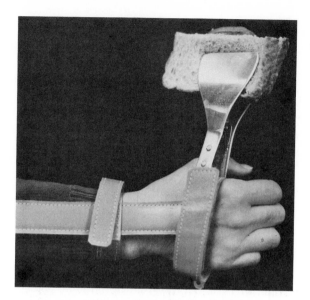

FIGURE 11–5 ■ A splint may be added to stabilize the wrist, pictured here with a sandwich holder.

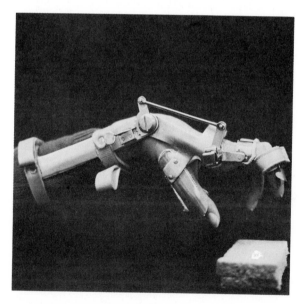

FIGURE 11–6 ■ A dynamic splint converts movement of the wrist into a pincher grasp, enabling this person to pick up a sandwich.

ity and allow sideways movement to bring food to the mouth. Such support systems may take the form of an overhead suspension system or of bilateral swivel arm supports attached to the sides of the wheelchair. Patients who sustain injury at the C_{1-4} level must rely on others to feed them.

The quadriplegic person will also require assistance with kitchen design for wheelchair living. More adaptations will be needed to contend with upper extremity weakness, which makes opening containers, cutting food, and handling household items more difficult.

LONG-TERM IMPLICATIONS

Long-term nutritional management for disabled people is similar to that for the general population. Good nutrition is essential to good health. The same nutrients are required; the caloric need simply decreases with less activity. People with spinal cord injuries require constant adequate fluid intake to promote urinary function and plenty of roughage to regulate bowel elimination.

A community health nurse must be alert for a variety of problems. For example, homemaking tasks may become too burdensome for one reason or another. Consultation and referral may be necessary to initiate appropriate interventions: perhaps an occupational therapist to update skills, some actual assistance in the home, or a community weight loss program.

SELECTED REFERENCES

Burke, D., and Murray, D. 1975. *Handbook of Spinal Cord Medicine.* London and Basingstoke: Macmillan. *Introductory overview of gastrointestinal complications in Section 6; includes paralytic ileus, acute gastric dilatation, acute peptic ulceration, bowel obstruction, and acute abdomen.*

Colley, R., and Wilson, J. 1979. Meeting patients' nutritional needs with hyperalimentation: part I. *Nursing '79* 9 (5): 76–83; part II. *Nursing '79* 9 (5): 59–61. *Comprehensive clinical guide with photostory.*

Griggs, B., and Hoppe, M. 1979. Update nasogastric tube feeding. *American Journal of Nursing* 79: 481–485. *Review of improved tubes, equipment, and formulas; includes related nursing care, step-by-step guide to tube insertion, and helpful overview of potential complications.*

Holloway, N. 1979. *Nursing the Critically Ill Adult.* Menlo Park, Calif: Addison-Wesley, Chapter 12. *Presents nutritional assessment, planning, and implementation; includes abdominal assessment and focuses on TPN.*

Kewalramani, L. 1979. Neurogenic gastroduodenal ulceration and bleeding associated with spinal cord injuries. *Journal of Trauma* 19 (4): 259–269. *A review of 24 patients; signs and symptoms, management, and updated exploration of etiological factors.*

Peiffer, S., et al. 1981. Nutritional assessment of the spinal cord injured patient. *Journal of American Dietetic Association* 78 (5): 501–505. *Study of nutritional status of 18 patients with spinal cord injury, which showed that these patients are nutritionally at risk.*

Pollock, L., and Finkelman, I. 1954. The digestive apparatus in injuries to the spinal cord and cauda equina. *Surgical Clinics in North America* 34: 259–268. *Examines the normal and altered motor, sensory, and secretory functions of the digestive tract.*

Wieman, T. 1978. Nutritional requirements of the trauma patient. *Heart Lung* 7 (2): 278–285. *Reviews altered nutritional needs and symptoms of deficiency, advantages and disadvantages of feeding tubes and gastrostomy tubes, nutrients in liquid feeds, and hyperalimentation.*

Wilmot, C., and Walsh, J. 1973. Abdominal emergencies in acute spinal cord injuries. *Proceedings from Veterans Administration Spinal Cord Injury Conference* 19 (Oct.): 202–205. *Includes incidence, causes, and types of abdominal trauma and signs and symptoms emphasizing how diagnosis, not treatment, is the greater problem.*

SUPPLEMENTAL READING

General

Arlin, M. 1979. Controversies in nutrition. *Nursing Clinics of North America* 14 (2): 199–213. *A brief review of the continuing debate of dietary habits in North America; includes information on sugar, salt, and fiber intake among others and presents current dietary goals for the United States.*

McConnell, E. 1977. Ensuring safer stomach suction with a Salum Sump tube. *Nursing '77* 7(9): 54–57. *Explains advantages of air-vented tubes.*

Meiners, C. 1976. *How to be Healthier Through Proper Nutrition.* Published by the National Paraplegia Foundation and the NPF Allied Health Committee. Available through the National Spinal Cord Injury Foundation. *General nutritional information related to special needs of people with spinal cord injuries; detailed information on dietary fiber and acid-ash intake as it relates to bladder management.*

Assessment

Guyton, A. 1976. *Textbook of Medical Physiology.* 5th ed. Philadelphia: W. B. Saunders. *Classic text detailing neuroanatomy and physiology, including the gastrointestinal system.*

Keithley, J. 1979. Proper nutritional assessment can prevent hospital malnutrition. *Nursing '79,* February, pp. 68–72. *Includes explicit tables on signs suggesting malnutrition, ideal weight for height, body frame type (determined by simple wrist measurement), and standards and measurement instructions for mid-upper-arm circumference and triceps skin fold.*

Naftchi, N. 1980. Metabolic dysfunctions. *Spinal Cord Injury Digest* 2 (Winter): 17–27. *Concise overview of the dysfunctions of bone mineral metabolism and the endocrine system and autonomic nervous system following spinal cord injury. Describes common problems and complications related to these dysfunctions.*

Patient assessment: examination of the abdomen. 1974. *American Journal of Nursing* 74: 1697–1702. *Programmed instruction in inspection, auscultation, percussion, and palpation of the abdomen.*

Nutritional Supplements

Buergel, N. 1979. Monitoring nutritional status in the clinical setting. *Nursing Clinics of North America* 14 (2): 215–227. *Reviews risk factors for hospitalized patients and evaluation, and provides concise tables of information on nutritional support products (liquid formula and chemically defined diets and nutrient supplements). Defines nurse's role.*

Lumb, A. D., et al. Aggressive approach to intravenous feeding of the critically ill patient. *Heart Lung* 8 (1): 71–80. *Describes modified techniques for the use of hyperalimentation when the patient has multisystem failure or shortage of catheter insertion sites; includes recommendations for monitoring and management protocols.*

Potential Problems

Burke, D. 1973. Resuscitation and parenteral nutrition in patients with acute spinal cord injuries and associated injuries. *Proceedings from Veterans Administration Spinal Cord Injury Conference* 19 (Oct.): 177–188. *An overview of acute management including an in-depth look at the complication of paralytic ileus; includes assessment, resultant metabolic disturbances, detailed replacement therapy, and other management techniques.*

Epstein, N., et al. 1981. Gastrointestinal bleeding in patients with spinal cord trauma. *Journal of Neurosurgery* 54 (1): 16–20. *The effect of steroids, cimetidine, and minidose heparin on the frequency and degree of bleeds was examined in 131 patients with spinal cord injury. Overall incidence of 21% did not appear to be affected.*

Tibbs, P., et al. 1979. The problem of acute abdominal disease during spinal shock. *American Surgeon* 45 (6): 366–368. *Examines the value and ease of peritoneal lavage in diagnosis when lack of sensation and reflex activity masks classic signs and symptoms of abdominal distress.*

Long-Term Implications

Klinger, J., comp. 1978. *Mealtime Manual for People with Disabilities and the Aging.* 2d ed. Published by Campbell Soup Co., Box (MM) 56, Camden, New Jersey 08101. *Directed toward disabled homemakers; includes meal-planning and kitchen-tested techniques and recipes, current supplies, prices, and other information. Specific sections for the homemaker who uses a wheelchair, has upper extremity weakness, or lacks sensation. Very useful.*

Mahan, L. 1979. The obese patient. *Nursing Clinics of North America* 14 (2): 230–245. *Comprehensive assessment techniques and recommendations for program design encompassing educational techniques for management of eating behavior and for increasing physical activity.*

Owen, A., et al. 1979. Counseling patients about diet and nutritional supplements. *Nursing Clinics of North America* 14 (2): 247–303. *Reviews elements of nutritional services in clinical and community settings; discusses the need for knowledge about behavioral change theories in counseling; and offers current information about vitamin supplements with a view to eliminating confusion about their use and abuse.*

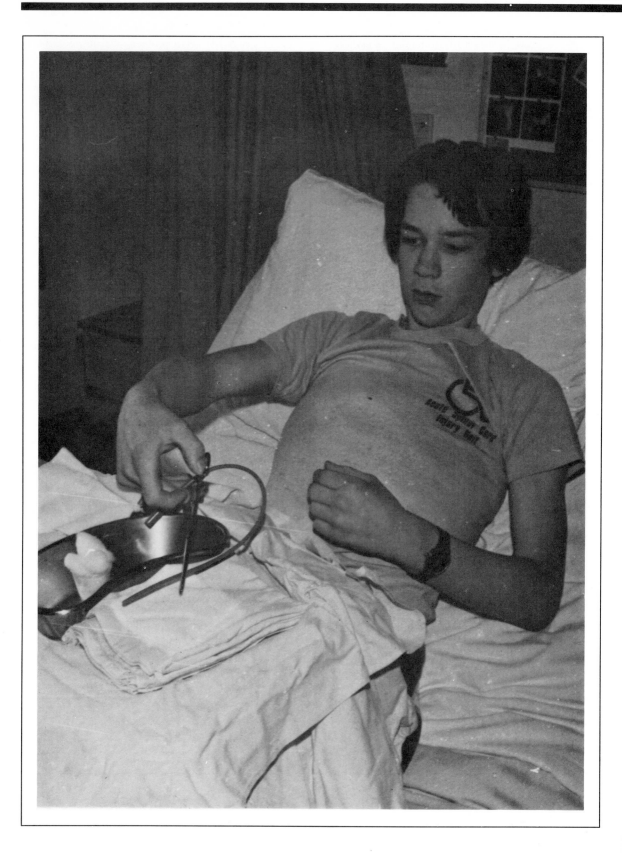

Chapter 12

Maintaining Urinary Function

CHAPTER OUTLINE

OBJECTIVES

- To identify health care goals of urinary care
- To describe anatomy and neural control of the urinary tract
- To specify the expected dysfunctions of voiding as they correlate with level of injury
- To describe assessment and diagnostic tests for urinary dysfunctions during both initial postinjury period and recovery from spinal shock
- To describe methods of bladder management used in the initial postinjury period and during recovery

- To present nursing interventions for patient who, in addition to spinal cord injury, has urinary infection, calculus formation, and autonomic dysreflexia due to urinary complications
- To develop an educational program to teach appropriate self-care skills to patient and family
- To describe long-term implications and follow-up care for spinal cord injured patients with neurogenic bladder dysfunction
- To discuss alternate methods of bladder management.

GOALS OF HEALTH CARE

The term *neurogenic bladder* describes a number of dysfunctions caused by lack of neural control over voiding. Almost all patients with spinal cord injuries experience partial or complete, temporary or permanent loss of control of bladder function. This loss of control can embarrass patients or disrupt their daily activities and sometimes leads to complete social isolation. Moreover, until recently, severe renal problems were the major cause of death in patients with spinal cord injuries. This threat is no longer as great, but it is still present. Hence the management of the urinary system is of the utmost importance in a comprehensive care program. Management requires detailed assessment, diagnostic investigations, and establishment of an individual treatment plan. The success of the plan directly depends on consistent care by skilled personnel and the involvement of patient and family in planning and education.

The goals of the health care are:

- To preserve the function of the upper urinary tract
- To prevent bladder overdistension

- To ensure adequate bladder filling and as complete emptying as possible to avoid stasis of urine
- To prevent or control infection and other complications
- To achieve a reliable and socially acceptable bladder management program that patients can manage independently or can teach others to perform
- To educate patients and families in essential components of long-term bladder care

ASSESSMENT OF URINARY FUNCTION

Pathophysiology of Voiding After Injury

The urinary system

The urinary tract, or system, consists of the kidneys, ureters, bladder, and urethra.

Each of the two *kidneys* is located in the retroperitoneal area on either side of the midline, at the point where the last rib joins the spine.

The kidneys separate waste products from the blood and maintain essential body substances at the constant level. They excrete and conserve nutrients according to body need, regulate volume and composition of body fluids by excreting water, and influence blood pressure by controlling blood volume (which largely depends on the sodium content) and vascular space (which is affected by hormonal production).

After formation in the kidneys, *urine* passes into the collection system through the *ureters,* in which wavelike contractions propel the urine into the bladder. The point at which the ureters join the bladder is called the *ureterovesical junction,* a muscular one-way valve that prevents backflow or reflux of urine.

The *bladder* is a highly elastic muscular container that collects, stores, and expels urine. Its wall is composed mainly of smooth muscle layers collectively known as the *detrusor urinae.* Although this muscle functions automatically, it is controlled by higher centers. The triangular floor of the bladder or *trigone* admits the ureter and urethral openings.

The *urethra* leads from the bladder neck to the outside of the body. The urethra is much longer in males than in females.

Urethral sphincters are muscular structures also involved in the voiding process. The *internal sphincter* is the first valve in the bladder outflow tract at the base of the bladder. It is not a distinct anatomical structure but an elastic mechanism formed by bladder muscle fibers that pass around the origin of the urethra at the bladder neck. These structures close the bladder neck in the resting state, maintaining continence. The *external sphincter* is a well-defined ring of strong, striated skeletal muscle surrounding the urethra. This structure provides voluntary control of voiding. In the male it lies around and below the prostate gland. In the female, it surrounds the middle of the urethra. The striated muscles of the pelvic floor also have a valvular action in voluntary control. An important factor in normal bladder emptying is the ability of these muscles and sphincters to relax.

Neural control of voiding

Neural supply to the bladder musculature has both a voluntary and an involuntary component. Voluntary control is achieved by the brain communicating via upper motor neurons with the sacral portion of the spinal cord, which contains the *reflex voiding center.* The reflex voiding center is located in the S_{2-4} cord segments and is composed of lower motor neurons that transmit stimulation from the bladder to the cord and return a response.

Three areas of the nervous system supply nervous stimulation to the bladder: the $T_{11}-L_2$ segments provide sympathetic stimulation; S_{2-4} segments provide parasympathetic stimulation and a final pathway for voluntary motor control; and finally micturition centers in the pons and hypothalamus provide ultimate cerebral control. Relatively new information indicates that the sympathetic nervous system plays an important role in filling the bladder and contracting the internal bladder neck sphincter. In addition, the sympathetic system provides innervation for vasomotor control, sphincter closure, and ejaculation in the male. It thus appears that a combination of the parasympathetic, sympathetic, and central nervous systems controls the micturition cycle. See Figure 12–1.

Micturition can be described as a sequence of events involving sensory input when the bladder fills with urine, activation of the spinal reflex voiding center, stimulation and provision of cerebral control, and progression and termination of actual voiding.

Sensory input is received from stimulation of the stretch receptors in the detrusor muscle when the bladder fills with urine. This stimulus enters the spinal cord via the dorsal root of the lower motor neurons of the pelvic nerves. In the adult, a sensation of filling first occurs when the bladder contains 175 to 250 mL. An urge to void occurs when the bladder contains 350 to 400 mL of urine.

At this point the reflex voiding center is activated by tension within the bladder wall, and simultaneous communication with the brain occurs. Reflex bladder contractions and relaxation of the internal sphincter are achieved by the parasympathetic motor response returning to the bladder via the ventral root of the lower motor neuron reflex arcs. This reflex activity subsides if voiding is not appropriate but may become powerful enough to override cerebral control.

The brain receives *stimulation* via the upper motor neurons of the spinal cord and interprets it as the desire to void. If voiding is appropriate,

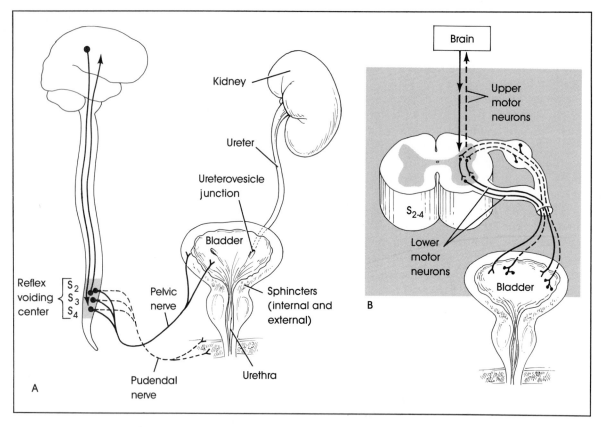

FIGURE 12–1 ■ Neural control of the urinary system. (A) Innevervation from the sacral cord segments to the urinary tract is shown. The pelvic and pudendal nerves are specific spinal nerves (formed from lower motor neurons) innervating the bladder. (B) Upper and lower motor neurons are shown in relation to the reflex voiding center.

response to the reflex voiding center stimulates the parasympathetic nervous system and allows voiding.

The dorsal root of the lower motor neuron arcs provides a final common pathway for voluntary motor and parasympathetic response. The pudendal nerve is the main pelvic spinal nerve carrying this innervation to the bladder.

When the sensation of fullness occurs in infants, transmissions to the sacral segment of the spinal cord cause the detrusor muscle to contract reflexly, resulting in spontaneous, involuntary urination. As the child develops, the brain assumes control over the reflex voiding center located in this sacral segment of the spinal cord. In the adult, cerebral inhibition suppresses the reflex, and individuals void only when the time and place are suitable.

Voluntary relaxation of the external sphincter and pelvic floor initiates voiding by decreasing resistance to the urine flow through the urethra. Muscle fibers of the bladder wall contract reflexly, pulling open the internal sphincter. The increase in bladder or intravesical pressure and the decrease in urethral resistance allow voiding to progress.

Voiding may be interrupted by voluntary contraction of the external sphincter and perineal muscles, which initiates a reciprocal reflex action that closes the bladder neck. This allows the bladder to return to its original or resting position. The same process occurs at the end of spontaneous voiding.

In summary, normal bladder function is a cyclical, coordinated balance between retention and expulsion forces. The normal bladder has sensation indicating filling and the need for micturition. Residual urine (the amount left in the bladder) is normally nil and there is the ability to interrupt or initiate the stream of urine.

Dysfunctions after injury

The kidney is not directly affected by a spinal cord injury because the nervous connections do not appear to play an important role in kidney function. Production of urine is essentially unchanged. The bladder and sphincters, however, are composed of muscular tissues under autonomic and central nervous system control, and any disruption of those systems directly affects bladder sensation and function.

Interruption of communication pathways between the bladder and the reflex voiding center or between the reflex voiding center and higher cerebral centers will cause bladder dysfunction. The location of actual injury has a profound affect on the type and degree of neurogenic dysfunction. An upper motor neuron paralysis of the bladder results when the level of lesion occurs above the reflex voiding center in the sacral cord, and a lower motor neuron paralysis of the bladder results when injury to the sacral portion of the cord involves the reflex voiding center itself. Interruption of the upper motor neurons causes loss of voluntary, coordinated control over the reflex voiding center. An *upper motor neuron,* or *spastic,* automatic bladder results. See Figure 12–2. During the spinal shock phase a spastic bladder will not be evident due to temporary loss of all reflex activity below the level of lesion.

Patients with spastic bladder are unaware of bladder filling and unable to control voiding. When enough urine fills the bladder, stimulating the stretch receptors in the detrusor muscle, the simple reflex arcs contract independently, causing uncontrolled, spontaneous voiding. A common problem, though, is spasm of bladder sphincters, which prevents expulsion of urine and causes overdistension of the bladder.

As the sacral segments of the spinal cord relate to the T_{12} vertebra, fractures causing upper motor neuron damage usually occur above the T_{11} cord segment, leaving the simple reflex arcs intact.

Interruption of the lower motor neurons causes destruction of the simple reflex arcs and

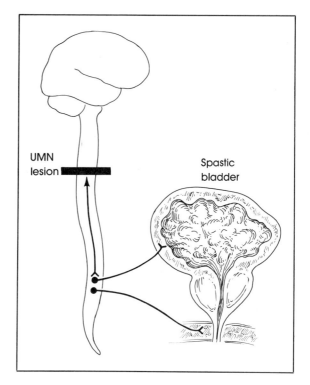

FIGURE 12–2 ■ Dysfunction associated with upper motor neuron damage causes the bladder to become spastic (an automatic bladder).

loss of the reflex voiding center, breaking pathways of communication to the intact upper motor neurons. All reflex activity and bladder tone are destroyed, which cause a *lower motor neuron,* or *flaccid, autonomous bladder.* See Figure 12–3. The patient is unaware of bladder filling and is unable to initiate voiding. The bladder continues to fill with urine, but the patient is unable to void. Again, overdistension results.

As the sacral segments of the spinal cord relate to the T_{12} vertebra, fractures causing lower motor neuron damage are usually at the T_{12} cord segment and below. The upper motor neurons remain intact, but communication to the bladder and sphincters is incomplete and no final pathway is formed by the intact simple reflex arcs.

Incomplete lesions may leave some neurons intact, preserving elements of motor or sensory functioning below the level of injury. For this reason, patients may be aware of bladder fullness yet have no voluntary control or only lim-

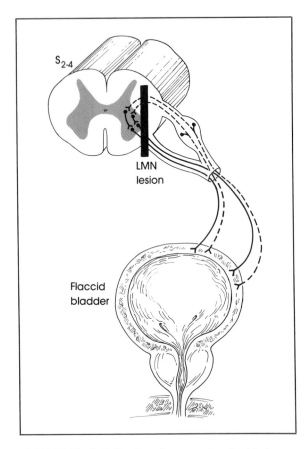

FIGURE 12–3 ■ Dysfunction associated with lower motor neuron damage causes the bladder to become flaccid (an autonomous bladder).

ited control over voiding. Many patients with incomplete injuries, for example, those with Brown-Séquard syndrome, or central cord injury, eventually regain bladder control.

Injuries occurring at the conus-cauda equina junctions are more complicated, resulting in a *mixed*, or *spastic/flaccid*, *bladder*. A combination of spastic involvement of the external sphincter and flaccid involvement of the bladder, or the reverse, is possible. For example, preserved reflex activity in the pudendal nerve but not in the pelvic nerve may cause strong contractions of the external sphincter, preventing weaker detrusor muscle contractions from emptying the bladder.

A simplified classification of a neurogenic bladder due to spinal cord injury is outlined in Table 12–1. In addition to classifying the type of

bladder found after spinal cord injury, it is important to classify the type of sphincteric injury, because this influences treatment and prognosis greatly. One can classify the sphincter as either spastic, normal, or flaccid. Classification also depends on level of lesion, complete or incomplete injury, and the time since injury. Neurogenic bladder classification can be extremely difficult. Factors influencing diagnosis (which cannot be made accurately by segmental level of lesion alone) are cord edema, hemorrhage, ischemia, and thrombosis causing temporary or permanent damage in ascending or descending tracts within the spinal cord.

History

Level and extent of injury

The level and extent of cord injury diagnosed indicates the type of neurogenic bladder dysfunction to expect. It is necessary, however, to remember that spinal shock causes a flaccid bladder in all patients immediately after injury.

Associated injuries

Associated abdominal injuries rupturing visceral organs or even the bladder itself often occur with fractures of the thoracic spine, high-velocity accidents, and sometimes seat belt injuries. Any patient with multiple injuries experiencing signs of hemorrhagic shock has decreased urinary output.

Preexisting urinary complications

It is important to note any preexisting urinary complications, including frequency, urgency, dysuria (painful or difficult voiding), burning sensation on voiding, and retention or incontinence. Also include a medication history.

Common causes of urinary problems are related to outflow obstructions, calculi formation, infections, or systemic problems affecting urinary production and output. For example, an enlarged prostate gland is a common cause of urinary obstruction in males. The female is more prone to bladder infections due to a much shorter urethra. Genitourinary and gynecological problems are common in the elderly and are sometimes complicated by diabetes or anemia.

TABLE 12–1 ■ CLASSIFICATIONS OF NEUROGENIC BLADDER DYSFUNCTION FOLLOWING SPINAL CORD INJURY

Upper Motor Neuron Dysfunction (Automatic, spastic, reflex bladder dysfunction)	Lower Motor Neuron Dysfunction (Autonomous, flaccid dysfunction)	Mixed Dysfunction
Level of lesion occurs above the reflex voiding center in the sacral cord.	Level of lesion damages the sacral portion of the cord involving the reflex voiding center.	Level of lesion damages a portion of the reflex voiding center.
Generally associated with fractures of the T_{12} vertebra (T_{11} cord segment) and above.	Generally associated with fractures to the lumbar and sacral spine (T_{12} cord segment and below).	Generally associated with fractures of the lumbar spine causing conus–cauda equina junction injuries.
Communication pathways between the brain and reflex voiding center are interrupted; communication pathways between the reflex voiding center and the bladder are preserved (reflex activity is maintained after the passing of spinal shock).	Communication pathways between the reflex voiding center and the bladder are interrupted (loss of reflex activity); hence communication pathways to the brain are interrupted.	A combination of upper motor neuron/lower motor neuron dysfunction exists; for example, an upper motor neuron paralysis of bladder sphincters and a lower motor neuron bladder paralysis may exist concurrently.
The patient is unaware of the sensation to void and may experience uncontrolled spontaneous voiding when enough urine fills the bladder to stimulate a reflex (spasmodic) contraction of the detrusor muscle.	The patient is unaware of the sensation to void and does not experience spontaneous voiding; when urine fills the bladder, the bladder becomes overdistended, because there is no reflex activity.	The patient is unaware of the sensation to void and may or may not experience spontaneous voiding.

Note: An incomplete injury to the spinal cord results in varying degrees of preserved motor and/or sensory function below the level of lesion sustained. For example, the patient may be aware of the sensation to void but has limited or no control of micturition.

Physical Examination

The physical examination reveals the patient's current renal status and provides information pertinent to bladder function and potential for retraining. Examination includes assessment within the first few hours of injury and continuous assessment throughout the recovery phase from spinal shock. The neurological picture changes dramatically as spinal shock passes; this ongoing assessment cannot be stressed too strongly.

During the initial postinjury period

Early examination includes assessment of the abdomen, inspection of the perineal and genital area, measurement and observation of urinary output, and assessment of other related body systems.

Assessment of the abdomen Techniques used to assess the chest, that is, visual inspection, palpation, percussion, and auscultation. The following assessment information pertains to bladder function.

- Inspection of the abdomen. Inspect the abdomen visually for asymmetry, localized swelling, inflammation, or lacerations or bruises. Closely observe patients with fractures of the thoracic spine, because such fractures are usually caused by high-velocity accidents, which are commonly associated with abdominal injuries. Also note any scars that may indicate previous trauma or surgery.
- Auscultation of the abdomen. Auscultation is of limited value in assessment of urinary system function unless severe internal trauma or venous malformations are suspected. Bruits, swishing, or blowing sounds are abnormal. Remember that loss of bowel sounds occurs with paralytic ileus.
- Palpation of the abdomen. Normally the abdomen is soft when palpated. When empty, the bladder lies behind the pubic bone; when full, it can be palpated in the lower abdomen. If distended, the bladder can expand to the umbilical region. In a patient without sensation, gentle palpation may cause referred pain if the area is traumatized internally. Assessment by palpation is often restricted for fear of causing further damage when the patient is without sensory warning mechanisms.
- Percussion of the abdomen. Percuss the suprapubic area. If dullness rather than tympany occurs, the bladder is probably distended.

Inspection of the perineum and genital area

Inspect the perineal and genital areas for evidence of trauma—bruising, swelling, bleeding, and, particularly, urethral bleeding or discharge—that may indicate internal problems. Also note any evidence of infection. (Remember that infection in any paralyzed part of the body is more difficult to heal, and vigorous treatment for minor irritations is necessary to prevent complications.)

If the patient is male, examine the penis and scrotal folds carefully for skin ulceration and general cleanliness. Retract the foreskin in uncircumcised males to expose the glans penis.

If the patient is female, examine for evidence of vaginal infection or menstruation. (Often the menstrual cycle is delayed by injury. It is a good idea to obtain the dates of the last menstrual period and obtain a menstrual history.)

When the female is in the supine position, it is safe to bend her knees gently, place her ankles together, and separate her legs (supporting the outer portion of the legs on pillows) to complete your examination.

Measurement and observation of urinary output

Perhaps the best indication of renal function and bladder status is the volume and nature of urinary output.

- *Measurement of urinary output.* Accurate and detailed measurement of intake in relation to output is of utmost importance during the first 48 to 72 hours after injury. On the patient's admission to the emergency room or intensive care unit, be sure to obtain and record the exact amount and type of fluid intake and any output measured during transport. This information is vital in preventing fluid imbalances, particularly overload, which may prove fatal. An indwelling catheter should be inserted immediately if not already in place to avoid the high risk of bladder overdistension and to monitor hourly urine output and specific gravity. Be alert for periods of diuresis, either natural or forced, or low urinary output during the first 48 hours when acute tubular necrosis may occur due to hypotension. A healthy adult's average hourly output of urine is 60 mL.
- *Measurement of residual urine volume.* When intermittent catheterizations are first begun and before manual techniques are successful, residual urine refers to the total amount of urine obtained from a single catheterization. As spontaneous voiding, incontinence, or voiding induced with manual techniques occurs, the residual urine is the amount of urine obtained by catheterization after the bladder has been emptied by other means. To obtain a true residual volume, catheterization must take place immediately after voiding. A normal volume of residual urine in a person without neurogenic bladder dysfunction is 0 mL.
- *Observation of urine.* Note the color, odor, and concentration of urine. It is also possible to detect hematuria, sediment, or mucous plugs on visual inspection. Simple tests (reagent paper strips) at the bedside can show the pH and protein content of urine. There is also a bedside test for approximate specific gravity. Lab-

oratory analysis is discussed in the section on Diagnostic Tests.

Assessment of other related body systems Inadequate renal function can be reflected by altered function of other body systems, and examination of the cardiovascular and central nervous systems in particular should be included in the general assessment of the urinary system. Due to spinal shock, and sometimes to hypovolemic shock caused by multiple injuries, all patients experience an initial fall in blood pressure. Should severe hypotension decrease renal perfusion and cause acute tubular insufficiency, acute renal failure may result. If unchecked, uremia can cause drowsiness, confusion, altered thought processes, and irritability that may progress to twitching and convulsions. Patients with a history of diabetes or hypertension or those prone to transfusion reactions should be monitored closely.

During recovery from spinal shock

The assessment techniques described below may be applied at any time after injury when a bladder retraining program is being considered. These techniques are summarized in Table 12–2.

Prognosis based on level and completeness of injury As previously discussed in this chapter, it is possible to make a simplified estimate of expected bladder function based on the level of injury to the spinal cord. However, patients may experience some motor or sensory preservation if the injury is incomplete. This makes forming a prognosis a highly individual and complex process.

The passing of spinal shock and return of reflex activity make it possible to obtain a permanent bladder profile. Many patients begin to have some success with bladder retraining, or reconditioning, around eight weeks after injury. If not, extensive urological diagnostic procedures may be carried out. Surgical intervention is generally delayed for a year or so, until the bladder profile is stable.

It is possible to predict bladder function fairly accurately by completing a detailed physical examination of the saddle area and the bulbocavernosus reflex. This is usually completed by the physician and recorded in the doctor's notes.

- *Saddle sensation* (referring to the portion of anatomy in contact with a saddle when riding a horse) "is checked for intactness by means of light touch and pinprick of the penile skin, scrotal skin and portions of the adjacent thighs and buttocks. If there is any sensation present, the lesion is incomplete, and the sensory afferents (neurons) are relaying impulses to the brain" (Felder 1979: 98). This may be significant enough to establish some bladder control or at least a sensation of bladder fullness and awareness of the need to void.
- The *bulbocavernosus reflex* (see Figure 7–5) "is elicited by squeezing the glans penis or clitoris or by pulling gently on an indwelling catheter for a few seconds while a lubricated finger is in the rectum. In a positive test, as it is normally, the rectal sphincter can be felt to contract" (Johnson 1980: 300). Although the bulbocavernosus reflex is not the same as the voiding reflex, innervation is at the same level in the spinal cord. A positive reflex suggests the voiding re-flex is intact. This test may be hyperactive in the spastic (automatic) bladder and is absent in the flaccid (autonomic) bladder.

Fluid intake and voiding patterns Ideally an intermittent catheterization program is begun a few days after injury. When this is the case, an assessment of voiding patterns is not included. The following assessment data can be used before beginning an intermittent catheterization program at any time after injury and can be used during an intermittent catheterization program to reduce the number of catheterizations necessary. The information is based on Johnson (1980) and Whittington (1980) and includes detailed observation of fluid intake and output patterns, plus information about motor control or sensory appreciation of the patient.

- Observation of fluid intake pattern. Compile a 24-hour record of fluid intake over a three- or four-day period. The amount and time of fluid intake aids in estimating voiding responses and is verified by the time and amount voided. Be alert for periods of increased intake, for example, at meal times.

TABLE 12–2 ■ BLADDER RETRAINING

Assessment Skill	Signs and Symptoms	Implications
Sensory testing of the saddle area	Absent sensation	Predictive of accompanying loss of sensation to the bladder; no sensation of bladder fullness; no control over voiding
	Present (or limited) sensation	Predictive of accompanying bladder sensation; partial to full awareness of bladder fullness perhaps significant enough to establish voiding control
Testing of the bulbocavernosus reflex	Positive (or hyperactive)	Predictive of an intact reflex voiding center; suggestive of an upper motor neuron neurogenic bladder dysfunction
	Negative	Predictive of damage to the reflex voiding center; suggestive of a lower motor neuron neurogenic bladder dysfunction
Observing fluid intake pattern over a 24-hour period	Unregulated intake with periods of excessive intake followed by little or no intake	Fluctuating voiding responses, difficulty in controlling and detecting bladder fullness; poses an ever-present threat of overdistension
Observing voiding pattern over a 24-hour period	Incontinence with continual leakage of urine or sudden passing of large amounts of urine	Indicative of an unregulated drinking pattern; inadequate timing of intermittent catheterizations or use of other techniques to induce voiding; urinary tract infection; incontinence with complications such as detrusor-sphincter dyssynergia
Measuring residual urine	Unacceptable residual volume greater than 20% of bladder capacity	Unbalanced bladder; overdistension with susceptibility to reflux of urine and bladder infections

• Observation of voiding pattern. Compile a 24-hour record of output, accurately recording both volume and frequency. If the patient is incontinent, urine amounts can be approximated as follows (Stryker 1977: 89):

Diameter of Stains	Amount Voided
9 inches	50–75 mL
12 inches	100–125 mL
18 inches	150–175 mL
24 inches	200–300 mL

A patient may be incontinent and continually leak urine or may suddenly pass large amounts of urine. Incontinence may be associated with stress, such as straining or coughing. Measure the amount voided (or estimate the amount of urine lost through incontinence) and the immediate postvoid residual urine to obtain an idea of the patient's bladder capacity.

• Observation of motor control or sensory appreciation. Note any voluntary control of voiding. Since innervation to the anal sphincter is at the same level in the spinal cord as innervation of the voiding center, contraction of the anal sphincter on command suggests some voluntary control over initiating or stopping the urinary stream. Also question the patient on use of other methods to initiate voiding, such as abdominal pressure, manual expressions, or cutaneous stimulation. (These methods will be described more fully in the section on General Nursing Interventions.) Be sure to note any awareness the patient has of bladder fullness or spontaneous voiding. The quadriplegic, for example, may perspire more when the bladder is full. Positioning often affects the patient's awareness of bladder fullness and ability to void. In particular the supine position inhibits voiding.

Practical aspects related to bladder retraining A number of factors affect the outcome of a bladder retraining program:

- Assessment of physical abilities. In the early stages, an intermittent catheterization program may be instituted while the patient is on bedrest. As mobilization begins, it is desirable to have the patient void in the normal sitting position. At this point the patient's balance, coordination, and tolerance to the upright position must be considered. To determine possible self-care skills, the occupational therapist will complete an in-depth assessment in collaboration with the nurse. Although people with paraplegia have the physical potential to become independent with bladder care, the initial use of thoracolumbar braces makes manual techniques to induce voiding and self-catheterizations more difficult. Quadriplegic patients require a detailed assessment of hand and arm function and adaptive aids.
- Assessment of potential for cooperation. The key to success in a bladder retraining program is the rigid implementation of scheduled intake and output times. The patient needs to comprehend and participate fully in all aspects of care. Motivation, reliability, learning ability, and receptiveness are all important factors. Denial of this condition can lead to a lack of cooperation that might impede the goals of the program.

Another important factor is the support of knowledgeable staff and family members who will be involved in implementing the schedule, particularly if the patient will be totally dependent for bladder care.

Diagnostic Tests

Diagnostic findings produce more sophisticated data on bladder function and generally include the standard procedures discussed below.

Urine examinations

Urine is a most important body fluid. The body must excrete urine to maintain its delicate balance of water and electrolytes and get rid of waste products. Frequently performed laboratory tests are urinalysis and urine culture and sensitivity. The following information is based on the work of French (1980).

Urinalysis A routine urinalysis usually includes a description of appearance, pH value, specific gravity, and protein and sugar content. Microscopic examination of the sediment and screening for various other abnormal constituents are also included. Since constituents of urine deteriorate rapidly on standing, a specimen not analyzed within the hour should be refrigerated. This is a most important nursing responsibility.

Normal urine is clear and may range from pale yellow to dark amber depending on the concentration. Diet, fluid intake, and certain drugs can cause changes in the appearance. Urine may be clouded by crystals, casts, blood cells or pus, or bacteria. Urine pH values from 4.5 to 7.5 or 8 are normal; however, normal urine is usually slightly acidic. Repiratory or metabolic acidosis causes the urine to be acidic (pH below 6). An alkalosis or infection causes the urine to become alkalotic (pH above 6). Control of urinary pH may be desirable to prevent infection and calculi formation.

The specific gravity (SG) or urine ranges from 1.010 to 1.025. The SG is an indicator of urinary concentration. It depends on kidney function to concentrate or dilute urine and on the patient's status of hydration.

The SG can be measured approximately at the bedside by use of a hydrometer that works on the theory of displacement. At least 20 mL of urine are required, which may be a problem to collect if urinary output is low. Laboratory analysis does not require as much volume and osmolality measurements are more accurate, but they take longer to complete. It is important to remember that such tests as an IVP using contrast media will produce false elevations of the SG for 24 hours or so following the procedure.

If anything is abnormal in the urinalysis the physician will probably order other renal function tests.

During the bladder retraining program a urinalysis should be done weekly, or at the first sign of infection or other problems.

Urine culture and sensitivity Urine cultures are used at frequent intervals to monitor any type of bladder retraining or maintenance program. Bacteruria is a constant, serious threat to patients with spinal cord injuries. Some physicians recommend culturing urine with each catheterization (this may be several times a day); others believe in prophylactic screening such as taking a weekly specimen. Certainly all physicians support culturing the urine when an infection is suspected. Observe urine carefully for sediment, odor, or cloudiness that can indicate infection, and monitor the systemic temperature.

A most important nursing responsibility is the collection and care of the specimen. Extreme caution must be taken to avoid contamination during specimen collection. Main sources of contamination are penile or vaginal secretions, cleansing fluid preventing bacterial growth in the specimen, and improper handling of the specimen before laboratory analysis. Be sure to refrigerate the specimen immediately or ensure prompt delivery to the laboratory. The less expensive, more convenient dip slide technique is gaining popularity.

Catheterized specimens are the most common in patients with spinal cord injuries. A midstream urine is almost impossible to collect, because the patient has neurological impairment of voiding control. Early morning specimens are recommended for the most accurate analysis, because urine is most concentrated at this time.

BUN and creatinine levels

Urine is 95% water with electrolytes, bacterial toxins, certain pigments, hormones, and ni-

trogenous waste broken down from the metabolism of protein. The most plentiful waste products are *urea* and, to a lesser extent, creatinine. Urea nitrogen and creatinine both circulate in the blood, but are largely excreted in the urine. The amounts excreted are proportional to the rate of production and the glomerular filtration rate. The following information is based on the work of Stark (1980).

Blood urea nitrogen (BUN) is normally 11 to 23 mg/100mL. When urea is not being excreted adequately, the BUN level will rise. This is a helpful indicator when assessing renal function. However, several other factors unrelated to kidney function can cause an increase or decrease in BUN values:

- Protein metabolism is not constant and can be affected by poor nutritional status, infection, trauma, surgery, hepatic dysfunction, or certain medications such as corticosteroids or tetracyclines.
- The urea excretion rate can be altered by dehydration, vomiting, diarrhea, infection, surgery, and hypovolemia, all of which alter blood volume and reduce the glomerular filtration rate.

The BUN is therefore examined with the creatinine level to give a more exact reflection of kidney function.

Creatinine blood levels are normally 0.6 to 1.2 mg/100 mL. Creatinine is an end product of muscle metabolism. Since the muscle mass of the body seldom changes rapidly, creatinine levels are generally constant unless kidney failure has begun.

Carefully observe the BUN/creatinine ratio. This is normally 20:1. When the BUN rises, but the creatinine remains normal, look for any physiological reason that can cause decreased blood flow to the kidney, which will reduce the glomerular filtration rate or increase protein catabolism. Be alert for low fluid intake, chronic hypotension, and urinary infection as causes of volume depletion and low perfusion of the kidneys. Also consider depleted nutritional status, fever, bleeding from stress ulcer, and corticosteroid therapy as possible causes of increased protein catabolism. Reaction to trauma or surgery may cause BUN levels to vary. When the BUN and creatinine both rise, suspect kidney disease with nephron damage. Note any early signs of uremia such as weakness, fatigue, nausea and vomiting, headache, weight loss, and tremors. Confusion, disorientation, or convulsions that may develop will require seizure precautions and an airway ready for emergency use.

Intravenous pyelogram

The intravenous pyelogram (IVP) is considered a diagnostic cornerstone, because it gives more overall information about the urinary system than any other single test. In the early stages, as soon as the patient's condition stabilizes and transportation to the X-ray department is safe, an IVP will provide baseline data for future comparisons and rule out any gross abnormalities of the urinary system. In an emergency, when trauma to the kidneys, ureters, or bladder is suspected, the procedure can be carried out at the bedside.

An IVP is a series of X rays in which the "absence, presence, location, size, and configuration of each kidney as well as of the filling of renal calyces, pelves, and outlines of ureters can be determined. Some idea of the lower urinary tract is also obtained" (Winter and Morel 1977: 65–66).

Preparation for the patient should include an explanation of the procedure, its purpose, and the reason for physical preparation. This usually includes omission of food and fluids from midnight on the night before the procedure to improve concentration of the opaque contrast medium in the urinary system and produce a clearer X ray. Bowel evacuation is also necessary as the kidneys lie retroperitoneally. Fecal material or gas may cause shadows on the film. Many physicians routinely order vigorous laxatives such as castor oil and cascara combinations. Such cathartics are contraindicated for people with neurogenic bowel, because their strong effects can cause nausea, vomiting, fainting, and even blackouts or signs of autonomic dysreflexia. Scheduling the test on a day of routine evacuation or use of a rectal suppository on that day is usually satisfactory.

The patient is placed on a full-length X-ray table in the supine position. Care must be taken to maintain spinal alignment while transferring the patient. A mobilizer stretcher or surgilift (described and illustrated in Chapter 4) works well.

The table must be padded with one-inch foam rubber or a soft sheet to protect the bony prominences.

A plain X-ray film of the kidneys, ureters, and bladder is taken first. The physician then injects a radiopaque contrast medium intravenously to outline anatomical structures. During this time the patient must be observed for any allergic reactions. Serial X rays are then taken over a 20-minute period. If delayed films are necessary, the patient should be moved back to bed for comfort measures and protection against skin breakdown during the intervals between X rays.

Urodynamic studies

Cystometry The cystometrogram (CMG) is a urodynamic procedure used to aid in diagnosing the nature and extent of neurological impairment to the bladder. To document abnormalities of the urethra and muscles surrounding the urethra that create the internal and external bladder sphincters, further studies such as the urethral pressure profile and electromyography are needed.

The principles of the CMG are:

- As fluid is instilled through an indwelling urinary catheter, the bladder reacts as if it were naturally filling with urine.
- When the fluid volume is increased, the normal bladder will eventually respond by contracting to expel the fluid.
- Detrusor muscle action produces measurable increases in pressure within the bladder itself.

These pressures and other observations of sensation and reflex activity are recorded and interpreted by the physician to assist in determining the exact classification of neurogenic bladder. This procedure can be performed at the bedside, but many hospitals have more sophisticated cystometry equipment in the urological endoscopic procedure areas. Bladder volume and pressure measurements are determined electronically. Both fluid and gas media are used to fill the bladder. Carbon dioxide, a rapidly absorbed gas, is used rather than fluid, because it is a more rapid method of assessing bladder profile. (The gas flow rates of insertion are 100 to 200 mL/min.)

The normal bladder response is the ability to

perceive "(1) temperature and entrance of fluid; (2) the point at which a desire to void is experienced; and (3) the stage at which pain or distress is first felt, as well as the point of severe pain beyond which no further bladder filling can be tolerated. . . . until a massive contraction empties the bladder" (Chusid 1979: 270).

Full understanding of the abnormal results of cystometric testing requires a clear understanding of the concept of lesions involving upper motor neurons as contrasted with lesions involving lower motor neurons at the voiding center.

In a person with an upper motor neuron (spastic) bladder dysfunction, after spinal shock subsides a cystometrogram will reveal many uninhibited contractions in response to bladder filling. See Figure 12–4(A). Eventually, one contraction will be strong enough to expel some of the fluid. This usually occurs at a lower-than-normal bladder capacity (approximately 250 to 300 mL). A large residual amount of urine is often left. Many patients do not have either desire to void or a feeling of bladder fullness but an involuntary urinary stream may be elicited by various trigger methods.

In a person with lower motor neuron (flaccid) paralysis of the bladder a cystometrogram will show no uninhibited bladder contraction because the reflex arcs to the voiding center are damaged. See Figure 12–4(B). A person experiencing spinal shock will also demonstrate this flaccid bladder profile. No sensation or desire to void is present. The bladder cannot expel urine. Manual expression or catheterization is required to empty the bladder. Overflow incontinence as a result of bladder overdistension must be avoided at all costs.

During cystometric tests insertion of warm or cold fluids may be used to test sensation. Insertion of ice-cold fluid into the bladder of a patient with an upper motor neuron (spastic) bladder will elicit a strong contraction causing expulsion of the solution. A patient with a lower motor neuron (flaccid) bladder will have no response. This is referred to as the "ice water test."

Sometimes medications are inserted into the bladder to assess bladder sensitivity and response to the drugs. For example, bethanecol chloride (Urecholine) may be introduced into a flaccid bladder to elicit contractions, or propantheline bromide (Pro-Banthine) may be used to inhibit uncontrolled contractions of a spastic bladder.

Urethral pressure profile Urethral pressure profiles (UPP) are used to measure pressures along the length of the urethra. The test is performed by slowly removing a small catheter at the same time as fluid or gas is infused. Pressures recorded reflect pressures along the length of the urethra.

Electromyography Muscular activity measurement of the external urinary sphincter and rectal sphincter may be recorded simultaneously with the CMG by sphincter-perineal *electromyography* (EMG). Electrically sensitive rectal plugs and uretheral catheter sensors are used to record electrical activity of the pelvic floor. Again, hyperactivity is suggestive of upper motor neuron damage; flaccidity of lower motor neuron damage.

GENERAL NURSING INTERVENTIONS

Surely one of the most disruptive problems facing a person with a spinal cord injury is the loss or alteration of bladder control. Maintaining bladder elimination is a major nursing responsibility requiring a special combination of knowledge, skill, and patience. "The knowledge, the conviction of its importance, the interest and the support of the nurse are essential factors for a successful program. Nursing intervention in this area needs to be *individualized, ingenious* and *rigorous* (emphasis added)" (Stryker 1977: 94). The urologist will consider a number of factors including the patient's history, physical assessment, and diagnostic findings before selecting an appropriate bladder management program. However, the techniques involved may be distasteful to some patients or impractical for others. Assessment must encompass the patient's capabilities during the psychosocial adjustment period, personal preferences, and physical limitations. The nurse has a valuable contribution to make in helping the patient and family accept the preferred methods of urological care.

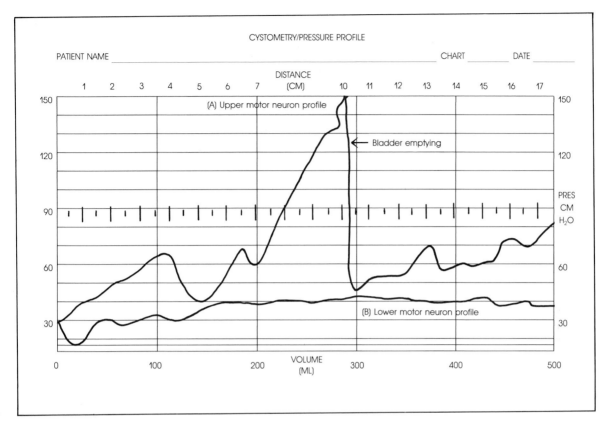

FIGURE 12–4 ■ Cystometrogram (CMG) results are graphed illustrating (A) an upper motor neuron profile showing several uninhibited contractions before one is finally strong enough to empty the bladder, and (B) a lower motor neuron profile showing total lack of any ability to contract the bladder.

A stable profile of bladder function evolves as the stage of spinal shock passes and reflex activity returns. Nursing care to help the patient maintain urinary elimination occurs in three broad stages: the initial postinjury period, the phase of recovery from spinal shock, and the long-term phase of bladder management. During the acute stage the nurse deals with the first two phases, which are discussed in this section. The last phase is discussed in the sections on Self-Care Skills and Long Term Implications later in this chapter.

Although bladder retraining continues to be a subject of much debate, during the past decade intermittent catheterization has gained worldwide acceptance as the preferred method of initial management. Many patients suffering neurogenic bladder dysfunction due to spinal cord injury have achieved a catheter-free state with this method. Numerous investigators have found considerable reduction in persistent bladder infections and prevention of the many serious problems associated with any form of indwelling catheter. Other advantages include better patient acceptance, since freedom from an indwelling catheter promotes independence, improves personal hygiene, and eases sexual relations.

The history of intermittent catheterization is an interesting one. Presently this concept is helpful for a variety of patients with neurogenic bladder dysfunction, but it was first introduced by Sir Ludwig Guttman in 1949, following his work with large numbers of British veterans of World War II with spinal cord injuries. Guttman used a scrupulous sterile procedure performed only by physicians, but more recently a clean procedure, often performed by patients, has gained acceptance. However, for the most part, a sterile procedure is adopted when the patient is hospitalized to reduce the ever-present hazard of cross-contamination.

Many larger spinal injury centers in the United States have catheterization teams composed of a group of technicians often led by RNs or nursing assistants. Bladder management is their exclusive duty. Part of the rationale for this specialization is to eliminate any contact with the gross contamination encountered in general nursing care duties. The other aspect is mainly ease of training for fewer staff members. However, the patient population does not always support such an approach, and more and more centers consider repeated catheterizations an integral part of nursing care. Existing literature does not clearly correlate infection rates with categories of staff performing the catheterizations. In one study a group of rehabilitation nurses integrated intermittent catheterizations with other aspects of nursing care (Kuhn et al. 1974). The infection rates and numbers of patients catheter free at the time of discharge achieved by this nurse delivery system compared favorably to results achieved by alternative delivery systems.

At any rate many general critical care areas and specialized neurological facilities support an intermittent catheterization regime soon after initial injury. To ensure success and avoid complications, the staff must have a high level of interest, motivation, and skill. One point that is often discussed is the subject of female nurses catheterizing male patients. Experience has shown there is no particular problem with this providing the nurse is adequately trained in the technique. Many patients feel that bowel accidents or procedures are far more distasteful or embarrassing than a "clean" medical procedure such as catheterization.

Maintaining Elimination During the Initial Postinjury Period

The initial postinjury period may generally be considered as the first 72 hours after injury.

Providing continuous drainage

Although an intermittent catheterization regime is the method of choice in the management of neurogenic bladder dysfunction in patients with spinal cord injuries, it is almost always necessary to insert an indwelling catheter to establish continuous drainage for the initial 24- to 72-hour postinjury period. If the patient's general condition is unstable for any reason, continuous drainage may be necessary for a longer period, and an intermittent catheterization regime will be delayed accordingly.

The acutely ill patient needs a detailed hourly intake and output record when urinary output is low, as with hypotension from neurogenic or hypovolemic shock or dehydration, or abnormally high, as with overhydration or diuresis. An indwelling catheter may be required for a prolonged period during the acute phase to monitor these parameters in a seriously ill patient with associated injuries or severe respiratory difficulty.

During the early stages of spinal shock, the tone of all tissues, including blood vessels, is reduced and the pressure of a catheter in the urethra can produce ischemia and lead to formation of abscesses or fistulae very quickly. For patients with spinal cord injuries, the presence of an indwelling catheter for a week or more is invariably associated with infection and a tendency toward bacterial urethritis and prostatitis in male patients (Pearman and England 1973). In the United States today, indwelling catheters are the greatest cause of hospital-acquired infections and the most common factor leading to fatal gram-negative septicemia (Kunin 1974). The patient with neurogenic bladder dysfunction is in double jeopardy of developing complications. During this period diligent nursing care is required to minimize these risks. See Procedure 12–1 and Figure 12–5.

Initiating intermittent catheterizations

An intermittent catheterization program is based on the concept of evacuating the bladder at regular intervals by inserting a straight (non-retaining) urethral catheter every few hours to drain the bladder of urine. For most patients with spinal cord injuries, the ultimate goal of bladder retraining is to become catheter free.

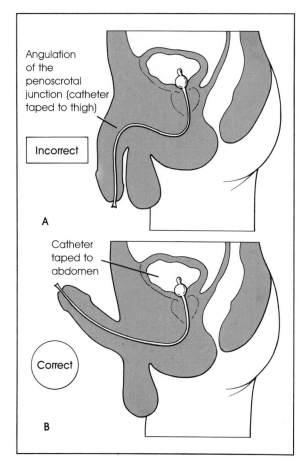

FIGURE 12–5 ■ Positioning an indwelling catheter to the abdomen of a male patient straightens the angulation of the penoscrotal junction and reduces pressure exerted by the catheter.

To ensure success the nurse must clearly understand the principles of an intermittent catheterization regime.

- It is vital to avoid overdistension of the bladder. Overstretching the bladder wall ruptures detrusor muscle cells. Resultant fibrosis, associated with loss of contractility, may permanently impair bladder tone and function. Overdistension significantly decreases the blood supply to the urethra, bladder, ureters, and kidneys and weakens resistance to infection. Furthermore, the increased pressure of chronic overdistension causes ureterovesical reflux allowing ascending infection to infiltrate the ureters and kidneys. Preservation of the upper urinary tract is vital to life. Prevention of overdistension is thought to be the key to preventing urinary tract infection.
- The bladder must be emptied completely and frequently to reduce the residual medium in which bacteria may rapidly multiply.
- Strict aseptic technique must be followed when the patient is hospitalized to reduce the risk of cross-contamination and hospital-induced infection.
- The catheter must be inserted with the utmost care to prevent urethral trauma.
- Finally, intermittent catheterization eliminates the need for an indwelling catheter, which acts as a chronic foreign body, inciting inflammatory reaction and allowing bacterial invasion.
- Early initiation of intermittent catheterization is believed to accomplish faster retraining results and reduces the inevitable infections associated with an indwelling catheter. One to three months after injury is a reasonable time to estimate for return of detrusor activity in patients on an intermittent regime, as compared with three to six months for those treated with indwelling catheters (Burke and Murray 1975).

Keeping these principles firmly in mind, nurses can work closely with physicians to begin intermittent catheterization programs as outlined in Procedure 12–2. See also Tables 12–3 and 12–4.

Maintaining an intermittent catheterization program

The information in this section is summarized in Table 12–5.

Regulating fluid intake The fact that the detrusor muscle responds with more powerful contractions when the bladder is full is important during bladder retraining (Pearman and England 1973). A drinking pattern is necessary to develop the desired relationship between timing and amount of fluid intake, and timing and amount of voiding or catheterization volumes. Intake should be maintained at approximately 2000 mL/day and strictly monitored to 150 to 180 mL/hour from early morning until after supper.

Reduction of intake in evening hours leads to reduction of urinary output at night. Initially,

PROCEDURE 12–1 ■ CARE OF A PATIENT REQUIRING A CONTINUOUS DRAINAGE SYSTEM

Purpose

The purpose of caring for a continuous drainage system is to provide unobstructed drainage while avoiding trauma to the urethra and bladder neck and preventing infection.

Equipment and Supplies

- Size #14 or #16 (French) indwelling catheter
- Standard sterile catheterization set
- Additional set of sterile forceps
- Urinary collection system (tubing and bag)

Action

1. Select a catheter no larger than a size #16 (French) for males and no larger than a size #14 (French) for females. Do not inflate balloon beyond 8–10 cm.

2. Lubricate the catheter *liberally*.

3. Follow strict sterile technique when catheterizing patient. After donning sterile gloves, use one set of forceps to hold the cotton balls for cleaning genital area and an additional set of forceps to manipulate catheter for insertion. Secure tip of the catheter with forceps; control end of the catheter by placing between third and fourth fingers.

4. If there is any difficulty passing the catheter, try a curve-tipped (Coudé) catheter, which can be gently rotated to maneuver past the penoscrotal angle or circumnavigate any narrowing of urethra or resistance at bladder neck.

5. Secure catheter with tape. Tape catheter to inner thigh of a female; tape upward on abdomen of a male. If a patient is on a regular bed, tape catheter in a central position on the abdomen so tubing can be placed to either side when patient is turned. If patient is on a Stryker frame, pad catheter tubing with gauze and place it just above iliac crest before turning to prone position. If patient is sitting, catheter can be taped more to side of the abdomen to promote drainage.

6. In early stages, while patient is on bedrest, secure catheter with a strip of lightweight paper or non-allergic tape.

7. Coil excess tubing at level of the patient's bladder and secure the collection bag at a lower level. *Never*

Rationale

Avoid larger sizes that dilate the urethra and sphincters unnecessarily.

To minimize urethral trauma, especially when patient is without sensory warning mechanisms. Also, male patient, because of the larger urethra, requires additional lubricant.

This "no-touch" technique is recommended to minimize the risk of introducing infection. There is a risk of contaminating the sterile glove when cleaning, even though forceps are used.

To avoid urethral trauma, *never* force introduction of a catheter; notify the physician if any difficulty arises.

Taping prevents any pulling on the urethral mucosa or the bladder neck. When the penis rests in a downward position, there is sharp anatomical angulation at the penoscrotal junction. If the catheter is taped on the thigh, excessive pressure causes irritation and greatly increases the risk of penoscrotal fistula. Taping the catheter upward onto the abdomen straightens the urethra at the penoscrotal angulation, relieves undue pressure, and reduces risk of complications. See Figure 12–5.

This tape is sufficient and less traumatic to newly desensitized skin.

To provide continual gravity. Assisted drainage to promote constant urinary outflow.

(Procedure continues)

PROCEDURE 12–1 ■ (continued)

Action	Rationale
lift the drainage bag above level of patient's bladder when turning or transferring. Be alert for a solid column of urine in the drainage tubing indicating obstructed flow. Air bubbles should always be present. Low urine output may be another indication that urinary flow is obstructed. Catheter may simply need to be changed or if continual obstruction is a problem, bladder irrigations may be necessary. Routine irrigation of catheters is not recommended.	
8. Clean entire perineal area, particularly external urinary meatus. Gently wash the perineum with soapy water twice daily. Rinse and dry well. Avoid use of powders and lotions in the perineal area. These tend to become trapped in the skin folds.	To prevent accumulation of bacteria at the point where catheter enters body. Because of its proximity to the bladder, this is a significant site of possible infection.
9. Observe entire perineal area, including gluteal fold, for reddened, irritated areas. Clean and dry. Directing a flow of oxygen (available from standard wall outlet) over perineal area for 15 min several times a day may sufficiently dry area. Try to alleviate cause. If you suspect that soap is irritating, clean with normal saline instead.	When female patient is in supine position cleansing solutions tend to run down and accumulate in gluteal fold. Be sure to check area thoroughly. It is necessary to turn patient to do so. It cannot be overstressed that reddened areas on desensitized skin with compromised circulation will rapidly break down unless dealt with immediately.
10. If infection is suspected, swab area for a culture and apply appropriate topical antibiotics as ordered by physician. Crusted secretions around the meatal opening can be removed with hydrogen peroxide. Neomycin ointment may be applied to meatal opening twice daily as a prophylactic measure.	
11. Care for the urinary collection system. When patient is on bedrest, change urine collection bag only when catheter is changed unless it is accidentally contaminated or leaking. Sediment or odor indicates need for a change. To obtain a urine specimen from rubber catheter, swab puncture area with alcohol and aspirate the urine with needle and syringe.	Even though modern drainage tubing and collection bags incorporate drip chambers, one-way flutter valves, and vents that have drastically reduced possibility of urinary backflow and contamination when emptying, this equipment is still a major source of ascending infection. Any opening of system increases the risk of infection.
12. Change catheter routinely every one to two weeks. To check for crystal formation, roll catheter between fingers. If there is grit in the catheter, change it and report it to physician.	Rubber catheters will deteriorate, absorb fluid, and swell.
13. Provide adequate fluid intake. Generally 2500 to 4000 mL every 24 hr is recommended, but in acute stage, fluid intake may be restricted for other priorities. Use of urinary antiseptics and acidifying agents are delayed until patient can tolerate fluids administered orally.	

PROCEDURE 12–2 ■ BEGINNING AN INTERMITTENT CATHETERIZATION PROGRAM

Purpose

The ultimate goal for most patients with spinal cord injuries is to become catheter free. During the intermittent catheterization program goals of management are (1) to prevent overdistension of the bladder; (2) to prevent introduction of infection; and (3) to control infection by complete and frequent emptying of the bladder.

Action	Rationale
1. Assess general condition of the patient.	To determine if it is possible to begin intermittent catheterization when patient: • Has stable blood pressure, pulse, and respiratory rate and a normal body temperature • Produces adequate amounts of normal urine *consistently* (approximately 60 mL/hr over a 24-hour period) • Is free from associated trauma or preexisting conditions that would make repeated catheterizations difficult and traumatize the urethra Intermittent catheterizations are contraindicated when: • Monitoring of hourly urinary output is required • Natural or forced diuresis is present
2. Regulate fluid intake to total of approximately 2000 mL/24 hr. Encourage patient to follow a drinking pattern of approximately 150 mL/hr during waking hours or adjust intravenous fluids to flow at 75–80 mL/hr. Decrease infusion rate if fluids are tolerated by mouth.	This avoids large amounts of urine from overdistending the bladder. Unregulated fluid intake causes fluctuating voiding responses and difficulty in detecting and controlling bladder fullness. Regulating fluid intake becomes a major patient responsibility as rehabilitation progresses.
3. Schedule catheterizations. Begin every 4 hr around the clock. Remove the indwelling catheter in the early morning hours. A convenient schedule to start with is 1000, 1400, 1800, 2200, 0200, and 0600 hr.	This facilitates close observation of patient throughout the day. Try to avoid catheterizations when the ward is particularly busy, such as mealtime or change of shift.
4. Use a small, red rubber catheter, a size #12 or #14 (French). The catheter should be soft and pliable.	This prevents urethral dilatation and trauma. Repeated sterilization tends to make rubber catheters brittle. When this occurs they should be discarded.
5. Perform catheterizations. Follow a strict sterile technique.	The "no-touch" technique in Procedure 12–1 (step 3) is preferred. A new disposable kit developed at the Rehabilitation Institute of Chicago, which is basically a catheter contained in a narrow plastic drainage bag, has significant advantages and is particularly suitable for intermittent catheterizations of male patients (Wu et al. 1980).
6. Withdraw the catheter slowly and apply a firm, downward pressure over the suprapubic area. Female nurses will probably have to use a closed fist to exert enough pressure.	This ensures complete bladder emptying and elimination of residual urine.
7. Observe the patient closely for overdistension. Initially check the abdomen for palpable distension every 1–2 hr. Catheterize immediately if distension is suspected.	This minimizes overdistension of bladder with subsequent loss of bladder tone and susceptibility to infection. *(Procedure continues)*

PROCEDURE 12-2 ■ (continued)

Action	Rationale
8. Maintain bladder capacity of less than 500 mL. If the volume is greater than 500 mL reevaluate intake regulation. If diuresis is present, resume continuous drainage.	The volume of urine obtained at any catheterization should never exceed 500 mL. If it does, contact the physician to reevaluate the situation. It is not practical to catheterize more frequently than every four hours. If, despite controlled intake, the volume is persistently greater than 500 mL at each catheterization, diuresis should be suspected. This is common during the first week after injury. Delay the intermittent catheterizations temporarily.
9. When intravenous fluids are discontinued, schedule catheterizations at 6-hour intervals. Maintain bladder capacity at approximately 450 mL. If bladder capacity exceeds this volume, resume 4-hour schedule.	If complications are not present, regulating oral intake should control bladder capacity.
10. Record intake and output.	Conventional fluid charts, which are tallied at the change of each shift, do not lend themselves to recording an intermittent catheterization program. Table 12-3 is an example of a chart record that may be used throughout the program, and Table 12-4 is an example of a corresponding bedside record.

this enables early discontinuation of night catheterizations and allows uninterrupted sleep. If bladder care is unnecessary during the night, it is more convenient for patients to manage self-care.

With intense rehabilitation activities, it is difficult to regulate hourly intake, and patients must avoid large amounts of fluid at any one time. It is helpful to have drinks available during physiotherapy sessions. Fluids delivered to the bedside when the patient is not there are of no value to anyone. Alternative arrangements may have to be made involving dietary service.

As with all aspects of care, involving patients in decision making will immeasurably improve the chances for success. In the beginning it is helpful to prepare a sample record outlining goals for intake patterns to use as a guide at the bedside. Place in clear protective cover or envelope where the patient can see, reach, and use it. Be prepared to encounter some difficulty regulating fluid intake due to loss of appetite from physical and emotional adjustments. During the early stages gentle persuasion is more successful than outright forceful confrontation.

Avoid excesses of caffeine-containing drinks and carbonated and alcoholic beverages, which tend to irritate the bladder.

Manual techniques to induce voiding During the recovery phase from spinal shock continual assessment is necessary in order to begin appropriate manual techniques to elicit a voiding response. Intermittent catheterizations, by allowing filling and emptying of the bladder, facilitate manual techniques because they stimulate existing spinal cord reflexes; stimulate both internal and external sphincters; and assist in maintaining bladder tone.

Although these techniques are used while a patient is on bedrest, any means of voiding is improved when the sitting position is assumed, which promotes gravity drainage. Therefore early mobilization is encouraged when the patient gains orthopedic stability.

The manual techniques are trigger voiding, straining to void, and manual expressions (Credé maneuver). A fourth technique, anal sphincter stretch, is specifically practiced to overcome the problem of detrusor-sphincter dyssynergia and will be described later in this section.

TABLE 12–3 ■ AN INTERMITTENT CATHETERIZATION PROGRAM SAMPLE CHART RECORD

Part A: A numerical recording of fluid intake and output

- Begin recording fluid in and out, making sure to use the appropriate space for the entry. Enter the date in the margin beside the appropriate day. In other words, do not record in the first horizontal section unless it is a Monday.
- The *time* column permits a maximum of six separate entries, enough spaces to accommodate recording of intermittent catheterizations performed every four hours over a 24-hour period (Example 1). When catheterizations are reduced, for example, to every six hours as shown in Example 2, record data in the first four consecutive spaces.
- Calculate fluid intake for the time interval between catheterizations, rather than the standard practice from shift to shift. For this reason, it is essential to accompany this chart record with a corresponding bedside record as shown in Table 12–4. Enter fluid intake in the second column.
- Next record the amount of urine voided in between or before catheterizations. This amount refers to output obtained when voiding is spontaneous or is induced by trigger techiques or straining to void.
- Use the Credé column to record the amount of urine expressed manually.
- The urinary output obtained via catheter is the residual volume of urine obtained.
- Total the urinary output from all sources.

P. 1

DATE	TIME	INTAKE	VOIDED	CREDÉ	CATHETER	OUTPUT	SPECIMENS	COMMENTS
MON. Record correct date here.	*Commence this form on the correct day. Do not start recording at the top of this page unless it is a Monday.*							
	TOTAL	■				■		
TUE.								
	TOTAL	■	*Example: q 4h program* ↓			■		
WED.	0200	400	—	—	300	300	*Admission*	
	0600	400	—	—	300	300	*urinalysis*	
Sept. 10, 1983:	1000	500	—	—	300	300	*C & S*	
	1400	500	—	—	500	500	*taken*	
	1800	300	—	—	350	350		
	2200	300	—	—	350	350		
	TOTAL	■ 2400				■ 2100		

(Table continues)

TABLE 12–3 ■ (continued)

Part A: A numerical recording of fluid intake and output

DATE	TIME	INTAKE	VOIDED	CREDE	CATHETER	OUTPUT	SPECIMENS	COMMENTS
THU.								
		Example: q 6 h program						
	TOTAL		↓					
FRI.	0600	280	—	200	250	450		Incontinent
	1200	800	50	250	100	400		
Oct. 1, 1983	1800	750	300	200	200	700		See nursing
	2400	280	400	—	100	500		notes.
	TOTAL	2110				1950		
SAT.								
		Example: BiD program						
	TOTAL		↓					
SUN.	0900	Total	250	150	75	475		Voiding
		intake						spontaneously
Nov. 3, 1983	2100	only	300	150	10	360		
		↓			Total remaining, output			Leg bag emptied
		↓				1065		× 4
	TOTAL	2500				1900		

(Table continues)

TABLE 12–3 ■ AN INTERMITTENT CATHETERIZATION PROGRAM SAMPLE CHART RECORD (*continued*)

Part B: A corresponding graphic record of urinary output (*see opposite page*)

- Begin recording output data on the correct day. Note Example 1 is entered on a Wednesday to correspond with Example 1 as shown in Part B.

- The numbers *1* through *6* in the horizontal Treatment column refer to the number of catheterizations performed during a 24-hour period. In Example 1, the number *1* refers to the first catheterization of the 24-hour period, which was performed at 0200 hr (as recorded in Part A); the number *2* refers to the second catheterization of the 24-hour period, which was performed at 0600 hrs. In Example 3, the number *1* refers to the first catheterization of the 24-hour period, which was performed at 0900; the number *2* corresponds to the second catheterization, which was performed at 2100 hr.

- The graphic record allows the viewer to interpret at a glance progress toward achieving a balanced bladder. Initially, the broken line, which indicates the amount of residual urine obtained from each catheterization, is superior on the graph. As the intermittent catheterization program proceeds and more urine is expelled from the bladder either by spontaneous voiding or as a result of techniques to induce voiding, the amount of residual urine (obtained by catheterization) gradually decreases. The broken line graphically illustrating the amount of residual urine then becomes inferior. At the same time, the solid line representing the total amount of urine expelled from the bladder gradually becomes superior. To present this concept clearly Examples 1, 2, and 3 have been linked to show a condensed version of progress over a two-month period.

(Table continues)

1. *Trigger voiding.* A number of maneuvers are used to stimulate so-called trigger areas by eliciting a strong reflex or spasm in the detrusor muscle of the bladder, which expels urine and efficiently empties the bladder. The reflex contractions that occur spontaneously from the filling of the bladder usually do not empty the bladder completely. The patient finds a "trigger point" to augment the voiding contraction (Burke and Murray 1975). See Procedure 12–3.

Trigger voiding is successful only when the reflex arcs to the sacral voiding center are intact. As previously mentioned the reflex voiding center is located in the S_{2-4} segments of the spinal cord, which relates to the T_{11-12} and L_1 vertebrae. A patient sustaining injury above this level will probably experience an upper motor neuron (spastic) bladder and have success with trigger voiding. A patient injured at this level may find trigger voiding of some value if a portion of the reflex arcs are left intact and a mixed neurogenic bladder exists. Trigger voiding is of no use if the patient has a lower motor neuron (flaccid) bladder.

2. *Straining to void.* When straining to void, the patient strains as if attempting to have a bowel movement, by taking a deep breath and bearing down. Straining requires strong abdominal muscles. As these muscles are innervated by the T_{6-12} cord segments, patients with injury sustained at

TABLE 12–3 ■ (continued)

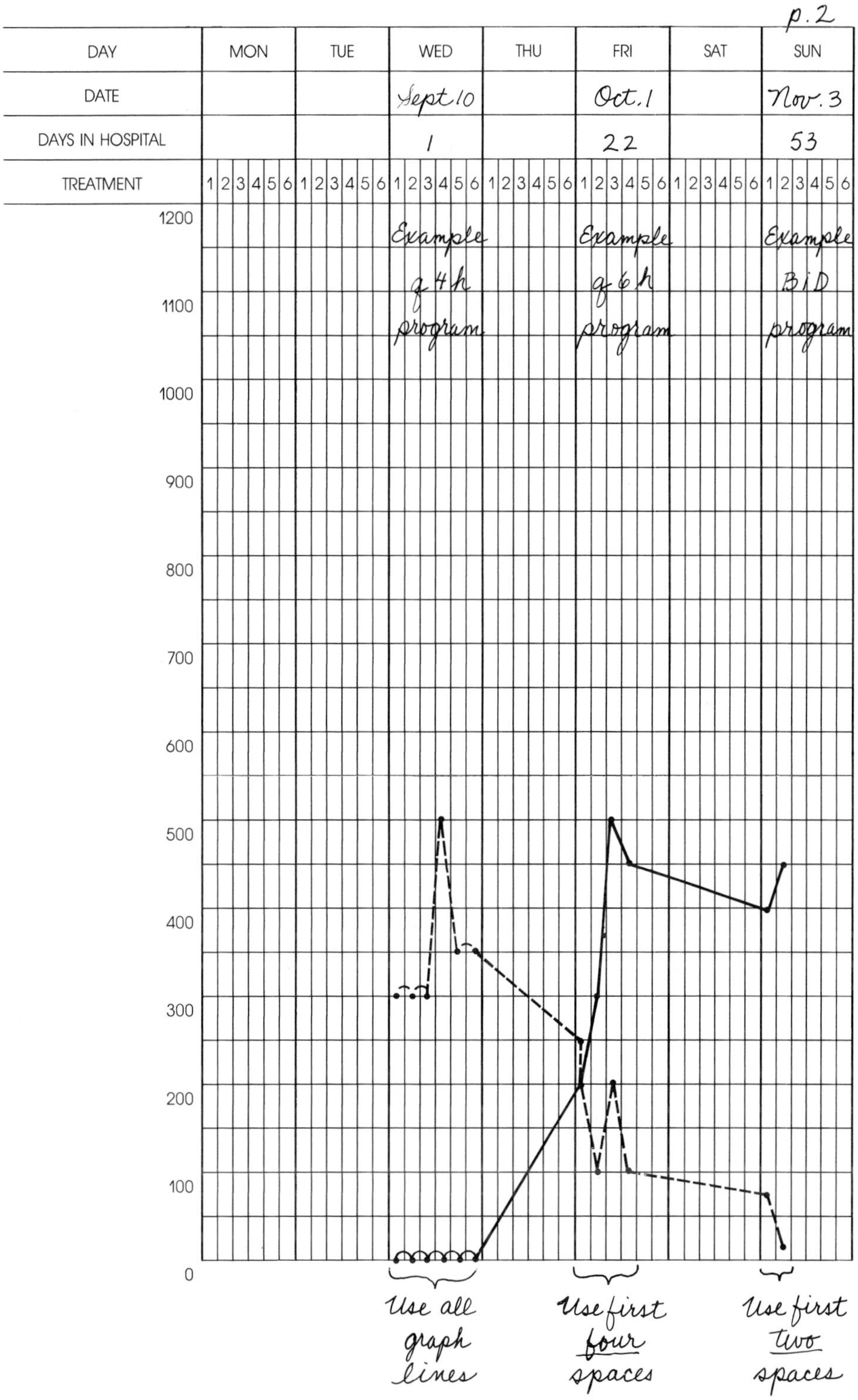

p. 2

DAY	MON	TUE	WED	THU	FRI	SAT	SUN
DATE			Sept 10		Oct. 1		Nov. 3
DAYS IN HOSPITAL			1		22		53
TREATMENT	1 2 3 4 5 6	1 2 3 4 5 6	1 2 3 4 5 6	1 2 3 4 5 6	1 2 3 4 5 6	1 2 3 4 5 6	1 2 3 4 5 6

Example q 4h program

Example q 6h program

Example BiD program

Use all graph lines

Use first four spaces

Use first two spaces

TABLE 12–4 ■ A SAMPLE FLUID INTAKE AND OUTPUT RECORD USED AT THE BEDSIDE DURING AN INTERMITTENT CATHETERIZATION PROGRAM

A staff member or patient can enter information on this bedside worksheet designed to accompany a chart record as shown in Table 12–3. It is important to calculate fluid in and out between catheterizations, rather than the usual practice of calculating amounts only at the end of each shift.

Fluid Measurements	Time	Intake		Output
		Oral	Intravenous	Urine Output
Yellow paper cup 150 mL Large blue paper cup 240 mL Coffee mug 240 mL	(2200 0200)	(10 p.m.–2 a.m. NOTHING TO DRINK) Goal = 0 mL		Voided Credé Catheter
	Total			
China cup 190 mL Tumbler 180 mL Small cream 70 mL Large cream 100 mL	0600	(AFTER 2 a.m. MAY HAVE GLASS OF FLUID) Goal = 200 mL		Voided (Catheter at 1000 hr will likely have most mL in Credé bladder.) Catheter
	Total			
Tea pot 240 mL Soup bowl 120 mL Soup cup 150 mL Blue feeder cup 210 mL	1000	(BREAKFAST AND NOURISHMENT) Goal = 600 mL		Voided Credé Catheter
	Total			
Blue water carafe 750 mL Carafe top 90 mL Wide mouth water jug 800 mL Top to wide mouth water jug 100 mL	1400	(LUNCH AND NOURISHMENT) Goal = 600 mL		Voided Credé Catheter
	Total			
	1800	(DINNER) Goal = 400 mL		Voided Credé Catheter
	Total			
	2200	(AFTER DINNER 2 SMALL GLASSES) Goal = 200 mL		Voided (Goal for 24-hr Credé period = 2000 mL) Catheter

TABLE 12–5 ■ MAINTAINING AN INTERMITTENT CATHETERIZATION PROGRAM: A SUMMARY OF INFORMATION

Action	Rationale
1. Establish a pattern of regulated fluid intake.	This promotes more effective bladder emptying. Reduction of fluid intake during evening hours results in reduction of urine output during the night. Rest and sleep are promoted. Complete patient and family health education regarding regulation of fluids and avoidance of fluids that irritate the bladder.
2. Introduce appropriate manual techniques to induce voiding.	For most spinal cord injured patients these techniques are used to achieve a catheter-free state. Using these voiding techniques emphasizes the need for: • Continual assessment to detect the passing of spinal shock (when reflex activity returns) • Knowledge of the characteristics of the neurogenic bladder dysfunction exhibited • Manual skills to use voiding techniques correctly Perform, or, when appropriate, teach the patient to perform, the following techniques: • Trigger mechanisms • Straining to void (a Valsalva maneuver) • Manual expression (Credé maneuver) • Anal stretch technique Also when appropriate teach the patient (and possibly the family) to perform catheterizations.
3. Help the patient achieve a "balanced bladder."	Continual assessment is needed to prevent overdistension and ensure complete emptying of the bladder. • Maintain bladder capacity of 300–400 mL using combined techniques of catheterizations and maneuvers to induce voiding. • Reduce catheterizations to q6h; when residuals are less than 400 mL for 2 days reduce to q8h; when residuals are less than 300 mL for 2 days reduce to postvoid residual checks as designated. • When residuals are consistently less than 100 mL collaborate with physician to terminate catheterizations.
4. Evaluate effectiveness of program.	Observe for return of neurological function and kidney function. Compare serial diagnostic tests with baseline data: • Neurological examination • Urinalysis (weekly) • Urine for ciulture and sensitivity as indicated • Blood urea nitrogen and serum creatinine levels • Intravenous pyelogram • Urodynamic studies Be alert for infection (note early signs of elevated systemic temperature and urinary pH above 6). Detect high residual urine volumes (over 2 to 3 month period) and collaborate with physician to diagnose specific problem.

PROCEDURE 12–3 ■ TRIGGER VOIDING

Purpose

The purpose of trigger voiding is to stimulate effective reflex bladder emptying.

Action	Rationale
1. Observe for leg spasms, reflex erections, which commonly occur during catheterizations, or a positive bulbocavernosus reflex to indicate that trigger voiding attempts may be successful.	Reflex voiding is one of the last functions to return as spinal shock passes in an ascending manner. If the bulbocavernosus reflex is not present do not frustrate patient by attempting trigger voiding.
2. Ensure that patient is in a comfortable position. If in bed, flex patient's hips slightly and elevate the head of the bed if possible.	This position facilitates voiding and reduces the chance of causing leg spasms. The abdomen must be relaxed for stimulation to reach the bladder.
3. Firmly tap, stroke, or gently pinch the lower abdomen and inner thigh. Alternatively gently pull on the pubic hair, stimulate the rectum, or apply gentle suprapubic pressure.	Of these methods, tapping is probably the most successful and most patients with quadriplegia will eventually be able to perform the technique themselves.
4. If successful, trigger mechanisms will start the urinary stream within a minute or so.	
5. Once the best trigger point or points are located, *show* the patient the exact site.	Due to lack of sensation the patient will be unable to feel the trigger point.
6. Record the location and effectiveness of mechanisms used.	

or above the lower thoracic vertebrae will not find this technique helpful for bladder evacuation. See Procedure 12–4.

3. *Manual expression (Credé maneuver).* This maneuver involves application of strong external pressure over and around the bladder so that pressure within the bladder builds and overcomes the resistance of the bladder neck and urinary sphincters. Urine is literally forced to pass. Manual expression is used when other methods of stimulation are unsuccessful, that is, when a flaccid bladder exists. See Procedure 12–5.

Reducing frequency of intermittent catheterizations As output is obtained from the use of various manual techniques previously described or spontaneous voiding occurs, the number of catheterizations per day may be reduced. Whatever the combination of methods used, adhere to the principles of maintaining bladder capacity at 300 to 400 mL, avoiding overdisten-

sion, and ensuring complete emptying of the bladder.

Manual techniques or spontaneous voiding should be attempted in between and prior to scheduled catheterizations. For example, if catheterizations are scheduled for 0800 and 1400 hours, trigger voiding should be performed just before 0800, again at 1100, and just before 1400 hours. Eventually trigger voiding alone will be effective enough to empty the bladder at timed intervals and replace catheterizations.

The following criteria are recommended for use as a general guideline when the number of catheterizations required is being reduced (Kuhn 1974):

• When the residuals are less than 400 mL for two days, reduce intermittent catheterizations to every six hours.
• When the residuals are less than 300 mL for two days, reduce intermittent catheterizations to every eight hours.

PROCEDURE 12–4 ■ INSTRUCTING THE PATIENT TO STRAIN TO VOID

Purpose

The purpose of straining to void is to use the abdominal muscles to exert pressure on the bladder for more effective emptying.

Action	Rationale
1. Select patients with strong abdominal muscles who can successfully and safely try this technique.	Patients with any history of coronary artery disease should avoid this technique. This Valsalva maneuver, or holding the breath against a closed epiglottis, should not be used when patient is on bedrest as it is associated with increased incidence of deep vein thrombosis (see Chapter 10).
2. When about to void, instruct patient to take a deep breath, hold it, and bear down. Ask patient to strain throughout the voiding process until the bladder is empty. The patient may rest for a minute or so and repeat technique if necessary.	This enhances bladder emptying.
3. Warn patient that hyperventilation or a bowel movement may occur.	
4. Later in the rehabilitation process, snugly apply a lumbosacral corset.	When a hyperextension brace or body cast is no longer required for orthopedic stability, a lumbosacral corset may be used to produce greater intra-abdominal pressure.

- When the residuals are less than 100 mL for two days, discontinue the formal catheterization program. Perform a postvoid residual every two days for a week, then every three days for a week, then once the next week, and finally once a month for two months. Catheterization checks may be discontinued completely if the residual urine is less than 100 mL and the physician feels that adequate evacuation is being maintained.
- When adjusting the number of catheterizations, monitor the patient's tolerance and response. Again, adhere to the principles of avoiding overdistension and ensuring complete emptying of the bladder. Check for palpable bladder distension, especially during the night. This can be achieved at routine turning times without excessively disturbing the patient. It may be necessary to "tap" or manually express the patient every two hours. The urine output may double during the night when the patient resumes the supine position.
- Observe the patient with quadriplegia closely. Many are unable to tolerate three hours without voiding and may experience nausea, headache, chills, or signs of autonomic dysreflexia should voiding techniques fail. Catheterize immediately in these situations.
- Catheterization should be rescheduled taking into account patient preferences and planned therapy sessions. Night catheterizations may be omitted first to promote rest and sleep. For example if catheterizations were scheduled every four hours at 0200, 0600, 1000, 1400, 1800, and 2200 hours, schedule catheterizations every six hours at 0600, 1200, 1800, and 2300 or 2400 hours.
- To assess the degree of bladder emptying accurately, obtain postvoid residuals immediately following spontaneous voiding or expression, before the bladder starts to fill with urine again.
- Should manual techniques begin to fail and the residual urine volume increase, check the

PROCEDURE 12–5 ■ MANUAL EXPRESSION (CREDÉ MANEUVER)

Purpose

The purpose of manually expressing the bladder is to empty it as completely as possible.

Action	Rationale
1. Select patients with a flaccid bladder who will be able to safely use this technique.	This technique is most successful when patient is free from resistance imposed by preserved abdominal muscles and is free from urinary outlet obstruction (as a result of a mixed neurogenic bladder or from pre-existing disease). Avoid the use of manual expression for patients with spastic bladder because ureterovesical reflux or drainage to the urethra may occur if the external sphincter is in spasm and contracts, thus blocking urinary outflow.
2. Assess the abdomen to detect overdistension. If overdistension is suspected, perform a straight catheterization. Do not proceed with manual expression.	To avoid the risk of manual pressure forcing urine into the upper urinary tract.
3. If possible have patient sit on the toilet, lean forward, and perform this technique.	To achieve the best angle at which to apply pressure. Since a flaccid type of bladder exists with trauma to the sacral portion of the cord, patients will have good upper extremity strength and transfer potential, so independence in performing manual expression is usually achieved.
4. Ask patient to strain to void (optional).	These techniques used together may be helpful for some patients with partially preserved abdominal muscles.
5. To perform a manual expression, place one hand on top of the other or use a closed fist to apply firm pressure over the bladder. Press downward toward the pubic arch and repeat several times until the urine is passed. In the early stages avoid undue exertion of pressure on a fracture site of the lower spine. If a body cast is required, a "window" is needed in the suprapubic area to allow manual expression of the bladder.	Manual expression requires considerable strength and is a potentially dangerous technique. If the pressure exerted is too vigorous or is applied in the wrong direction, urine may be forced back up the ureters, thereby damaging the ureterovesical valves and threatening the entire upper urinary tract. This is especially true if the technique is performed while the patient is supine or if the bladder is full.

patient's drinking pattern and types of fluids taken and be alert for any signs of bladder infection. Bowel irregularity can also play havoc with bladder function and schedules.

• Observe patients carefully on return from day and weekend passes. Although early outings are most valuable, problems related to bowel and bladder care tend to increase during them.

It must be stressed that the preceding information is a *general* guideline. When assessing the program, the physician will be interested in helping the patient achieve a balanced bladder. Assessment does not depend on the actual residual volume alone, but must include consideration of the relationship of residual volume to the bladder capacity or total volume of urine stored in the bladder.

A state of balance is expressed in percentages or ratios. The goal is a minimum requirement of 5:1 ratio, 5 parts urine voided or expressed to 1 part residual. In other words the residual is 20% of the total volume of urine in the bladder. A normal bladder residual is 0 mL. For example, when a patient voids or expresses 375 mL urine, a postvoid residual of 75 mL is considered acceptable. The bladder is balanced:

$$\frac{375 \text{ mL voided/expressed}}{75 \text{ mL residual}} = \text{ratio 5:1 or 20\%}$$

However, if a patient voids or expresses 225 mL urine, a postvoid residual of 75 mL would be considered unacceptable, despite the fact that the actual volume of residual is the same in both cases. In this case, the bladder is unbalanced:

$$\frac{225 \text{ mL voided/expressed}}{75 \text{ mL residual}} = \text{ratio 3:1 or 33\%}$$

Obtaining or preparing the patient for diagnostic tests Throughout the recovery phase, any number or combination of physical examinations and diagnostic tests may be required to establish baseline or accumulate comparative data.

Preliminary examination usually includes examination of the saddle area for any preserved sensation; testing of the bulbocavernosus and anal sphincters; urinalysis and urine for culture and sensitivity; blood urea nitrogen (BUN) and serum creatinine and electrolyte levels; an intravenous pyelogram (IVP) within the first two weeks after injury; and possibly a cystometrogram. Throughout the intermittent catheterization program the patient should be monitored closely for urinary tract infection. A daily systemic temperature should be taken and weekly urinalysis specimens obtained. The pH of urine can be easily checked with reagent strips at each catheterization. A rise in pH above 6 is almost always associated with positive urinary tract infection in patients who are maintained on methenamine mandelate (Mandelamine) and ascorbic acid (Perkash 1978). Culture and sensitivity studies can be performed weekly or at any suspicion of infection.

If the patient still has high residuals after intermittent catheterizations have been maintained for two months, or at the physician's discretion, detailed urodynamic studies will be added. For those with flaccid bladder involvement Perkash (1974) recommends an IVP be re-peated in three months to detect any ureteral dilatation, which would probably indicate indiscriminate (too vigorous) use of manual expression.

Some problems to consider Attention must be directed to a number of problems that make it difficult to achieve a balanced bladder. For the patient with a spastic bladder, *detrusor-sphincter dyssynergia* represents a major obstacle to bladder retraining. This occurs when the detrusor muscle and the external urethral sphincter contract at the same time. It can occur spontaneously or when trigger voiding is attempted. The expulsion action of the detrusor muscle is blocked when it is unable to overcome the resistance of the contracted sphincter. One action counteracts the other. A combined cystometrogram (CMG) and electromyelogram (EMG) is valuable for evaluation of this condition. For some it may be possible to overcome the dyssynergia, empty the bladder completely, and maintain continence between voidings by the use of the anal sphincter stretch technique. The external anal and urethral sphincters relax when manual distension of the anal sphincter is sustained. See Procedure 12–6.

Other problems include: a weak contractile force of the detrusor muscle; incontinence secondary to irritability and hyperactivity of the detrusor muscle; and spasticity of the skeletal muscles of the external urinary sphincter and the pelvic floor. See Table 12–6 for an outline of these problems and relevant interventions. Drug therapy and surgical measures as well as other special techniques have been used to overcome these difficulties with varying degrees of success (Johnson 1980).

Medication As the reflex voiding phase develops in the patient with a spastic bladder, an unbalanced bladder with high residual urine volumes may persist. This may be manifested by a constant, dribbling incontinence or by an inability to void despite the use of manual techniques. Imperfect emptying may be caused by poorly coordinated, weak, or irritable expulsion forces (bladder detrusor muscle contractions) poorly balanced against stronger or spasmodic forces of the external urethral sphincter and muscles of the pelvic floor.

When urinary retention is due to hyper-

PROCEDURE 12–6 ■ TEACHING A PATIENT THE ANAL SPHINCTER STRETCH TECHNIQUE

Purpose

The purpose of teaching the anal sphincter stretch technique is to overcome the problem of detrusor-spincter dyssynergia. Although a staff member can perform this technique, the patient must accomplish it to provide a workable solution to this problem.

Action	Rationale
1. Collaborate with occupational therapist and possibly physical therapist to assess toilet transfer ability, balance, and hand function. Patients must demonstrate capabilities in each of these areas to be able to use this technique.	This technique is best accomplished when patient is able to perform a toilet transfer and maintain adequate balance. Adequate hand function is also needed. For this reason it is much easier for people with paraplegia, although selected quadriplegic people can manage the technique by using an adapted aid for finger insertion (Donovan et al. 1977).
2. Instruct the patient to: • Bend foward on the toilet • Place one gloved hand behind the buttocks • Gently insert one or two gloved fingers just far enough in to stretch the anal sphincter • Pull in the posterior direction or spread the fingers apart.	Warn patient that too vigorous stimulation of the rectal mucosa may result in a bowel movement and traumatize the rectum.
3. Have patient strain while voiding (optional).	Some patients find this helpful to aid in the opening of the bladder neck.
4. Have patient with high paraplegia try a corset.	Greater intra-abdominal pressure may help some patients to void.

activity of the detrusor muscle, without evidence of urinary outflow obstruction, effective bladder contractions can be produced by administering bethanechol chloride (Urecholine). This drug is a cholinergic or parasympathomimetic agent that strengthens bladder contractions and initiates voiding. Bethanechol chloride also stimulates the gastrointestinal tract, so nausea, vomiting, or abdominal cramping are possible side effects. It may be necessary to reduce the dosage or discontinue the drug. As reflex voiding becomes well established it may be discontinued altogether. Bethanechol chloride is not recommended for patients in spinal shock or with spastic bladders. It stimulates the external striated muscular sphincter and may exacerbate any previous obstruction at this level. This creates a situation in which the bladder and sphincters are hyperactive, causing such complications as ureterovesical reflux, ruptured bladder, and dysreflexia.

When incontinence is secondary to hyperactivity of the detrusor muscle, dryness can be achieved by administering propantheline bromide (Pro-Banthine). This drug blocks the effect of the parasympathetic system (an anticholinergic agent) to diminish the frequency of uninhibited bladder spasms. Possible side effects of propantheline bromide include dryness of the mouth and constipation. Although side effects are generally not severe, some patients cannot tolerate the drug. Some patients may require propantheline bromide on a long-term basis for practical management of incontinence.

Spasmodic activity of the external urinary sphincter and muscles of the pelvic floor may cause obstruction to urinary outflow. Medications such as diazepam (Valium) may be selected for their generally relaxing effect on skeletal muscles. Suppressing sphincter and pelvic floor muscle spasms decreases resistance to urinary outflow. Diazepam (Valium) is used with extreme caution because it is a central nervous system depressant and is addictive. Observe for slow mentation, drowsiness, or a dazed appearance as an indication that dosage must be reduced. Patients must be warned that alcohol augments the effect of diazepam. Diazepam has not been found to be effective against spasm of the external sphincter. Better medications include phenoxybenzamine hydrochloride and prazosin hydrochloride (Minipres). These drugs interfere with sympathetic stimulation of the external smooth muscle sphincter.

Medications have little effect on the autonomic nervous systems of patients with flaccid bladder, because the reflex arcs are not intact. If a mixed bladder is suspected, a trial course of medication may be useful. An unbalanced bladder may exist simply because successful manual expressions are delayed by immobilization measures required for orthopedic stability. Certainly the physician will attempt to achieve bladder control with medication before contemplating surgical intervention.

Surgical intervention when intermittent catheterizations are unsuccessful Surgical intervention may be contemplated when there is evidence of an obstruction in the bladder outlet system at either the bladder neck or level of the external sphincter. Vesical outlet obstruction occurs in approximately 30% of all patients with spinal injuries. Some physicians approach surgery very conservatively, avoiding intervention for a year after injury until the effects of spinal shock completely subside and a true neurogenic profile exists. Others advocate surgical intervention if intermittent catheterization (in those with a complete lesion) is prolonged over 20 weeks (Perkash 1978).

Bladder outlet obstruction is characterized by difficulty in maintaining a urinary stream, persistent high residuals, severe bouts of autonomic dysreflexia, persistent urinary tract infection, evidence of obstruction on cystometry and electromyography, and radiographic evidence of reflux.

Transurethral operations performed on male patients with spinal cord injuries include transurethral prostatic resection around the internal sphincter at the bladder neck and external sphincterotomy. Second operations are sometimes needed to increase results. Detrusor-sphincter dyssynergia is the most important reason for surgical intervention for those with spastic bladder. Transurethral resection of the bladder neck may be selected for those with flaccid bladder when straining to void or manual expressions are not successful.

Although surgical intervention is quite successful in relieving bladder outlet obstruction, it can also be associated with temporary or even permanent loss of erection ability. It may also cause total incontinence, which necessitates external catheter drainage that was not previously needed. The patient must be fully aware of the possibility of these consequences and they are often a matter of great concern to patients and care givers. Discussion with the surgeon and the sexual health counselor is appropriate.

Caring for the patient requiring an external urine-collection system

Many patients with spinal cord injuries can ultimately become catheter free. However, even though adequate spontaneous voiding can be achieved, inability to predict or control urinary flow may necessitate some method of protection against incontinence.

A patient with a spastic bladder may experience an accidental triggering of a voiding response from general physical activity, such as during transfers, or even the slight irritation from a piece of clothing. A patient with a flaccid bladder may accidentally induce voiding by increasing abdominal pressure. This can result from bending forward during the course of daily activities or even laughing. For some, constant dribbling of urine can be a problem. For others, even though an urge to void can be appreciated, the urgency may be so great that it is often impossible for them to reach appropriate facilities in time.

There are some fairly successful external

TABLE 12–6 ■ POTENTIAL PROBLEMS AND KEY INTERVENTIONS OF AN INTERMITTENT CATHETERIZATION REGIME

Classification of Dysfunction	Potential Problems	Signs and Symptoms	Intervention
Upper motor neuron (spastic) bladder profile	Urinary retention due to hypoactivity of the detrusor muscle (without evidence of outflow obstruction)	• Unbalanced bladder with persistent high volume residuals • Inability to void	Administer cholinergic (parasympathomimetic) agent, such as bethanecol chloride (Urecholine) to strengthen bladder contractions and initiate spontaneous voiding.
	Incontinence due to hyperactivity of the detrusor muscle	• Constant dribbling incontinence	Administer an anticholinergic (sympathomimetic) agent, such as propantheline bromide (Pro-Banthine) to diminish frequency of uninhibited bladder spasms.
	Obstruction of urinary outflow due to spasmodic activity of the external urinary sphincter and muscles of the pelvic floor	• Unbalanced bladder with persistent high volume residuals	Administer skeletal muscle relaxants, such as diazepam (Valium) to suppress spasms and decrease resistance to urinary outflow.
	Detrusor-sphincter dyssynergia occurring wen the detrusor muscle and external sphincter contract at the same time	• Unbalanced bladder with persistent high volume residuals • Evidence of dyssynergia on cystometrogram and electromyogram	Assist and instruct the patient to perform the anal sphincter stretch technique (to influence the external sphincter muscle to relax simultaneously). If nonresponsive, surgical intervention may be necessary.
	Severe obstruction in the bladder outlet system (at the bladder neck or level of the external sphincter) unresponsive to nonsurgical management	• Unbalanced bladder • Persistent high volume residuals • Difficulty maintaining urinary stream • Persistent urinary tract infection • Evidence of obstruction on cystometrogram and electromyogram • Radiological evidence of reflux	Transurethral operations (on the male patient) include: • Transurethral prostatic resection around the internal sphincter at the bladder neck • External sphincterotomy
Lower motor neuron (flaccid) bladder profile	Urinary retention due to loss of bladder tone	• Inability to void spontaneously • Overflow incontinence	Generally unresponsive to drug therapy. Permanent practice of intermittent catheterizations is treatment of choice. Selected patients may have success with straining to void and/or manual expression of urine. Transurethral resection of the bladder neck is possible for selected patients, if bladder outlet obstruction is a problem.

catheter (condom) drainage devices available to men. No satisfactory device has yet been developed for women, so they must currently rely on absorbent padding.

External catheter drainage device In general, in an effort to avoid bladder infections and trauma to the urethra with resultant complications, external catheter drainage systems have replaced the use of indwelling catheters in the management of male urinary incontinence.

A wide variety of condoms and drainage systems are available. However, whatever system is selected, it must be applied and cared for to ensure that:

• An unrestricted drainage system is provided.
• The penile skin is free from the effects of pressure and chemical irritation.
• A reliable, convenient, and economical system is established.

An external catheter drainage system basically consists of a condom, attached to a two-inch connector, which is inserted into a leg bag or, when the patient is in bed, a standard drainage system.

The leg bag assembly consists of latex rubber tubing, cut to the desired length, that extends from the two-inch connector to the leg bag. The leg bag can be disposable plastic or rubber. See Figure 12–6.

Most external drainage systems differ at the point where the condom is attached to the connector. The two most popular systems today seem to be the "Texas" catheter system and the disposable condom catheter with a reinforced tip.

The *Texas catheter* uses a small half-inch rigid plastic insert to secure the perforated end of the condom to a short length of latex rubber tubing to fit the connector. See Figure 12–7. As these inserts are reusable, this version is less expensive. However, the main disadvantage is the tendency of these condoms to twist at the connection site causing leakage or ballooning of the condom.

The newer disposable *condom catheter with a reinforced tip* extending into a large-diameter tubular construction that attaches directly to the connector is probably the best. See Figure 12–8. It is a more successful system, less easily twisted, and easier to assemble, but it is more expensive.

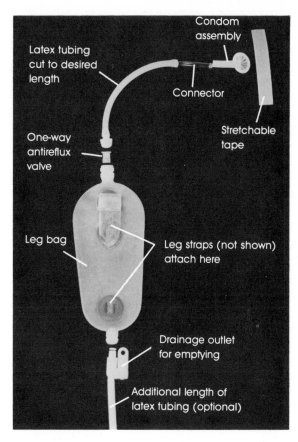

FIGURE 12–6 ■ An external catheter (condom) drainage system.

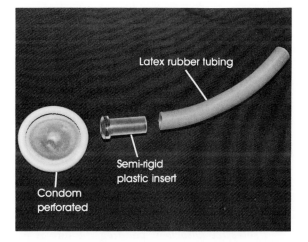

FIGURE 12–7 ■ A Texas catheter assembly, including a condom with semirigid insert attached to a short length of rubber tubing (to fit the connector).

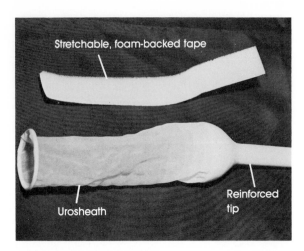

FIGURE 12–8 ■ A condom with a reinforced tip (attaches directly to the connector).

The condom can be secured by tape, or by using a type of skin adhesive, or both. Adhesives used are surgical glues, cements, or sprays, similar to those used for colostomy care.

Condoms are available in small and large sizes. Occasionally however, a patient may have a penis that is too short or retracted to make condom drainage a feasible, or even possible, method of management. The use of permanent intermittent catheterizations in conjunction with medications to achieve dryness may be considered as an alternative.

The problem of long-term exposure of the penile skin to continuous moisture, medical adhesives, and rubber chemicals predisposes the patient to skin breakdown. Good personal hygiene to ensure cleanliness and drying or airing of the genital area are imperative to avoid complications. See Procedure 12–7.

It is one skill to apply a condom; another to get it to stay on; and yet quite another to avoid complications. This seemingly simple procedure requires meticulous care, individual adaptation, and almost always some experimentation to develop a reliable system. During this time the patient needs much support, encouragement, explicit instructions, and help with problem solving.

Protective absorbent padding   There is no effective external collection device to handle the problem of incontinence in women. The idea of using some type of vulvular suction cup to provide a waterproof seal is currently being studied,

but the device exerts undue pressure when a woman is sitting up, and associated vaginitis is still very much a concern. The use of sanitary napkins or disposable toddler-size diapers secured with plastic panties seems to be the only workable alternative. (Do not unfold the diapers, just place between the legs.) However, these pads are unable to absorb much urine, and every time the patient changes position the pads seem to need adjusting. Plastic panties can be fashioned with side snap or velcro openings; these panties can be made at home or purchased. The woman with quadriplegia has the most difficulty changing pads as it is time consuming and/or requires assistance from others. Many women equate the use of absorbent padding with diapering and find it distasteful. It is important not to reinforce this idea by using the word *diaper*.

Although beset with a number of practical problems, the correct use of external padding is desirable to prevent infection of the upper urinary tract. General nursing care measures include prompt changing of wet pads with careful and frequent skin inspection and maintaining as dilute a urine as possible. Sleeping without plastic panties (just absorbent pads on a water-proof surface) helps dry the skin and prevent maceration. Daily bathing is the best way to ensure complete cleanliness and freedom from odor.

An intermittent catheterization regime with the use of medication to obtain desired retention may be an alternative. Again, quadriplegic women with limited hand function will likely not be able to self-catheterize, find it too time consuming, and/or require assistance from others. Many physicians resort to an indwelling catheter to overcome these problems. Fortunately, an indwelling catheter poses fewer complications in women than men because the female urethra is shorter and without angulation.

Caring for a patient requiring a long-term indwelling catheter

During the phase of recovery from spinal shock, it may become quickly evident that a patient needs a permanent indwelling catheter. For example, there may be preexisting bladder complications. For others, a bladder recon-

PROCEDURE 12–7 ■ APPLICATION OF AN EXTERNAL CATHETER (CONDOM) DRAINAGE SYSTEM

Purpose

The purpose of applying an external drainage system is to provide a reliable, convenient, and economical system of unrestricted urine drainage without leakage or skin problems.

Equipment

- Basin, soap and water, wash cloths, and a towel
- Skin Preparation* and/or tincture of benzoin (optional)
- Skin cement (glue)
- Stretchable tape (optional)
- Blunt-tipped scissors
- Preassembled condom drainage system (Figure 12–6) including a condom or condom assembly; 2-inch plastic connector; latex rubber tubing cut to the desired length (to reach from the condom tip to the leg bag); a leg bag with straps (or standard collection bag)

Action	Rationale
1. Wash hands	This minimizes risk of cross-contamination.
2. Thoroughly wash genital area with soap, rinse with clear water, and dry well. If necessary, retract penile foreskin to clean. Leave area open to air (about 30 min daily). Then if patient is uncircumcised, pull foreskin toward head of penis before applying condom.	This minimizes the accumulative effects of chemical irritants, bacteria, and moisture, which render the skin more susceptible to pressure and excoriation. Allowing the penile skin to dry is single most important defense against skin excoriation. Avoid using petroleum-based preparations to protect skin as they tend to interact with condom material. Powders tend to cake and be messy.
3. Apply adhesives if necessary.	When necessary to remove condom every few hours, as during an intermittent catheterization regime, taping may be quite sufficient. However, most active patients need skin adhesives and sometimes additional tape.
• Before using any adhesives on penile skin, perform a patch test on inner thigh.	To check for an allergic response to any chemicals.
• Protect pubic hair with a paper towel (simply tear a small hole in center and place over penis).	Adhesives are difficult to remove from pubic hair and add to infection potential. Clipping pubic hair around base of penis is also helpful.
• Spray Skin Preparation* on shaft of penis (optional). Allow 30 seconds to dry and become "tacky" before proceeding.	Skin Preparation dries as a plastic film to provide a waterproof seal. It peels off easily and helps protect delicate skin (especially in early stages when skin tolerance is building). It may be used by itself, or cement or glue may be applied on top. If, during a retraining period, condom will be removed frequently for intermittent catheterizations, Skin Preparation and taping may be sufficient and least irritating.
• Apply tincture of benzoin (optional) or a skin cement to penile shaft. (It may be easier for some to paint shaft near head of penis first and begin applying condom befoer putting cement over whole shaft.) Paint 1–4 in. of shaft of penis. Do not apply skin cement over reddened areas.	This is a matter of personal preference. Generally, the more coverage, the more confident patient feels about avoiding accidental removal. Skin Preparation or tincture of benzoin is not usually necessary once skin has toughened (6–12 months after injury).

(Procedure continues)

PROCEDURE 12–7 ■ APPLICATION OF AN EXTERNAL CATHETER (CONDOM) DRAINAGE SYSTEM (*continued*)

Action	Rationale
4. Before applying condom, unroll slightly to leave 3/4–1 in. free space between end of condom and tip of penis.	This prevents plastic insert or end of reinforced condom tip from causing pressure or irritation on penis. If too much space is left, condom tends to twist, blocking urine drainage. This also prevents backflow of urine inside the condom.
5. Unroll condom sheath slowly onto penis.	Unrolling slowly helps avoid trapping air bubbles under condom. Bubbles can be pressed out with finger.
6. Clip off ring at top of condom with blunt-tipped scissors.	This prevents pressure from ring on the thigh and scrotum. Use blunt-tipped scissors to avoid scraping skin.
7. Spiral 1/2 in. stretchable adhesive tape around penis (optional, avoid if possible). Do *not* stretch tape tight. Fold tape end back on itself to make a tab.	This reduces risk of condom peeling off. Spiral application of stretchable tape allows for reflex penile erection and adequate circulation. The greatest danger in using tape is applying it too tightly, which is in effect like applying a tourniquet. This constriction of penis reduces circulation and can lead to severe problems. Always use stretchable tape, never plain adhesive, silk, or paper tape. Tape tab facilitates removal.
8. Assess circulation to penis now and, most importantly, within half-hour of application. Look for penile swelling or change in color.	To fit correctly, a condom must be applied snugly enough to prevent leakage but not so tightly to impair circulation. One key point to remember is to allow for reflex erections. Often manipulation of penis required when applying the condom results in a reflex erection.
9. Select appropriate drainage system. Use a standard collection bag when patient is in bed (while in hospital); use a leg bag assembly when patient is up.	Avoid using a leg bag assembly when patient is in bed because it is difficult to achieve a gravity-assisted flow of urine. For this reason, always connect condom assembly to a standard collection bag when patient returns to bed. When at home a length of tubing draining into a variety of containers can be used as an alternative to more expensive collection bags.
10. Connect condom assembly to drainage system. • Insert connector between condom and rubber tubing leading to leg bag. • If a standard collection bag is used while patient is in bed (mostly for night drainage) ensure gravity-assisted flow of urine. Check that all connections are secure.	This prevents leakage.
11. Attach rubber tubing to leg bag; secure leg bag to inner calf with soft, pliable straps and adjustable buttons supplied. • Do not attach straps too tightly.	It should be emphasized that function of tape and/or adhesive is to provide a watertight seal; correct placement and security of leg bag keep condom from pulling off. This will create a tourniquet effect and obstruct circulation.

(Procedure continues)

PROCEDURE 12–7 ■ (continued)

Action	Rationale
• Position drainage tubing carefully. • Do not cut tubing too long or too short.	Any twisting will obstruct drainage. Tubing cut too long will aggravate twisting; cut too short it will cause pulling pressure on the condom.
12. Change condom drainage system daily, or at least every other day.	This maintains cleanliness, and helps eliminate odor and reduce accumulation of bacteria at external urinary meatus. Changing system is most convenient and best accomplished during bathing or showering.
13. Inspect skin when the condom is changed. Be alert for inflammation of glans penis, skin excoriation, ulceration, or flaking. Should this occur: • Air the area. • Do not apply adhesives directly. • Leave condom off overnight. A urinal (preferably one with flattened sides as opposed to rounded urinal) may be propped against patient to handle incontinence. If extremity spasms cause urinal to tip, absorbent padding may be used (even placed in a shower cap!). • Obtain a swab of area for culture and sensitivity if infection is suspected and apply topical antibiotic ointment as ordered.	Patient may develop contact dermatitis or allergic responses at any time. If these measures are not successful, intermittent catheterization or use of indwelling catheter may have be resumed temporarily. Constant irritation or inflammation of foreskin may necessitate circumcision for long-term management.
14. Care for reusable leg bag assembly:	Although care and cleaning or supervision of leg bag and equipment is eventually within the patient's capability, in an acute setting disposable equipment, though expensive, is more convenient. Leg bags do not stand up well to usual methods of hospital sterilization.
• Label each bag with patient's name. • Thoroughly wash with lathering antiseptic soap and rinse. A syringe or small funnel will make pouring easier. Many wards have narrow gooseneck taps that are idea for this purpose. • Check tubing and connectors every few days for mineral buildup from the urine. Soaking in a 25% acetic acid (vinegar) solution in water overnight is most effect method of removing these accumulations. If crusting is still evident, discard equipment. • Located at the top of the leg bag is a flutter valve to prevent reflux of urine into tubing. To check patency of this valve, invert bag. If fluid leaks down tubing, discard bag.	This decreases risk of cross-contamination.

* This aerosol adhesive, made by Dow Corning, is universally recommended (Nanninga and Rosen 1975, and Bransbury 1979) because it is hypoallergenic and easy to remove, which reduces trauma to the skin. Unfortunately it is relatively expensive.

ditioning program may be deemed unsuccessful after a period of time. The woman with quadriplegia may present the classic problem: incontinence between catheterizations that cannot be controlled or intermittent catheterizations that are just too cumbersome. In these cases, an indwelling catheter becomes the only practical option.

The ultimate goal of an indwelling catheter is to provide unobstructed drainage while avoiding infection and trauma to the urethra and bladder neck. Infection and trauma predispose the patient to a host of other complications. Despite the potential hazards, an indwelling catheter is the method of choice for long-term bladder management for some patients with spinal cord injuries. With diligent care, complications can be averted. See Procedure 12–8.

Other systemic factors   Provision of adequate fluid and dietary intake, activity, and compliance with medications are other key factors in avoiding problems of the urinary tract when a catheter is in place.

Fluid intake should be maintained from 2500 to 4000 mL/day. A variety of fluids and foods should be offered to maintain a balance of the effects of each. Drinks containing caffeine have a diuretic effect, large quantities of carbonated beverages are very irritating to the bladder, and excessive fruit juices tend to alkalize the urine, enhancing calculi formation, and may also cause diarrhea.

To combat urinary stasis, encourage as much activity as possible within the limits of orthopedic stability. When the patient is able, sitting should be encouraged.

SPECIFIC NURSING INTERVENTIONS FOR POTENTIAL COMPLICATIONS

Infection

Although intermittent catheterization has considerably reduced its incidence, paralysis of the bladder following spinal cord injury renders the bladder susceptible to infection as a result of gross interference with the natural defense mechanisms that normally protect it against bacteria. This predisposition to infection extends throughout the acute and late phases and may be present for the remainder of an individual's life (Pearman and England 1973).

A urinary tract infection is indicated by the following:

- A systemic illness with pyrexia
- An oral temperature of 37.5°C (99.5°F) or a rectal temperature of 38°C (about 100°F) for more than eight hours
- A white blood cell count greater than 10,000/cu mm
- Presence of one or two pathogenic organisms in the urine greater than 100,000 org/mL (More than two would be interpreted as a mixed growth due to a contaminated specimen)
- Presence of 20 or more pus cells in the urine as measured by urinalysis
- A low urinary output of concentrated, cloudy, or foul-smelling urine

Patients with neurogenic bladder dysfunction usually have some bacterial growth in the urine. The urinary bladder somehow establishes a local relationship with these bacteria and, in the absence of high residual urines or reflux, their growth is partially controlled by and is confined to the bladder. There are no systemic effects (Burke and Murray 1975). A very confusing question remains: What constitutes a bladder infection that must be treated? In other words, what degree of bacteruria is acceptable? From a review of the literature, it is difficult to compare results and identify the most successful techniques used for bladder care because the variables are so great. For example, prophylactic use of urinary antiseptics, antibiotics, and local irrigating solutions varies greatly, and the frequency and method of obtaining culture specimens to monitor infection also differ.

Goals of care
- To identify patients at risk of developing bladder infection
- To inhibit bacterial growth by preventing overdistension of the bladder

- To prevent the introduction of bacteria into the urinary tract
- To recognize the onset of bladder infection
- To control infection to preserve upper urinary tract function and avoid systemic involvement

Nursing interventions

1. Minimize the risk of overdistension. Assist patient to empty the bladder frequently and completely to remove multiplying bacteria. During the initial postinjury period, do not initiate intermittent catheterizations if the patient is diuresing. During an intermittent catheterization regime do not allow the volume of urine to exceed 500 mL at any given time; adjust fluid intake or reschedule catheterizations accordingly. Apply external suprapubic pressure toward the end of each catheterization procedure to avoid accumulation of urine in the bladder neck area. Ensure that bladder is adequately emptied when using techniques of trigger voiding, manual expression (Credé maneuver), straining to void (a Valsalva maneuver), and/or the anal stretch method by accurately measuring output voided and obtaining postvoid residual measurements immediately. Ensure that patient is taught, understands, and demonstrates competence in bladder management techniques before intensive supervision is withdrawn. If the patient has an indwelling catheter, ensure that unobstructed, gravity-assisted drainage is constantly maintained.

2. Prevent introduction of bacteria into the urethra and bladder. Follow strict aseptic technique when catheterizing and when caring for sterile drainage equipment, and ensure adequate and regular disinfection of external catheter (condom) drainage equipment. Select appropriate types and sizes of catheters to minimize urethral irritation, which predisposes the patient to infection.

3. Administer prophylactic medications as ordered. Methenamine mandelate (Mandelamine) is a urinary antiseptic, and vitamin C (ascorbic acid) is an acidifying agent that retards bacterial growth. These maintenance drugs are usually well tolerated. Prophylactic use of antibiotics is not recommended. Cautious and specific use is necessary to avoid developing resistance to a drug that may be badly needed in the long-term management ahead.

4. Observe and record the volume and nature of urinary output. Be alert for foul-smelling, clouded urine and/or a low output of concentrated urine. Unusually high residuals, frequency or increased incontinence, an increase in bladder or extremity spasms, and bypassing of urine around an indwelling catheter may also be less obvious signs of early infection.

5. Monitor weekly urinalysis specimens as a routine measure. Be sure to refrigerate the specimen if not delivered to the laboratory within the hour, because urine decomposes relatively rapidly. As an indicator of infection, be alert for alkalotic urine shown by a rise in the pH to 7.5 or 8. A rise in the pH above 6 is considered significant when a patient is maintained on methenamine mandelate (Mandelamine) and vitamin C. An increase in specific gravity above the normal range of 1.010 to 1.025 for concentrated urine and the presence of more than 20 pus cells on microscopic examination are also considered significant.

6. Monitor urine culture and sensitivity reports. For some patients, routine cultures are considered necessary every week. A urine culture should be obtained immediately for all patients at the onset of a suspected infection. Be sure to avoid contamination of the specimen when collecting. Refrigerate the urine or deliver promptly to the laboratory. The specimens are examined qualitatively for kinds of bacteria, and quantitatively for the maximum number of bacteria per mL of urine. After incubation a colony count is taken. A colony is 1000 organisms. A colony count of 10,000/mL, that is, 100,000 (10^5) organisms/mL, is generally considered a significant growth indicating a probable urinary infection. Once organisms are identified, they are tested for susceptibility or sensitivity to specific antibiotics. Common organisms causing urinary tract infections are *E. coli*, *Klebsiella*, and *Pseudomonas*. Patients with *Serratia marcescens*—a gram-negative rod, aerobic and motile—should be isolated. If more than two pathogenic organisms are present in the urine at a greater concentration than 100,000/mL, a mixed growth due to contamination is likely.

Purpose

The purpose of this procedure is to provide unobstructed drainage while avoiding trauma to the urethra and bladder neck and preventing infection. Trauma and infection predispose the patient to subsequent (often severe) complications.

Action	Rationale
1. Introduce silastic (silicone) or silicone-treated catheter. Teflon and some plastic catheters are also available.	The development of these newer catheters has introduced into long-term bladder management the principle of a smoother, nonadherent or noncling surface designed to reduce urethral irritation and discourage crystal and, therefore, calculi formation.
2. For general use select catheter no larger than a size #16 (French) for males, and no larger than size #18 (French) for females. Balloons should not be inflated beyond 8 to 10 cm.	If urine bypasses catheter, it is usually due to bladder spasm. Selection of a larger catheter or larger balloon will not solve problem. An increased incidence of spasms is an indication of irritation from a noxious focus, and there should be a thorough investigation into cause. Often leakage can be early sign of bladder infection. If infection is not apparent, physician may order medication to subdue bladder irritability.
3. Insert and secure catheter with tape as outlined in Procedure 12–1.	
• Use an antiseptic lubricant as ordered by physician.	Lower portion of urethra itself, especially in patients who are permanently catheterized, tends to harbor bacteria that may be pushed back into bladder when catheter is introduced.
• Particularly when catheterizing male patient, anticipate difficulty in passing catheter if external sphincter goes into spasm on contact with catheter. Maintain gentle pressure on catheter, and often sphincter will relax in a few minutes and allow catheter to pass.	In long-term management, bladder spasms are not uncommon.
• Replace nonallergic tape with adhesive tape to secure catheter.	Precautions should be taken when applying tape to desensitized skin, but as patient becomes more active and skin builds up tolerance, adhesive tape can be used and left in place for a week or so at a time. Surgical tie tapes work well to tie catheter assembly securely in place for males.
• Check for pressure areas, even inside a woman's labia, and alternate taping of the catheter from side to side.	This minimizes the risk of building pressure areas. Sometimes leg spasms can produce rubbing or pulling on a woman's catheter.
4. Use leg bag assembly when patient is up in a wheelchair. Insert a 2-in. connector between catheter and length of rubber tubing leading to leg bag. Swab all connections with alcohol before insertion.	The physically active patient, who is mobilized early, may greatly appreciate use of a leg bag within one to two weeks after injury. Although most nurses are thoroughly familiar with precautions necessary for indwelling catheter connected to a standard closed drainage system, leg-bag assembly requires further care to minimize risk of infection.
5. Use standard drainage system when patient is in bed.	This promotes gravity-assisted drainage, which is difficult to achieve when patient wears leg bag in bed. This minimizes risk of infection.

(Procedure continues)

Action	Rationale
6. Care for urinary collection system:	
• Maintain sterile technique when changing from standard collection system, which patient needs at night or while resting in bed, to leg bag assembly, which is used when patient is up. When system is not in use, protect tips of tubing with sterile caps. These may be soaked in alcohol at bedside. Swab end of catheter and all tubings with alcohol before connecting.	
• Discard plastic disposable systems every 24 hours, when alternating between leg bag and standard urinary collection systems.	Leg bags are available in disposable plastic or reusable rubber designs similar to those used for condom drainage. Disposable bags are recommended for hospital use, to reduce risk of cross-contamination. In most acute settings, there is no feasible method of adequately disinfecting an individual reusable system, because standard methods of sterilization will ruin the rubber. It is always important to explain these extra precautions to patients, so when it is time to prepare for home, they will be receptive to different techniques. This also minimizes risk of infection.
• If drainage system remains closed, that is, if the patient is on bedrest for a few days, do not change standard collection system unless you change catheter.	
• Clean rubber reusable leg bag assembly. Thoroughly wash with lathering soap; rinse with aid of a syringe, funnel, or gooseneck tap; soak overnight in 25% acetic acid (vinegar) solution to remove accumulations.	Reusable leg bags do not stand up well to usual methods of sterilization. Cared for in the described manner, leg bag assemblies should last about 4 months.
• Label equipment with patient's name; order two complete leg bag assemblies, and alternate use.	
7. Clean perineal area with soap, particularly external urinary meatus, and rinse with clear water twice daily. Dry thoroughly; do not use powders or lotions. Remove crusted secretions around meatus with hydrogen peroxide; apply neomycin ointment (as ordered by physician) prophylactically. If infection is suspected, obtain a swab for culture and sensitivity. Tub bathing with catheter in situ is also recommended.	Because of its close proximity to the bladder, the external urinary meatus is a significant potential source of infection. Powders, lotions, and strong soaps can become trapped in folds and irritate the skin.
8. Change catheter routinely:	
• Change rubber or latex catheters every one to two weeks.	Rubber will deteriorate in this time; rough surface may precipitate crystal formation.
• Roll catheter between fingers to check for grit, which indicates need for an immediate change.	
• Change Silastic, silicone-treated, teflon, or plastic catheters every 4 to 6 weeks.	These firmer catheters with noncling, nonadherent surfaces are designed to discourage crystal formation so routine changes can be safely delayed. Even though these new catheters are considered nonreactive with human tissue, some patients still develop contact allergy and are unable to tolerate them.
Watch for contact allergy when in use, and note any bubbling, peeling or cracking of catheter, which indicates need for an immediate change.	

7. Observe the systemic signs of urinary tract infection: pyrexia (with an elevated temperature over 38°C (100°F) for more than 8 hours); systemic illness manifested by general malaise, loss of appetite, chills, tremors, nausea, and vomiting; disturbance in voiding patterns; and additional signs of painful catheterization or dysuria in patients with preserved sensation.

8. Administer antibiotics or sulfa drugs as ordered. The physician should be notified of culture results as soon as possible to order the specific drug to which the organism is sensitive.

9. Administer antipyretics and analgesics as ordered to control symptoms.

10. Encourage a regulated fluid intake of 2000 mL for a patient on intermittent catheterizations. For a patient with an indwelling catheter at least 3000 mL is recommended.

11. Ensure adequate bladder emptying. Intermittent catheterizations are not contraindicated in the presence of infection. In fact, the physician may wish to resume a four-hour schedule during the course of the infection to minimize the risk of urinary stasis and overdistension. In patients with septicemia, it is preferable to stop intermittent catheterization and place an indwelling catheter until the episode is over.

12. Be aware of possible ascending infection to the upper urinary tract caused occasionally by reflux of urine into the ureter and kidney resulting in pylonephritis. Observe for a high, spiked fever, usually over 40°C (104°F), severe chills, with loin pain or tenderness. Clinical signs and symptoms tend to be more severe and slower to respond to drug therapy. Be alert for presence of casts, protein, or occult blood in the urine, indicating kidney infiltration or impairment; elevated BUN and serum creatinine; and, in the later stages, evidence of dilatation of the ureters or hydronephrosis on an IVP examination.

13. Watch for signs of septic shock. Bacteremia or sepsis is due to a rare complication of urinary tract or other systemic infection whereby gram-negative bacteria are released into the bloodstream and cause production of fatal endotoxins. Observe for sudden onset of signs and symptoms of respiratory distress, a decrease in level of consciousness, and other signs of central nervous system depression, such as a fall in blood pressure, pulse, and urinary output. It may be necessary to initiate advanced life-support measures. Every effort is made to locate the entry source of the bacteria and eradicate or control the cause. Treatment usually consists of massive doses of IV antibiotics and corticosteroids and blood volume replacement.

14. Evaluate the effectiveness of treatment according to level of outcome criteria reached:

- Bladder capacity so regulated as not to exceed 500 mL at any given time without evidence of retention or increased bouts of incontinence
- Clear urine of normal color and odor, free from infective organisms
- Urinary pH, specific gravity, and microscopic examination within normal limits for patient
- BUN and serum creatinine levels within normal range
- Patient comfortable without signs or symptoms of systemic illness and body temperature within normal limits for patient
- IVP clear without evidence of reflux, dilatation of upper tract, or deterioration when compared with baseline data obtained immediately after injury.

Calculi Formation

Although the formation of urinary calculi or renal stones may be considered a more long-term complication, effective prevention must begin during the acute stage. Multiple factors predispose patients to renal stone formation, including hereditary tendencies, metabolic imbalances, urinary stasis, and urinary infection. Stones form when the constituent of the stone is highly concentrated or when inorganic substances in the urine precipitate around a nidus or nucleus. This central focal point may be bacteria, urinary crystals, or a foreign body such as the balloon on an indwelling catheter.

Patients with spinal cord injuries experience hypercaluria when calcium is mobilized from the bones and concentrates in the urine as a result of paralysis and immobilization. About 90% of stones contain calcium or magnesium in combination with mineral salts and other substances. The patient is also prone to urinary stasis, mucosae inflammation of the bladder wall, and chronic infected urine. These factors place the paralyzed person at much greater risk of developing calculous uropathy, particularly when the patient has an indwelling catheter.

It should be pointed out that early mobilization, better control of infection, and intermittent catheterizations have greatly reduced the incidence of renal calculi formation.

The following is based on the work of Shields (1980) and Burke and Murray (1975).

Goals of care
- To identify the patients at risk of developing renal calculi
- To inhibit formation of calculi
- To recognize presence of calculi in the urinary tract
- To assist with appropriate treatment

Nursing interventions
1. Reduce the risk of calculi formation. Take measures to prevent or control urinary infection as previously outlined and maintain unobstructed drainage to reduce stasis of urine.

2. Maintain acidic urine by administering urinary antiseptics and ascorbic acid as ordered. A low urinary pH (around 5) discourages aggregation of calcium salts, which form best in alkaline urine. The patient may need to be taught how to check urinary pH routinely. If the pH is greater than 6 the physician should be notified and medications adjusted.

3. Maintain adequate fluid intake of 2000 mL/day, or up to 4000 mL/day if the patient has an indwelling catheter. A high fluid intake dilutes the urine, which then has a better "wash-out" effect. "Eggshell" calculi tend to form around the balloon of an indwelling catheter where the urine is most stagnant at the base of the bladder.

4. Help the patient develop and follow an acid ash diet if recommended by the physician. This is mainly a high-protein diet low in fruit. This includes meat, whole grain products, eggs, cheese, and cranberries or dried fruit (such as prunes or plums). The restriction of milk and dairy products to reduce calcium intake is not as controversial as in the past. Most physicians now recommend a normal but not excessive intake.

5. Change the indwelling catheter at regular intervals (the latex catheter every one to two weeks; the Silastic catheter every four to six weeks). Check for grit in the tubing or catheter and report findings.

6. Encourage as much activity as possible, to combat skeletal calcium loss from immobilization. This is a most important measure.

7. Recognize that stones may exist when urine bypasses an indwelling catheter or there is a general increase in spasticity or profuse sweating. Also watch for hematuria. The classic renal colic pain will not exist in a patient without sensation, but referred pain and other signs may occur depending on the level of injury.

8. Observe abnormal results of diagnostic tests. Note the presence of red or white blood cells, crystals, or casts in the urinalysis. A positive urine culture, particularly of a proteus species, can produce urea-splitting organisms that are more apt to create "infection stones." The majority of calculi are detected by X ray, either on plain abdominal films or IVP.

9. Assist the physician to maintain unobstructed urinary outflow. Small stones may pass through the catheter or irrigation may be needed and ordered specifically. Surgical intervention by transurethral crushing and removal may be required.

10. Urge routine follow-up care. Calculi have a tendency to recur, particularly in patients with indwelling catheters. This must be monitored by a physician every three to six months.

11. Evaluate effectiveness of treatment according to level of outcome criteria reached:

- Clear urine of normal color and volume, free from sediment, and without evidence of dehydration or hematuria
- Acidic urinary pH of around 5
- Urine free from infective organisms, particularly *Proteus* or urea-splitting organisms

- Continuous, unobstructed drainage from indwelling catheter without urine bypassing
- Adequate bladder emptying for those on intermittent catheterizations
- Good systemic health without chills, profuse sweating, increased spasms, or referred renal colic pain
- Patient active and complying with follow-up care

Autonomic Dysreflexia (Hyperreflexia)

Autonomic dysreflexia or hyperreflexia is most frequently precipitated by an overdistended bladder or urinary complications. It is commonly encountered during routine bladder care. Every RN, nursing assistant, and orderly should be familiar with the onset of autonomic dysreflexia. Symptoms can quickly progress to dangerous or even fatal levels, thereby creating a medical emergency. A patient is more prone to developing autonomic dysreflexia during the first year after injury, but a danger persists throughout life.

Autonomic dysreflexia is mainly characterized by a sudden, severe headache secondary to an uncontrolled elevation of blood pressure. It is caused by a variety of abnormal stimuli creating an exaggerated response of the sympathetic nervous system. Bladder-related problems that can trigger abnormal stimuli are associated with visceral distension or irritation. This condition occurs when the injury is sustained at the T_{4-6} levels or higher and control from the higher nervous system centers is impaired. To review the mechanism of autonomic dysreflexia in detail, see Chapter 10.

Goals of care
- To identify patients at risk of developing autonomic dysreflexia
- To prevent an overdistended bladder or other urinary complications from triggering an exaggerated sympathetic nervous system response
- To recognize immediately the onset of this condition and initiate measures to relieve the cause

- To gain control of the elevated blood pressure to avoid fatal complications such as cerebral hemorrhage

Nursing interventions
1. Practice measures to minimize risk of bladder overdistension. During an intermittent catheterization regime, maintain general nursing care measures to ensure that the amount of urine in the bladder at any given time does not exceed 500 to 600 mL. Caution the patient against drinking several glasses of fluid at one time. When the patient has an indwelling catheter, promote unobstructed, gravity-assisted drainage at all times.

2. Take measures to prevent urinary infection, reflux, and calculi formation that could serve as a focus for abnormal stimuli.

3. Closely observe the patient with quadriplegia or high paraplegia. The patient may experience an isolated incident of autonomic dysreflexia or develop autonomic dysreflexia signs following certain procedures. Check the history.

4. Observe the postoperative patient closely. Following any invasive diagnostic procedures or surgery involving the urinary tract, hemorrhage or clots may block a catheter and cause overdistension of the bladder.

5. Be alert for the following signs and symptoms, indicating the onset of autonomic dysreflexia:

- Headache of a pounding, severe, and sudden onset due to elevated blood pressure. Thoroughly investigate complaints of *any* headache.
- Elevated blood pressure. Compare with baseline data. A blood pressure of 140/90 may be considered high for some; others may experience obvious extremes of blood pressure, such as 300/160.
- Bradycardia (low pulse rate), which is most common, or tachycardia (high pulse rate) may be experienced by extremely high quadriplegics.
- Profuse sweating, flushed face, and blotchiness of skin above level of lesion and goose bumps.

- Nasal stuffiness or obstruction.
- Apprehension.

6. Return the patient to bed and elevate the head of the bed or hold the patient in the sitting position to lower the blood pressure. Postural hypotension is induced in the sitting position. Avoid keeping the patient in a chair as it will be more difficult to check the possible source of stimuli. During a crisis situation, care will require two or three staff members to monitor the blood pressure every few minutes and check for possible cause.

7. Remove the source of causative stimuli if possible. First, check the bladder for over-distension (the most frequent cause). If the patient is on an intermittent catheterization program, catheterize immediately regardless of how recently the last procedure was performed. If the patient has an indwelling catheter, examine the tubing for kinks, plugged connections, or a full leg bag, which cause back pressure, or anything that may obstruct the urinary flow (Taylor 1974). If the obstruction persists, immediately irrigate or change the Foley catheter. Second, check the lower bowel for the presence of stool. Bowel problems often cause onset of autonomic dysreflexia during routine evacuation measures. Gently and gradually try to remove stool manually. If symptoms persist, stop the procedure. Resume when symptoms subside.

8. Consult the physician promptly if "first aid" treatments are not successful. Although the techniques mentioned are usually effective, miscellaneous problems need to be identified and treated. For example, if profuse bleeding and clotting occur following a urological procedure, the patient will probably have to return to the operating room for surgical intervention.

9. Administer ganglionic blocking agents as ordered, monitor the patient's blood pressure, and provide psychological support.

10. Reconsider the causative factors contributing to the onset of autonomic symptoms. The physician may order a course of propantheline bromide (Pro-Banthine) should a patient experience headache, a rise in blood pressure, and diaphoresis every time voiding is

imminent. These may be described as "autonomic signs." Pro-Banthine is used to quiet the hyperactivity of bladder contractions.

11. Evaluate effectiveness of treatment according to level of outcome criteria reached:

- Blood pressure and pulse within normal limits for patient, usually 90/60 mmHg for a person with quadriplegia in the sitting position
- Patient comfortable without signs of headache, diaphoresis, flushed face, or nasal stuffiness during routine bladder management
- Bladder capacity maintained at 450 to 500 mL with adequate bladder emptying
- Continuous urinary drainage without obstruction if there is an indwelling catheter

SELF-CARE SKILLS

It is quite possible to introduce self-care skills within the first few weeks of injury. However, most patients approach such activities as physiotherapy much more enthusiastically than the mundane tasks required for bladder care. Depression, anger, and aversion—feelings that any of us might experience if we had lost bladder control—may surface quickly. Frustration levels are easily reached, because these tasks, unlike gross motor activity, create rather than relieve anxiety.

Although obstacles can be encountered with patients experiencing denial or depression, early involvement gives patients some control over their environment and reinforces the idea that they will eventually be responsible for their own care. Perhaps the greatest incentive for achieving independence with bladder care is the early opportunity of a day or weekend pass. It is important for both the patient and the nurse to realize that bladder rehabilitation usually takes weeks, even months to accomplish. The patient often becomes discouraged by continued incontinence and needs much encouragement to continue the program. Patients gain motivation as they realize that bladder care is an integral part of reaching the goal of maximum independence.

In fact, protecting upper urinary tract function evolves as the single most important factor in terms of life-preserving measures. As the patient gains strength, mobility, and independence, it is necessary to do a complete clinical assessment including interest, reliability, and physical capabilities. The nurse and the occupational therapist must then collaborate to develop a self-care program to meet individual needs. The "marriage" of skills required goes far beyond arranging convenient times to work with the patient. For example, it is far more meaningful for patients to learn how to apply condom drainage during morning care on the ward than for them to get dressed and go "down to O.T." to learn about it. Another distinct advantage of performing activities at the bedside is the facilitation of more thorough interdisciplinary communication about current progress or related problems.

Basically nursing responsibilities involve teaching patients the essential anatomy and function of the urinary tract in relation to their disability; the importance of fluid and dietary management; appropriate techniques to empty bladder; skin care; and how to prevent, recognize, and treat bladder infection and other complications. The nurse must be thoroughly familiar with application and care of all types of urinary drainage systems. Whether physical limitations allow patients to perform the task themselves or whether their responsibility is instructing others in doing so, patients will need to know this information.

The occupational therapist's responsibilities include assessing hand function and upper body strength and coordination, as well as transfer abilities, degree of balance when sitting, accessibility of toilet, and appropriateness of clothing; adapting or fabricating equipment for the patient's individual use; suggesting alternative positions; altering clothing for easier removal or exposure of the perineal area; providing resources for available supplies; and instructing patients and families when appropriate. Eventually home assessment will be necessary.

To ensure optimum bladder management, the selected self-care skills should not impose an unnecessary burden on patients or families or curtail work, school, or social life. Above all, the techniques involved must be reliable and personally acceptable to patients if they are expected to become totally responsible for carrying on successfully.

The Paraplegic Patient

Patients with paraplegia have the physical potential for independence with all aspects of bladder care and many progress very quickly. Compared with patients with quadriplegia, their physical illness is less difficult to contend with, and their preserved upper body strength and hand function improve their tolerance, balance, transfer techniques, and ability to perform procedures. However, during the first six months after injury the required orthopedic thoracolumbar appliances may hamper ability to void by restricting access to the suprapubic area and preventing bending forward on the toilet.

Self-catheterization is probably the most difficult technique to learn, but most paraplegic people are able to accomplish this. Even if catheterizations are required for only a few months during the bladder retraining period, most patients find self-catheterization convenient, especially when planning activities outside the hospital. Self-catheterization should be encouraged as soon as possible in the acute setting to promote independence and reduce the hazards of cross-contamination. See Procedure 12-9. Some physicians recommend a sterile procedure while in hospital, but most agree that a clean procedure is more practical, economical, and likely to be followed when the patient is at home.

The Quadriplegic Patient

Patients with quadriplegia vary greatly with their abilities to become independent. Most patients with quadriplegia can learn to induce voiding by using trigger techniques and can apply and empty condom drainage systems by using aids and adaptive devices. See Figure 12–9. Some quadriplegic patients can learn to catheterize themselves. Review Procedure 12–9.

The patient sustaining injury from C_1 to C_4 will be totally dependent on others for all aspects of bladder care. Patients with C_5 to T_1 lesions

PROCEDURE 12–9 ■ TEACHING SELF-CATHETERIZATION

Purpose

The purpose of teaching self-catheterization is to empty the bladder regularly and completely. The ultimate goal of an intermittent catheterization regime for many patients with spinal cord injuries is to become catheter free. For those with lower motor neuron neurogenic bladder dysfunction, lifelong practice of intermittent catheterizations is the treatment of choice.

When teaching this procedure to a patient it is vital to reinforce the following concepts:

- The importance of regular and frequent emptying to prevent overdistension of the bladder, which weakens its resistance to infection.
- The necessity of performing catheterizations on time to control bacterial growth in the bladder. Stress that the washout effect of frequently emptying the bladder to remove multiplying bacteria, rather than the sterility or cleanliness of the technique used, is the major defense against infection. Complete bladder emptying is also important to inhibit the growth of bacteria.

Part A: Female Patient

Equipment and Supplies

- Catheter: a short metal catheter with a slightly curved, nondilating tip, or a 6-in. plastic disposable catheter (preferred); a size #12 or #14 (French) catheter of red rubber or clear plastic may be used
- Sterile towel (for use in hospital only)
- Waterproof pad (if performed in bed)
- Antiseptic wipes for hand washing (while in hospital)
- Antiseptic wipes or cotton balls for cleaning perineum (while in hospital)
- Water-soluble lubricant (optional)
- Collecting device for measuring urine (during early stages); a large plastic or paper cup (500 to 1000 mL), kidney basin, or bedpan may be used
- Mirror (first few times only)
- Washcloth and towel for genital hygiene following procedure
- Covered container with antiseptic solution for storing reusable catheters (while in hospital)
- Storage bag or container (for home use)

Action	Rationale
1. Before teaching actual technique, explain principles (concepts) supporting intermittent catheterization.	
2. Help patient assemble equipment. Show most convenient arrangement by using a table beside bed or toilet. (When in hospital, cover table with a sterile towel.)	
3. Have patient assume a well-balanced, comfortable position in bed. Position patient at a 60-degree angle with knees spread apart (possibly supported with pillows) and heels placed together (frog position). Place waterproof pad under buttocks. Or have patient sit on toilet or forward in wheelchair. When on toilet (or balanced forward in wheelchair) a rigid device to spread the legs may be used if maintaining correct position is difficult due to spasms.	It is usually easier to begin teaching with patient in bed. This position improves vision of perineum and eases catheter insertion and drainage.
4. Ask patient to wash hands. When in hospital, septic wipes are recommended. At home, hand washing with mild soap and water is sufficient.	This minimizes risk of cross-infection and is convenient.

(Procedure continues)

PROCEDURE 12–9 ■ TEACHING SELF-CATHETERIZATION (*continued*)

Action	Rationale
5. Show patient how to open sterile towel, catheter package, or container and to apply lubricant to catheter tip (optional).	Use of lubricant is optional because of natural secretions in female urethra. However, until patient is proficient with self-catheterization, use lubricant to minimize risk of trauma.
6. Clean inner labia and urethral opening with downward strokes, from pubic area to anus, of an antiseptic towelette or cotton balls soaked in antiseptic solution or normal saline, if antiseptic is too irritating.	While in hospital, added precaution of cleaning perineum is preferred to reduce risk of infection. At home, antiseptic cleaning is unnecessary.
7. Instruct patient to:	
• Spread labia using her *nondominant hand.*	This leaves dominant hand free to manipulate the catheter.
• Using her third finger, locate urethral opening just below clitoris (which is easier to feel) and above vagina.	Use a mirror (for first few times) to show her anatomical structures. *Feeling* for urinary opening becomes the easier and more reliable method.
• Lift third finger off opening while keeping other fingers in place.	
• Grasp catheter 1–3 in. from tip.	The firm plastic or metal catheters are easier to direct; a soft, pliable catheter may have to be held nearer tip.
• Gently insert into urinary opening (about 2 in.) until urine flows.	
Be sure to tell woman to insert catheter in an upward motion to follow natural anatomical curve. If resistance is met, taking a few deep breaths may help overcome sphincter spasm.	
8. Remind patient to check that end of catheter is in the collection container.	A length of IV tubing can be used as an extension if needed.
9. Instruct patient to remove catheter slowly. Show patient how to press gently downward on bladder (manual expression or Credé maneuver) during removal of catheter.	This ensures complete emptying of bladder.
10. Remind patient to pinch catheter or place finger over open end before removing.	This avoids wetting clothes or bedding from urine left inside catheter.
11. Encourage patient to wipe herself well with a damp washcloth and dry perineal area.	This will remove any irritating solutions, lubricant, or urine that might make the skin more susceptible to the effects of pressure and excoriation.
12. Teach patient to measure and record urinary output on a bladder retraining flow chart.	Recording progress is essential during early stages of intermittent catheterization program. It is also wise to monitor urinary output for a few weeks after discharge. Measurement of residual urine is a valuable diagnostic aid throughout life for patient with a neurogenic bladder dysfunction.

(*Procedure continues*)

PROCEDURE 12–9 ■ (*continued*)

Action	Rationale
13. Teach patient how to care for equipment:	
• If the catheter is a reusable metal one patient should run tap water through it and store it in a covered container in a mild antiseptic solution, while in hospital. Solution should be changed twice weekly, at which time metal catheter could be sterilized as an added precaution. At home, a reusable catheter can be stored in containers such as a paper towel, a plastic toothbrush case, a cosmetic bag, or a ziplock plastic bag. No solution is necessary. The home care of standard red rubber catheters is discussed in Part B.	
• Disposable catheters should be discarded after each use.	

Part B: Male Patient

Goals

The methods and goals of self-catheterization for male patients are similar to those for female patients.

Equipment

- Catheter: a soft, pliable size #12 or #14 (French) catheter, of red rubber or clear plastic; feeding tubes may be used for children
- Sterile towel or waterproof pads for lap (for use in hospital only)
- Antiseptic wipes for hand washing (while in hospital)
- Antiseptic solution for cleaning penis (while in hospital)
- Water-soluble lubricant
- Collecting and measuring device (during early stages)
- Washcloth and towel for genital hygiene following procedure
- Storage bag or container (for home use)

Action	Rationale
1. Help patient assemble and arrange equipment. A urinal can be hooked in a variety of places for convenient collection and measurement.	
2. Have patient assume a comfortable, well-balanced sitting position in bed or wheelchair or on toilet.	During early stages a person with paraplegia is able to assist a staff member with sterile intermittent catheterization program as soon as he is able to sit at a 45-degree angle in bed. At first patient may assist nurse with steps involved in sterile procedure. Then as mobility and strength increase and transferring to toilet is possible, procedure can be modified.
3. Remind patient to use manual techniques to induce voiding before catheterizing.	Patient with an upper motor neuron bladder dysfunction may successfully use trigger voiding, manual expression, straining to void, or anal stretch technique. Those with lower motor neuron dysfunctions may plan on lifelong use of intermittent catheterizations.

(Procedure continues)

PROCEDURE 12–9 ■ TEACHING SELF-CATHETERIZATION (*continued*)

Action	Rationale
4. Ask patient to wash hands well with an antiseptic soap. Penis may also be cleaned with an antiseptic solution or washed with soap and water. If patient is uncircumcised, instruct him to pull back foreskin before cleaning. A sterile towel or disposable pad may be placed over the lap. At home, good personal hygiene is essential to prevent gross contamination. Washing hands and penis with a mild soap and water is usually sufficient.	This reduces risk of cross-contamination and hospital-induced infection.
5. Show patient how to open the catheter package (almost completely) and generously lubricate the tip and almost entire length of catheter with water-soluble jelly.	Unlike female urethra, male urethra lacks natural secretions. Lots of lubricant is needed to minimize risk of trauma to long urethra.
6. Instruct patient:	
• To hold penis, with nondominant hand, in an upward position (at a 60-degree angle to thighs) and apply a slight stretch.	It is easier to manipulate catheter with dominant hand.
• To grasp catheter firmly about 3 in. from tip and slowly and gently insert it about 6 in. until urine flows.	
• To maintain a continuous gentle pressure on catheter; taking a few deep breaths or slightly twisting the catheter will help overcome resistance.	Slight resistances are normally encountered at internal and external urethral sphincters. With upper motor neuron dysfunction stronger resistance from sphincter spasms is common. Stop and wait for spasm to pass.
• Never use force to overcome a major resistance.	
7. Remind patient to direct catheter end toward collection container.	
8. Instruct patient to remove catheter slowly. Show him how to press gently downward on bladder (manual expression or Credé maneuver) during removal of catheter.	This ensures complete emptying of bladder.
9. Encourage patient to clean and dry genital area thoroughly.	This will remove any irritating solutions, lubricant, or urine that might render skin more susceptible to effects of pressure and excoriation.
10. Teach patient to measure and record urinary output on a bladder retraining flow chart. Be sure to include any output obtained from manual techniques to induce voiding.	Recording progress is essential during early stages of an intermittent catheterization program. It is also wise to monitor urinary output for a few weeks after discharge. Measurement of residual urine is a valuable diagnostic aid throughout life for patient with a neurogenic bladder dysfunction.
11. Teach patient how to care for equipment:	
• While in hospital, a fresh sterile catheter should be used each time.	

(*Procedure continues*)

PROCEDURE 12–9 ■ (continued)

Action	Rationale
• For home use, a variety of carrying containers (similar to those used by women) can be used for catheter storage. Following each use, run tap water through catheter. Red rubber catheters can be boiled (for 10 minutes) once weekly to sterilize. Sterile catheters can be stored in the refrigerator in individual ziplock bags along with lubricant for convenient future use.	Risk of cross-contamination is considerably less at home. Storage in refrigerator helps retard bacterial growth.
Warn the patient to discard a rubber catheter when it becomes brittle or is deteriorating.	This procedure will keep catheters soft, pliable, and free of debris. With care, a dozen catheters will last about a year. Disposable catheter sets designed specifically for intermittent catheterization, although more expensive, are an attractive alternative.

may become independent with adaptive aids for condom application, leg bag assembly and emptying, and trigger methods to induce voiding. Selected patients with injury to the lower cervical region (C_6–T_1) may use adaptive aids to self-catheterize and to perform an anal-stretch technique if detrusor-sphincter dyssynergia is a problem.

For the patient with low quadriplegia (C_5–T_1) the greatest loss of muscle power is in the hand with varied limited movements of the shoulder, elbow, and wrist depending on the level of injury. Those with adequate hand control may not require adaptive aids. Some may use natural tenodesis or pressure of the palms together; others may need orthoses (specifically the flexor-hinge splint) to create a pincer grasp. Generally when the flexor-hinge splint is needed to achieve some of these skills it meets with better success and patient acceptance later in the rehabilitation period. See Chapter 16 for discussion of splinting.

The natural progression of skills to be learned is generally as follows:

• *Trigger voiding* can be achieved by the use of the ulnar side of the hand for tapping. Tell the patient where the most effective spots are. Tapping is easiest when sitting at 45 degrees in bed or up in the wheelchair. It is difficult to move arms against gravity while lying in bed.

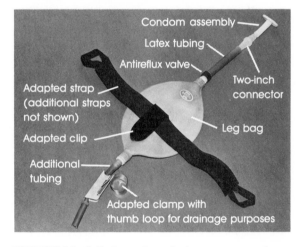

FIGURE 12–9 ■ A condom drainage system adapted for independent use.

• If the patient has adequate hand control, *condom application* can be attempted next. (The skills required to manage and empty the leg bag may be easier but balance and ability to resume an upright position is also necessary and this is most difficult in the early stages.) A plastic mirror, adapted glue and spray cans, and a groin shield are necessary equipment. Different ways of using hand control is also possible. See Figure 12–10.
• *Leg bag assembly and emptying* is possible with the aid of adapted straps and clips. The leg bag

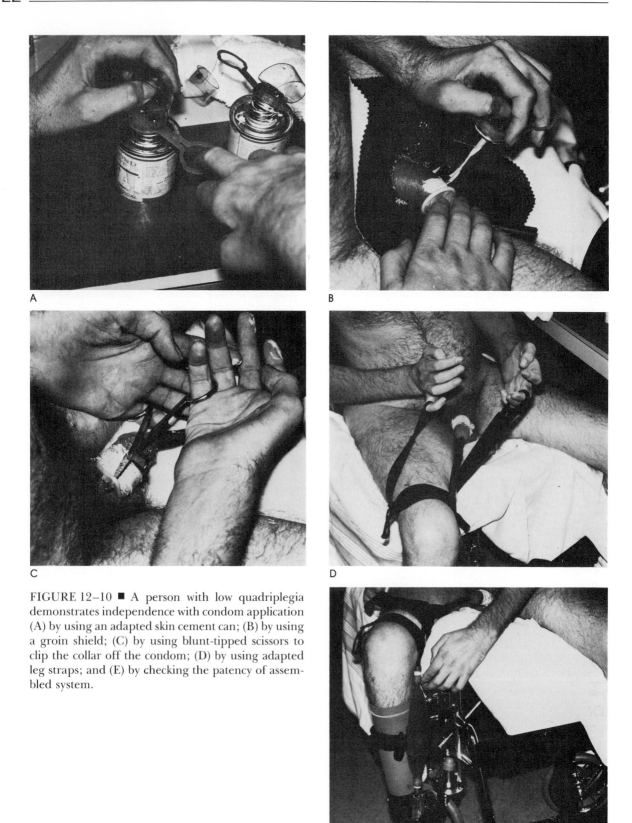

FIGURE 12–10 ■ A person with low quadriplegia demonstrates independence with condom application (A) by using an adapted skin cement can; (B) by using a groin shield; (C) by using blunt-tipped scissors to clip the collar off the condom; (D) by using adapted leg straps; and (E) by checking the patency of assembled system.

may be emptied into the toilet or into a urinal or other container.

- Intermittent *self-catheterization* is possible for selected patients with injury at the C_6 to T_1 cord segments. The sterile insertion procedure required for an indwelling catheter is not possible, but a sterile procedure for irrigation is. This is a most complex task requiring much time, patience, and individualized adaptation during the final stages of rehabilitation.
- The method to follow when teaching a patient to use the *anal stretch technique* to overcome detrusor-sphincter dyssynergia has been described previously. Patients with C_{6-7} quadriplegia, who are able to transfer to the toilet and maintain adequate balance, may use an adaptive aid made for finger insertion to provide adequate stretch.
- Adaptations and aids for the toilet are described in Chapter 13.

It is possible for a person with paraplegia to achieve independence in a three-month period; a person with quadriplegia in a six-month period. When patients are discharged to the home setting they must be fully aware of their individualized bladder program, from fluid requirements to care of equipment in the home and from prevention of complications to recognition and initiation of early treatment. Some excellent and creative literature for patient and family education is described in the reference material at the end of this chapter. When discharged, however, the patient must have a *resource person* to contact. This may be the urologist, the public health nurse, the family practitioner, or a rehabilitative outpatient service. If the patient has doubts or difficulties, a simple telephone call may solve both large and small problems.

LONG-TERM IMPLICATIONS

Precise bladder care is essential throughout a patient's lifetime to preserve the delicate and precious function of the upper urinary tract. Urinary tract complications are still the major cause of mortality in patients with spinal cord injuries (Pearman and England 1973).

Alternate Methods of Bladder Management

When conservative measures fail and the urinary system is threatened, there are a number of surgical interventions/urinary diversions and electrical methods of stimulating the bladder to empty.

Surgical interventions/diversions

Suprapubic cystostomy The suprapubic cystostomy is a direct opening made into the bladder through the abdomen to allow passage of a catheter. A standard Foley catheter may be used for continuous drainage or a cystocatheter with a three-way stopcock may be used for intermittent emptying.

A suprapubic cystostomy is selected in some rehabilitation centers as an alternative to intermittent urethral catheterization when labor and financial resources are limited. With meticulous care it is possible to prevent infection, and the use of fine-gauge, nonreactive silastic tubing decreases the chance of precipitating stone formation. Aspiration is necessary to empty the bladder satisfactorily and occasionally irrigation of the cystocatheter or advancing and retracting the tubing through the puncture site may be necessary to ensure unobstructed drainage (Donovan, Kiviat, and Clowers 1977).

An indwelling suprapubic catheter may be used as a temporary measure to bypass the urethra when strictures may urethral catheterization impossible, or during the course of treatment for ailments such as penoscrotal fistula or abscess or epididymitis. Suprapubic drainage may also be selected as a permanent measure to avoid the use of a perineal catheter in women, for example. As the suprapubic catheter introduces a route for ascending bacteria, nursing care measures are similar to those needed with a regular Foley catheter. The suprapubic catheter should be anchored to the abdomen with tape to prevent any direct trauma to the bladder or stoma.

Ileal conduit The ileal conduit (ureteroileostomy) or ileal loop diversion is an extreme measure used to divert urine from the bladder in cases of persistent or progressive hydronephrosis when conservative measures have failed (Hackler 1978–79). The ureters are implanted into the ileum (the lower third of the small intestine). The ileum is fashioned into a tubular pouch with an opening on the surface of the abdomen. A bag is attached for urine collection with a waterproof seal to the skin. Consultation with an enterostomal therapist is invaluable when providing care. At one time this was considered the safest way to avoid upper urinary tract involvement when bladder emptying was unsatisfactory. During the last decade, however, extensive follow-up indicates that even more renal damage is being caused through deterioration of the stoma and devices.

Continent vesicostomy The continent vesicostomy, or dry urinary diversion, may be a more successful alternative for some patients with a persistent unbalanced bladder. To create a continent vesicostomy a flap from the anterior bladder wall is fashioned into a tube, one end of which becomes a stoma on the external abdominal wall and the other, a valvelike structure on the inside bladder wall. This valve intussuscepts or folds back on itself from the increased intravesical pressure as the bladder fills with urine. Incontinence is prevented and a drainage pouch is not necessary. However, intermittent catheterization through the stoma is required every four to six hours. The fact that the ureterovesical junctions are left intact and the ability of the bladder to act as a reservoir is preserved allows more normal bladder defense mechanisms to exist.

A suprapubic catheter is used postoperatively to drain the bladder continuously, and a Foley catheter is maintained in the vesical stoma until the operative site is healed in about six weeks. Both catheters drain urine into a standard closed system and while in hospital the surrounding skin should be cleaned, rinsed, and covered with a light gauze dressing. Catheter irrigation may be required. When intermittent catheterization is taught, the principles stressed previously apply. A sterile procedure is recommended in hospital, while a clean procedure is acceptable for home use.

Patients with flaccid bladders are good candidates for continent vesicostomy. Lifelong practice of intermittent catheterization, however, has largely replaced the continent vesi-

costomy. Patients with spastic bladders are poor candidates for this operation, because they tend to develop severe pain or bladder spasms after creation of the bladder pouch.

Electrical stimulation

The use of electrical stimulation to control voiding is still largely in the research and experimental stages. Stimulation may be applied directly to the bladder or to the reflex voiding center in the spinal cord.

One approach activates the voiding reflex by electronic stimulation of a permanently implanted spinal electrode. The reflex arcs in the conus medullaris must be intact; that is, the patients must have a spastic bladder to be candidates for this procedure. A total laminectomy is performed to expose the dura, where the electrode is implanted, and the receiver is placed subcutaneously in the abdominal wall. Another approach involves stimulation through a receiver implanted in the bladder.

These methods of stimulation enable the patient to void at will, thus enhancing independence. However, numerous problems—including the need for surgery, postoperative complications, the risk of infection, pain, and the necessity of a cumbersome apparatus—make electrical stimulation neither feasible nor practical for all patients (Ince, Brucker, and Alba 1977). Some further research is being done using noninvasive electrical stimulation to the abdomen or inner thigh, coupled with classical conditioning of psychological responses.

Follow-Up Medical Services

Follow-up medical services go hand in hand with good bladder care. It is universally recommended that patients with spinal cord injuries have an intravenous pyelogram and kidney function studies annually. During the first two years after injury the urologist may wish to do these tests every six months. Serious upper urinary tract involvement may occur, especially when the patient is catheter free, even if the patient is completely asymptomatic (Nanninga and Rosen 1975). The physician may wish to see urinalysis and culture specimens and residual volumes every few months.

The most common urinary tract complication is infection, and the most important defense against the spread of infection to the upper urinary tract is an intact ureterovesical valve, the one-way valve located at the point where the ureters enter the bladder, to prevent reflux of urine up the ureter into the kidney. Damage to this valve is caused by overdistending the bladder as a result of increased intravesical pressure from high residuals, infrequent emptying of the bladder, or obstruction to urinary outflow. Unchecked, infection can progress from *ureteritis* to dilatation of the ureters (*hydroureter*) and can eventually ascend to the kidney and cause *pyelonephritis* and *hydronephrosis*.

When assessing a patient who has had neurogenic bladder dysfunction for some time, always be alert for signs of infection. Anticipate a chronic low-grade bacteriuria. The patient should be free from "significant" infection. In other words, a urine culture should not show more than two organisms in concentration of 100,000 organisms/mL. There should be no systemic signs of illness. Also watch for calculi formation and upper urinary tract involvement. Collect baseline data for assessment as described at the beginning of this chapter.

One of the major obstacles encountered during follow-up care is the time and inconvenience involved for the patient and family. This is especially true for those living some distance from major centers. Some Regional Spinal Cord Injury Centers coordinate medical services with local resources. Tests can be done in the home or by the local physician or hospital, and information can be relayed to special centers for interpretation. Other centers are developing outreach programs using mobile interdisciplinary teams to provide specialized services to those in rural areas. However achieved, follow-up care is vital to the patient's well-being.

SELECTED REFERENCES

Breen, S.; Clements, G.; and Mellalieu, C. 1981. Incidence of urinary tract infection in conventional intermittent catheterization technique as compared to touchless catheter technique in a patient population with neurogenic bladder dysfunction. Unpublished study. Shaughnessy Hospital, Vancouver, BC. *Includes parameters to define bladder infection.*

Burke, D., and Murray, D. 1975. *Handbook of Spinal Cord Medicine.* London and Basingstoke: Macmillan Press, pp. 38–53. *Concise overview of neurogenic bladder dysfunction, bladder training, and potential complications. Excellent introductory resource.*

Chusid, J. 1979. *Correlative Neuroanatomy and Functional Neurology.* Los Altos, Calif: Lange Medical Publications, Chapter 20. *Helpful illustrated section on the diagnosis and pathophysiology of neurogenic bladder dysfunction.*

Donovan, W.; Clowers, D.; Kiviat, M.; and Macri, D. 1977. Anal sphincter stretch: a technique to overcome detrusor-sphincter dyssynergia. *Archives of Physical Medicine and Rehabilitation* 58 (July): 320–324. *An updated review of this technique, which illustrates methods, describes criteria for selection of patients, and examines results; includes introduction of a simple finger prosthesis for independent use by selected quadriplegic patients.*

Donovan, W.; Kiviat, M.; and Clowers, D. 1977. Intermittent bladder emptying via urethral catheterization or suprapubic cystocath: a comparison study. *Archives of Physical Medicine and Rehabilitation* 58 (July): 291–296. *A study primarily undertaken to determine infection rates; includes helpful information on procedures and equipment.*

Felder, L. 1979. Neurogenic bladder dysfunction. *Journal of Neurosurgical Nursing* 11 (2): 94–104. *Comprehensive overview of all types of neurogenic bladder dysfunctions as a result of brain and spinal cord damage; includes chart to correlate classification, signs and symptoms, sensation, and principles of nursing management.*

French, R. 1980. *Guide to Diagnostic Procedures.* 5th ed. New York: McGraw-Hill, Chapter 6. *Tests for specific kidney function and related nursing care.*

Hackler, R. 1978–79. When is an ileal conduit indicated in the spinal cord injured patient? *International Journal of Paraplegia* 16:257–262. *Based on long term. Explains why ileal loop diversion is only considered when conservative bladder management has failed; includes descriptions of complications.*

Ince, L.; Brucker, B.; and Alba, A. 1977. Conditioning bladder responses in patients with spinal cord lesions. *Archives of Physical Medicine and Rehabilitation* 58 (Feb.): 59–65. *A technical article exploring psychological techniques used to condition physiological responses of the spinal cord, in this case urination.*

Johnson, J. 1980. Rehabilitative aspects of neurologic bladder dysfunction. *Nursing Clinics of North America* 15 (2): 293–307. *Comprehensive review of neurogenic bladder dysfunction emphasizing nursing assessment and intervention in conjunction with drug therapy, intermittent catheterization, and surgical measures to maintain optimal urinary function.*

Kuhn, H., et al. 1974. Intermittent catheterization as a rehabilitative nursing service. *Archives of Physical Medicine and Rehabilitation* 55 (Oct.): 439–442. *This study of a nurse delivery system describes how intermittent catheterizations were integrated with other aspects of patient care and demonstrates favorable results.*

Kunin, C. 1974. *Detection, Prevention and Management of Urinary Tract Infections.* 2d ed. Philadelphia: Lea and Febiger. *Basic theoretical and practical considerations for clinical management of the urological patient.*

Nanninga, J., and Rosen, J. 1975. Problems associated with the use of external urinary collectors in the male paraplegic. *International Journal of Paraplegia* 13: 56–61. *Cites complications of inflammation of the penis, skin breakdown, and urethral fistula with some recommendations for management.*

Pearman, J., and England, E. 1973. *The Urological Management of the Patient Following Spinal Cord Injury.* Springfield, Ill.: Charles Thomas. *Includes normal bladder function; neurogenic dysfunctions, diagnosis and treatment throughout all phases of care, and guidelines for procedures. An Australian perspective primarily.*

Perkash, I. 1974. Intermittent catheterization: the urologists' point of view. *Journal of Urology* 111: 356–360. *Discusses the successful results of intermittent catheterization in 86 patients to establish a catheter-free status; includes helpful description of methods and materials.*

———. 1978. Intermittent catheterization failure and an approach to bladder rehabilitation in spinal cord injury patients. *Archives of Physical Medicine and Rehabilitation* 59 (Jan.): 9–17. *An overview of variables and diagnostic procedures used to assess progress and determine problems in an intermittent catheterization regime; includes early indications for transurethral surgery as an adjunct to treatment.*

Shields, L. 1980. Urinary function. In *Comprehensive Rehabilitation Nursing.* N. Martin, N. Holt, and D. Hicks (Eds.). New York: McGraw-Hill, pp. 187–222. *Superb clinically relevant reference on all aspects of neurogenic bladder management. Highly recommended.*

Stark, L. 1980. BUN/creatinine—your keys to kidney function. *Nursing '80* 5: 33–38. *Explains how to interpret laboratory findings and relate information to nursing care.*

Stryker, R. 1977. *Rehabilitative Aspects of Acute and Chronic Nursing Care.* Philadelphia: W. B. Saunders, Chapter 8. *Brief section on bladder training, intermittent catheterization, and indwelling catheter care.*

Taylor, A. 1974. Autonomic dysreflexia in spinal cord injury. *Nursing Clinics of North America* 9 (4): 717–725. *Detailed but concise review of pathophysiology, signs and symptoms, nursing and medical management, and patient and family education.*

Whittington, L. 1980. Bladder retraining. *The Canadian Nurse,* June, pp. 26–29. *An overview of normal bladder functioning, and upper motor and lower motor neurogenic dysfunction from a variety of causes; includes related nursing care and a step-by-step technique focusing on regulation of intake.*

Winter, C., and Morel, A. 1977. *Nursing Care of Patients with Urologic Disease.* 4th ed. St. Louis: C. V. Mosby. *Comprehensive text, which contains helpful information on neurogenic bladder disease in Chapter 17; discusses acute stage, recovery from spinal shock, and retraining following spinal cord injury. Also contains helpful information on infectious neuropathy and neurogenic bladder disease.*

Wu, Y.; King, R.; Hamilton, B.; and Betts, H. 1980. RIC-Wu Kit: new device for an old problem. *Archives of Physical Medicine and Rehabilitation* 61 (Oct.): 455–459. *Photostory of Diamed's unique, disposable catheter kit for sterile intermittent catheterization with comments on clinical evaluation. Highly recommended.*

SUPPLEMENTAL READING

General

Beaumont, E. 1974. Product survey, urinary drainage systems. *Nursing '74* 4 (1): 52–60. *Discussion of pros and cons, nursing likes and dislikes of disposable catheter trays, special-purpose catheters, and collection and irrigation sets. (Silastic catheters not included.)*

Boyarsky, S., et al. 1979. *Care of the Patient with Neurogenic Bladder.* Boston: Little, Brown. *An outstanding handbook written by a team of experts in urology, nursing, and rehabilitation. Explains anatomy and physiology of the normal urinary tract, then deals in detail with the pathophysiology of the neurogenic bladder. Other chapters contain evaluative procedures, therapeutic and drug management, medical and surgical intervention, sexual problems, and common urologic problems.*

Feustel, D. 1976. Voiding with an autonomous neurogenic bladder: the role of the rehabilitation nurse specialist. *Association of Rehabilitation Nurses Journal,* September–October, pp. 5–7. *A practical approach to nursing management of flaccid (lower motor neuron) neurogenic bladder dysfunction. Highly recommended.*

Guttman, L. 1973. *Spinal Cord Injuries Comprehensive Management and Research.* Oxford: Blackwell Scientific Publications. *A classic, multifaceted reference text on spinal cord injuries. Includes historical background information; general statistics; legal aspects; detailed anatomy and neuropathology of cord trauma and effect on all body systems; regeneration; fractures and dislocations, gunshot injuries, and stab wounds; and neurophysiological and clinical management aspects. Extensive bibliography.*

Horsley, J. 1981. *Closed Urinary Drainage Systems.* New York: Grune & Stratton. *An excellent reference for conducting a research project. Outlines protocols and research bases. Includes useful appendices.*

Wu, Y., and Hamilton, B. 1980. Safe emptying interval and bladder graph: a new look at the bladder defense mechanism against infection. *Abstracts Digest.* Sixth Annual Scientific Meeting, American Spinal Injury Association, May 8–11, New Orleans, La.

Assessment

Guyton, A. 1976. *Textbook of Medical Physiology.* 5th ed. Philadelphia: W. B. Saunders. *Classic text detailing neuroanatomy and physiology, including that of the urinary system.*

Morel, A., and Wise, G. 1979. 2d ed. *Urologic Endoscopic Procedures.* St. Louis: C. V. Mosby. *A nurse's guide to procedures and care; includes chapters on cystoscopy, urethroscopy, and urodynamic procedures, with information on cystometry, and sphincter electromyelography.*

Netter, F. 1975. *The CIBA Collection of Medical Illustrations. Volume I: The Nervous System.* New York: CIBA Pharmaceutical Co. *Superbly illustrated reference including neurological innervation to the urinary system.*

Piotrowski, M. 1980. Functioning of the normal and neurogenic bladder—programmed instruction. *Association of Rehabilitation Nurses Journal,* March–April, pp. 13–20. *Instructional unit designed for nurses, physicians, and paraprofessionals to understand basic concepts and indications for management. Highly recommended.*

Roberts, S. 1979. Renal assessment: a nursing point of view. *Heart Lung* 8: 105–113. *Renal assessment in a critical care setting with a nursing regime described as applied to the FANCAP concept (fluids, activity, nutrition, communication, aeration, and pain).*

Intermittent Catheterization

Dailey, J., and Michael, R. 1977. Non-sterile self-intermittent catheterization for male quadriplegic patients. *American Journal of Occupational Therapy* 31 (2): 86–89. *An illustrated guide for a patient with C_{6-7} quadriplegia; assessment, procedure, and adaptive aids described.*

Donovan, W., et al. 1977. A finger device for obtaining satisfactory voiding in spinal cord-injured patients. *American Journal of Occupational Therapy* 31 (2): 107–108. *Fabricated device that enables C_7 quadriplegic patients to perform anal stretch technique to overcome detrusor-sphincter dyssinergia.*

Maynard, F., and Dionko, A. 1980. Clean intermittent catheterization in the management of the neurogenic bladder of traumatic spinal cord injured patients: a critical review. *Abstracts Digest.* Sixth Annual Scientific Meeting, American Spinal Injury Association, May 8–11, New Orleans, La. *Report on extensive follow-up, which concludes that clean technique is safe and satisfactory with the added advantages of patient acceptance and compliance. Stresses the need for careful follow-up similar to other methods for management of neurogenic bladder dysfunction.*

Sperling, K. 1978. Intermittent catheterization to obtain catheter-free bladder function in spinal cord injury. *Archives of Physical Medicine and Rehabilitation* 59 (Jan.): 4–8. *A comprehensive overview justifying the use of intermittent catheterization programs.*

Yarnell, S., and Checkles, N. 1978. Intermittent catheterization: long-term follow-up. *Archives of Physical Medicine and Rehabilitation* 59: 491–496. *Retrospective evaluation of 100 patients with spinal cord injuries, 94 of whom were discharged catheter free. Analyzes data, concurs that intermittent catheterization is the best available method, and presents suggestions for prospective studies to evaluate more effectively this concept of neurogenic bladder management.*

External Appliances

Baum, M. 1978. I want to be dry! *Nursing '78*, February, pp. 75–78. *Selection, fitting, and related nursing care for a male pediatric urinary collection device.*

Condom Drainage

Bransbury, A. 1979. Allergy to rubber condom urinals and medical adhesives in male spinal injury patients. *Contact Dermatitis* 5 (5): 317–323. *Describes several products, cites common problems; recommends ideal qualities to look for when selecting adhesives for condom application.*

Hirsh, D., et al. 1979. Do condom catheter collection systems cause urinary tract infections? *Journal of American Medical Association* 242 (4): 340–341. *A study that concludes that the use of condom drainage does not increase the risk of upper urinary tract infection if the patient is cooperative with personal care.*

Lawson, S., and Cook, J. 1977. Condom urinals. *Nursing Mirror*, December, pp. 19–21. *Practical overview of condom application techniques and precautions.*

Manual Expression

Smith, P., et al. 1972. Manual expression of the bladder following spinal cord injury. *International Journal of Paraplegia* 9: 213–218. *Provides cautionary implications for nursing practice when using manual techniques (Credé maneuver) to empty bladder; cites complication of dilatation of upper urinary tract among others.*

Urinary Infection

DeGroot, J. 1976. Catheter induced urinary tract infections: how can we prevent them? *Nursing '76* (9): 34–37. *Includes step-by-step procedure on a Foley catheterization technique, specimen collection, and security of drainage system and a section on common practical concerns.*

Donovan, W., et al. 1978. Bacteriuria during intermittent catheterization following spinal cord injury. *Archives of Physical Medicine and Rehabilitation* 59 (Aug.): 351–357. *Describes incidence and nature of bacteriuria, which implies a decrease in host resistance during the initial one to five weeks after injury and stabilization thereafter.*

Merritt, J. 1976. Urinary tract infections, causes and management, with particular reference to the patient with spinal cord injury: a review. *Archives of*

Physical Medicine and Rehabilitation 57 (Aug.): 365–373. *Reviews natural host defenses and causative organisms; examines antimicrobial sensitivities, properties, and resistance; discusses relapse versus reinfection; and emphasizes preventive measures. Highly recommended.*

Newman, E., and Price, M. 1977. Bacteriuria in patients with spinal cord lesions: its relationship to urinary drainage appliances. *Archives of Physical Medicine and Rehabilitation* 58 (Oct.): 427–430. *Examines incidence, types, and sources of bacteriuria evident in follow-up care with implications for patients and family health education.*

Patient and Family Health Education

Engstrand, J., and Stuart, B. 1979. *Patient Handbook of Self-Care Procedures.* 2d ed. Birmingham, Ala: Spain Rehabilitation Center of the University of Birmingham. *Presents numerous home care procedures, including detailed suprapubic catheter changes and bladder irrigations and the making of saline and vinegar irrigation solutions.*

Ford, J., and Duckworth, B. 1974. *Physical Management for the Quadriplegic Patient.* Philadelphia: F. A. Davis, Chapters 4 and 7. *Chapters describe toilet transfers and illustrate use of adaptive equipment for condom drainage assembly.*

Goldfinger, G., and Hanak, M., Eds. 1981. *Spinal Cord Injury, a Guide for Care.* New York Regional Spinal Cord Injury System, New York University Medical Center, pp. 13–23. *Illustrated home guide incorporating principles of bladder management with step-by-step procedures for male and female catheterization, condom application, bladder irrigation, and information on care of collection equipment.*

Hartman, M. 1978. Intermittent self-catheterization. *Nursing '78* 11:72–75. *Includes illustrated patient teaching aid.*

King, R.; Boyink, M.; and Keenan, M. 1977. *Rehabilitation Guide.* Medical Rehabilitation and Research Training Center No. 22. Chicago: Northwest University and Rehabilitation Institute of Chicago. *Section on urinary system (pp. 8–51) presents definitions; anatomical drawings and explanations; diagnostic tests including testing for pH and*

residual urine; and principles and a guide to home care procedures for an indwelling or suprapubic catheter, intermittent catheterizations, and condom drainage. Also includes problem-oriented format for care of urinary tract infection, urinary stones, infection of the testicles, hydronephrosis, and autonomic dysreflexia.*

Norris, W. C.; Noble, C. E.; and Strickland, S. B. 1981. *Spinal Injury Learning Series.* Jackson, Miss: University Press of Mississippi. *Educational program purchased on a fee-for-service basis; currently offers education on bowel, bladder, and skin care with plans to expand and continually update content.*

Virginia Spinal Cord Injury Care and Teaching Manual. 1980. Copyright The Virginia Spinal Cord Injury System, University of Virginia Center and Virginia Dept. of Rehabilitation Services, Woodrow Wilson Rehabilitation Center, Box W-279, Fisherville, Va. 22939. *Presents neurogenic bladder functioning, self-catheterization, and condom application home guide and medication checklist.*

Long-Term Implications

Barret, N. 1979. Continent vesicostomy: the dry urinary diversion. *American Journal of Nursing* 79: 462–464. *Reviews and illustrates operative procedure, preoperative and postoperative nursing care including illustrated procedure to assist in teaching self-catheterization of the stoma.*

Gault, P. 1978. How to break the kidney stone cycle. *Nursing '78* 8 (12): 24–31. *Reviews information on stone formation, signs and symptoms, and prevention in long-term care.*

Self, L. 1979. Micturition control system for paraplegics. *Association of Operating Room Nurses Journal* 29 (7): 1289–1301. *Describes electrical stimulation to control voiding by means of an electrode implanated on the spinal cord; includes preoperative assessment and preparation, implantation procedure, and postoperative and follow-up care.*

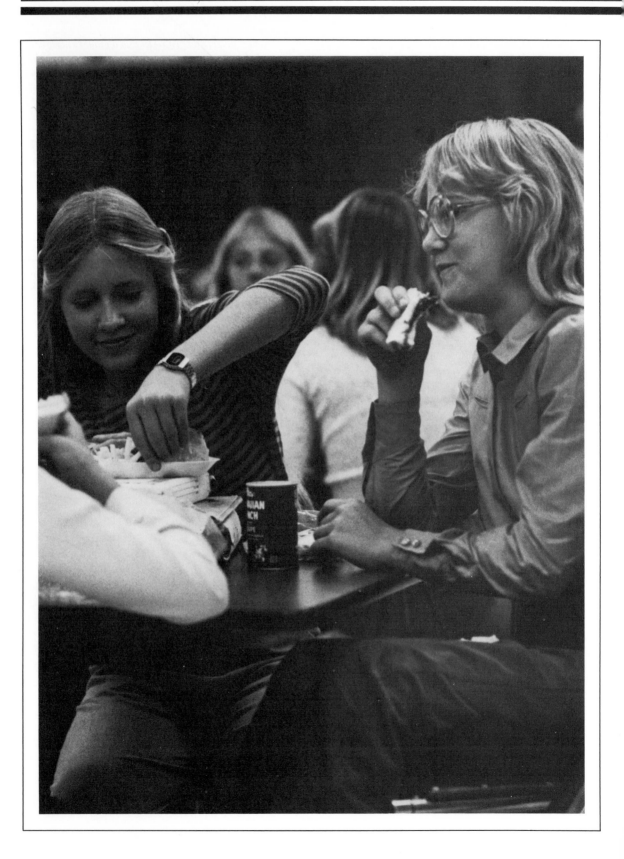

Chapter 13

Establishing Bowel Control

CHAPTER OUTLINE

OBJECTIVES

- To identify health care goals of reestablishing bowel control
- To describe bowel function and neural control
- To correlate dysfunctions of bowel control with level of injury diagnosed
- To discuss the relevance of the patient's history to postinjury bowel dysfunction
- To describe a physical examination for bowel dysfunction

- To describe the development of a bowel management program
- To discuss care of patients with spinal cord injuries suffering from constipation, diarrhea, hemorrhoids or rectal bleeding, and autonomic dysreflexia
- To discuss how to teach patient and family principles of good bowel management and self-care skills
- To describe long-term implications associated with neurogenic bowel dysfunction

GOALS OF HEALTH CARE

A good bowel management program, so often relegated to a minor role, is as important as any other aspect of care for patients with spinal cord injuries. Understanding the significance of a preinjury history of bowel habits, the current nutritional, emotional, physical and functional status, and the type of neurogenic bowel dysfunction exhibited, together with knowledge and appropriate skills to stimulate defecation, will help you in devising reliable methods to regulate bowel evacuation.

A *bowel program* is simply a fixed time to stimulate bowel evacuation to take place of the normal response, which is to defecate when the urge is felt. With complete loss of sensation and movement following spinal cord injury, voluntary expulsion and normal control over bowel activity is no longer possible. Once established, a good bowel program will regulate bowel movements; avoid "accidents"; and prevent constipation, diarrhea, and resulting complications. A bowel program sometimes takes months to establish and requires careful management to maintain. The goals of the health care team are:

- To ensure adequate elimination to preserve bowel function
- To help patients produce a softly formed stool according to an individual plan and regular pattern on a consistent bases

- To help patients avoid the embarrassment and inconvenience of involuntary evacuation
- To prevent constipation and other complications
- To teach patients and families principles of good bowel care
- To devise a reliable and convenient bowel program that patients will be able to perform or teach others how to manage
- To assist the patient with appropriate modifications of the home bathroom

ASSESSMENT OF BOWEL CONTROL

Bowel Dysfunction After Spinal Cord Injury

The large intestine

The large intestine or colon extends from the *ileocecal valve* (which connects to the small intestine) to the *anus*. See Figure 13–1. The *cecum*, a pouchlike structure located in the right lower quadrant of the abdomen, forms the beginning of the large intestine. The *appendix* is a short outgrowth attached to the cecum. The colon then basically consists of three straight portions—the ascending, transverse, and descending sections—arranged around the abdominal perimeter. The descending colon continues downward to the pelvic brim ending in an S-shaped segment called the *sigmoid colon*. The sigmoid colon leads to a short section of bowel called the *rectum,* which terminates the intestinal tract at the anus. Two sphincters control the anal canal. The *internal anal sphincter* is a thickened portion of circular muscle surrounding the canal just inside the anus. This sphincter remains tonically contracted to maintain continence. The *external anal sphincter* is the visible portion of the anus. The *levator ani* muscles also act as a sphincter of the intestine and support the rectum and pelvic floor. The unique feature of the two latter structures is the ability to contract and relax them voluntarily to control bowel evacuations.

The primary functions of the large intestine are to complete the digestive process by absorbing water and electrolytes from the undigested residue and to store fecal matter until it can be expelled. The proximal half of the large intestine is concerned mainly with absorption; the distal half with storage.

Motility in the large intestine is normally sluggish and includes mixing movements to aid in digestion and propulsive movements to push fecal matter toward the anus. Circular constrictions of each pocket of the large bowel (*haustral contractions*) cause further mechanical breakdown of contents to promote absorption. Unlike the continual peristaltic movements of the small intestine (described as bowel sounds), strong peristaltic movements, called *mass movements,* occur a few times each day and push the fecal material large distances in a few seconds. Such a mass movement frequently occurs following a meal when the filling of the stomach and duodenum increases the activity of the entire colon. This action is referred to as the *gastrocolic reflex* and is generally strongest following the first meal of the day—an important fact to remember when initiating bowel retraining. Eventually, when the rectum is distended with feces, the urge to defecate is felt. The residue from any given meal is normally eliminated in 24 to 48 hours.

Neural control of bowel function

The nerve supply to the large intestine includes an intrinsic component (located entirely within the bowel); autonomic nervous stimulation; and, similar to mechanisms involved in voiding, an element of central nervous system

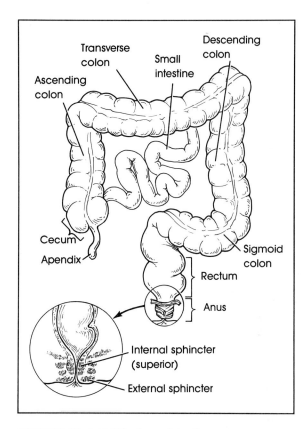

FIGURE 13–1 ■ The large intestine.

innervation to control the actual act of defecation.

Intrinsic control is achieved by networks of nerve fibers within the walls of the large bowel that respond to local stimulation. When the bowel becomes overdistended with fecal material peristalsis is stimulated. Because of this intrinsic factor, it is difficult to interrupt nervous stimulation, so bowel function is maintained even after severe injury to the autonomic nervous system.

The autonomic nervous system provides both parasympathetic and sympathetic stimulation to the bowel. Parasympathetic fibers emerge from the vagus nerve and sacral (S_{2-4}) outflow to terminate in the colon, rectum, and internal and external anal sphincters. Sympathetic fibers emerge from the lower thoracolumbar (T_6–L_3) outflow to innervate the same areas. The parasympathetic influence is more important to daily regularity. Parasympathetic stimulation increases motility and peristalsis, maintains tone, stimulates secretions, and

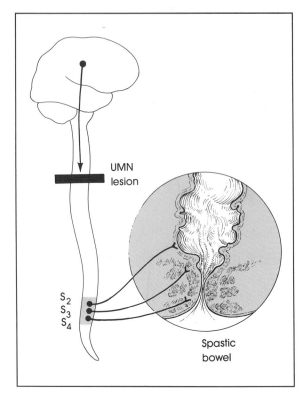

FIGURE 13–2 ■ The thoracic and sacral cord segments innervate the abdominal musculature and the rectal sphincters.

usually relaxes sphincter activity; sympathetic stimulation provides antagonistic control to decrease motility, slow peristalsis, inhibit secretions, and generally contract sphincters (Chusid 1979).

Defecation is controlled by communications from the brain, via the sacral spinal cord (S_{3-4}), to the external anal sphincter. When the urge to defecate is felt, and if it is convenient to do so, voluntary relaxation of the external anal sphincter allows stool to be passed. If it is inappropriate to defecate, however, the external anal sphincter is kept tonically contracted until the defecation reflex is suppressed and disappears for several hours. At an appropriate time the person can stimulate the defecation reflex by abdominal straining, but this is not usually as effective as a natural reflex.

Actual elimination of stool may be aided by straining the abdominal muscles. This is accom-

plished by a *Valsalva maneuver* when the person takes a deep breath and attempts to exhale against a closed glottis while at the same time tightening the abdominal muscles. This action may be described as "bearing down" and requires intact innervation to the lower thoracic cord (T_{6-12}) to stimulate these accessory muscles. The actual increase in intra-abdominal pressure forces stool into the rectum.

In summary, the complex mechanisms of defecation require the combined action of the intrinsic and spinal reflexes, aided by voluntary actions. See Figure 13–2.

Loss of bowel control after injury

The location and completeness of cord injury determines the extent to which control of defecation is altered. Basically spinal cord injury can damage either the upper motor neurons, located above the defecation reflex center in the cord, or the lower motor neurons, which destroy the defecation reflex center. In either case voluntary control is impaired or lost due to interrupted communication with the brain.

Tests that determine perineal sensation and activity may help determine the type of neurogenic bowel dysfunction following injury.

If the patient can appreciate any sensation in the *saddle area* of the perineum, it indicates that some sensory function remains at the sacral spinal level. Any ability to sense the urge to defecate will help establish bowel control. This is most valuable information for the patient with an incomplete lesion, such as a central cord injury or sacral sparing. Sensation will be absent in patients with a complete lesion.

A positive bulbocavernosus reflex indicates that the reflex activity of the sacral cord is intact. This reflex causes a palpable and visible contracture of the anal sphincter when pressure is applied to the glans penis or clitoris. The bulbocavernosus reflex is usually present very soon after injury, before spinal shock fully subsides. It indicates an upper motor neuron bowel dysfunction.

The anal reflex, or anal "wink," if present, also indicates an upper motor neuron bowel dysfunction. This reflex causes a visible contraction of the external anal sphincter in response to a pinprick.

Although techniques involved in the management of each are similar, the patient with upper motor neuron damage is a little easier to regulate. In addition, it must be stressed that neural damage alone does not dictate bowel habits; dietary intake, activity, and medication are important variables on which to capitalize when attempting to regulate bowel activity.

Upper motor neuron damage Upper motor neuron damage occurs when injury to the cord is sustained above the conus medullaris (Figure 13–3). As this sacral portion of the cord (specifically S_{2-4} segments) corresponds to the T_{12}–L_1 vertebrae, the patient sustaining a thoracic or cervical fracture will probably experience an upper motor neuron injury. This causes spastic paralysis with inability to control defecation caused by reflex activity of the bowel. Reflex activity is uninhibited because paralysis causes lack of sensation and movement. Ascending sensory signals are interrupted and the patient is unable to feel the urge to defecate; descending motor signals are interrupted blocking the normal control of external anal sphincter activity. (Fortunately, the spastic contraction of this sphincter discourages leakage of stool.)

Lower motor neuron damage Lower motor neuron damage occurs when injury is sustained directly to the sacral cord segments in the conus medullaris or the sacral nerve roots in the cauda equina. These injuries are generally associated with fractures of the lumbosacral spine below the T_{12} level. The lower motor neurons, which are responsible for the defecation reflex center, are destroyed, causing a flaccid paralysis, including total loss of anal tone. See Figure 13–4. Even though intrinsic contractile responses remain, peristaltic movements are quite ineffective without the support of the spinal reflex. Fecal retention and oozing of stool through the flaccid sphincter are associated with lower motor neuron damage. As the final pathway for sensory and motor signals is interrupted, the patient loses the ability to appreciate an urge to defecate and exercise voluntary control of the external anal sphincter. Table 13–1 summarizes the characteristics and management techniques involved with both types of neurogenic bowel dysfunction.

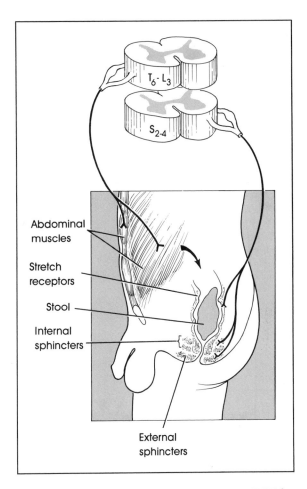

FIGURE 13–3 ■ An upper motor neuron (UMN) lesion results in spastic bowel function.

History

As the patient's general condition stabilizes, the nurse will question the patient about past elimination patterns, nutritional and fluid intake, reaction to loss of bowel control, and any associated injuries that may negatively affect reestablishment of bowel control. If the patient's bowel habits were healthful, every effort should be made to duplicate them; if not, reeducation and modifications will be needed (Cannon 1980). The bowel history is added to the general nursing history to provide information to people working with the patient and to ensure continuity when implementing the bowel program.

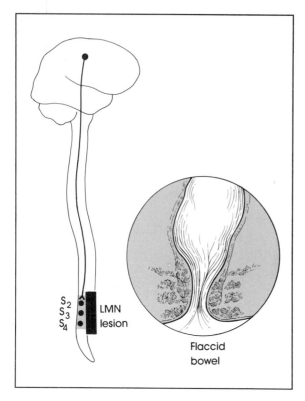

FIGURE 13–4 ■ A lower motor neuron (LMN) lesion results in flaccid bowel function.

Associated injuries

Associated abdominal injuries occasionally present problems. For example, a traumatic pancreatitis may cause early constipation and later diarrhea. If prolonged nasogastric feedings are required for any reason, diarrhea is a common problem.

Past elimination patterns

Many patients are almost unaware of elimination patterns before injury. As bowel habits are a very personal and private concern, some patients may be embarrassed to discuss them. However, explaining the value of a bowel history to establish a program that will control incontinence usually overcomes this problem.

It is important to note the *frequency* of bowel movements. The definition of *normal* has a wide range. A daily bowel movement is not necessary for everyone; elimination may occur twice a day, every second day, or even every third day.

The *consistency* of the stool is much more important than the frequency of bowel movements. Therefore the nurse should ask about the nature and amount of stool. The time of day most convenient for defecation will help determine the most suitable time for a bowel program later on. Other necessary questions include those about anything that stimulates bowel action, such as exercise, hot drinks, fruits, or spicy foods; whether the patient is prone to constipation or diarrhea; and the use of laxatives, suppositories, and even enemas on a regular basis. Older patients may have preexisting bowel problems because gastrointestinal system motility generally slows with age. Occasionally preexisting bowel disease or complications may be evident.

Nutritional history

Nutritional and fluid intake is the single most important factor in achieving bowel control. Therefore it is imperative to take a detailed history assessing nutritional adequacy, food preferences, fiber content, fluid intake, cultural implications, and excessive intake of undesirable foods such as greasy ones or those high in calories but low in food value. For further discussion of nutritional data collection, see Chapter 11.

Reaction to loss of bowel control

During the early stages the nurse must assume almost total responsibility for maintaining bowel elimination. This can be a most unpleasant and degrading experience for the patient, producing feelings of helplessness, depression, or loss of sexuality. Nurses must make every effort to be sensitive to these feelings. As the rehabilitation process unfolds, self-care is encouraged. Again, adjustment to injury may elicit feelings of anger or depression, which may interfere with learning and coping abilities, and nurses may have to resume responsibility for the bowel program temporarily. Acknowledgment of feelings and concerns will help patients resume participation, which will increase the likelihood of a successful bowel program.

TABLE 13–1 ■ CLASSIFICATIONS OF NEUROGENIC BOWEL DYSFUNCTION FOLLOWING SPINAL CORD INJURY*

Upper Motor Neuron Dysfunction (Spastic Bowel Dysfunction)	Lower Motor Neuron Dysfunction (Flaccid Bowel Dysfunction)
Level of lesion occurs above the defecation center in the sacral cord.	Level of lesion damages the sacral cord involving the defecation center.
Generally associated with fractures of the T_{12} vertebra (T_{11} cord segment) and above.	Generally associated with the lumbar and sacral spine (T_{12} cord segment and below).
Communication pathways between brain and reflex defecation center are interrupted; communication pathways between reflex defecation center and bowel are preserved (reflex activity is maintained after passing of spinal shock). Patients are unaware of sensation to defecate.	Communication pathways between reflex defecation center and bowel are interrupted (loss of reflex activity); hence, communication pathways to the brain are interrupted. Patients are unaware of sensation to defecate.
Bulbocavernosus and anal reflexes are positive.	Bulbocavernosus and anal reflexes are negative.
Spastic contraction of anal sphincter discourages leakage of stool.	Tendency toward fecal retention with oozing of stool through flaccid anal sphincter.
Evacuation may be planned for every 2 or 3 days.	Daily planned evacuation is necessary to minimize leakage of stool.
Medications and suppositories have slower than normal action but produce desired results.	Medications and suppositories tend to be less effective on a flaccid bowel.
Digital stimulation technique used to initiate a reflex bowel evacuation.	Manual removal of stool is necessary. Bearing down (a Valsalva maneuver) is helpful because patients have strong abdominal muscles and can force stool out. Digital stimulation is of no value.

* Note: An incomplete injury to the spinal cord results in varying degrees of preserved motor and/or sensory function below the level of lesion sustained. For example, the patient may be aware of sensation to defecate but have limited or no control over bowel movements.

Physical Examination

The physical examination reveals the patient's current status. During the 72 hours immediately following the injury, the abdomen, lower bowel, and rectal area will be assessed in the general physical examination to monitor neurological status and detect onset of complications such as a paralytic ileus. However, as nursing intervention to provide bowel evacuation is not usually necessary during this time, this chapter will describe only assessment meaningful to bowel management.

Assessment of the abdomen, lower bowel, and rectal area

It is helpful for the nurse to be familiar with the patient's history and physical assessment as recorded on the medical record and by communication with other team members. Awareness of previous bowel and nutritional health will help the nurse identify and evaluate potential problem areas. The physical examination should include assessment of the abdomen, assessment of the lower bowel and rectal area, examination of the stool, diagnostic findings, observation of physical activity, and functional skills. See Procedures 13–1 and 13–2.

Examination of the stool

A normal stool is softly formed and has a characteristic odor caused by the bacteria present in the large bowel to aid digestion. A normal stool is composed of 75% water and 25% solid materials, such as undigested roughage and other digestive wastes. Note any hard, dry stools that are difficult to pass or any loose, watery stools. During the first four weeks after injury, when gastric ulceration is most frequent, be alert for dark, tarry stools (melena).

Diagnostic findings

An X-ray examination of the abdominal organs shows the condition of the intestinal pathways and the extent and locale of any distension. Orally administered contrast media or a contrast enema is rarely necessary (Paeslak 1966). To determine intestinal motility, especially slowed function, radiopaque markers administered orally may be monitored as they pass through the intestinal tract (transit time).

Chemical and microscopic examination will determine the presence of occult blood or actual composition of the stool. If diarrhea is present a Gram's stain, stool culture, or stool for ova and parasites is useful to pinpoint the source of an infective process. The normal digestive flora in the bowel can be greatly reduced in patients requiring long-term administration of antibiotics.

Observation of physical activity

Early activation is a most important consideration when promoting elimination. Regular turning of patients and range of motion exercises during the early phases are just as important as general physical activity when orthopedic stability allows.

Functional skills

Since gravity assists bowel evacuation in the sitting position, some thought must be given to toileting activities as mobility and strength are regained. Sitting tolerance, trunk balance, and ability to transfer to a commode or toilet will need to be assessed. In addition, the quadriplegic patient's hand function and ability to use arms need to be assessed before introducing self-care skills such as suppository insertion or digital stimulation. This usually requires the combined efforts of the patient, the nurse, and the occupational and physical therapists.

GENERAL NURSING INTERVENTIONS

The nurse observes, on a daily basis, the effectiveness of the bowel program and collaborates with the physician to establish a reliable program for each patient. Patient cooperation is also needed to achieve this goal. A bowel program is a planned approach to avoid incontinence (Cannon 1980: 224). The objective is to produce a planned, predictable bowel movement. In other words, a fixed time pattern—the same time each day, every other day, or every third day—takes the place of normal voluntary control to avoid accidents. An individualized bowel program is based on a thorough nursing assessment and knowledge of the type of neurogenic bowel dysfunction exhibited. The patient's general state of health, altered physiology of the lower gastrointestinal tract, activity, functional skills, and ability or willingness to participate in the program are all aspects that must be taken into account.

Measures discussed in this general section describe methods to promote bowel elimination while the patient is on bedrest or during early mobilization. As the rehabilitation period progresses, the patient's participation must dramatically increase to ensure success. Consideration must also be given to the convenience and practicality of the designed program for use at home.

Assisting with Bowel Evacuation Immediately After Injury

When strong bowel sounds have returned, the patient may begin with clear fluids and progress from a light to a full diet. A minimum

PROCEDURE 13–1 ■ ASSESSMENT OF THE ABDOMEN

Purpose

The purpose of abdominal assessment is to help determine the status of the patient's gastrointestinal system, especially to detect paralytic ileus and constipation.

Action	Rationale
1. Place patient supine and remove clothing or bed covers.	
2. Auscultate entire abdomen to listen for bowel sounds.	Complete auscultation before percussing and palpating the abdomen. These latter techniques tend to activate bowel sounds and therefore give false impression.
• During the first 7 to 15 days after injury, be alert for occasional or absent bowel sounds.	Lack of bowel sounds indicates that paralytic ileus has not yet subsided. With the exception of manual removal of stool from rectum, it is dangerous to proceed with any laxatives, suppositories, or enemas if paralytic ileus is present.
• Note any hyperactive sounds in the small bowel.	These indicate impending diarrhea.
3. Inspect abdomen for distension. If distension is suspected, measure abdominal girth at level of umbilicus and obtain serial comparisons daily.	Always obtaining serial measurements at the umbilical level facilitates continuity for more accurate comparisons of serial data.
4. Be alert for abdominal signs of constipation:	With neurogenic bowel dysfunction, there is a definite tendency toward constipation.
• A dull sound on percussion of descending colon • Hardness or resistance of abdomen on palpation, especially on right side • Rigidity or hard stool felt in any bowel section • Referred pain, especially aggravated by assessment techniques • Increased leg spasms aggravated by assessment techniques	These signs are caused by accumulation of fecal material, usually in the descending colon.

fluid intake of 2000 mL/day is recommended. Oral intake is usually possible on the second or third day after injury, unless prolonged paralytic ileus or other complications have set in. As most patients will be suffering from spinal shock at this time, a flaccid bowel can be expected.

Procedure 13–3 outlines certain measures, which, if initiated early, can avert serious problems. However, due to frequent paralytic ileus, immobilization, and lack of oral intake, it is not unusual for the patient to be without a substantial bowel movement for five to seven days.

Frequent enemas are not necessary during the early stages. Enemas cause dilatation of the lower bowel; frequent dilatation overstretches the bowel musculature and causes loss of bowel tone. This is the complete opposite of the desired effect.

Administering Medications

Laxatives are greatly abused by the general public and health professionals alike, and there are many erroneous ideas concerning constipation. However, during the acute postinjury period, laxatives are essential to maintain bowel elimination for most patients.

PROCEDURE 13–2 ■ ASSESSMENT OF LOWER BOWEL AND RECTAL AREA

Purpose

The purpose of assessing the lower bowel and rectal area is to help determine the type of neurogenic bowel that exists and to detect complications.

Action	Rationale
1. Observe external anal area for any skin excoriation and also for hemorrhoidal tissue.	Development of hemorrhoids is common for people with spinal cord injuries. Causes and treatment of this complication are discussed later in this chapter.
2. Use well-lubricated gloved finger to complete internal examination. Check for presence of stool in rectum. Sometimes internal hemorrhoids can be felt.	This minimizes irritation, or even trauma, to desensitized rectal area.
3. Check if patient can appreciate any sensation in *saddle area* of the perineum; also check status of *bulbocavernosus* and *anal* reflexes.	Tests that determine perineal sensation and reflex activity help determine type of neurogenic bowel dysfunction present. Their status of reflexes has implications for nursing care. Table 13–1 summarizes types of neurogenic bowel dysfunction.

Medications helpful in establishing bowel programs include bulk-forming laxatives, stool softeners (emollient laxatives), and stimulant laxatives. (Harsh cathartics should be avoided.) There is a wide and confusing variety of laxatives but little rationale to support their use and insufficient data to compare their properties. It is difficult to recommend exact medications and effective dosages, but a few general concepts are useful:

- Carefully consider the effect of medications and their action time. The paralyzed bowel is insensitive and seems to take approximately 24 hours longer to respond than a normal bowel. Increasing the dosages at the regular suggested time interval often results in unpleasant cumulative reactions that are difficult to control. Generally, start out with the minimum recommended dosages and gradually increase until effective.
- Plan bowel evacuation to coincide with peak effectiveness of oral medications.
- Remember adequate fluid intake is essential for bulk-forming laxatives and stool softeners to work. If intake is not sufficient they will cause constipation.
- Should medications need adjusting, change

only one element of the bowel program at a time and allow sufficient time to evaluate results (at least three days).
- Some stimulant or irritant laxatives can cause harsh side effects, such as signs and symptoms of autonomic dysreflexia; others, such as osmotic agents, may cause electrolyte imbalance. Side effects of all medications may be hard to detect, especially in quadriplegic patients, who cannot feel cramps due to lack of sensation but may experience nausea and general malaise.
- Laxatives tend to lose their effectiveness when used on a long-term basis, so dietary control and good fluid intake must take their place. Sticking to regular evacuation times is most important. Generally the need for medication decreases as activity increases.

Maintaining High Fluid Intake

To keep the formation of stool soft requires a daily intake of 2000 to 3000 mL. This intake must be regulated according to the requirements of the bladder program. When stool softeners or bulk-producing laxatives are used, a high fluid intake is mandatory to prevent constipation. Stools will become elastic if these laxative dos-

PROCEDURE 13–3 ■ ASSISTING WITH BOWEL EVACUATION IMMEDIATELY AFTER INJURY

Purpose

The purpose of this technique is to eliminate fecal material from the bowel and prevent constipation.

Action	Rationale
1. Position patient on right side if possible. If Stoke-Eggerton bed is in use, place bed flat and manually logroll patient. Alternate positions are: • Supine with knees flexed and supported with pillows • Prone, if patient is on a turning frame	This position is preferable to provide gravity-assisted evacuation. Although bowel evacuation is possible in supine position on a turning frame, prone position allows better access to rectal area and therefore minimizes risk of inadvertent trauma to desensitized area.
2. Protect bed linen with soft waterproofed pads. *Never use bedpan.*	This avoids any possible pressure or trauma to skin.
3. Insert a well-lubricated gloved finger into rectum. Gently and slowly remove fecal material.	Generous lubrication minimizes risk of trauma for patient without rectal sensation.
4. Note amount and *consistency* of stool.	
5. If stool is not too hard (and it usually isn't within a few days of injury), administer a small-volume commercially prepared enema, with aid of an ordinary, well-lubricated rectal tube attached to nozzle.	Placement of enema must be high in bowel, as lack of sphincter tone makes it impossible for patient to "hold" fluid. This method is usually effective.
6. If stool is dry and hardened, or if impaction higher in the bowel is suspected, administer an oil retention enema.	When stool is softened and dislodged, it can be more easily removed from rectum.
7. Give oral laxatives as needed. Start with mild stimulant laxative on third or fourth evening after injury.	This controls stool consistency and stimulates peristalsis.

ages are too high or, more commonly, if fluid intake is too low.

Encouraging Intake of High-Fiber Foods

Dietary fiber is a complex carbohydrate that is not completely broken down by the digestive process. Fiber not only adds bulk to the stool but also promotes normal peristalsis. Table 13–2 contains a recommended high-fiber diet.

Fiber aids in stool formation by absorbing many times its own weight in water. This makes a larger and softer stool that is more easily passed and thus helps prevent constipation. In North America many foods are prepared with refined flour and sugar, which are low in fiber. A diet restricted in fiber will result in formation of very firm, often dehydrated stools that are difficult for the bowel to pass. Natural elimination is also assisted by a high intake of dietary fiber because it stimulates the muscle lining of the colon to move stools along.

The chief sources of fiber are the *bran* of whole grain breads and cereals and the *cellulose* of fresh raw fruits and vegetables with skins and seeds. Nuts are another good source.

To avoid cramping or discomfort, natural laxative foods must be introduced *gradually*. It is wise to start with cereal or cereal products and then increase the amounts of cooked fruits and vegetables before introducing raw ones. Un-

TABLE 13-2 ■ SHAUGHNESSY HOSPITAL HIGH-FIBER DIET

Patient's Name:	Dietitian:
Date:	Phone:

General Instructions

1. This diet is based on Canada's Daily Food Guide.
2. At least three regular meals each day are important to establish good bowel habits and to prevent constipation.
3. Whole grain cereals and breads must be used in place of refined cereals and breads.
4. Fruits and vegetables, cooked or raw, must be used in liberal amounts. Prunes, figs, and flax contain substances that are natural laxatives, and their use is recommended.
5. Normal amounts of liquids must be consumed each day (approximately 6 to 8 cups).
6. Excess use of concentrated sweets must be avoided.
7. Milk and milk products should be consumed as recommended by the Daily Food Guide.

Foods to Emphasize

1. All unrefined foods.

   Breads—whole grain breads, e.g., 100% whole wheat bread and bran muffins.

   Cereals—coarse whole grain and bran cereals, e.g., granola and all bran.

   Cookies—made from coarse whole grain flours and/or fruit and nut filled, e.g., graham wafers, digestives, or oatmeal.

   Fruit—preferably raw and dried fruits. The skins of apples, peaches, and pears should be eaten.

   Nuts and seeds.

   Soups—preferably made with fresh coarse vegetables and whole grains, e.g., barley, corn, dried peas, brown rice.

   Vegetables—preferably raw and green, leafy, e.g., carrot sticks, all salad greens, and tomatoes; potato with skin.

2. Fats such as butter, cream, gravies, margarine, oils, salad dressings, and sauces should be included with each meal.

Foods to Restrict

1. All highly refined foods.

   Breads—white bread, refined melba toast.

   Cereals—cream of wheat, puffed rice.

   Cookies—arrowroots, social teas, plain sugar.

   Sweets—candies, rich desserts, honey, jam, jellies, and syrups.

2. Excessive amounts of fried foods.

3. Excessive use of seasonings and spices.

Suggested Meal Pattern

Refer to the lists of Foods to Emphasize and Foods to Restrict so that you can vary your menu daily.

Breakfast	Lunch	Supper
Fruit	Egg, cheese,* meat, or meat alternate	Egg, cheese,* meat or meat alternate
Whole grain cereal and/or bread	Whole grain bread and/or potato	Whole grain bread and/or potato
Fat	Fat	Fat
If desired, egg, cheese, meat, or meat alternative	Vegetable	Vegetable
Milk	Fruit	Fruit
Beverage	Milk	Milk
	Beverage	Beverage

(Table continues)

TABLE 13–2 ■ (continued)

Between-meal nourishment, if desired, may be selected from any of the foods listed under Foods to Emphasize.

Your friends and family want to bring some food for you? Please ask them to select among the items below. These foods are nutritious and also contribute to increasing your fiber intake.

1. Fresh fruits: apples, peaches, pears, bananas, oranges, plums.

2. Nuts and seeds: dried fruits such as prunes, raisins, dates, and apricots; trail mix (mixture of dried fruits and nuts).

3. Granola bars.

4. Date square; banana/carrot/nut/dried fruit loaves; peanut butter and oatmeal cookies; fruit crisps; cinnamon rolls made with whole wheat flour; bran muffin; muffins made with dried fruits or nuts or whole wheat flour.

* An additional iron source must be chosen when cheese is substituted for egg, meat, or meat alternate.

Source: Shaughnessy Hospital, Vancouver, B.C.

processed bran may also be added. Generally, one to two ounces daily will be sufficient for an adult. Bran can be sprinkled on cereals, taken in yogurt, used in baking, or added to casseroles and sauces. Prune juice and orange juice are well-known natural laxatives. One or two tablespoons of a fruit laxative (a mixture of one-third each dates, prunes, and figs, blended with a little water) may also be given.

Eating at regular times and incorporating many high-fiber foods in the diet will help the patient attain the goal of more predictable, natural bowel training. Dietary measures to control stool consistency, maintain bowel tone, and prevent constipation are of great value to maintain a healthful, long-term bowel management program (Meiners 1976).

Maintaining Physical Activity

Encourage as much activity as orthopedic stability will allow. Inactivity reduces food needs and slows muscular and physiological responses. When patients are on bedrest, vigorous exercises to unaffected limbs and range of motion exercises to paralyzed limbs help prevent sluggish bowel activity that leads to constipation. Encouraging patients with skills such as feeding, dressing, grooming, and pushing their own wheelchairs promotes rehabilitation activities that will improve general bowel function.

Selecting Consistent Time for Evacuation

Planning a consistent time for evacuation each day is vital to successful bowel retraining. Unless the same hour is used each time, defecation will take longer to stimulate and constipation may occur more easily.

To begin with in an acute setting, a bowel program established every other morning is usually sufficient and most convenient. To take advantage of the *gastrocolic reflex,* plan bowel stimulation 30 to 60 minutes after breakfast.

As the rehabilitation period progresses it is wise to review the timing of the bowel program to consider preinjury habits and discharge plans. While in the rehabilitation setting the patient will begin to realize how difficult it is to stick to a rigid schedule. There are times when establishing bowel control must take priority over early morning therapy class or evening recreational activities. When changing the bowel routine from a morning to an evening schedule, it will take two or three weeks to reestablish regularity.

Providing Privacy

Privacy is an important issue in developing a bowel regulation plan. Bowel procedures are distasteful to most patients and heighten feelings of asexuality, regression, and helplessness. Patients are most aware of the sounds and odors created when they are on bedrest and others are around in the room. To minimize the patient's embarrassment:

- Place a few drops of a strong liquid deodorizer on a paper towel at the bedside.
- Turn the radio up.
- Drape the patient fully.
- Pin the curtains closed to avoid interruptions.
- Avoid having a staff member of the opposite sex assist with bowel procedures.

Family members may also be a source of embarrassment for the patient. Many patients cannot accept having a family member, particularly a spouse, learn about such procedures. This should not be pushed for the sake of gaining independence in the home. Alternate arrangements should be made for care if the patient will not be able to manage independently.

It is hard to believe that some nurses insist on "getting the bowel record straight" during visiting hours and are insensitive to this invasion of the patient's privacy. At a summer camp for disabled adults, to be aware of the bowel functions of the "camper" population, the nurse posted a sign in the corridor asking the counselors to check on and record the campers' "performance." During the night the list was replaced with graphic details of the counselors' bowel habits—the nurse's at the top of the list! Message received.

Positioning the Patient

Methods to position patients in bed are described in Chapter 14. In general, having the patient positioned on the left side promotes absorption of suppositories or enemas by using gravity to assist the anatomical structure of the sigmoid colon; conversely, positioning the patient on the right side aids in evacuation of stool.

The sitting position takes the most advantage of gravity assistance in bowel evacuation and the patient who can sit on the toilet in the bathroom gains privacy. *Initiate toilet transfers* (see Figure 13–5) when spinal stability is achieved or protected adequately with braces; and balance and tolerance are adequate to allow completion

of the procedure (30 to 60 minutes). This generally means the patient can tolerate two to four hours up in the wheelchair. Bowel procedures can be exhausting, especially for the quadriplegic patient who has an initial tendency to faint with the additional stress of these procedures. Collaborate with the physiotherapist to determine transfer capabilities and with the occupational therapist to determine use of aids in the bathroom.

Care must be taken when placing the patient on the toilet. It is important not to part the buttocks, which will cause tension on the cleft of the gluteal crease. On the other hand the buttocks must not be compressed, which would inhibit evacuation (Ford and Duckworth 1974). Especially for the heavier patient, placement of a towel underneath the thighs helps the nurse transfer the patient to the toilet, because the towel makes it easier to grip and control the patient. Also be cautious on bathroom floors that may become wet, slippery, and unsafe.

A raised toilet seat improves access to the anal area for suppository insertion, digital stimulation, or manual evacuation of stool. It also makes transfers easier becaue of the compatible height with the wheelchair. Commode chairs or a shower chair that doubles as a commode chair can also be used, but generally they are not as sturdy; good arm, foot, and back supports are essential for safety and comfort. If the commode has castors, it can be wheeled over the toilet, but reliable brakes are essential. Some models have side openings that improve access to the perineal area.

To protect the patient's skin, the toilet seat must be *padded*. Padded backrests are also available. Powdering the seat will prevent the patient from "sticking." Patients must not remain sitting too long, especially patients who are thin and without sensation. Decreased circulation can cause both pressure areas and hemorrhoids.

To aid with balance, a footstool is needed because of the added height of the toilet seat. Grab bars are also useful for assisting with transfers and maintaining balance.

Be constantly aware of *safety*. Using the toilet for bowel elimination is desirable but not always practical. Tolerance must be developed. If balance is poor or spasms may cause a loss of posi-

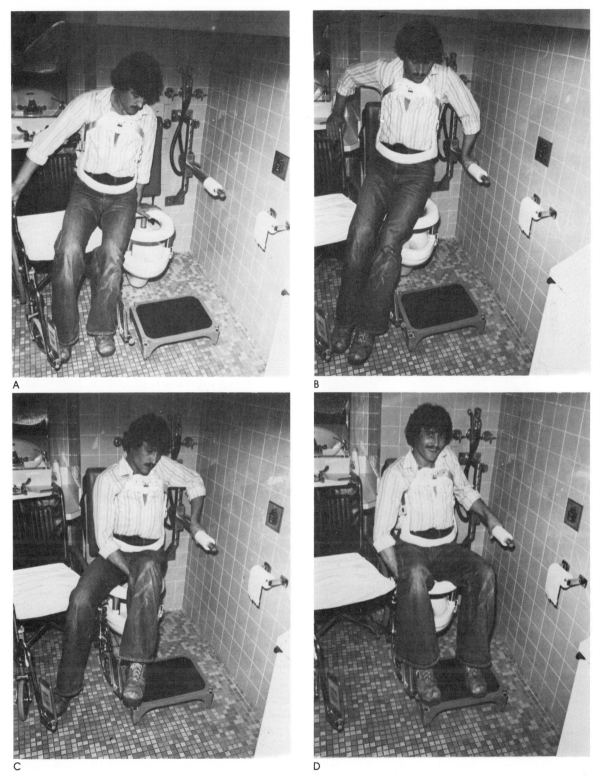

FIGURE 13–5 ■ A paraplegic patient performs a toilet transfer. Note the padded raised toilet seat, the grab bar, and footstool used as aids.

tion, additional stability can be attained by securing the patient to the backrest or commode with a safety buzzer or some other way to notify staff quickly and easily in the event that problems develop.

Other Factors that Facilitate Bowel Evacuation

Patients who have strong abdominal muscles (innervated from T_{6-12}) can "bear down" (Valsalva maneuver) to initiate defecation. Clockwise massage of the abdomen may stimulate stool evacuation. Also to increase intra-abdominal pressure, instruct patients to lean forward if their balance is sufficient and movement is not restricted by braces.

In general, use any stimulating agents, such as hot liquids, that have been helpful to the patient in the past, and avoid things that have led to constipation.

Stimulation Techniques

Although many measures, such as nutritional management and maintaining physical activity, are common to all patients with spinal cord injuries, actual stimulation techniques differ slightly. The following information is partially based on the work of Emerick (1979) and Cannon (1980).

Upper motor neuron dysfunction

To determine the passing of spinal shock, which indicates a transition from a flaccid to a more spastic bowel, carefully observe patients with fracture sites above the T_{12} vertebra for leg spasms; reflex erections, especially during catheterizations; and a positive bulbocavernosus or anal wink reflex. If these signs are present, an upper motor neuron dysfunction is indicated and the techniques given in Procedure 13–4 apply.

Lower motor neuron dysfunction

When the patient exhibits a flaccid paralysis of the extremities and/or the bulbocavernosus and anal wink reflexes are absent, a lower motor

neuron dysfunction exists. This may be temporary, as in spinal shock; or permanent, when the patient has a conus medullaris or cauda equina injury (generally associated with fractures at or below the T_{12}–L_1 vertebrae). See Procedure 13–5 for special techniques.

Recording

Accurate and comprehensive recording of bowel program results is often difficult in an acute care setting. Standard clinical records provide only a small space to check whether bowel movements have occurred, and collected data frequently become "lost" when charted in the nurse's notes. To meet this need, a clinical flow sheet may be devised or adapted, or a rehabilitation unit within the hospital may already have developed a suitable form. From the legal point of view it is unwise to add forms without appropriate consent.

Many rehabilitation centers have developed bowel program records to include information about medication, stimulation techniques, facilities used, stool consistency, and results obtained. Detailed records may be necessary only during the beginning stages of retraining or for problem solving. Asking the patient to keep the menu and record nutritional intake for a few days is often sufficient to detect causes of problems.

Evaluation

Patient involvement in continual evaluation is essential to a successful program. Education is not something that begins when discharge is a few weeks away. Ensuring the patients' understanding will help them cooperate. Keep patients well informed about their progress, any necessary adjustments to the program, and the reason for change. Explain the relationship between fluid and dietary intake and stool consistency; and between physical exercise and bowel motility. Provide information about medications and suppositories, including action time (the time between intake or insertion and bowel movement), dosage, side effects, and changes necessary.

PROCEDURE 13–4 ■ STIMULATION OF THE DEFECATION REFLEX FOR A PATIENT WITH UPPER MOTOR NEURON DYSFUNCTION (DIGITAL STIMULATION TECHNIQUE)

Purpose

The purpose of the defecation reflex includes use of suppositories and the digital stimulation technique to adequately evacuate stool from the lower bowel. Eventually it is desirable to use digital stimulation alone to produce reflex elimination.

Action	Rationale
1. Stimulate defecation reflex at a planned time, usually every other day:	
• Insert suppository against rectal mucosa.	Contact with rectal mucosa is essential for absorption; this is not possible if suppository is directly inserted into stool.
• Insert suppository 15 to 30 min ahead of planned evacuation time, usually just before breakfast.	This takes advantage of the gastrocolic reflex, which naturally stimulates defecation.
• Try glycerine suppository first (medium strength). If it is ineffective, try stronger bisacodyl (Dulcolax) suppository, but watch for signs of autonomic dysreflexia.	Starting with weaker medication can prevent undesirable accumulative effects.
2. Ask patient to:	
• Attempt evacuation on toilet if possible.	These measures assist with defecation.
• Bear down (Valsalva maneuver) if abdominal muscles are strong.	
• Massage abdomen in clockwise manner.	
• Lean forward, if possible.	
3. If no bowel movement has occurred within 15 to 30 min, attempt *digital stimulation*:	
• Insert a well-lubricated gloved finger into rectum.	Generous lubrication minimizes risk of traumatizing rectum. Digital stimulation is contraindicated if any rectal bleeding or hemorrhoids are present.
• Move it from side to side in a circular motion. (Simple insertion may be enough for one patient; a full massage may be necessary for another.)	This stretches and relaxes anal sphincters.
• Do not stimulate for more than 5 min.	
• Stop if severe spasms of the anal sphincter occur or if signs of autonomic dysreflexia appear.	
• Once sphincter is relaxed, allow stool to pass. Resume until all stool has passed.	Again, "bearing down" and abdominal massage may be helpful.
4. If no bowel movement has occurred, repeat entire procedure next day. If this is not successful, take measures to treat constipation.	Assessment and interventions to alleviate constipation are detailed later in this chapter.
5. Evaluate timing of the program.	To begin program some may prefer a daily evacuation until a reliable bowel pattern is identified. A consistent pattern of a large, soft stool one day and a small, soft stool the next signals that an every-other-day program would be appropriate. If stool consistency remains soft, an every-third-day program may be attempted. Twice weekly may be sufficient for some, but not good if patient develops lethargy, poor appetite, or autonomic dysreflexia during evacuation.

A successful bowel program will result in:

- An adequate amount of softly formed stool
- Stimulation of defecation at regular and predicted intervals to ensure adequate bowel elimination
- Freedom from bouts of constipation and diarrhea

SPECIFIC NURSING INTERVENTIONS FOR POTENTIAL COMPLICATIONS

Constipation

Constipation may be described as difficult or infrequent passing of hard stools. The longer the stool is retained in the colon, the drier it becomes, because water is continually absorbed by the colon. Constipation is the most common complication encountered with neurogenic bowel dysfunction. Interrupted defecation mechanisms result in sluggish movement of fecal material through the bowel. This may be aggravated by insufficient bulk in the diet, low fluid intake, inactivity, immobilization, and inconsistent bowel management techniques.

Progressive accumulation of feces may result in *impaction*—a mass of stool that blocks the bowel. Signs and symptoms of impaction are similar to those of constipation. As nursing goals and interventions are also similar, the two conditions will be discussed together.

Goals of care

- To identify patients at additional risk of developing constipation or impaction
- To recognize early signs of constipation and initiate corrective treatment
- To assist patients with evacuation of constipated stool or relieve impaction
- To evaluate and adjust bowel program to prevent recurrence

Nursing interventions

1. Promote regular evacuation of a large amount of softly formed stool. For example, en-

sure that patients eat an adequate amount of high-fiber foods. If patients are unable or unwilling to eat sufficient quantities, substitute a bulk-forming laxative. Maintain a regulated fluid intake of at least 2000 mL/day to keep stools soft. If the stool remains a bit hard, add a stool softener to help the fecal mass absorb water. If the patient has missed a bowel evacuation at the planned time, try a night-before stimulant laxative to obtain results.

2. Closely observe patients at additional risk of developing constipation—the elderly; those with preexisting difficulties; and, especially, those with lower motor neuron bowel dysfunction. Lower motor neuron loss is more serious in many ways and regulation is difficult to achieve. The destruction of the sacral segments or roots causes loss of spinal reflex activity and, in turn, an atonic bowel with diminished muscle tone. The colon does not automatically respond to distension of its walls with feces, and peristalsis is not stimulated as it is for patients with higher lesions.

3. Look for signs and symptoms of constipation, such as loss of appetite, abdominal discomfort or referred pain (quadriplegic patients may feel unusually irritable or experience headache or diaphoresis, nausea, and even vomiting), and a hard or distended abdomen. If the patient is continually oozing liquid or loose stool, impaction is a possible cause.

4. Check the bowel program record for number of days since the last bowel movement, the quantity of stool produced, and fecal consistency. Be sure to clarify this information with the patient; some will insist they are constipated if only one day has been missed.

5. Institute vigorous treatment if no bowel movement has occurred for four or five days. The sooner interventions are started, the more effective they will be. Emerick (1979) suggests some of the following measures. Perform a rectal examination to determine presence of stool in the lower bowel. Gently break up and manually remove any stool in the rectum. If the patient is oozing stool around an impacted fecal mass, it may be possible to feel such a mass and proceed with manual removal. A mineral oil re-

PROCEDURE 13–5 ■ EVACUATION METHODS USED FOR A PATIENT WITH LOWER MOTOR NEURON DYSFUNCTION

Purpose

The purpose of using suppositories and manual removal of stool is to adequately evacuate stool from the lower bowel. Eventually it is desirable to use suppositories alone to stimulate defecation and avoid frequent manual removal, which tends to traumatize the rectum.

Action	Rationale
1. Time program according to patient's activity. While patients are on bedrest every other day is usually sufficient, but when mobilization begins, a daily bowel program is recommended.	When patient is active any stool in rectum may be expelled whenever the intra-abdominal pressure is increased (e.g., during transfers). Accidents can be prevented by evacuating any stool in rectum before periods of activity. In addition, though, a major evacuation should be carried out daily.
2. Ask patient to: • Transfer to toilet, if possible. • Bear down (Valsalva maneuver). • Massage the abdomen. • Lean forward, if possible.	These measures are all helpful to initiate defecation. Strong abdominal muscles and measures to increase intra-abdominal pressure help force stool through flaccid anal sphincters.
3. If these measures are ineffective, manually remove stool from rectum with generously lubricated gloved finger.	This must be done with caution to avoid trauma to the desensitized rectum.
4. After removing stool from lower rectum, insert a strong stimulant suppository (such as Bisacodyl or senna preparations) as high as possible against rectal wall.	This stimulates colon (via intrinsic or local reflexes) to empty stool into rectum, where it can be expelled or removed manually.
5. Examine stool consistency.	Stool consistency is a vital factor for these patients, as loose stools leak through a flaccid anal sphincter and hard stools are difficult to remove.
6. If these techniques are ineffective, repeat entire procedure next day. If this is not successful, take measures to treat constipation.	Measures to assess and treat constipation are outlined later in this chapter.

tention enema may be used before manual removal of stool to soften the fecal mass or a small-volume cleansing enema may be placed high in the bowel following the procedure. Throughout these procedures be constantly alert for the onset of autonomic dysreflexia in the high paraplegic and quadriplegic patient.

6. Administer a stimulant laxative if impaction is located above the rectum. Medication, such as large doses of senna (Senokot) tablets—four tablets twice a day for one or two days—are usually well tolerated and effective in moving stool to the rectum where it can be expelled or manually removed.

7. Ensure the bowel is empty before restarting the program. Reassess the effectiveness of diet, fluids, medications or suppositories, activity, time of planned evacuation, and stimulation techniques used, and initiate appropriate changes. Remember to alter only one aspect of the bowel program at a time to allow accurate evaluation.

8. Pain, tension, surgical intervention, and emotional upsets may slow bowel activity. Identify the relationship of these additional stresses to bowel elimination, and initiate appropriate interventions to relieve the cause.

9. Evaluate the program daily until regularity is achieved.

10. Evaluate effectiveness of treatment according to level of outcome criteria reached:

- Bowel movement of normal color, amount, and consistency at planned evacuation times (at least twice a week)
- Daily bowel movement of adequate formed stool for those with lower motor neuron bowel dysfunction
- Good appetite
- Abdomen soft and flat without evidence of discomfort, referred pain, or distension
- No signs or symptoms of autonomic dysreflexia

Diarrhea

Diarrhea may be described as the frequent passing of watery stools. The frequency and, to a lesser extent, the fluidity of bowel movements is relative to the habits of each individual. For some, three bowel movements a day is quite normal. For patients with neurogenic bowel dysfunction, diarrhea usually reflects an upset in the gastrointestinal system rather than an infective process, although the latter possibility should not be ruled out. Diarrhea is often related to ingestion of different foods or alcohol or excessive use of laxatives. The possibility of impaction must always be investigated. Diarrhea cannot be treated without determining the cause.

Goals of care

- To identify patients at risk of developing diarrhea
- To recognize onset and initiate early corrective treatment
- To prevent skin breakdown of perineal area
- To evaluate and adjust bowel program to prevent recurrence

Nursing interventions

1. Take measures to avoid diarrhea. Foods and fluids that stimulated diarrhea in the past will do so after injury. Spicy foods and too many fruit juices can interrupt a well-regulated bowel program. If constipation is suspected, refrain from increasing laxatives too quickly and always begin with minimal dosages. Remember cautious adjustments to the bowel program will prevent accumulation of undesired effects that are difficult to control. Closely observe patients with pre-existing tendencies to develop diarrhea.

2. Avoid harsh laxatives at all costs. Strong cathartics such as castor oil are routinely used before certain X-ray procedures, such as the intravenous pyelogram. Although the bowel must be cleared to visualize the urinary tract, this type of routine should be modified for patients with spinal cord injuries. For example, you might schedule the diagnostic procedure after a routine bowel evacuation. Otherwise uncontrolled diarrhea, with all its other ramifications and patient discomforts, may persist for one or two weeks.

3. Carefully observe the patient's drug profile. Many antibiotics and certain antacids have side effects that can contribute to diarrhea.

4. Determine whether the patient is impacted. Check the bowel program record for previous signs of constipation. Perform a rectal examination to determine if a fecal mass is blocking normal passage of stool. If such a mass cannot be felt rectally, palpate the abdomen over the area of the large intestine to feel any hardened areas. Abdominal distension, discomfort, or referred pain with loss of appetite or nausea and vomiting may also be present. Collaborate with the physician to follow measures for relief of impaction. Remember that with neurogenic bowel dysfunction, diarrhea, resulting from liquid stool oozing past the blockage of fecal matter, is a common sign of impaction.

5. Determine whether diarrhea is the result of an infective process. Observe for systemic signs of a fever. Stool may be an abnormal color or foul smelling. Obtain stool specimens as ordered for culture, ova, and parasites. A complete blood count and differential may show abnormality. In bacterial infection the white blood count will be elevated. In extremely rare cases septicemia—characterized by a decrease in consciousness level, persistent high fever, and signs of hypovolemic shock—may ensue. Follow interventions as ordered by physician and take measures to isolate the patient to stop spread of infection.

6. Replace fluid and electrolyte loss if patient has become dehydrated. Watch for decreased amounts of concentrated urine or dryness of skin and mucous membranes. The patient may have to return temporarily to a four-hour intermittent catheterization schedule to compensate for a higher fluid intake. Soups and broths are recommended for their high sodium and potassium content. Milk, fruits, and high-roughage foods should be avoided for a few days.

7. Administer palliative drugs as ordered by physician if diarrhea persists. Lomotil or kaolin with pectin may be useful.

8. Ensure the bowel is empty before restarting the program. Reassess the effectiveness of diet, fluids, medications or suppositories, activity, time of planned evacuation, and stimulation techniques, and initiate appropriate changes. Remember to alter only one aspect of the bowel program at a time to allow accurate evaluation.

9. Evaluate program daily until regularity is achieved.

10. Evaluate effectiveness of treatment according to level of outcome reached:

- Bowel movement of normal color, odor, and consistency at planned evacuation times
- Stool cultures negative
- CBC and electrolytes within normal limits
- General condition satisfactory without evidence of infection, dehydration, or loss of appetite
- Abdomen soft and flat without evidence of distension or firmness

Hemorrhoids

Hemorrhoids are varicosities of the veins around the rectal and anal area. These dilated blood vessels may occur outside the anal sphincter or within the sphincter but beneath the mucous membranes. In the general population straining with constipated stool is a common cause. For patients with spinal cord injuries a number of additional factors may impair venous circulation from the rectal area. Changes in the autonomic nervous system tend to produce a general passive state of vasodilation, which hampers venous return to the heart. Lack of position change, extended time periods spent on the toilet, and, occasionally, rough manual stimulation of the bowel will cause local trauma to the rectal area. Bowel irregularity and sometimes preexisting tendencies will aggravate the situation.

Goals of care

- To identify patients at additional risk of developing hemorrhoids
- To recognize the condition and take measures to alleviate cause
- To heal the affected areas and arrest any bleeding
- To prevent secondary infection
- To minimize risk of recurrence

Nursing interventions

1. Promote circulation to the rectal area. Ensure pressure relief by position changes every half-hour when the patient is up in the wheelchair. Do not let patients sit on the toilet too long during a bowel program. The entire body weight against the toilet seat can rapidly diminish circulation to the area. Pressure relief lifts are a good idea if the patient is able to perform them. One hour should be the maximum toilet time.

2. Closely observe patients who are at additional risk: those with preexisting occurrence; those who tend to become constipated; and, especially, those with lower motor neuron damage. The degree of vasodilation tends to be greater with flaccid paralysis, and these patients require more manual manipulation of the rectal area to evacuate stool. Generously lubricating the gloved finger will minimize trauma to the rectal wall. When patients are learning manual techniques, too vigorous stimulation may be a problem if they become frustrated or angry. Emphasize the importance of gloving (or use of finger cot) for added protection, even if in a hurry and stool evacuation is frequent.

3. Observe stool and cleaning tissue for blood—a most common sign of internal hemorrhoids. (External hemorrhoids are easily identified). Although pain and itching may not be felt, an increase in leg spasms in patients with higher lesions may be a clue.

4. Stop or proceed very gently with bowel procedures. It may be possible to reinsert external hemorrhoids with the use of a lubricant when the patient has returned to bed. Warm daily baths may also help to promote circulation. Ice packs should be used cautiously, as they can easily burn the skin.

5. Administer anti-inflammatory suppositories or topical ointments as ordered. Occasionally the physician may incise or inject the hemorrhoidal tissue. In rare instances anal fissures or fistulas may develop.

6. Clean and dry the rectal area thoroughly following each bowel movement or every eight hours to prevent secondary infection.

7. Reassess the effectiveness of the bowel program. Take measures to avoid constipation. Collaborate with the dietitian to alter diet and add stool softeners to bowel medications (as ordered) to produce a softer stool if necessary.

8. Evaluate effectiveness of treatment according to level of outcome criteria reached:

- No evidence of external hemorrhoids or rectal bleeding
- Bowel program well established
- No evidence of aggravated leg spasms in those with higher lesions

Autonomic Dysreflexia

Autonomic dysreflexia or *hyperreflexia* is mainly characterized by a sudden, severe head-ache secondary to an uncontrolled elevation of blood pressure, which, if untreated, may progress to fatal complications, such as cerebral hemorrhage or myocardial infarction. As signs and symptoms may be precipitated by routine bowel evacuations, the nursing staff, particularly assistants who are involved in bowel care, should be familiar with its onset and treatment to avoid a medical emergency.

Autonomic dysreflexia is a potential risk for high paraplegic and quadriplegic patients who have a spinal cord injury above the T_{4-6} levels. The mechanisms involved in this unusual autonomic nervous system response are usually triggered by abnormal stimuli from the abdominopelvic region. Chapter 10 outlines this pathophysiology in detail. Although the most frequent source of abnormal stimuli is bladder overdistension, rectal stimulation and a blocked bowel are also common causes. Autonomic dysreflexia can be an isolated incident precipitated by a full bowel or may recur during routine bowel procedures.

Goals of care

- To identify patients at risk of developing autonomic dysreflexia
- To establish an effective bowel program to minimize risk of abnormal stimuli triggering an exaggerated autonomic nervous system response
- To recognize immediately the onset of this condition and initiate measures to lower the blood pressure
- To be aware of patients who have a tendency to develop autonomic dysreflexia and take measures to avoid recurrence

Nursing interventions

1. Take measures to avoid constipation and impaction and to maintain a normal, soft stool consistency.

2. Carefully observe patients wigh high thoracic and cervical fractures resulting in cord damage at or above the T_6 level. Check the history to find out if the patient has a tendency to develop autonomic dysreflexic signs, such as headache, diaphoresis, or general tension during routine evacuation measures. If so, a local anesthetic such as Nupercainal ointment may be instilled 10 minutes before the procedure.

3. Be alert for the following signs and symptoms, indicating the onset of autonomic dysreflexia:

- Headache (secondary to elevated blood pressure) of a pounding, severe, and sudden onset. Thoroughly investigate complaints of *any* headache.
- Elevated blood pressure. Compare with baseline data. Blood pressure of 140/90 may be considered high for some; others may experience obviously high pressures of 300/160.
- Bradycardia (low pulse rate), which is most common; or tachycardia (high pulse rate), which may be experienced by high quadriplegics.
- Profuse sweating, goose bumps, and blotchiness of skin about the level of the lesion.
- Nasal stuffiness or obstruction.
- Unusual apprehension.

4. Return patient to bed and elevate 45 degrees if possible. Two or three staff members should monitor and check symptoms simultaneously. Be sure to check for an overdistended bladder that may be the cause. Also monitor the blood pressure and pulse every three to five minutes.

5. Stop bowel procedures until signs and symptoms subside (as the added stimulation may just raise the blood pressure further). Resume cautiously. This may require instillation of a local anesthetic 10 minutes before resuming.

6. Consult the physician immediately if first aid treatment does not work. The techniques mentioned are usually effective.

7. Administer ganglionic blocking agents as ordered and collaborate with physician to evacuate bowel contents.

8. Monitor vital signs every four to eight hours for 24 hours, because the nervous system tends to remain unstable if the attack has been severe. Mild autonomic dysreflexia signs frequently occur when the bowel is being evacuated. Monitor vital signs closely and proceed with caution.

9. Provide psychological support. The exaggerated sympathetic response is accompanied by an increased circulation of catecholamines, which are known to increase anxiety. The patient may feel apprehensive and agitated and find it difficult to rest. Explain the body's reaction and make the patient comfortable to promote sleep.

10. Reconsider the causative factors contributing to the onset of autonomic dysreflexia, and initiate nursing actions to prevent further episodes if possible. Teach the patient and family the relationship between the bowel program and this abnormal neural response. It must be stressed that prevention is the best treatment.

11. Evaluate effectiveness of treatment according to level of outcome criteria reached:

- During bowel evacuation procedures, blood pressure and pulse within normal limits for patient without signs of headache, profuse sweating, or blotchiness of skin
- Bowel program regular and effective
- Patient aware of preventive measures, first aid treatment, and action to take in emergency

SELF-CARE SKILLS

Patients must be taught principles of good bowel management. To achieve regularity and control stool consistency, emphasis is placed on maintenance of a high fluid intake, a high-fiber diet, and as much physical activity as possible. Prolonged use of laxatives irritates the bowel, which results in decreased tone; the laxatives then become less and less effective.

The Paraplegic Patient

The patient with paraplegia is physically capable of becoming totally independent with all aspects of bowel care. Good arm function and upper body strength enable the patient to perform toilet transfers and cope with suppositories, digital stimulation, and manual extraction of stool with relative ease. Occupational therapists can help patients organize bowel equipment and, following a home assessment, recommend bathroom alterations. Often only additional hand rails are needed; a padded, raised toilet seat may not be necessary.

The Quadriplegic Patient

Bowel care is much more difficult for quadriplegic patients, because of poor dexterity, weak arms, and difficulty balancing on the toilet.

For independent bowel care patients must be able to transfer to the toilet or commode or assume a side-lying position in bed. Equipment may be needed for digital stimulation. A loop attached to a wrist device and tension applied to isolate the middle finger for insertion or a smooth plastic digital stimulator may be necessary. Some patients will require suppository inserters. Handles can be individually designed for optimal angle insertion, or a compression ejector device may be needed. Patients will require some wrist strength or wrist splinting to maneuver most devices. Arm placement must, of course, be adequate to reach the rectal area. Following bowel procedures, cleanliness must be considered. Most patients will probably need to return to bed to wash the perineal area, or they may take a shower if convenient. The buttocks should be washed with mild soap and water and thoroughly dried to prevent odor and skin breakdown. Close collaboration with the occupational therapist is essential to teach this independent living skill, and home bathroom renovations, often using a commode, will likely be more extensive.

The very high quadriplegic patient (C_{1-4}) will be unable to maintain a safe balance when on the toilet and to proceed with manual skills. Such people will require assistance.

LONG-TERM IMPLICATIONS

When assessing the patient who has been paralyzed for some time, keep in mind that planned and regular evacuation is a realistic goal, although there is always a tendency toward constipation. Should problems occur, nothing but the thorough history taking and current physical assessment outlined here will identify the problems accurately. Based on that assessment nurses can help patients continue with current practice, provide appropriate intervention, or refer patients to other resources, such as a nutritional counselor or rehabilitative facility, to update their skills. Be alert with the patient who has bouts of constipation. Underlying depression, inactivity, or lack of social or vocational opportunities may be the major contributing factor.

Common problems are deliberate constipation to avoid bowel procedures, unpalatable laxatives, and bowel programs that are impractical because they are too time-consuming. Aim for a program of 30 minutes.

It is wise to follow the patient closely for the first month following discharge from a rehabilitation facility, for this is when "accidents" are most likely to occur. If the bowel program was well established in the hospital, reassure patients that it will probably settle down as they adjust to home life and routines become more established. Many people with spinal cord injuries agree that fear of having a bowel accident or failure to achieve bowel management can lead to social isolation.

SELECTED REFERENCES

Cannon, B. 1980. Bowel function. In *Comprehensive Rehabilitation Nursing*. Eds. N. Martin, N. Holt, and D. Hicks. New York: McGraw-Hill, pp. 223–241. *Normal and altered function of neurogenic bowel disease, assessment, management, and common complications. Highly recommended.*

Chusid, J. 1979. *Correlative Neuroanatomy and Functional Neurology*. 17th ed. Los Altos, Calif.: Lange Medical Publications, Chapter 6. *Describes physiology and effects of the autonomic nervous system on the gastrointestinal system and defecation.*

Emerick, C. 1979. Nursing management of the neurogenic bowel. *Association of Rehabilitation Nurses Journal* 4 (Jan.–Feb.): 15–16. *Excellent reference on altered physiology, the effects of diet and medications on a bowel program, and related nursing care.*

Ford, J., and Duckworth, B. 1974. *Physical Management for the Quadriplegic Patient*. Philadelphia: F. A. Davis, Chapter 8. *Includes independent skills for suppository insertion, positions in bed and on toilet, and various other adaptive aids.*

Meiners, C. 1976. *How to be Healthier Through Proper Nutrition.* Published by the National Paraplegia Foundation and the NFP Allied Health Committee. Available from the National Spinal Cord Injury Foundation. *General nutritional information related to specific needs of people with spinal cord injuries; includes detailed information on dietary fiber, sources, and recommended intake.*

Paeslak, V. 1966. Disorders of bowel function in spinal lesions. *International Journal of Paraplegia* 4: 250–254. *Neural and functional pathology; physical assessment skills; and bowel-training techniques.*

SUPPLEMENTAL READING

General

Bergstrom, D. 1968. *Care of Patients with Bowel and Bladder Problems: A Nursing Guide.* Minneapolis, Minn.: Sister Kenny Institute. *Includes diagrammatic explanations of neurogenic bowel disorders and offers clear, concise, and practical management strategies.*

Bertholf, C. 1978. Protocol: acute diarrhea. *Nurse Practitioner* 3 (3): 17–20. *Review of assessment, differential diagnosis, and related nursing care; focus on an infective process.*

Connell, A. 1967. The physiology and pathophysiology of constipation. *International Journal of Paraplegia* 4 (Feb.): 244–250. *Review of normal and altered bowel habits and defecation patterns following spinal cord injury.*

Devroede, G., et al. 1979. Traumatic constipation. *Gastroenterology* 77: 1258–1267. *Examines four ambulatory patients with trauma to the lumbar spine resulting in chronic constipation; includes detailed explanation of diagnostic aids—marker studies to measure transit time in the bowel and rectal pressure and reflex studies.*

Frankel, H. 1967. Bowel training. *International Journal of Paraplegia* 4 (Feb.): 254–258. *Principles of bowel management during and after spinal shock.*

Guttman, L. 1976. *Spinal Cord Injuries Comprehensive Management and Research.* 2d ed. London: Blackwell Scientific Publications. *A classic, multifaceted reference text on spinal cord injuries. Includes historical background information; general statistics; legal*

aspects; detailed anatomy and neuropathology of cord trauma and resultant effects on all body systems; regeneration; fractures and dislocations, gunshot injuries, and stab wounds; and neurophysiological and clinical management aspects. Extensive bibliography.

Guyton, A. 1976. *Textbook of Medical Physiology.* 5th ed. Philadelphia: W. B. Saunders. *Classic text detailing neuroanatomy and physiology, including that of the gastrointestinal system and functional disorders.*

Jones, F. 1972. *Management of Constipation.* London: Blackwell Scientific Publications. *Informative chapters on physiology of the colon and therapeutic agents.*

Rogers, E. 1976. Management of the neurogenic bladder and bowel. *Queen's Nursing Journal,* August, pp. 133–138. *Includes overview of bowel program.*

Thompson, W. 1976. Constipation and catharsis. *Canadian Medical Association Journal* 114: 10. *A general pharmacologic review.*

Patient and Family Health Education

Goldfinger, G., and Hanak, M. 1981. *Spinal Cord Injury: A Guide for Care.* New York Regional Spinal Cord Injury System, pp. 27–30. *Concise review of practical considerations for management including procedures and supplemental medication.*

King, R.; Boyink, M.; and Keenan, M., eds. 1977. *Rehabilitation Guide.* Medical Rehabilitation Research and Training Center No. 20. Chicago: Northwest University and Rehabilitation Institute of Chicago. *Detailed section on understanding and managing a bowel program; guide to home management with problem-solving format includes information on medications; procedures; and problems of constipation, impaction, diarrhea, and changing routine.*

Norris, W. C.; Noble, C. E.; and Strickland, S. B. 1981. *Spinal Injury Learning Series.* Jackson, Miss: University Press of Mississippi. *Educational program purchased on a fee-for-service basis; currently offers education on bowel, bladder, and skin care with plans to expand and continually update content.*

Virginia Spinal Cord Injury Care and Teaching Manual. 1980. The Virginia Spinal Cord Injury System, University of Virginia Center and Virginia Dept. of Rehabilitation Services, Woodrow Wilson Rehabilitation Center, Box W-279, Fisherville, Va. 22939. *Concise and clear presentation, including factors to consider when setting up and maintaining a bowel program, helpful tips, aids, medication, and problem solving.*

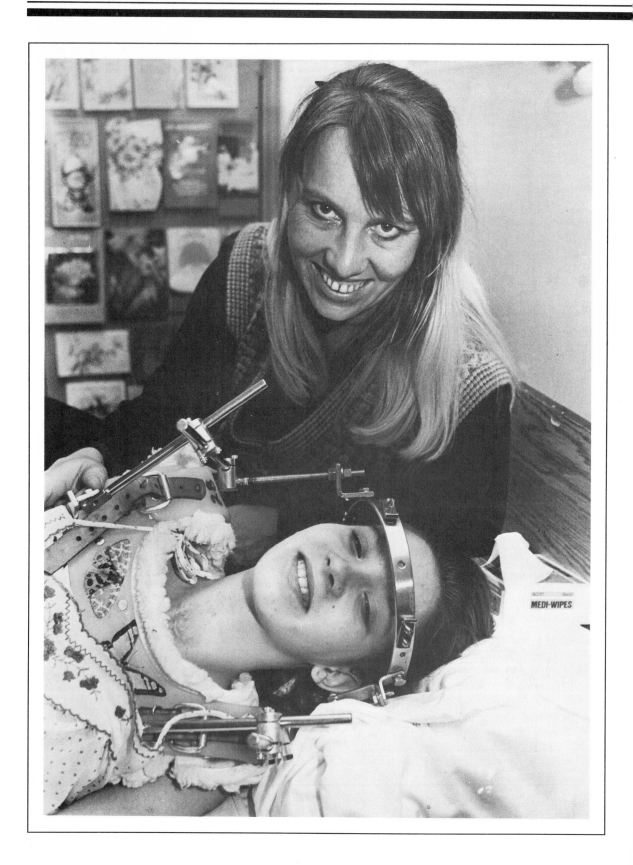

PART V

REESTABLISHING
MOBILITY AND
INDEPENDENCE

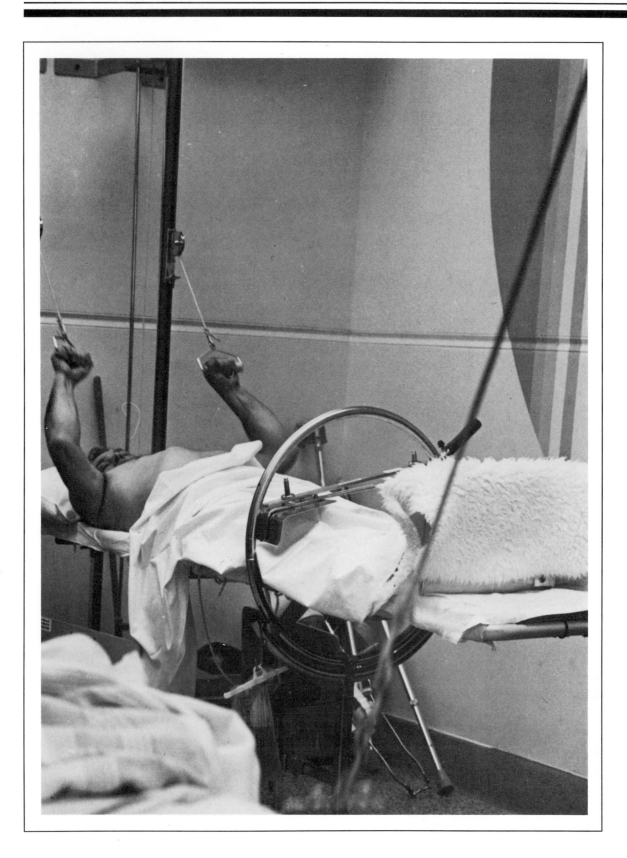

Chapter 14

Maintaining Skeletal System Integrity

OBJECTIVES

- To identify health care goals for maintaining skeletal system integrity
- To explain the philosophy of early mobilization
- To define correct body alignment
- To discuss measures that achieve correct alignment and promote circulation
- To describe care requiring specialized beds and cervical traction
- To describe care requiring cervical or thoracolumbar orthoses
- To discuss general goals and indications involved with surgical management
- To describe preoperative and postoperative care for the patient requiring spinal surgery
- To describe care for the patient with associated skeletal injuries and heterotopic bone formation
- To explain how to teach patients and families appropriate self-care skills
- To describe long-term implications of damage to skeletal system integrity

GOALS OF HEALTH CARE

Management of bony injury to the spinal column is a most important aspect of acute care for patients with spinal cord injuries. There is growing recognition that ultimate surgical management of spinal cord injuries is best achieved by collaboration between an orthopedic surgeon and a neurosurgeon. After emergency measures have been taken, the health care team will select a total treatment approach that accommodates the patient's general condition, stabilizes the fracture site, and facilitates any potential neurological recovery. Early mobilization to prevent physiological and psychological complications associated with bedrest is a key consideration influencing this decision-making process.

Maintaining good body alignment is vital during all stages of care. This requires not only understanding basic principles but also acquiring numerous manual skills to move patients safely and care for immobilization equipment and orthotic devices. The goals of skeletal system care are:

- To prevent further neurological damage and/or facilitate potential neurological return
- To provide complete stability to the injured spine, ensuring early and adequate immobilization of the spine throughout the acute phase to prevent long-term complications such as spinal curvatures
- To support a philosophy of early mobilization
- To maintain correct body alignment and ensure adequate position change, preventing skin breakdown, muscle fatigue, contractures, and nerve or joint damage and minimizing patient discomfort and spasm
- To restore as much functional activity as possible

ASSESSMENT OF THE SKELETAL SYSTEM

Assessment of the skeletal system begins with a review of the patient's history to note any preexisting factors that would, in addition to the spinal cord injury, influence skeletal system integrity. Awareness of previous osteopathic changes is imperative. Conditions, such as arthritis, resulting in abnormal spinal alignment or in a compromised spinal canal may have predisposed the patient to the initial spinal cord trauma. Normal course of aging also causes changes in the physiological function and physical appearance of the skeletal system.

The physical examination of the skeletal system should include observation of the head and neck to detect any abnormal spinal curvatures, examination of the fracture site, and observation of body alignment.

In-depth assessment of skeletal system integrity depends largely on radiological findings. During the remobilization period, X-ray evaluation is used at specific intervals to monitor spinal stability, evaluate the degree of healing, and detect evidence of any developing malalignment. Flexion/extension views, often taken when the patient is sitting in a wheelchair, provide information to determine the degree of spinal mobility. Spinal mobility is directly related to the healing of ligamentous structures; if mobility is excessive, healing is probably incomplete. The physician will use this information in deciding when it is safe to replace a strong, inflexible brace with a brace that offers less support. X-ray information is also useful to predict what degree of stress the patient will safely tolerate with increased physical activity.

Preexisting conditions or abnormal findings necessitate additional precautions and modifications to the nursing care plan. For assessment techniques and an anatomical and physiological review of the skeletal system, see Chapter 5.

GENERAL NURSING INTERVENTIONS

To promote skeletal system integrity, nursing measures focus on maintaining correct body alignment, preventing muscle contractures, and preserving the protective functions of the skin.

Comprehensive nursing care can minimize pain or spasm and prevent skeletal deformity. Most importantly, though, is the skilled movement of the patient, which will prevent further neurological damage.

Considerable advancements in both surgical and nonsurgical management techniques have allowed earlier general mobilization of the patient while still protecting and immobilizing the spine. These advances have greatly reduced both the formerly lengthy periods of bedrest and the accompanying hazards of physical immobilization and psychological isolation. This means a shorter period of hospitalization and earlier return to community life.

Conservative or nonsurgical management has been improved by the continuing development of strong, light-weight braces that can be easily fitted to individual patients. The most outstanding breakthrough has been the Halo-thoracic brace, which has virtually eliminated months of bedrest for the quadriplegic patient.

Surgical management techniques have also improved. Adaptation of spinal instrumentation—insertion of metal rods into the vertebral column—is now used for thoracic and lumbar injuries. This surgery, in combination with bracing techniques, has provided earlier mobilization for the patient with paraplegia.

To most new staff members of all disciplines, the orthopedic component of spinal injury care is overwhelming. However, working with an experienced staff member develops skill and confidence. In-service education with active participation by staff members will ensure that all are familiar with equipment and procedures. For example, nurses should actually be turned in a turning frame or try on an immobilization brace. Especially when mobilization begins, nursing staff, physicians, and physical therapists will need to collaborate closely to coordinate physical activities.

Nursing care involved when the spine is immobilized will be discussed in three main areas: when spinal immobilization is achieved by *bedrest* (with or without traction); when spinal immobilization is achieved by the use of *orthoses*; and when *surgical intervention* is used to achieve stabilization. These techniques are often used in combination.

Immobilizing the Patient with Bedrest

Maintaining correct alignment

Nursing care measures to ensure correct positioning will help make the patient comfortable, enhance respiration, promote circulation, prevent gravitational edema, and preserve muscle function by preventing contractures. While the patient is in bed the side-lying, supine, prone, and sitting positions may be assumed; each has specific advantages.

Immediately after injury patients require a change of position every two hours around the clock, regardless of which immobilization bed or brace is used. Minor position changes are often required more frequently. Restlessness or increased pain or spasm may indicate this need. The schedule must be adjusted to meet individual needs and as tolerance for selected positions increases. Eventually self-turns can be taught to patients with sufficient strength and mobility.

Side-lying position The side-lying position is used to minimize risk of aspiration during mealtime; mobilize secretions from dependent areas of the lung; relieve pressure on the sacral area; and enable patients to see more of their surroundings. See Figure 14–1. Care must be taken to avoid undue curvature of the cervical or thoracic spine, to protect bony prominences and the nerve plexus in the shoulder, and to support and separate skin surfaces of the extremities. See Table 14–1 for a summary of potential problems and measures associated with this position.

- *Head/neck.* For the patient with a new cervical injury place a small, flat pillow or one-inch foam pad under the head (as ordered by physician). Be sure to protect the ear with surrounding padding. The ear is a vulnerable pressure point when the patient can only be *tipped* toward the side as opposed to a full lateral (side-lying) position, for example, the patient requiring cervical traction. A small pillow may also be more comfortable for those with high thoracic lesions. Most patients with thoracic and lumbar injuries prefer a regular pillow. Correct neck support prevents lateral flexion of the cervical spine and prevents fatigue of sternocleidomastoid muscles, which significantly aid respiration.

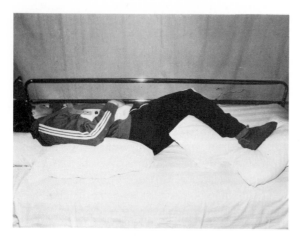

FIGURE 14–1 ■ Maintaining secure support with pillows in the side-lying position.

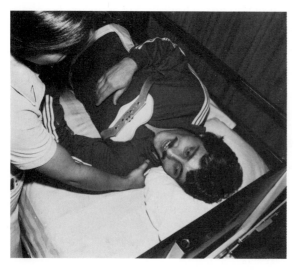

FIGURE 14–2 ■ Relieving pressure on the shoulder is important.

• *Trunk*. Support the back with a rolled pillow to maintain *secure* support. Place the pillow lengthwise against the patient's back, tuck the pillow edge snugly between the patient and the mattress, grasp the other edge, and firmly roll and secure this edge underneath the pillow itself.

Loss of correct position, which easily occurs when the patient has little or no trunk control, causes malalignment of the spine and limbs, contributing to back discomfort and extremity spasms.

• *Extremities*. Correct positioning of the extremities is extremely important for the patient with paralysis and loss of sensation. First, pull the bottom shoulder through to relieve pressure and find a comfortable position. See Figure 14–2. Then support the top arm with a pillow to prevent internal rotation and shoulder adduction, promote chest expansion, separate skin surfaces, and facilitate circulation. If the paralyzed arm is left dangling, gravitational edema will develop. Also elevate the bottom arm on a pillow to avoid this problem. Splints may be required to maintain functional alignment of the wrist and hand.

Generally for patients with cervical injuries extend arms in a comfortable position to prevent flexion contractures and subsequent loss of function. Most quadriplegic patients are able to flex but not extend their arms; therefore flexion contractures are the more common danger. This is especially true if the level of lesion is C_5 or C_6. These patients are able to flex but not extend the arms. Patients position themselves with elbows flexed. Therefore their arms should be positioned in full extension two out of every eight hours. A loose tie around the arm secured to the bed will remind the patient to maintain this position. Extension contractures of the elbows, though less common, can occur in patients with higher lesions where elbow flexors are absent. It is also important to maintain shoulder range. For these patients *without* arm movement, alternate positions of flexion and extension are necessary to avoid contractures in either direction.

Flex both legs slightly, the top one more, and place pillows lengthwise between the legs for balance and comfort, to relieve pulling force on the injured spine, and to prevent internal rotation and adduction of the hip. To prevent foot drop support both feet at a 90-degree angle to the ankles using padding or pillows kept in place by sandbags or footboard. Always separate ankles with padding to avoid pressure areas over bony prominences. See Figure 14–3.

Supine position The supine position is desirable for many general nursing functions such as bathing or catheterizations. See Figure 14–4. Because this position is assumed so frequently, it

TABLE 14–1 ■ SIDE-LYING (LATERAL) POSITION

Potential Problems	Supportive Measures for Patients with Cervical Injuries	Supportive Measures for Patients with Thoracic or Lumbar Injuries
Excessive lateral neck flexion; fatigue of sternocleidomastoid muscles	One-inch foam pad or small, flat pillow placed under head of newly injured patients	Regular pillow under head (high thoracic injured patients may be more comfortable with a small pillow)
Pressure area on ear	Soft protective padding surrounding ears	
Loss of correct position; subsequent malalignment of spine and limbs contributing to discomfort and extremity spasm	Rolled pillow positioned securely behind back	Rolled pillow positioned securely behind back
Skin excoriation under arms; limited chest expansion; compromised circulation to and gravitational edema in paralyzed arms; and internal rotation and adduction of the shoulder with contractures of arm musculature	Pillow under top arm and bottom forearm to support them in good alignment*	Pillow under arms to support in position of comfort
Hip internally rotated and adducted; loss of correct positioning contributing to back discomfort and extremity spasms	Pillows placed lengthwise between legs to maintain good alignment, balance, and comfort	Pillows placed lengthwise between legs to maintain good alignment, balance, and comfort
Foot drop, which complicates sitting in wheelchair	Padding or pillows kept in place with sandbags or footboard to support feet in 90-degree position	Padding or pillows kept in place with sandbags or footboard to support feet in 90-degree position
Pressure areas developing over bony prominences	Padding to separate ankles	Padding to separate ankles

* For most quadriplegic patients position arms in extension to avoid flexion contractures of the elbow. If the patient has a high-level cervical injury with *no* arm movement, alternate flexion and extension positions to avoid contractures.

is better to schedule turns from side to side (and not from side to back to side) to avoid the patient spending prolonged periods of time on the back. Patients with limited neck movement will need prism glasses to see and observe activities around them. Nurses must take measures to avoid rotation of the neck, support natural body curvatures, protect the sacral area and heels from pressure areas, and support feet to prevent foot drop. See Table 14–2 and Figure 14–4 for a summary of potential problems and measures associated with this position.

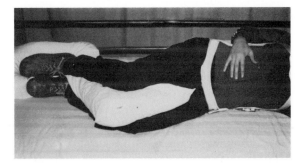

FIGURE 14–3 ■ Supporting the legs and feet in side-lying position.

TABLE 14-2 ■ SUPINE POSITION

Potential Problems	Supportive Measures for Patients with Cervical Injuries	Supportive Measures for Patients with Thoracic or Lumbar Injuries
Excessive flexion or extension of the head and neck exerting undesirable pressure on injury site	One-inch foam pad or small flat pillow placed under head of newly injured patient	Pillow of suitable thickness placed under head
Flexion of lumbar curvature with undue pressure contributing to back pain and possibly increased neurological deficit	Optional padding or small pillow to support lumbar curvature	Hyperextension padding to support lumbar curvature and promote reduction of injured spine
Compromises of circulation; gravitational edema of forearms and hands; and elbow contractures	Pillows elevating forearms and hands*	Support not required except as comfort measure
Hyperextension of knees; impaired circulation; and tension on the lower spine	Small pillow or padding under lower thigh to flex legs slightly (optional if full-length padding is used on bed)	Small pillow or padding under lower thigh to flex legs slightly (optional if full-length padding is used on bed)
Foot drop	Pillows or padding and footboard to flex feet at a 90-degree angle	Pillows or padding and footboard to flex feet at a 90-degree angle

* Position most quadriplegic patients with arms extended to avoid flexion contractures of the elbow. If the patient has a high-level cervical injury and *no* arm movement, alternate flexion and extension positions to avoid contractures in either direction.

- *Head/neck.* For the patient with a cervical injury place a small pillow or one-inch foam pad under the head as ordered by physician. This padding relieves pressure on the occiput and maintains a neutral position of the neck. An unsupported head causes slight hyperextension of the neck; a regular pillow would cause too much flexion. Place sandbags (with soft covering) on each side of the head to restrict neck rotation.

  Most patients with thoracic and lumbar injuries prefer a regular pillow. Patients with high-level thoracic injuries may require a small pillow or foam pad to avoid flexion of the neck, which would exert a pulling force on the injured part of the spine.

- *Trunk.* There is no need to use a small pillow or roll to support the lumbar curvature. Usually full-length padding, such as synthetic sheepskin, is quite sufficient. Numerous small

pads tend to be easily misplaced and become an undesirable source of pressure on another area of the body.

Hyperextension padding may be specifically ordered by the physician for thoracolumbar injuries to support normal curvature of lumbar spine and promote reduction of the injured spine.

- *Extremities.* Extend the arms of patients with cervical injuries and support on pillows to prevent contractures and gravitational edema. Again, for patients with high cervical cord injuries with no arm movement, alternate flexion and extension positions to avoid contractures in either direction. Splints may be necessary to maintain wrists and hands in functional alignment.

  Place small pad or pillow under lower thigh to flex legs slightly and relieve tension on the lower back. The popliteal artery, which

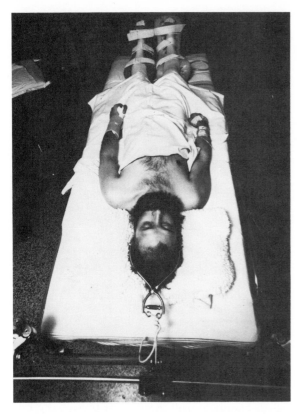

FIGURE 14–4 ■ A patient with a cervical injury is correctly supported and aligned in the supine position. Note the covered sandbags on either side of the head to prevent neck rotation; extension of arms to prevent flexion contractures; application of long opponens splint on the left arm to preserve functional hand position; and "moon boots" to prevent foot drop.

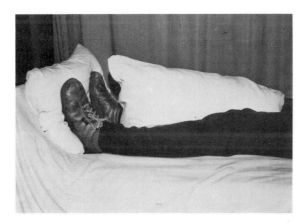

FIGURE 14–5 ■ Padding, pillows, and footboards can be used to prevent foot drop later in the rehabilitation period.

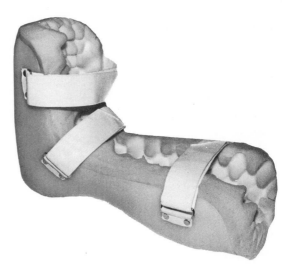

FIGURE 14–6 ■ "Moon boots" are used to preserve a 90-degree angle between feet and ankles. These are made out of platizote and lined with egg crate foam.

sup-plies the lower limb, is very close to the skin surface and circulation may be impaired by padding placed directly under the knee. Support ankles to prevent pressure on heels and support feet in a 90-degree angle to prevent foot drop by using pillows, padding, and footboard or special "moon boots." See Figures 14–5, and 14–6. The patient frequently has to be moved down in bed to reach the footboard. Supporting the legs and feet in such a way will combat the tendency of the legs to rotate externally.

Prone position   The prone position is especially valuable to counteract prolonged periods of hip flexion and to provide pressure relief for the buttocks following long periods of sitting in a wheelchair.

Check with the physician before placing the patient in the prone position and check again when different orthoses are used. For example, a patient in a Halo may tolerate the prone position well, but when the brace is removed and replaced by a less protective neck brace, the position may be quite unsafe. Check with the physician when thoracolumbar braces are removed. Rotational movements may still need to be restricted.

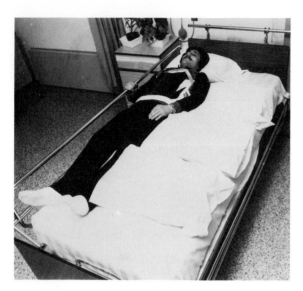

FIGURE 14–7 ■ Placement of pillows, while the patient is in the supine position, is completed before turning the patient prone.

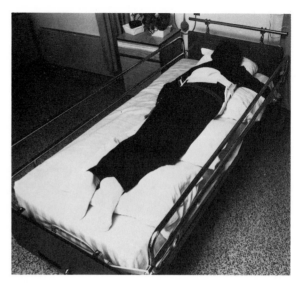

FIGURE 14–9 ■ The patient is supported by the pillows in the finished prone position.

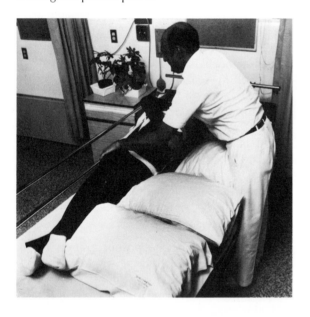

FIGURE 14–8 ■ The patient is rolled toward the pillows. To ease the move the left arm is at the patient's side and the right arm and right leg are crossed over the patient's body.

Turning the patient prone can be simplified by practicing the following techniques. Move the patient to the side of the bed in the supine position, and arrange pillows in the desired position beside the patient. See Figure 14–7. Prepare the patient for turning prone by placing the op-

posite arm and leg across the body; if turning the patient toward the left, position the right arm and right leg. Tuck the left arm down by the patient's side or place above the head. See Figure 14–8. Finally logroll the patient toward the pillows. See Figure 14–9.

Many patients are apprehensive about trying this position because they fear difficulties with breathing or discomfort. For this reason, it is advisable to do a "trial run" of proning during the day, before attempting to include it in the night routine. Building a tolerance for proning can eventually allow undisturbed rest in that position throughout the night.

Care must be taken to avoid undue curvature of the cervical or thoracic spine; to position arms comfortably; to protect male genitalia, iliac crest bones, and knees; and to prevent foot drop. See Table 14–3 for a summary of possible problems and supportive measures associated with this position.

- *Head/neck.* Patients with cervical injuries must avoid rotation, extension, or flexion of the neck until the spinal fracture site is stable. It is possible to support the forehead and the chin with padding to allow a "breathing space" when the patient is wearing a variety of neck supports. Be sure to check with the surgeon for specific positioning orders.

TABLE 14–3 ■ PRONE POSITION

Potential Problems	Supportive Measures for Patients with Cervical Injuries	Supportive Measures for Patients with Thoracic or Lumbar Injuries
Rotation, flexion, or extension of an unstable neck fracture site with subsequent interruption of bony healing and possible loss of function	Padding to support the chin and forehead and allow a "breathing space"	
Loosening of brace with loss of immobilization resulting in interrupted bony healing and possible loss of function	One or two pillows to support chest and relieve pressure on bars of the Halo-brace	
Hyperextension of lumbar curve; undue pressure on iliac crests and male genitalia; pressure on female breasts; and difficulty breathing	Pillow placed under abdomen	Pillow placed under abdomen
Hyperextension of knees, undue pressure on knees and toes, and foot drop	Pillow placed under lower legs to flex legs slightly, relieve pressure on knees, and promote plantar flexion	Pillow placed under lower legs to flex legs slightly, relieve pressure on knees, and promote plantar flexion
Brachial plexus damage and impaired circulation	Place arms in comfortable position alleviating pressure on shoulders	Place arms in comfortable position alleviating pressure on shoulders
Undue pressure on toes; foot drop	Position feet between mattress and footboard	Position feet between mattress and footboard

The prone position is of great value for the patient in a Halo-thoracic brace. Support the chest with one or two pillows to avoid excessive pressure on Halo bars. No other padding around the face or forehead is needed. See Figure 14–10.

- *Trunk.* Sometimes it is necessary to support the entire length of the body with pillows to "bridge" certain areas where it is important to relieve pressure. When the chest is supported with a pillow, it relieves pressure on the shoulders (to protect the brachial plexus) and, used with a pillow under the thighs, will bridge the genital area for the male patient. A pillow placed across the abdomen, just below the diaphragm, will ease breathing. The soft surface still protects the iliac crests and male genitalia.

- *Extremities.* For patients with cervical injuries, slightly flex or extend arms in position of comfort. Use hand splints to maintain functional alignment. Flex the knees slightly and support with padding above and below. Place the feet between the mattress and footboard. See Figure 14–11. Avoid pressure from footboard or padding touching the soles of the feet.

Sitting position Patients with cervical injuries, once braced, are encouraged to move in bed as tolerated. Orthopedic surgeons will specifically order the sitting position for patients with thoracic and lumbar injuries. (Elevation of the head of the bed will be stipulated from 30 to 90 degrees.) Sitting is limited mostly to mealtimes or short periods of 20 to 30 minutes, because it increases the load on the healing spinal

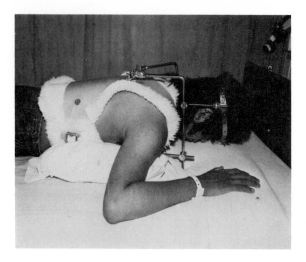

FIGURE 14–10 ■ One or two pillows placed under the chest supports the patient in a Halo-brace in the prone position. Additional padding around the face or forehead is not necessary.

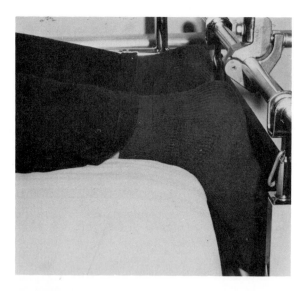

FIGURE 14–11 ■ In the prone position, the feet may be carefully placed between the mattress and the footboard to achieve a 90-degree angle position without pressure on either tops or soles of feet.

fracture site and causes excess pressure on the buttocks. The position is also difficult to maintain for any length of time without slipping.

Nurses must take measures to maintain the patient's balance; prevent rotational trunk movement; protect the sacral skin; and, above all

for the patient with paraplegia, avoid undue pressure on or curvature of the lumbar and thoracic spine. See Table 14–4 for a summary of potential problems and supportive measures associated with this position.

- *Head/neck.* During the early stages patients with cervical injuries will need the support of neck orthoses. Be sure to apply braces before the patient sits up to avoid any neck movement.
- *Trunk.* During the early stages patients with cervical injuries may need to be supported by pillows at the side to prevent loss of balance.

  Patients with thoracic or lumbar injuries must avoid any rotational movement of the trunk. Be sure patients are instructed accordingly. For example, they should avoid reaching for objects on the bedside table.
- *Extremities.* Always support the paralyzed upper extremities of patients with cervical injuries at the elbow and wrist with the palms of your hands when moving. Support arms with pillows to avoid gravitational pulling, which can cause considerable shoulder pain, impair circulation, and cause gravitational edema.

  Support the knees of patients with thoracic or lumbar injuries with pillows placed lengthwise. This will cause *slight* flexion of the legs to relieve pull on the back. See Figure 14–12. Avoid actually bending knees, which

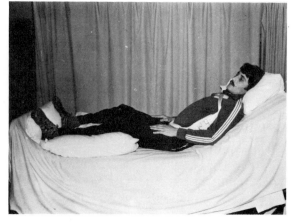

FIGURE 14–12 ■ A paraplegic patient sitting in bed at a 45-degree angle. Pillows placed lengthwise flex knees slightly to prevent back strain and support feet.

TABLE 14–4 ■ SITTING POSITION IN BED

Potential Problems	Supportive Measures for Patients with Cervical Injuries	Supportive Measures for Patients with Thoracic or Lumbar Injuries
Loss of neck immobilization with interrupted healing of the bone and possible decrease in function	Position neck orthosis before attempting to sit up	
Loss of position; possibility of falling	Pillows placed at patient's sides to maintain balance	
Shoulder pain; impaired circulation; gravitational edema of forearms and hands	Pillows placed under arms for support	
Strain on fracture site of lower spine	Padding under knees not necessary	Pillow placed under knees to relieve pull on lower spine; eventually long sitting (without supports) allowed
Pressure area on heels; foot drop	Padding under ankles to relieve pressure on heels; footboard to maintain plantar flexion	Padding under ankles to relieve pressure on heels; footboard to maintain plantar flexion

will impair circulation and predispose the patient to thrombus formation. Remember to place pillows *before* raising the head of the bed. Allow full extension of the legs (long sitting) when specifically ordered. See Figure 14–13. Remove padding at the knees to allow long sitting when the spine is more stable.

Support the ankles to prevent pressure on heels and support feet in the 90-degree position with padding. Avoid pressing feet hard on the footboard because this increases spasm or clonus and may damage the skin.

Special immobilization beds

This section will describe the two beds most widely recommended during the acute stage: the Stoke-Eggerton turning and tilting bed and the Wedge-Stryker turning frame. The Keane Roto-Rest bed, which continually rotates the patient to relieve pressure, is also suitable for acute care. The CircOlectric bed is also a device that

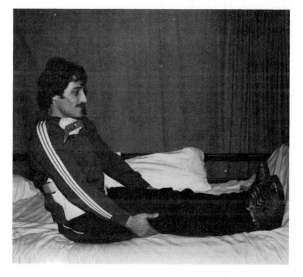

FIGURE 14–13 ■ A paraplegic patient is allowed to use the "long sitting" position as spinal stability increases. The position facilitates lower extremity activities such as dressing.

assists with turning, but experts agree that it should be avoided during initial management because it may cause excessive axial loading on the fracture site and postural hypotension due to a rapid progression to the upright position.

Many physicians prefer to have patients with complicated injuries in regular beds, relying on diligent and cautious turning and avoiding the prone position required on turning frames. Other specialized beds that minimize pressure (for example, water, air-fluidized, or MUD beds) may be specifically indicated later for the prevention or treatment of pressure sores. Refer to Supplemental Readings at the end of this chapter for more information.

The Stoke-Eggerton bed The Stoke-Eggerton turning and tilting electrical bed was designed by Sir Ludwig Guttman in Britain especially for the acutely injured patient with a high-level injury or associated injuries. It is a device that smoothly turns the patient from the supine to the side-lying position by simple electric controls. See Figure 14–14.

The mattress platform and the mattress itself are divided into three longitudinal sections and supported on a tubular frame that houses the electrical motors. When you wish to turn the patient to a side-lying position, operate the electrical control on the side of the bed toward which the patient will be turning. (This is an added safety feature; the motors that control the movable portions of the bed operate independently and the patient will always be turned toward you.) The mattress section nearest to you will remain flat while the middle and opposite sections will operate as one unit to elevate that side of the bed up to 70 degrees. Take advantage of the full 70 degrees when the patient is in the side-lying position to ensure maximum weight shift and relief of pressure. Next, walk to the opposite side of the bed and operate the control to elevate the flat portion of the mattress 30 degrees. This provides a "trough" for the patient to lie in, which adds to security and comfort. (This maneuver may actually be performed first.) Another important safety measure is to secure all tubing before and after each change of position. If possible attach the catheter bag to the foot of the bed. If it is overlooked and remains attached to the elevated side, urinary backflow will occur quickly.

Position the patient in basic alignment and schedule turns from side to side every two hours. A full-length synthetic sheepskin is an excellent adjunct to this bed. Although the mattress is made of foam, some protective covering should be added to keep it clean. Position the patient as follows:

1. *Side-lying.* The advantages, precautions, and nursing care measures previously described also apply when the patient is on a Stoke bed.

- *Head/neck.* A traction unit may be added for a patient with a cervical injury. The head of the bed tilts upward, so countertraction is possible. See Figure 14–15. The cervical traction unit is currently limited to a straight horizontal pull; a more flexed position of the neck is not possible. To prevent neck movement while turning and in the side-lying position, two steel arms with horseshoe-shaped pads extend from the head of the bed to fit over the ear. They have a tendency to slip and some patients find them dreadfully uncomfortable. Instead, it is best to support the patient's head with both hands during turning and immobilize it with some padded sandbags. Be sure to consider these measures *before* turning the patient.
- *Trunk.* If the patient has a tendency to slip forward, especially those with movement of the upper torso, a rolled pillow may be placed in front of the chest. A large restraint belt may be used for additional safety.
- *Extremities.* For patients with cervical injuries, support the bottom arm in an extended position on the arm board attachment (see Figure 14–16) and the top arm with pillows. Sometimes it is necessary to tie the supporting pillow to the bed frame with a cloth restraint to maintain the position of the paralyzed arm. A footboard attachment is also available.

2. *Supine.* The advantages, precautions, and nursing care measures previously described also apply when the patient is on a Stoke bed.

It is necessary to logroll the patient manually two or three times during a 24-hour period to change the sheets, inspect the skin, wash the back, and perform bowel procedures.

If it is necssary to *transport* the patient, remember that the additional width makes the Stoke bed difficult if not impossible to move

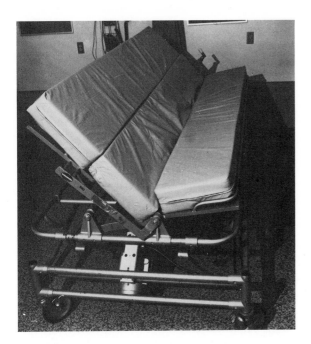

FIGURE 14–14 ■ The Stoke-Eggerton bed is an electrically controlled turning and tilting device. Note the movable longitudinal sections that create a "trough" to support the patient.

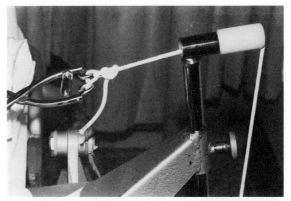

FIGURE 14–15 ■ A cervical traction unit.

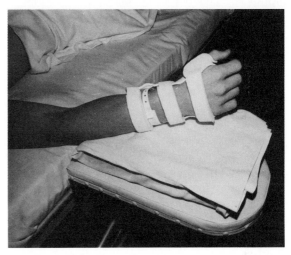

FIGURE 14–16 ■ An attachable arm board.

through standard room and elevator doors. The additional weight also makes it cumbersome to move. If the patient is to be moved to another surface for special diagnostic or operative procedures, choose the mobilizer, if possible, since the standard surgilift does not fit under the tubular frame of the bed. A three- or four-person lift is the only alternative.

The Stoke bed has several distinct advantages: caring for the critically ill or unconscious patient with associated chest or other injuries is easier, safer, and more comfortable for the patient, and only one nurse is required to turn the patient. The greatest disadvantage is the larger size and weight of the bed. With engineering advancements, however, some of these problems will no doubt diminish on subsequent models.

The Stoke bed can be disassembled for shipping. To meet individual electrical standards, it should be examined and approved within each institution.

The Wedge-Stryker Frame The turning frame most widely used at the present time is the Wedge-Stryker frame. It is noted for its wedge or

"pie" shape formed by the anterior and posterior frames for added protection against movement of the spine when turning; simplicity of operation (requiring only one person to complete the turn); and lightweight but sturdy structure. See Figure 14–17.

The Stryker frame is most suitable for patients with uncomplicated low cervical or thoracic or lumbar injuries. It is unsuitable for obese patients (check the manufacturer's recommended weight limit—usually not over 200 pounds); unconscious patients; or patients with respiratory complications or severe restlessness from head injury, a psychiatric condition, or alcoholic state.

Several adjustments are available to help meet individual requirements. A padded metal

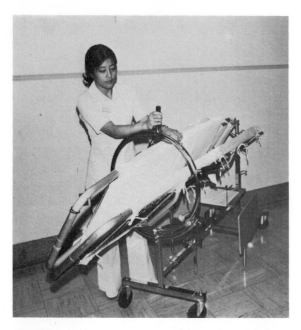

FIGURE 14–17 ■ The Wedge-Stryker frame offers simplicity of operation. Note the wedge shape formed by the frames for maximum security when turning the patient.

face mask can be attached to minimize neck rotation for patients with cervical injury, but without additional foam padding it fits poorly and is usually very uncomfortable. Face straps are attached to the frame for patients with thoracic or lumbar injuries. Adjustable arm boards and a footboard are available. The canvas on the anterior frame can be lengthened or shortened according to the patient's height. (When the patient is prone, the tops of the feet should just clear the canvas to dangle over the edge at a 90-degree angle.) There is also an adjustment, located on the circular turning ring, to press the frames more closely together to accommodate thinner patients.

To turn the patient, secure the frame to a single point at the head of the bed; clamp the circular ring in place; secure safety straps (two or three); complete the turn; and lock the frame into position. (Detailed instructional steps should be provided by the manufacturer and institution.) For the quadriplegic patient it is most convenient to attach the top frame and close the circular ring before removing the arm boards. Weak arms can then be supported on the arm boards until the last minute before securing with the safety straps.

Another safety feature is to secure all tubing just before and after each turn. Stop to visualize the exact route the IV tubing will follow. Should the IV bag be passed under the frame or over the top? Be sure the catheter bag is placed on the side toward which the patient is turning. It is a good idea to use a loosely fastened safety strap to restrain patients who are restless or experiencing spasms or who have an incomplete injury.

Position the patient in basic alignment and schedule turns every two hours. It is possible to adjust the time to three hours prone and one hour supine or vice versa for special needs. A one-inch continuous foam mattress can be designed to cover both anterior and posterior canvases. Again, a full-length sheepskin is an important adjunct. Padding of this thickness eliminates the need for numerous smaller pads, which tend to be misplaced or slip.

1. *Supine.* The advantages, precautions, and nursing care measures previously described also apply to the Stryker frame. Arm boards that adjust to height and lateral position accompany the frame. A removable footboard attachment is also available.

If smaller pads are to be used, the natural curvatures of the head, back, knees, and ankles must be supported. Place a small roll under the neck of the patient with a cervical injury to make the patient comfortable and prevent neck fatigue. Narrow one- or two-inch foam pads are placed under the occiput, lumbar curvature, and lower thigh and above the ankles.

2. *Prone.* Again, general principles described previously apply, such as avoiding undue curvature of the spine and protecting the shoulders, male genitalia, iliac crest bones, knees, and feet. The prone position allows for maximum hand activities involved with self-care such as personal hygiene, reading, or writing. Eating is much easier although the patient may need straws and assistance with cutting meat. Bowel procedures should also be performed while prone. Removing a canvas strip to insert a bedpan is most dangerous, especially for lumbosacral injuries. The prone position improves visualization of the anal area, which is essential when using manual evacuation techniques.

- *Head/neck.* Traction and a cervical face piece can be added for patients with cervical injuries. Be sure the forehead and the chin are well protected to prevent skin breakdown. Additional foam pads with soft coverings are usually necessary. Countertraction is possible by tilting the head of the bed up.
- *Trunk.* If smaller pads are to be used, one- or two-inch narrow foam pads are best. They may be positioned between the shoulder and just above the nipple line; across the abdomen below the diaphragm and above the pubis; and above the knees and just above the ankles. This padding helps relieve pressure on the clavicle, ease body weight pressing on female breasts, enhance lung capacity, bridge the male genitalia, and relieve pressure on knees. It is also believed to be less fatiguing on back muscles.

  For the male patient an indwelling catheter can be padded with gauze and taped just above the iliac crest to promote drainage and avoid any pressure on the abdomen. Again, if sheepskin is used it is not necessary to add additional foam pads. If not, a one-inch foam pad can cover the iliac crests and, along with another pad on the thighs, will bridge the genital area.
- *Extremities.* Check the point at which the front of the shoulders touch the frame. This is especially important for patients with cervical injuries; those without sensation will be unable to feel numbness, tingling, or weakness in the arm indicating pressure on the brachial plexus. To avoid pressure on this area the arm boards should be elevated to the level of the frame and should be padded with pillows or foam and comfortable for the patient; the patient's arms should be extended upward or outward.

If it is necessary to transfer the patient to another surface, the surgilift is the method of choice as the mobilizer is not compatible with the turning ring of the Stryker frame. The only alternative is a three- or four-person lift. To use the surgilift correctly:

- Place the sheepskin and then canvas over the patient in the prone position before placing the top of the frame on the patient.
- Tuck straps in carefully so they will not interfere with turning the frame, and turn the patient.
- Lift with a metal frame or surgilift, pulling corresponding straps on each side simultaneously to avoid an uneven movement.

If transporting the patient on the frame, it is wise to use the supine position to promote patient observation. Surgery can also be performed while the patient is on the Stryker frame.

The Wedge-Stryker frame is advantageous for selected uncomplicated injuries for its ease in turning and maximal spinal immobilization. It is also convenient to move the frame freely around the ward to encourage socialization. Detachable traction devices, arm boards, and footboards are available. Its greatest disadvantage is that the patient may not be able to tolerate the prone position and the frame does not allow for a side-lying position.

Cervical traction

Skeletal traction in the treatment of cervical spine injuries is universal. Realignment of the spinal canal not only corrects the mechanical deformation and protects the cord and nerve roots from further compression but also may enhance vascular supply. Skeletal traction may be used to achieve both reduction and immobilization of the fracture. See Figure 14–18.

Various types of skull traction devices, tongs or calipers, may be used. See Table 14–5 and Procedure 14–1. The Halo-ring is being used more and more as an immediate skull traction device with the support vest being attached at a later date.

When cervical traction is in place, nursing care includes the following:

- Maintain a constant traction force at all times. Ensure that weights hang freely and do not touch the floor. Check this especially during postural drainage and chest physiotherapy. Also check that the knot on the traction rope tied to the skull fixation device is clear of the traction pulley or traction collar. If not, move

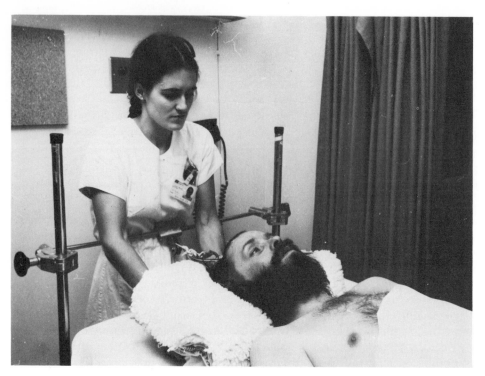

FIGURE 14–18 ■ Cervical traction.

the patient down in bed using a four-person lift with the patient in a supine position. If this is a continual problem, check with the physician to see if countertraction can be applied by raising the head of the bed.

If the tongs should be accidentally dislodged, immediately reapply traction by immobilizing the head and neck with your hands. Maintain a gentle, but firm, pressure on the jaw and occiput and summon the physician immediately. Application of a soft collar with sandbags will assist with immobilization. It is difficult to apply halter traction without manipulating the neck and therefore presents too much risk for the patient and the nurse. To prevent infection, clean and dress the original tong sights and look for leakage of cerebrospinal fluid (a clear, yellowish fluid that will leave rings on the bed linen and test positively for sugar on a reagent paper strip). A specimen of any fluid leakage should be collected for laboratory identification.

• Clean insertion sites regularly every four to eight hours. See Procedure 14–2.

• Turn and position the patient every two hours, regardless of what type of bed or frame is used, to combat the hazards of immobility. Chapter 4 contains a procedure for logrolling the patient. The person at the patient's head must reach around the traction device and place one or both forearms just behind the skull tongs with extended hands reaching the patient's shoulders. (In other words the elbows are placed flat along the bed.) If it is too difficult to place your arm or will be too difficult to remove your arm once the patient is turned, simply use one hand to guide the head and neck and extend the other arm and hand to the patient's shoulder to ensure alignment. Before turning times, explain the procedure carefully, as patients tend to be extremely apprehensive during this time.

Immobilizing the Spine with Orthoses

Orthoses are externally applied force systems (either braces or splints) that exert mechanical pressure on the body at prescribed points.

TABLE 14–5 ■ SKULL TRACTION DEVICES

Type	Description	Preparation for Application	Special Equipment
Crutchfield tongs	Small skull calipers that fit to the top of the head, just behind the hairline	Requires localized shave preparation and scalp incisions	Requires drill for application; tightening screw device attached directly to tongs for individual adjustment
Cone-Barton tongs	Larger skull calipers that fit to the side of the head, just above the ear, with pointed pins that insert directly into the skull	Requires localized shave preparation	A wrench (not interchangeable) accompanies each set of tongs to fit tightening device
Vinke tongs	Large skull tongs that fit to the side of the head, again just above the ear, with an interlocking device between the inner and outer tables of the skull for maximum stability; prevention of slipping or dislodging is the primary feature of these tongs	Requires localized shave preparation and scalp incisions	Specialized Vinke drill accompanies tongs for application
Gardner-Wells tongs	Large tongs that fit to the head just above the ear that feature large side knobs to grasp for insertion; Gardner-Wells tongs do not actually penetrate the skull; may be inserted by skilled paramedical personnel at the accident site	No shave preparation or incisions necessary	No drills or other equipment necessary

Spinal orthoses frequently apply pressure to the head or torso at some distance from the spine itself to limit movement and control position. Treatment focuses on achieving desirable position and limiting movement so that the spinal fracture site can heal in good alignment preventing long-term complications such as scoliosis or muscle contractures.

In the immediate postinjury phase rigid immobilization is warranted in the presence of serious instability to prevent irreversible neurological damage secondary to bony impingement on the spinal cord. As rehabilitation progresses, callus formation will eventually heal the bony injury and less rigid external support will be required to maintain alignment. While surgical intervention may realign the vertebral column, bone growth is still required to complete healing. For this reason a brace is required during the postoperative period. As a general rule of thumb rigid immobilization of a fractured spine is necessary for the first three months after injury and a less rigid support is needed for the next two to three months.

The *orthotist* works in close collaboration with the treatment team, particularly the orthopedic surgeon, to provide effective and comfortable suport to the damaged skeletal system. The orthotist measures, designs, and fabricates a variety of braces and may modify commercially

PROCEDURE 14–1 ■ APPLICATION OF SKULL TRACTION DEVICES

Purpose

The purpose of applying skull traction devices to produce cervical traction is to simply maintain alignment or, with additional weights added, reduce the fracture.

Equipment

- Immobilization bed of choice with traction setup
- Rope
- Selected weights
- Cardiac monitor (optional)
- Nasogastric tube (optional)
- Local anesthetic such as 1% lidocaine hydrochloride with a variety of syringes and needles
- Sterilized tray including appropriate devices, drills (optional), and specialized equipment (see Table 14–5)
- Razor and shaving equipment (optional)
- Sterile gloves for physician (optional)

Action	Rationale
1. Explain procedure to patient. Give presedation as ordered.	This is a painful procedure and can be frightening, especially when the skull is penetrated.
2. Place patient on the immobilization bed of choice and assemble appropriate traction equipment.	The cervical traction units on Stryker and Stoke beds have already been described. There are traction set-ups, with two supporting poles at either side and a crossbar with sliding pulley apparatus, that fit many regular beds or emergency stretcher beds. See Figure 14–18.
3. Provide continuous cardiac monitoring during procedure for severely traumatized, fatigued, and older patients.	The added stress of inserting skull traction devices may precipitate pulse irregularities, cardiac arrhythmias, and fainting.
4. If necessary, insert a nasogastric tube to evacuate stomach contents before proceeding.	The stress of this procedure can precipitate aspiration if the newly injured patient has recently eaten.

(Procedure continues)

produced braces. However, correct application is essential to provide their fullest benefit. This, and meticulous care of the skin at points where the brace applies pressure to the body surface, are major nursing responsibilities. If the contact force exceeds capillary pressure, blanching, then redness, and later ischemia will occur. Such pressure concentrations will normally cause extreme pain, which acts as a warning mechanism, but if the brace covers an area of the body that is without sensation, the nurse must be especially conscientious about skin care.

When the patient requires an orthotic device the nurse should be familiar with:

- The appearance and function of the brace
- The method of application (or donning)

- Specific safety precautions and procedures
- The contact points on the body where the brace exerts the greatest pressure
- The degree of physical activity allowed
- Measures for removing the brace

Cervical orthoses will be described in three broad categories: those that provide rigid immobilization (the Halo apparatus); those that provide moderate stabilization (neck poster appliances such as the Guilford brace); and orthopedic collars that limit neck movements minimally.

Thoracolumbar orthoses will be described in two categories: standard hyperextension braces (such as the Jewitt): and individualized trunk supports (such as body jackets or casts).

PROCEDURE 14–1 ■ (continued)

Action	Rationale
5. In most instances, assist physician to shave area surrounding tong insertion sites.	This minimizes risk of infection spreading to inner table of skull.
6. Clean insertion sites with antiseptic solution.	
7. In most instances, assist physician to infiltrate insertion sites with local anesthetic.	
8. When necessary, assist physician with scalpel incisions, drill penetration, and tong insertion.	
9. Secure selected weights, thread through a pulley or traction device, and tie to skull tongs or calipers to produce traction.	Traction may be held in a neutral, extension, or flexion position to counteract the mechanism of injury. Traction begins from 5 to 50 lb depending on the bony level of injury involved.
10. Ensure that weights hang freely and do not touch floor. Also the knot on traction rope tied to skull fixation device must be clear of pulley or traction collar.	This establishes a constant traction pull.
11. Following the procedure, assist with positioning patient for X-ray evaluation.	This helps to determine alignment and traction force. If closed reduction is being attempted serial clinical and X-ray evaluation is needed. Additional weights are added in 5-lb increments after 15-min intervals. The maximum amount of weight usually varies.
12. Anticipate discomfort at insertion sites, headaches, and neck discomfort. Give analgesics as ordered.	The patient needs to be continually evaluated for pain tolerance, especially if traction forces are increased.

The Halo-thoracic brace

The Halo apparatus has three main parts:

1. The halo-ring, which fits around the head and is fixed to the skull with metal pins
2. A plastic or plaster vest that suspends the weight of the apparatus around the chest
3. A metal frame of adjustable bars that connects the ring to the vest

See Figure 14–19. The Halo has virtually replaced skeletal traction, turning frames, and prolonged periods of bedrest formerly used to immobilize the cervical spine during bony healing. See Procedure 14–3 for method of application of this rigid immobilization device.

Care of the skin Care of the skin at the pin-site insertion points and under the vest is of utmost importance. Nursing care measures to maintain the protective functions of the skin include cleaning of the pin site areas and regular inspection of the skin, daily hygiene, and changing of vest liners when necessary. See Procedures 14–4 through 14–6. A synthetic sheepskin liner a few sizes larger than the vest will help protect the paralyzed patient without sensation from the hard edges of the brace. Synthetic sheepskin tends to be cooler and less irritating than natural wool sheepskin. Collaborate with the occupational therapist to design patterns and make liners.

Points of greatest pressure on the skin tend to be the vest edges, the tops of the shoulders, and the scapular blades. Pressure points can also occur over the spinous processes from T_1 to T_3. Using a bright flashlight the nurse can make a thorough skin inspection under the Halo vest with the patient in a side-lying position. Be sure to observe patients with unusual chest contours very carefully. Inspect the skin every eight hours for the first 48 to 72 hours after application of

PROCEDURE 14–2 ■ TONG SITE CARE

Purpose

The purpose of tong site care is to maintain cleanliness and prevent infection at tong insertion sites.

Equipment

- Face mask
- Sterile dressing tray
- Package of sterile cotton-tipped applicators
- Hydrogen peroxide
- Bacteriostatic solution

Action	Rationale
1. Put on face mask.	To minimize risk of infection.
2. Set up small dressing tray with sterile cotton-tipped applicators and small containers of sterile cleaning solution (hydrogen peroxide) and bacteriostatic solution (tincture of Savlon 1:30).	
3. Remove gauze wrapped around tong site.	
4. Observe condition of tissue surrounding each tong site, looking for any redness, swelling, skin tension, tenderness, or pruritis.	These signs may indicate infection.
5. Clean each tong site with a sterile applicator dipped in hydrogen peroxide. Clean in one sweeping motion around tong site; discard swab. Gently repeat until site is clean. Do not dab or prod with swab, even to remove crusting. This additional trauma is a major cause of tong site infection because it increases irritation.	Serous crusting is common. 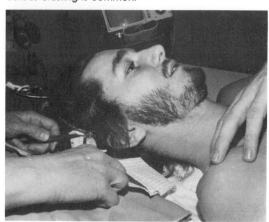
6. Apply a nonocclusive bacteriostatic solution (with or without dressings). A 2 × 2 in. gauze unfolded then refolded lengthwise and tied around the tong will stay in place best.	Sprays or ointments may cake around insertion sites and increase risk of infection.
7. If drainage is present obtain a wound culture.	Infection may be present and a course of antibiotics may be necessary. If infection cannot be controlled, traction device may have to be removed and reinserted to prevent more serious complications of abscess formation or osteomyelitis.
8. Wash patient's hair weekly or more often with a liquid antibacterial soap.	Bathrooms large enough for beds and equipped with long hose spray attachments are ideal.

the vest, then daily for one week, and twice weekly thereafter until the brace is removed (Figure 14–20). A practical way to monitor skin checks is presented in Table 14–6. Regular turning must be maintained, not only to prevent skin breakdown but also to relieve pressure on pin sites. Be alert for any strange odors that may indicate skin breakdown. If skin breakdown is evident, the vest must be removed and traction maintained on bedrest with the Halo-ring.

Maintaining cleanliness of the skin underneath the vest requires daily washing. It may also be necessary to change the vest liners every month or so, particularly since quadriplegic patients are prone to excessive sweating and are relearning eating skills. Trapped food particles quickly contaminate the liner and cause skin breakdown. (See Procedures on washing and changing Halo-vest liners for instructions.)

Activity   Once the Halo is donned and the physician is satisfied with the position and immobilization of the spine, a patient with quadriplegia can be mobilized in a wheelchair within days after injury. Mobilization is introduced gradually by elevating the head of the bed for longer and longer intervals. Postural hypotension causing dizziness or fainting is the major problem. As soon as patients can sit upright for 20 minutes, however, the physical therapist should assess their readiness for sitting in a wheelchair and will then perform the initial transfer. Modifications of basic transfer techniques are described in Chapter 16. Progression to mat activities and wheelchair management is considered next.

To prevent chest infections, which if left unchecked may necessitate removal of the vest to gain access to the chest, incentive spirometry to encourage deep breathing may be helpful. Assisted coughing and postural drainage are also possible when the Halo apparatus is in place. The Halo apparatus weighs about 25 pounds and does restrict chest expansion. See Procedure 14–7 for emergency removal of the Halo-vest.

Removal   Throughout the 10 to 12 weeks the Halo is in place, the physician will probably order periodic X rays to evaluate healing. Before planning final removal of the brace, flexion and extension views will be needed to ascertain ligamentous healing. The best films are obtained in the X-ray department (as opposed to portable

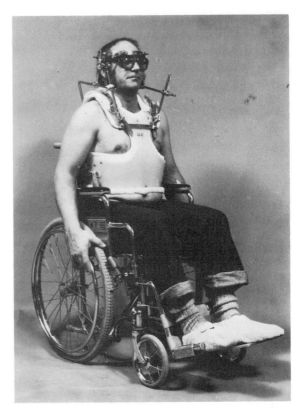

FIGURE 14–19 ■ The Halo device has created a breakthrough in medical management by allowing early mobilization for patients with cervical injuries.

films) with the patient sitting in a wheelchair. To accomplish this the vest is removed and the Halo-ring is left in place in case reapplication is necessary. Meanwhile a neck brace is applied for protection until X-ray evaluation can be completed. Thereafter a less restrictive cervical orthosis or soft collar is usually required.

The Guilford brace

The Guilford brace is an example of the "post" style cervicothoracic orthoses. These neck braces afford fairly good support limiting flexion and to a lesser extent extension and rotational movements. This type of orthosis is characterized by rigid metal supports between the chest plate and chin support anteriorly and between the back plate and occipital support posteriorly. See Figure 14–21. These posts are usually adjustable, and there are commonly two or four of them. Leather straps over the shoulders

PROCEDURE 14–3 ■ APPLICATION OF THE HALO-THORACIC BRACE

Purpose

The purpose of the Halo-thoracic brace is to provide rigid immobilization of the cervical spine. The Halo-ring may first be used as a traction device, or the ring and vest may be donned simultaneously following the removal of skull tongs or calipers.

Equipment

The application of the Halo-ring is a sterile procedure and the equipment needed is similar to that used for skull tong insertion:

- Local anesthetic such as 1% lidocaine hydrochloride with a variety of syringes and needles
- Sterilized tray including Halo-rings in several sizes, positioning plates, and four pins
- Gauze pads, forceps, and antiseptic solution for preparing pin sites
- Hair scissors or clippers (optional)
- Sterile gloves for physician to wear while screwing pins into place
- Variety of "Halo-tools" necessary for adjustments—torque screwdrivers for tightening skull pins, Allen, or L-shaped, wrenches to fit smaller sockets, and regular wrenches to fit larger sockets of the connecting bars between Halo-ring and vest

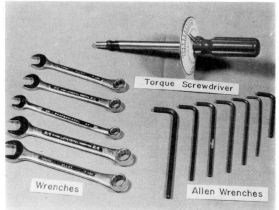

Tools for application and adjustment of Halo

Action	Rationale
Preparation and Selection of Equipment	
1. Collaborate with physician to assess patient's general condition, particularly respiratory status.	The Halo-vest tends to limit chest expansion and accessibility of chest wall. It may be necessary to delay application of Halo vest if frequent clapping and vibration is necessary to free lungs of secretions or if patient risks developing cardiopulmonary problems.
2. To obtain correct vest size, measure chest circumference at level of xiphoid process (at base of sternum).	Plastic vests with natural or synthetic sheepskin liners are available in a variety of sizes (34, 36, 38, and so on).
3. Note any irregular shape or bony protuberances of chest and back.	A plaster vest, shaped to individual, may be necessary to prevent undue pressure that might cause skin breakdown.
4. Plan time for procedure and explain it to patient. Give presedation as ordered.	Although actual procedure may not be that painful, it is usually quite frightening because of pressure felt on skull.
5. Position patient supine on a firm bed or stretcher with head just beyond edge. The head must be supported by an assistant's hands or a 4-in.-wide board placed under head and back. (A Stryker frame may be used following the same principles.)	This maintains skeletal alignment and guards against inadvertent movement of neck.

(Procedure continues)

PROCEDURE 14–3 ■ (continued)

Action	Rationale
6. Assist physician to measure head and select a Halo-ring that will allow $1\frac{1}{2}$ cm clearance all around head.	

Application of Halo-Ring

Action	Rationale
7. Clean scalp around each of four intended pin site areas with an antiseptic solution; two areas on forehead and two at back of head. Clip hair if necessary.	Hair may need to be trimmed if long or matted with blood or debris, but head need not be shaved.
8. Assist physician to infiltrate each of four pin sites with local anesthetic. The physician will then secure ring temporarily with positioning plates. When desired position is achieved, physician will don sterile gloves and screw each pin into place by hand. Posteriorly, the ring is placed about 1/8 in. above ear (not touching pinnae, which are very sensitive) and anteriorly, just above eyebrows.	
9. Provide torque screwdrivers to tighten pins, ideally used by two operators tightening opposite pins simultaneously. Final tension should reach about 5.5 to 6 kg/cm in adult (as measured by the dial on torque screwdriver). When desired tension is obtained, lock nuts are tightened with Allen wrenches to prevent pins from working loose.	

Application of the Halo-Vest

Action	Rationale
10. Assist physician to apply vest. Assemble vest and sheepskin liners. Generally posterior vest is placed on the back with patient logrolled to the side (head and neck well supported). The patient is returned to supine position and the anterior vest is placed. The metal framework is then loosely attached to connect vest and ring. When the apparatus is in proper alignment for desired degree of traction, physician will use various sizes of regular wrenches to tighten nuts and bolts connecting bars to the ring and then bars to the vest.	
11. Following the procedure, assist with positioning patient for radiological evaluation.	A cervical spine X ray to determine alignment or a skull X ray to check depth of skull pins may be ordered.
12. Be alert for the following problems and notify physician to make corrective adjustments if:	
• Discomfort persists for more than 24 to 48 hr.	Patients may have headaches for a day or two, which can usually be relieved with mild analgesics. Once established, the Halo is surprisingly comfortable.
• Persistent neck pain or swallowing difficulties occur.	These problems often indicate too much hyperextension.
• Patient cannot see straight ahead.	This problem indicates the apparatus is on slightly crooked.

This information is based on Young and Thomassen (1974) and Nickel (1977).

PROCEDURE 14–4 ■ HALO PIN SITE CARE

Purpose

The purpose of pin site care is to maintain cleanliness and prevent infection of pin sites.

Equipment

- 1 sterile bowl or medicine cup
- 2 packages of sterile cotton-tipped applicators
- Cleaning solution, such as hydrogen peroxide or liquid soap (Savlon solution 1:100)

Action

1. Gently clean each pin site separately with sterile applicator dipped in Savlon 1:100. Clean in one sweeping motion around pin site; discard applicator. Repeat until site is clean. Do not dab or prod with applicator even to remove crusting.
This additional trauma is a major cause of pin site infection from irritation.

Rationale

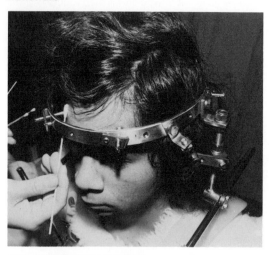

Cleaning solutions left on skin will cause excoriation.

2. In the same manner dry pin site with dry sterile applicator.

3. Repeat procedure for every pin site.

4. Observe condition of tissue around each pin site. Look for any redness, swelling, crusting, skin tension, tenderness, or pruritis.

These may indicate infection or a loose pin.

5. Repeat procedure every morning and evening, or more frequently if pin sites are crusty or infected.

6. Wash patient's hair with antibacterial soap weekly, or as needed. Protect vest with plastic sheeting.

Hair washing greatly minimizes risk of infection.

7. Tighten bolts on connecting framework weekly. Never pull directly on bars, framework straps, or vest when turning or transferring patient.

These measures protect brace from loosening, which could dislodge pins.

8. If a pin is loose, do not move patient. Summon physician to correct situation.

Nickel (1977) warns that pins should be tightened only when they become loose. Routine tightening of pins will hasten erosions and penetrations. If, on tightening, a pin appears to be penetrating too deeply, or if there is excessive inflammation around pin site, the pin should be replaced in an adjacent location.

PROCEDURE 14–5 ■ WASHING UNDERNEATH THE HALO-VEST

Purpose

The purpose of washing under the Halo-vest is to maintain cleanliness and prevent skin breakdown.

Equipment

- Washcloths (one wet and one dry)
- Basin of water
- Pillows to secure patient in recumbent position

Action	Rationale
1. Use water without soap.	This prevents irritants from accumulating on skin. It is also unwise to use lotions or powders.
2. Ring washcloth out thoroughly.	This minimizes risk that the liner will get wet. A wet lining will become matted, is difficult to dry (may take several days to do so), and can cause skin problems.
3. Wash patient by reaching under the vest. Securely support patient in a supine, prone, or side-lying position with pillows. Loosen lower straps to gain more access to chest and back. Take care not to stress framework.	Gentle handling prevents movement of the cervical spine.
4. Dry with washcloth in the same manner.	Towels are too bulky.

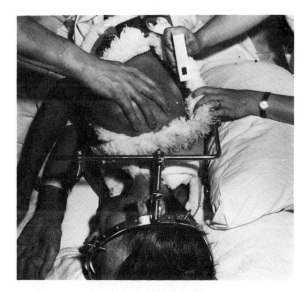

FIGURE 14–20 ■ With the patient in a side-lying position a skin inspection is performed with the aid of a bright flashlight.

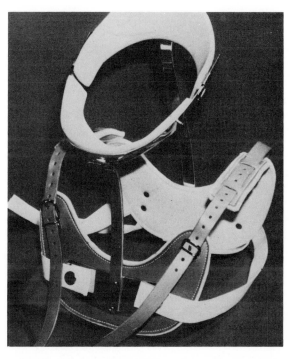

FIGURE 14–21 ■ The Guilford brace is an example of a cervical orthosis that provides moderate support.

PROCEDURE 14–6 ■ CHANGING HALO-VEST LINERS

Purpose

The purpose of this care is to protect the skin, to prevent skin breakdown, and to maintain personal hygiene.

Equipment

- A *firm* stretcher, table, or bed
- Three pillows
- Two clean liners (anterior and posterior)
- Additional sheepskin pieces (optional)
- Water, soap, face cloth, and small towel

Action and Rationale

1. Position patient prone on a firm surface with one or two pillows under chest. Place a third pillow under lower legs to relieve pressure on feet.
Front bars of brace must be well supported and well *balanced* to maintain alignment throughout procedure.

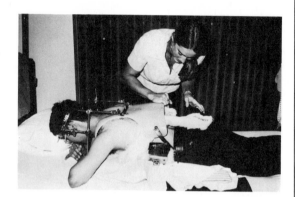

2. Release side buckles *only.* This will maintain maximum support to neck.

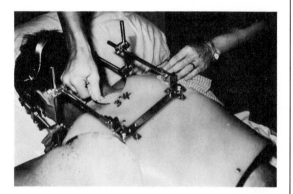

3. Beginning at the shoulders, loosen liner from vest by separating Velcro closures; roll liner downward to bottom of vest. This will move or lift vest as little as possible.

4. Inspect the skin and thoroughly wash and dry the back.

5. Slide a new liner into position under the vest. Once liner is in position, stick liner Velcro to vest Velcro. Ensure that a margin of sheepskin overlaps all edges of the vest. Overlapping is essential to provide adequate protection for the skin.

6. Tighten and buckle side closures in original position. Side closures must be secure before turning patient supine.

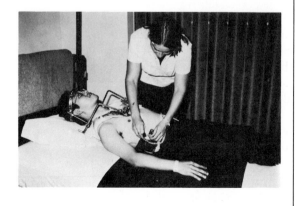

7. Position patient supine and change anterior liner in the same manner.

8. The liners must overlap underneath the side closures. If they do not, cut extra sheepskin 6 × 6 in. squares to cover this area. Squares smaller than 6 × 6 in. will not stay in place.

TABLE 14–6 ■ MONITORING SKIN CHECKS UNDER THE HALO-VEST*

Sunday	Monday	Tuesday	Wednesday	Thursday	Friday	Saturday
	1	2	(3) Halo Applied	(4)	(5)	(6)
(7)	(8)	(9)	(10)	11	(12)	13
14	15	(16)	17	18	(19)	20
21	22	(23)	24	25	(26)	27
28	29	(30)	31	1	(2)	3

* Skin checks are to be performed on days circled and recorded on a calendar. If designated days are missed, the omission can be easily detected and the skin inspected on the following day. Skin checks are to be performed daily for one week, then twice weekly until the brace is removed. If reddened areas are noted, resume daily inspection. This same procedure can be applied to other skin checks.

and around the chest connect the anterior and posterior structures.

The Guilford brace is described here because it is a simple style and easy to apply. The circular support structure for the head spreads the pressure on the skin surface, increasing patient comfort, and the shoulder straps make alignment adjustments easy.

Method of application The initial application and fitting is usually completed by the orthotist. Following application observe for any swallowing difficulties. Adjustment may be necessary. Initial X-ray evaluation may be ordered to check alignment. See Procedure 14–8.

The brace is designed to support weight in the sitting position and will cause uncomfortable pressure points otherwise. Therefore, the brace can generally be removed for short periods or at night when the patient is in the supine position. Prevent excessive flexion, extension, and rotation when the brace is removed, leaving the neck unprotected. Support the neck manually or with a soft collar when bathing or moving in bed. Instruct patients not to move their necks. An old brace can be worn while showering so that the good one remains dry. A soft collar must replace the brace during the night.

Care of the skin Points of greatest pressure on the skin are around the chin and occiput and under the straps and buckles, especially at the shoulders. For added protection, place the brace over a T-shirt. Examine the skin every two hours

PROCEDURE 14–7 ■ EMERGENCY REMOVAL OF THE HALO-VEST

Purpose

The purpose of emergency removal of the Halo-vest is to give cardiopulmonary resuscitation.

Equipment

- A firm surface
- Regular wrench (situated in a designated area and ready for emergencies)

Action	Rationale
1. Position patient supine.	Necessary position to perform cardiopulmonary resuscitation.
2. Unbolt (with a regular wrench) the two largest bolts in lowermost position on breast plate.	This is the quickest method to remove vest. Regular wrenches must be kept with routine emergency equipment.
3. Pull the two upright bars outward. The anterior portion of vest can then be unbuckled and removed without disturbing framework attached to ring.	The chest is then adequately exposed for cardiopulmonary resuscitation.

for a few days after application, then daily during morning and evening care. Daily bathing and, of course, turns or changes of position every two hours are needed to prevent general skin breakdown. It is dangerous to use the prone position.

Activity   When the fracture site requires this lesser degree of immobilization, the physical activity involved will be as full a program as the patient can tolerate, with occasional specified limitations.

Removal of the brace   X-ray evaluation is required before the brace is removed. After it is removed, patients often wear a soft collar.

The cervical collar

In its simplest form, the soft cervical collar is made of foam rubber covered with stockinette and is closed in the back. See Figure 14–22. More rigid collars are made of plastic and leather and often have two side closures. Whatever the construction, collars extend only from the chin and occiput to the shoulders and do not actually immobilize the neck. A cervical collar is applied whenever patients need a nonrigid support to remind them to be cautious with neck movements. (It is usually applied after removal

of other braces or when no bony injury has occurred.)

Method of application   Once the correct size and initial fitting has been completed (often by an occupational therapist) the collar can often be removed for short periods to provide nursing care. The same principles apply as when donning a neck brace: that is, major protection is needed during activity, so the collar should be removed and reapplied when the patient is in the supine position with the neck stabilized.

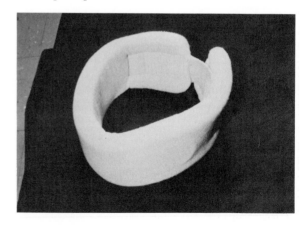

FIGURE 14–22 ■ A soft collar is used when minimal cervical protection is desired.

PROCEDURE 14–8 ■ DONNING THE GUILFORD BRACE (AN EXAMPLE OF A "POST" STYLE CERVICOTHORACIC DEVICE)

Purpose

The purpose of applying this brace is to provide support by limiting flexion and, to a lesser extent, extension and rotation of the cervical spine.

Action	Rationale
1. Assemble brace and check to make sure that buckles and straps are not broken or worn.	This is a safety precaution to prevent accidental movement when brace is in place.
2. Always don (and remove) brace when patient is flat in bed.	Donning the brace before patient sits up protects against major forces causing neck movement. This principle also applies to removal.
3. Logroll patient to one side keeping neck rigid. Put on back plate of the brace so occipital support fits snugly to base of skull. Extend straps and make sure they are not twisted. 4. Return patient to supine position.	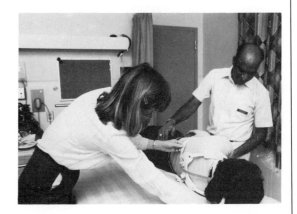
5. Put on chest plate so that chin support fits snugly.	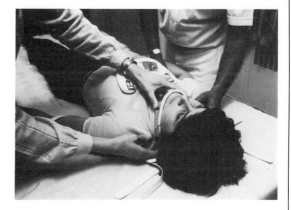
6. Secure under-the-arm and over-the-shoulder straps. Ensure that brace is snug and comfortable but not too tight.	The front and back pieces of the brace must fit securely to provide adequate support.
7. Mark straps with ink at the desired buckle closure.	Following adjustments, this ensures that correct position is then maintained.

Care of the skin A cervical collar exerts greatest pressure on the skin at the chin, occiput, and collar bone. The nurse should examine and wash the skin under the collar every day.

Activity Patients are generally allowed as much physical activity as they can tolerate.

Removal of the collar The soft collar is used primarily to provide some vertical support, which may reduce muscle spasm and neck ache. When discontinuing its use the physician will weigh this comfort aspect against the possibility of contributing to muscle atrophy from disuse of neck muscles.

Thoracolumbar orthoses

Fractures of the thoracolumbar spine are notoriously unstable. The physician will select a mode of management based on extent of neurological deficit, severity of spinal fracture, and general condition.

Immobilization with bedrest may be augmented by a brace to provide additional safety and comfort. Generally a six- to eight-week period of bedrest is required for soft-tissue healing and bony union. Following a sufficient period of bedrest, bracing is mandatory to provide spinal stability during gradual mobilization. When surgical reduction and internal fixation is carried out, bracing is still required but mobilization is generally more rapid.

The bracing is usually some type of individually molded body jacket, which can be removed for skin care, or removable hyperextension bracing. See Procedure 14–9. A permanently placed body cast may be applied when the patient has a low lumbar injury with preserved sensation over most of the torso. See Figure 14–23.

Method of application Body jackets are generally individualized braces fabricated by the orthotist. This involves application of a plaster body cast that is later cut up each side (bivalved) and used as a body cradle or as a mold to make anterior and posterior shells of various sturdier plastics. The shells are lined with removable sheepskin and joined together by straps at the level of the chest and abdomen.

Commercially made three-point fixation braces, such as the Jewett hyperextension brace, afford less stability but are widely used because they are much less expensive and can be individually adjusted to hip and body length. The anterior frame should be lined with sheepskin initially, and later worn over soft clothing. A back strap with a side closure secures the brace at the waist. Following initial application and fitting, the physician may allow removal for daily hygiene and, eventually, at night while the patient is in the supine position. Prevent any flexion, extension, or rotation movements when the back is unprotected by the brace, and caution patients against attempting to move the trunk.

Care of the skin Examine the skin under the brace every eight hours for one to three weeks after application and then daily until the brace is discontinued. Closely observe the underarms, iliac crests, small of back, and under buckles and Velcro straps. Regular change of position is necessary to prevent general skin breakdown. Once the patient can tolerate a full program of activity, a substitute brace can be used when tub bathing. It is a good idea to have former patients donate their braces when they no longer require them.

Activity Each stage of the progression of activity is specifically ordered for each patient, depending on clinical, surgical, and radiological findings, but the stages include:

- Bedrest in the recumbent position. (A longer period is required for conservative management.) During this time, the patient may use a self-propelling wheelchair-stretcher. The patient is positioned prone for propelling this equipment (pictured later in Figure 16–5).
- Gradual mobilization over seven days by elevating the head of the bed 45 degrees, flexing knees over the pillows placed lengthwise, and using the tilt table up to 70 degrees in physiotherapy.
- Increased mobilization over seven days by sitting in a wheelchair, assisting transfers at all times, avoiding trunk rotation, and avoiding long sitting.
- Full mobilization allowing all wheelchair activities, independent transferring, and using long sitting position for dressing.

The fracture site is evaluated regularly at the following intervals:

PROCEDURE 14–9 ■ DONNING THE JEWITT BRACE (AN EXAMPLE OF A HYPEREXTENSION THORACOLUMBAR ORTHOSIS)

Purpose

The purpose of applying this brace is to provide support by maintaining hyperextension and preventing flexion of the thoracic and lumbar spine.

Action	Rationale
1. Assemble brace and check that side closure is sturdy.	This is a safety precaution to prevent accidental movement when brace is in place.
2. Select a sheepskin liner (optional) that overlaps borders of anterior frame.	Overlapping is necessary to adequately protect skin. However, if brace is worn over soft clothing, sheepskin liner may not be needed.
3. Always don (and then remove) brace while patient is supine.	This avoids movements when patient is active.
4. Place the anterior shell low over torso.	
5. Logroll patient to one side and close back strap.	

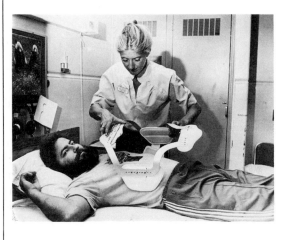 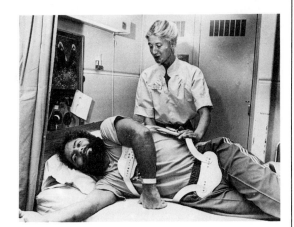

6. Ensure that brace fits snugly. It should be comfortable but not too tight.	
7. Check position of the brace when patient is sitting in wheelchair.	Braces have a tendency to ride up when sitting.

- Following application of the orthosis
- When the patient can tolerate a position of 70 degrees (with approximately seven days tilt table activity) (standing X rays)
- When the patient can tolerate a partial program of mobilization (seven days) (sitting X rays)
- After any accidental fall or with increased pain and spasm or neurological deterioration

Removal of the orthosis Radiological evaluation is continued at various intervals for four to six months before removal of the brace. The patient's clinical picture will be assessed, including any pain, before making a decision.

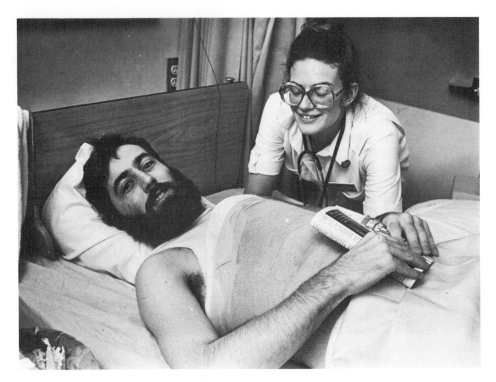

FIGURE 14–23 ■ A body cast.

Realigning the Spine with Surgical Intervention

Surgical management is a complex and controversial subject of international debate. In North America there is a tendency to favor an aggressive approach involving early surgical intervention to achieve internal skeletal stability, which promotes earlier mobilization. This is especially true for patients with thoracolumbar injuries.

The goals of any spinal operation are to achieve bony stability and healing of the spinal column and to promote and protect neural activity. There are no absolute indications for surgical stabilization of the spine. The possible gains must be weighed against the risks of operating on patients who often have multiple trauma and autonomic dysfunction with respiratory and cardiovascular instability. However there are *general* indications warranting surgical treatment in the acute and early stages (Carol, Ducker, and Byrnes 1979; Selecki 1979). Vertebral column injuries that cause severe fracture dislocations, facet-locking dislocations, or grossly unstable fractures (especially when the neurological injury is incomplete) frequently require surgery. Some indications for operative intervention are failure to achieve adequate alignment by closed techniques and bone fragments in the spinal canal. Progressive neurological deterioration is often considered an absolute indication for surgical intervention in selected patients.

Surgical management techniques

Open reduction is used to realign and stabilize the spine and to decompress the cord and nerve roots when possible.

The cervical spine is generally stabilized by a posterior fusion or a fusion and wiring. An anterior fusion may either be a bone refashioned to resemble and replace a vertebral body, or bone chips laid posteriorly around the neural arch. Graft sources are the iliac crest, fibula, or tibia. Wiring is secured in the strong, large spinous processes of the cervical spine.

The thoracolumbar spine is generally stabilized by inserting Harrington rods or other similar devices. These steel instruments are as thick and long as pencils and have cleats or hooks at each end. They are embedded in the neural arch, and the cleats are securely attached to a stable point (ideally the strong pedicles) one or two levels above and below the fracture site. Generally the surgeon performs a localized fusion at the fracture level at the same time. Wiring alone is not successful at this level as the spinous processes are too small to ensure stability.

Harrington rods are applied to provide a distraction force or a compression force. Most commonly the distraction rods are used to treat severe hyperextension injury of the lower thoracic and lumbar spine. Theoretically the rods stretch the posterior longitudinal ligament and each ligamentum flavum and therefore increase the diameter of the spinal canal (if the spinal canal was compromised by these structures). Compression rods are used to create the opposite effect; they draw together the neural arches to achieve alignment.

Most patients with thoracolumbar injuries are allowed up with additional supportive braces one to three weeks after surgery. This extra immobilization measure is needed to allow maximum healing of bone and avoid the long-term complications of spinal curvatures and pain. These operations can increase the risk of late complications if there is not skillful and careful monitoring during the early mobilization period. On occasion, the rods cause discomfort later and are removed once the spine is considered stable. This is possible because the rods act only as supportive struts, limiting bony movement and allowing the bone graft to become a physiological buttress.

For further information on recommended surgical procedures for various types of fractures at specific vertebral levels, refer to Perry (1977) and Ruge and Wiltse (1977).

Caring for patients requiring spinal surgery

Preparing patient and family for surgery   In addition to the general preoperative preparation and teaching required for any surgical patient, it is important to ensure that both patient and family have realistic expectations of the pending operation. It is important to assess their understanding after they have spoken with the surgeon. Often it is necessary to support the physician's explanation that bone structures can be repaired but the spinal cord cannot. Communicate any major problem to the physician for clarification. It may be helpful to contact the social worker, particularly if the family needs additional support. Postoperative psychological depression is often related to the realization that surgery is not a cure.

General postoperative care   Observe for excessive blood loss and monitor general reactions to transfusion, anesthetic gases, drugs, or fluid overload. Assess vital signs remembering that a patient with quadriplegia will normally have a lower blood pressure (90/60 mmHg) so an increasing pulse rate is a better indicator of hemorrhage. (The neural control of blood pressure, dysfunctions following spinal cord injury, and recognition of hemorrhagic versus neurogenic shock are described in Chapter 10.) The surgeon may order the patient to be kept supine for the first four hours to promote blood coagulation by increasing pressure on posterior cervical or lumbar incisions.

If an anterior approach has been used for a cervical fusion, closely observe the ease and rate of respirations. Distress may be caused by neck edema near the operative site.

Neurological status   The nurse should be familiar with the patient's preoperative level of movement and sensation to establish baseline data. During the immediate postoperative period neurological tests should be done hourly for serial monitoring. Any deterioration, which is rare, may be due to cord edema or possible hemorrhage at the operation site.

Correct positioning of patient   Turn and position the patient correctly every two hours. All the general measures to protect the patient from the hazards of immobility very much apply after surgery. For example, the patient with quadriplegia will need special supervision and possible assistance to keep the chest clear. It is also important to follow the protocol to prevent deep vein thrombosis formation. If anticoagulant therapy is ordered, anticipate added risk of hemorrhage from the surgical site. (These nursing measures are described in Chapter 10.)

Alleviating pain   Assess the level of pain and anxiety, which are often related to movement and turning of the patient in bed. Small doses of intravenous analgesics and antispasmodics are generally sufficient to relieve pain, muscle spasm, and tension. Try to anticipate needs; for example, medicate before physiotherapy treatments.

Caring for incision   The physician will likely replace the heavy initial dressing with a light pressure dressing after 72 hours. The dressing should then be changed daily until the sutures are removed in 10 to 14 days. A longer period may be necessary to prevent wound breakdown or evisceration.

Recovery period   Because of interference with the responses from the central and autonomic nervous systems, postoperative reactions of paralyzed patients tend to be more pronounced than those of other patients. When added to existing respiratory or circulatory problems, these heightened reactions usually slow recovery. The difficult psychological adjustment to disability may also delay recovery.

SPECIFIC NURSING INTERVENTIONS FOR POTENTIAL COMPLICATIONS

Associated Skeletal Injuries

With ever-increasing motor vehicle and high-velocity industrial and sports-related accidents, the incidence of associated skeletal injuries has been reported as high as 56% (Meinecke 1973). Skull injuries are the most common, followed by soft tissue or bony injury to the thorax, lower limbs, upper limbs, and the pelvis. Although some fractures are obvious, many are not, particularly if sustained in an area of the body that is without sensation. Lack of sensory warning mechanisms also hampers conventional treatments, such as casts or braces, due to the high risk of skin breakdown. Often surgical intervention to achieve early stabilization is warranted to avoid skin problems and prevent other hazards of immobility. If fractures are left untreated the patient may develop complications, such as osteomyelitis, soft tissue damage, muscle contractures, loss of joint mobility, and malalignment. It is just as important to restore skeletal function for the disabled patient as for the nondisabled. Even though limbs are paralyzed they maintain a supporting function in activities such as transferring, walking with braces, or even eating.

Goals of care

- To recognize bony injury to the skull, thorax, pelvis, and extremities
- To maintain good alignment for the injured part
- To achieve stability of the fracture and prevent additional soft tissue injury
- To reestablish full range of motion to joints and limbs
- To prevent skin breakdown and other long-term complications

Nursing interventions

1. Closely observe high-risk patients. For example the multiple traumatized patient runs a greater risk of sustaining associated injuries, and the patient with quadriplegia, who has larger desensitized areas, runs a greater risk of undetected associated injuries. Especially check patients with cervical cord injuries for head injury; those with thoracic cord injuries for rib fractures; and those with lumbar injuries for pelvic fractures.

2. Note any areas of localized heat, redness, and swelling. Always compare limbs bilaterally. With compound fractures, the skin will be broken and gross fractures of the extremities will cause obvious malalignment. Sensory or motor loss will make diagnosis more difficult and infection may set in. Osteomyelitis is characterized by skin inflammation and possibly muscle rigidity over the affected part, with fever, sweating, and chills as systemic signs.

3. Assist the physician to confirm diagnosis by positioning the patient for X ray.

4. Immobilize the site as ordered. Some fractures, such as those sustained to the ribs or pelvis, are treated with simple bedrest. Caution will be needed when turning, positioning, and mobilizing. Surgical intervention is the method of choice for long bone fractures of the extremities. As with any operative treatment, however, timing depends on the patient's general condition. If conservative management is needed, pillow splints, thick padded bandages (made of cotton batting, wadding, and elastic tensor bandages), or individualized splints lined with foam rubber should be used. Experts agree that plaster casts on desensitized skin invariably lead to skin breakdown. Although conservative treatment is less traumatic than surgery, difficult turning and frequent (daily) removal of supports for skin care often render these stabilization measures insufficient for fixation. Surgery may be needed at a future date. However as callus begins to form very soon in paralyzed patients, operations may become more difficult later.

5. Evaluate effectiveness of treatment according to the level of outcome criteria reached:

- Fracture site healed in good alignment without evidence of joint stiffness or muscle contractures
- Healthy skin over affected site without evidence of breakdown or localized inflammation
- Normal body temperature
- X-ray evaluation to show signs of healing

Heterotopic Bone Formation

Heterotopic bone formation, or more specifically *para-articular heterotopic ossification,* is misplacement, or an abnormal deposit, of new bone formation around joints of paralyzed limbs. The etiology is completely unknown, but it has been reported in approximately 15% to 20% of all patients with spinal cord injuries (Freehafer 1977). It is more common in higher level injuries, often involving the hip, knee, elbow, or shoulder joints. Calcification, which evolves into mature bone formation, causes swelling, stiffness, and limited function of involved joints. The process may last for a period of months.

Goals of care

- To recognize onset of heterotopic bone formation
- To maintain normal range of motion of involved joints
- To prevent permanent joint damage and muscle contractures

Nursing interventions

1. Carefully observe the quadriplegic patient, who runs the greatest risk of developing this complication. Onset is most common during the first year after injury.

2. Note characteristic signs: localized redness, swelling, or stiffness of joints, swelling of the involved extremity, systemic temperature elevation, and possibly discomfort or referred pain. Radiological evaluation will reveal bone formation and confirm diagnosis. Also the serum phosphatase is usually elevated.

3. Prepare the patient for bilateral X rays for comparison studies and a bone scan as ordered. Serial evaluations will monitor rate of bone formation.

4. Maintain activity as ordered by physician. Activation as soon as possible is the treatment of choice. Collaborate with the physiotherapist to provide gentle range of motion exercises at frequent intervals. Sitting with the hips and knees bent is desirable. Bedrest may cause stiff joints, which may eventually render sitting impossible. Fortunately, many patients respond satisfactorily with minor limitation of motion, which hampers transfer activities and lower extremity dressing. Eventually, however, when bone formation is mature, surgical removal may be necessary for some.

5. Evaluate effectiveness of treatment according to level of outcome reached:

- Full range of motion in involved joint without evidence of redness, swelling, or discomfort
- Normal body temperature
- X-ray evaluation within normal limits
- Serum phosphatase within normal limits

LONG-TERM IMPLICATIONS

When assessing the patient with paraplegia or quadriplegia who has been paralyzed for some time, the active or well-cared-for person will probably be able to maintain good body alignment without evidence of contractures.

Spinal curvatures may become evident relatively quickly during the first year after injury. This is often related to inadequte stabilization during the acute stage and perhaps to difficulty in maintaining alignment with extensive fractures, too much or too stressful activity too soon, or premature removal of orthoses.

Although many patients with heterotopic bone formation are able to complete a rehabilitation program, if ossification progresses it may cause joint immobility (ankylosis), which may lead to severe loss of function or prevent sitting in a wheelchair. Surgical removal may be necessary, but unless undertaken when bone is mature (one to two years) there is a definite incidence of recurrence (Stauffer 1977; Burke and Murray 1975).

Pathological fractures of the long bones are associated with osteoporotic changes accompanying paralysis. This increase in porosity and softness of the bones is related to disuse and is not sufficiently advanced until at least a year after injury to cause problems. Then a minor trauma, such as a careless transfer or a fall from a wheelchair, can cause a fracture, commonly in the leg bones. Observe for any localized swelling, abnormal alignment or mobility, crepitus, and possibly increased spasm. These fractures generally respond to conservative treatment and heal rapidly. Open reduction with internal fixation is rarely indicated (Stauffer 1977).

Encourage use of the *prone* position, especially as a natural sleeping position, as a prophylactic measure to prevent contractures (above all, hip and knee) and relieve pressure on buttocks to minimize risk of sacral skin breakdown.

Based on your assessment, help patients continue with preventive measures or refer them to a physician for further restorative management.

SELECTED REFERENCES

Burke, D., and Murray, D. 1975. *Handbook of Spinal Cord Medicine.* London and Basingstoke: Macmillan Press, Chapters 3 and 14. *Concise presentation of conservative and surgical management and of para-articular heterotopic ossification.*

Carol, M.; Ducker, T.; and Byrnes, D. 1979. Acute care of spinal cord injury: a challenge to the emergency medical clinician. *Critical Care Quarterly* (2): 7–21. *A clear guide to initial management, neurological assessment, types of spinal cord lesions, and treatment aspects with nursing implications.*

Freehafer, A. 1977. Long term management of lumbar paraplegia. In *The Total Care of Spinal Cord Injuries.* Eds. D. Pierce and V. Nickel. Boston: Little, Brown, pp. 135–164. *Multifaceted overview of management principles and potential complications.*

Meinecke, F. 1973. Pelvis and limb injuries in patients with recent spinal cord injuries. *Proceedings Veterans Administration Spinal Cord Injury Conference* 19 (Oct.): 205–212. *Incidence and rationale for prompt treatment of associated fractures to facilitate later rehabilitation.*

Nickel, V., 1977. The Halo. In *Spinal Disorders, Diagnosis and Treatment.* Eds. D. Ruge and L. Wiltse. Philadelphia: Lea and Febiger. *Describes the history* and development of the Halo-thoracic brace. *Outlines general care required and details common complications.*

Perry, J. 1977. Surgical approaches to the spine. In *The Total Care of Spinal Cord Injuries.* Eds. D. Pierce and V. Nickel. Boston: Little, Brown, pp. 53–80. *Includes illustrations and rationale for treatment.*

Ruge, D., and Wiltse, L., Eds. 1977. *Spinal Disorders, Diagnosis and Treatment.* Philadelphia: Lea and Febiger, Chapters 2–5, 34–37, 41–43. *Contains helpful information on anatomy and neurological and radiological evaluation; spinal cord injury and surgical management of the cervical and thoracolumbar spine; biomechanics of the spine and orthoses; spinal implants for the relief of pain; and neurosurgical management of spastic conditions.*

Selecki, B. 1979. Severe injuries to the cervical cord and spine: neurosurgical management in the acute and early stage. *Australia/New Zealand Journal* 49 (2): 267–274. *Presents diagnostic and early surgical management; includes detailed indications, contraindications, and techniques for surgical intervention. Clearly written.*

Stauffer, E. 1977. Long-term management of quadriplegia. In *The Total Care of Spinal Cord Injuries.* Eds. D. Pierce and V. Nickel. Boston: Little, Brown, pp. 81–102. *Multifaceted review of ongoing assessment, principles of management, functional goals of rehabilitation, and potential problems.*

Young, R., and Murphy, D. 1980. Hygiene care in the Halo vest. *Orthopaedic Review* 9 (2): 73–79. *Detailed, liberally illustrated guide, including washing skin, changing Halo vest liners, emergency removal, and other specific problems. Highly recommended.*

Young, R., and Thomassen, E. 1974. Step by step procedure for applying Halo ring. *Orthopaedic Review* 3 (6): 62–64. *Materials and illustrated application procedure.*

SUPPLEMENTAL READING

General

Attending Staff Association of Rancho Los Amigos Hospital Inc. 1972. Regional Spinal Cord Injury Rehabilitation Center. Final Report. Downey, California. *A detailed interdisciplinary perspective of acute and concurrent rehabilitative care.*

Guttman, L. 1976. *Spinal Cord Injuries Comprehensive Management and Research.* 2d ed. London: Blackwell Scientific Publications. *A classic, multifaceted reference text on spinal cord injuries. Includes historical background information; general statistics; legal aspects; detailed anatomy and neuropathology of cord trauma and resultant effects on all body systems; regeneration; fractures and dislocations, gunshot injuries, and stab wounds; and neurophysiological and clinical management aspects. Extensive bibliography.*

McKenzie, M. 1970. The role of occupational therapy in rehabilitating spinal cord injured patients. *American Journal of Occupational Therapy* 24 (4): 257–263. *Review of occupational therapy philosophy, goals, and treatment principles; delineates some obstacles; and examines vocational and avocational possibilities.*

Meyer, E., and Meyer, P. 1979. Initial management of the client with acute spinal cord injury. In *Current Perspectives in Rehabilitation Nursing.* Eds. R. Murray and J. C. Kijeck. St. Louis: The C. V. Mosby Company, pp. 55–75. *Discusses transport, neurological assessment, drug administration, principles of management, and related nursing care.*

Venier, L., and Ditunno, J. 1971. Heterotopic ossification in the paraplegic patient. *Archives of Physical Medicine and Rehabilitation,* October, pp. 475–479. *Comprehensive general review of this complication.*

Mobilization

Bergstrom, D., and Coles, C. 1971. *Basic Positioning Procedures.* Minneapolis, Minn.: Sister Kenney Institute. *Clearly present three basic concepts: the positioning plan; positioning procedures; and equipment for positioning.*

Calenoff, L., et al. 1979. Lumbar fracture-dislocation related to range-of-motion exercises. *Archives of Physical Medicine and Rehabilitation* 60 (Apr.): 183–184. *A report to increase awareness of precautions necessary with therapeutic ranging of the patient with neurological impairment.*

Ciuca, R.; Bradish, J.; and Trombley, S. 1978. Passive range-of-motion exercises. *Nursing '78* 8 (7): 59–65. *A photographic handbook of shoulder, hip, and foot exercises.*

Ford, J. 1980. *Wheelchair Handbook.* G. F. Strong Rehabilitation Centre, 4255 Laurel St., Vancouver, B.C., V5Z 2G9. *A guide to selection, cushions, accessories, and maintenance. Highly recommended.*

Mobilization (continued)

Ford, J., and Duckworth, B. 1974. *Physical Management for the Quadriplegic Patient*. Philadelphia: F. A. Davis. *Clearly illustrated manual with valuable sections on biomechanical principles of movement, transfers, bathing, dressing, bowel and bladder management, and care of the totally dependent patient. Gives insight into potential capabilities and skillful ways to assist patients. Highly recommended.*

Kaplan, P., et al. 1978. Calcium balance in paraplegic patients: influence of injury duration and ambulation. *Archives of Physical Medicine and Rehabilitation* 59 (Oct.): 447–450. *Research indicates that hypercalciuria (negative calcium balance) is significantly decreased with early ambulation; includes review of calcium metabolic balance determination studies and previous clinical and experimental data. Extensive bibliography.*

McGee, M., and Hertling, D. 1977. Equipment and transfer techniques used by C_6 quadriplegic patients. *Physical Therapy* 57 (12): 1372–1375. *Describes how electric double beds, wheelchair commodes, selection of wheelchair cushions, and modified transfer techniques, among others, enhance functional training.*

Odéen, I. 1979. Early mobilization of paraplegic patients following spinal cord injuries. *Physiotherapy Canada* 31 (2): 75–83. *Presents an excellent overview and guideline to early mobilization; describes bedrest activities for initial four-week period; tilt table and mobile stretcher or converted wheelchair activities; and adjustment to the upright position in the wheelchair. Highly recommended.*

Pepmiller, E. 1979. Selecting a wheelchair: helping your patient make the best choice. *Journal of Practical Nursing* 29 (Feb.): 12–13, 30. *Provides insight into wheelchair selection. Helpful overview with emphasis on nursing considerations.*

Orthoses

Bacon, G., and Olszewski, E. 1978. Sequential advancing flexion retention attachment. *American Journal of Occupational Therapy* 32 (9): 577–579. *A simple locking device added to the standard flexor-driven hinge splint to accommodate patients with weak wrist extension (eliminates the use of elaborate externally driven hand splints).*

Hart, D., et al. 1978. Review of cervical orthoses. *Physical Therapy* 58 (7): 857–860. *The characteristics of structure, ease of donning and adjusting, patient comfort, and general clinical applicability are described for cervical collars, poster-style orthosis, and the Halo traction system.*

Moratz, V. 1979. Adapting shirts to fit over a Halo vest. *American Journal of Occupational Therapy* 33 (8): 524–525. *Easy-to-follow pattern.*

Rutecki, B., and Seligson, D. 1980. Caring for the patient in a Halo apparatus. *Nursing '80* (Oct.): 19–23. *Photostory on preparation and application of a Halo apparatus and nursing care of an ambulatory patient.*

Specialized Beds

Green, B. 1975. *Keane Roto-Rest Turning Bed and Kinetic Nursing*. Continuing Education in the Treatment of Spinal Cord Injury, No. 5. Chicago: National Paraplegic Foundation. *Presents principles of design and general description of bed and related nursing care.*

Green, B., et al. 1980. Kinetic nursing for acute spinal cord injury patients. *International Journal of Paraplegia* 18(3): 181–5. *Review of 105 patients treated on a Roto-Rest Mark I hospital bed. This bed places the patient in perpetual motion while immobilizing the spine. Common complications were reduced.*

Keane, F. 1977–78. Pain and cervical traction variation during manual turning. *International Journal of Paraplegia* 15: 343–348. *Experimentally records variations causing bending forces in the neck which, together with variations in direction of traction, elicits pain. Presents rationale for the Roto-Rest bed.*

King, R. 1981. Assessment and management of soft tissue pressure. In *Comprehensive Rehabilitation Nursing*. Eds. N. Martin, N. Holt, and D. Hicks. New York: McGraw-Hill, pp. 242–268. *In depth review of specialized beds to relieve the effects of pressure included.*

Robertson, C. 1978. Life on a Stryker bed. *Nursing Times*, 4 May, p. 752. *Brief description from a patient's perspective.*

Rogers, E. 1978–79. Nursing management in relation to beds within the national spinal injuries centre for the prevention of pressure sores. *International Journal of Paraplegia* 16: 147–153. *Focus on nursing management of the patient on a Stoke-Eggerton turning and tilting electrical bed; includes step-by-step procedure for operating bed and instructions for positioning and manually lifting a patient.*

Surgical Management

Bedbrook, G. 1979. Spinal injuries with tetraplegia and paraplegia. *Journal of Bone and Joint Surgery* 61-B (3): 267–278. *A concise overview including acute skeletal system pathology and management.*

Croushore, T. 1979. Postoperative assessment: the key to avoiding the most common nursing mistakes. *Nursing '79* 9 (4): 47–51. *Systematic assessment focusing on common postoperative complications, charts on expected drainage from tubes and catheters, and early and late complications.*

Hamilton, R. 1980. Laminectomy. *Spinal Cord Injury Digest* 2 (Summer): 3–8. *Describes indications for and controversy surrounding laminectomies and cordectomies.*

Holdsworth, F. 1970. Fractures, dislocations and fracture-dislocations of the spine. *Journal of Bone and Joint Surgery* 52-A (8): 1534–1551. *Comprehensive review of classification of vertebral lesions; diagnosis of neurological lesion; X-ray characteristics; case histories; and stable and unstable injuries. Well illustrated.*

Pierce, D. 1977. Acute treatment of spinal cord injuries. In *The Total Care of Spinal Cord Injuries.* Eds. D. Pierce and V. Nickel. Boston: Little, Brown, pp. 1–22. *Illustrated guide to operative techniques.*

Yashon, D. 1978. *Spinal Injury.* New York: Appleton-Century-Crofts. *Detailed overview of various aspects of surgical medical management.*

Yosipovitch, Z.; Robin, G.; and Makin, M. 1977. Open reduction of unstable thoracolumbar spinal injuries and fixation with Harrington rods. *Journal of Bone and Joint Surgery* 59-A (8): 1003–1015. *Timing and principles of early open reduction; rationale for orthosis; and early mobilization. Well illustrated radiographically.*

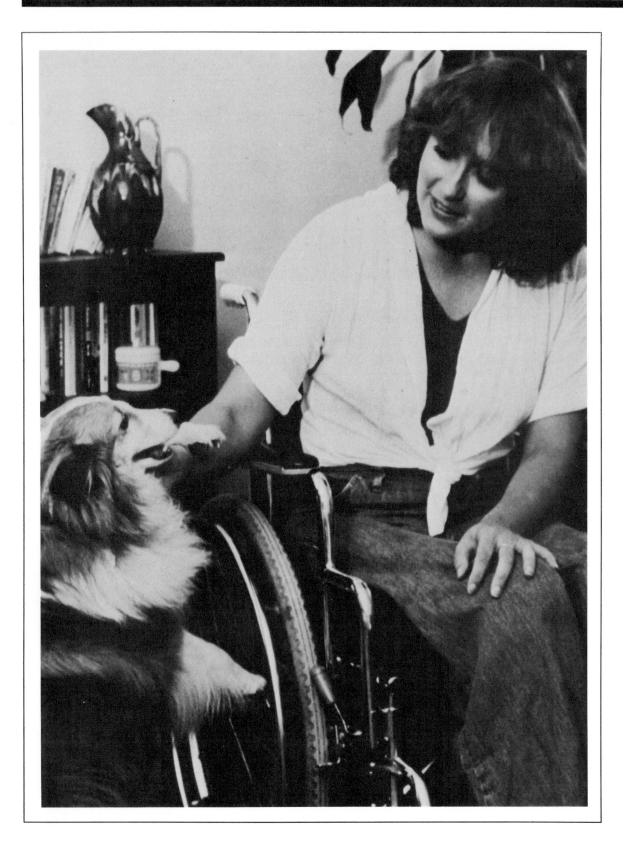

Chapter 15

Maintaining Protective Functions of the Skin

CHAPTER OUTLINE

OBJECTIVES

- To identify health care goals for maintaining protective functions of the skin
- To describe general functions of the skin, neural control, and dysfunctions following spinal cord injury
- To describe why patients with spinal cord injuries are prone to skin problems
- To describe how to assess a patient for possible skin problems
- To describe nursing care that helps patients avoid skin problems
- To describe care for a patient with a pressure area
- To explain how to teach patients and families principles of good skin care and self-care skills
- To describe long-term implications associated with care of the skin

GOALS OF HEALTH CARE

No single complication of spinal cord injury is as potentially preventable, as difficult to manage, or as much of a deterrent to the progress of a total rehabilitation program as skin breakdown. The process by which it occurs is fast and insidious. Efforts to prevent it must be planned and constant. [Thomas 1977: 258]

Currently nursing leaders are very much aware of the lack of well-designed research in the management of soft tissue pressure. Even though measures presented here may be "nothing new," the continuing failure of nurses and others to put them into practice is alarming.

Miller and Sachs (1974) posed the important question, Why do even conscientious nurses sometimes fail to deal effectively with the problem of pressure sores? Further study revealed that many of those who provide direct nursing care are unaware that they do not clearly understand the physiological and mechanical factors involved in the development of a pressure sore.

The way patients feel about themselves, general skin cleanliness, personal hygiene, nutritional status, and cardiopulmonary function are all important adjuncts to actual relief of primary causative forces that result in skin breakdown. A holistic approach to nursing care, combining basic knowledge and numerous manual and teaching skills, is essential to patients who must eventually assume the onus of responsibility for skin care. The goals of this holistic care are:

- To promote adequate circulation to soft tissue structures located over bony structures that support body weight
- To avoid primary factors of prolonged pressure, shearing forces, or local injury to the skin that cause skin breakdown
- To minimize secondary factors contributing to skin breakdown
- To design and implement an effective nursing care plan to meet individual needs
- To ensure cleanliness and personal hygiene
- To participate with the patient, family, and health care team to improve the patient's feelings of self-worth

- To teach the patient how to care for the skin to prevent skin breakdown

ASSESSMENT

The skin and its accessory structures—the hair and nails—comprise the *integumentary system*. The integumentary system fulfills an important role in perception of and protection from the environment. To understand the actual and potential problems that patients with spinal cord injuries may experience requires a review of the neurological, physiological, mechanical, and psychological factors involved. Intelligent nursing care often encompasses modification of standard treatment regimes to meet individual needs. Skillful adaptation is based on a clear understanding of the effects of pressure and an assessment of associated risk factors.

Changes in the Integumentary System Following Spinal Cord Injury

Skin, neural control, and dysfunctions

The skin protects the deeper structures of the body; regulates body temperature by controlling vasomotor activity and sweat production; prevents excessive water loss to the environment; and perceives sensations. Thus the skin helps protect the body from, and adapt it to, the environment; maintain normal internal homeostasis; and ensure the continued activity of individual cells (Spence and Mason 1979).

The entire skin surface of the body receives innervation from the central and autonomic nervous systems. Cutaneous distribution of this innervation is organized in dermatomes. A dermatome is simply a section or level of the body that is supplied by a cranial or spinal nerve. Each nerve branches out into many free nerve endings on the skin surface.

The central nervous system (in communication with the peripheral nervous system) provides sensory appreciation and motor control to each dermatome. Sensations of light pressure, pain, and temperature (hot and cold) are received from free nerve endings in the skin.

(Sensations of deep pressure and position sense are appreciated more in the muscles and joints.) Impulses are transmitted through the spinal nerves and cord to the brain.

The autonomic nervous system helps control body homeostasis and protects the skin from the environment by reflex activity. Stimulation to each dermatome provides vasomotor control of blood vessels and is thus a major influence over circulation. The autonomic nervous system also controls the sweat glands and thus influences excretion of body fluids and body temperature regulation. In turn, body homeostasis helps maintain healthy skin.

In response to sensory stimuli, a person moves to avoid unpleasant or painful sensations. This action may be as simple and automatic as withdrawing a hand from a hot stove; or it may require more complex actions, such as adjusting to a more comfortable position or changing clothes to suit outside temperatures. Reflex activity protects the body from extremely dangerous or painful stimuli.

People with spinal cord injuries lose sensory appreciation and voluntary motor ability below the level of lesion. Injury may also cause autonomic nervous system mechanisms to operate poorly, altering body homeostasis and circulation. Reflex activity may be preserved and become hyperactive or may be absent. The lack of sensory warning mechanisms, inability to move freely, and circulatory changes in people with spinal cord injuries pose major threats to the integumentary system. To identify areas susceptible to skin breakdown, it is essential to correlate the level of injury with the actual surface area (dermatome) of the body that is involved (see Figure 5–22). For example, a complete injury at the T_4 level will interrupt innervation to the skin below the nipple line on the body.

Factors associated with disruption of skin integrity

The cells of the integumentary system, like all cells, require constant oxygenation, nourishment, and elimination of waste products to remain functional. This is achieved only by good blood flow to all areas of the skin. Any prolonged blockage will quickly cause skin breakdown. The severity of this breakdown is directly related to the amount and duration of force and, to a lesser extent, a number of secondary factors.

Primary factors that predispose any patient to potential disruption of skin integrity are excessive *pressure; shearing forces;* or localized *trauma* or *skin irritation.* Obstruction of capillary flow and accompanying ischemia are widely recognized as the mechanisms responsible for skin breakdown or ulcer formation. Direct pressure and shearing forces can cause this obstruction. Trauma or other local irritations can also contribute, but by mechanical forces to the epidermis, rather than by ischemia (Mikulic 1980).

Pressure   If *pressure area, pressure sore,* and *pressure ulcer* are the accepted terms for skin breakdown, preventive and restorative measures may become more successful by adequately addressing the cause—pressure (Mikulic 1980).

Pressure develops through lack of movement of body weight. To avoid pressure, healthy people continually move their bodies in response to sensory stimuli, even during sleep. Areas of increased pressure may occur anywhere on the body, but pressure is most concentrated between bones and skin surfaces that support body weight. When soft tissue is compressed between a bone and another hard surface, such as a bed, wheelchair, or brace, blood is squeezed out of underlying tissue and the circulation is blocked. Altering position changes the pressure points.

The skin becomes red as a result of transient pressure, but this disappears when the pressure is removed. Relief of pressure following prolonged soft tissue compression results in a cellular reaction of edema and inflammation. If pressure is not relieved, sustained ischemia destroys cellular metabolism, which may lead to necrosis of fat, fibrous tissue, muscle, and even bone. Extensive involvement and undermining of deep fascia, muscle, bone periosteum, and nearby joint structures are evident. Large amounts of fluid and protein are lost from the wound. During this stage the patient may have multiple areas of skin breakdown and may develop dehydration, anemia, and toxicity, which can cause death.

There is a definite relationship between the duration and amount of pressure and the development of pressure sores. Usual pressures from body weight cause microscopic ischemic changes in capillary blood flow in less than 30 minutes. However, there is a critical interval of between one and two hours before pathological changes occur in both normal and denervated tissue. Experience has shown that these changes are reversible if pressure is relieved every two hours (Burke and Murray 1975). If the pressure force is greater than that caused by normal body weight, such as can be caused by wrinkles in the bed linen or an ill-fitting brace, irreversible changes can occur more quickly.

A *pressure sore* is an area of damage to the skin and/or underlying tissues created by inadequate circulation as a result of pressure. Resulting ischemic changes may progress to varying degrees of tissue death. A pressure sore is first manifested by a reddened area that does not disappear within 30 minutes or so after pressure is removed. Edema, inflammation, or blistering over a bony prominence may occur. See Table 15–1. If pressure is not relieved a superficial ulceration of the epidermis will form. All the measures suggested in this chapter, especially pressure relief, will prevent or reverse the process at this stage.

Shearing forces   Although not as great a factor as pressure, *shearing forces* can block blood flow significantly. Shearing forces occur when tissues rub or are pulled rather than compressed against each other. This can happen when a patient is slumped in a chair or bed. The soft tissues are pulled out of shape as the skin sticks to the chair back or mattress while the weight of the body slides to the foot of the chair or bed.

Localized factors   When skin nutrition and blood supply is compromised in a local area, by trauma or entrapment of moisture and heat, tissue resistance is decreased. The areas then become more susceptible to forces of pressure and skin breakdown, and infection occurs more easily. These factors also interfere with healing.

Traumas, such as cuts or bruising, and other forces, such as friction, may abrade the skin and interrupt blood flow. Friction may occur when a patient is slid rather than lifted up in bed or when bare skin comes into contact with a transfer board. Spasticity may be another source of friction.

TABLE 15–1 ■ CHARACTERISTICS OF A NEWLY DEVELOPED PRESSURE AREA

Reddened area
Reactive hyperemia appears as the first sign of a pressure area

Localized warmth

Hardened area

Localized area of edema or blistering

Bluish discoloration

Small open area
Ulceration of epidermis; possible inflammatory reaction affecting underlying soft tissue
With removal of pressure healing will occur in 48 to 72 hours

Entrapment of localized moisture and heat also contribute to pressure sore development. Dissipation of moisture and heat may well be impeded by the increased use of plastic incontinence padding and plastic or foam wheelchair cushions and mattresses.

Secondary factors can significantly contribute to this potential problem for patients with spinal cord injuries. Sensory deficit; motor impairment; circulatory changes; threatened nutritional status; hygiene problems especially associated with neurogenic bladder and bowel dysfunction; and psychological adjustment to disability can aggravate the situation.

History

Assessment of the skin should include information on general skin type, preexisting conditions that affect the skin, medications, and advanced age. If any unusual data are collected during history taking, general care regimes should be modified accordingly.

General skin type

Note tendency toward normal, oily, or dry skin. Dry skin is particularly troublesome, because it is inelastic and tends to crack, thus forming sites for ulceration. People with fair skin, especially those with red hair, generally have extremely sensitive skin.

Preexisting conditions

It is important to note any preexisting skin complications. Occasionally a definite dermatological disorder, such as eczema, or a circulation-related condition, such as diabetes, may be present.

Medications

A medication history is vital, particularly if the patient has a known allergy to any of the systemic or topically applied drugs used for a variety of disorders. Side effects may be skin dryness, pruritis, or rashes. Topical medications, especially if incorrectly applied, can actually burn the skin. One peculiar rash—a raised, reddened, pimply rash that occurs on the upper chest and back—is due to dexamethasone therapy, which is given frequently during the early stages after injury.

Advanced age

In the course of normal aging, the skin tends to become thin, wrinkled, dry, and occasionally scaly. The skin structures and subcutaneous fat are supported by an underlying network of collagen and other elastic fibers that give the skin its characteristic flexibility, elasticity, and strength. Changes in the skin due to aging—atrophy of all skin layers, decreased vascularity, and decreased elasticity—lead to loss of skin water, reduced sweating, decreased oil production, loss of hair, and pigmentation changes. Hair becomes grayer, and the skin has a more mottled appearance (Spence and Mason 1983).

Dermatitis often stems from frequent soap-and-water bathing, which is poorly tolerated by the fragile skin of the elderly and leads to the common problems of dryness and eczema. The vulvae and vaginal mucosa are particularly susceptible.

Physical Assessment

In-depth physical assessment is a major nursing responsibility. Assessment must encompass inspection of the skin, observation of circulatory changes, assessment of nutritional status, detailed observation during general illness, and assessment of functional skills.

Inspection of skin

Meticulous inspection of the skin is a crucial step in prevention of pressure sores. The skin must be checked at frequent and specific intervals. During the early stages skin inspection must be performed immediately following each turn when in bed and on return to bed from the wheelchair. It is also important to examine the skin carefully when a patient returns to the ward from diagnostic or radiological tests or operative procedures. These activities often necessitate positioning the patient on a hard surface, which increases pressure on bony prominences. As skin and wheelchair tolerance builds, skin inspection may be performed each morning before getting up and each night when returning to bed. This must become an integral part of the patient's daily life.

Skin assessment techniques combine visual observation and palpation for increased temperature in localized areas. The latter skill is particularly helpful for detecting hyperemic responses in dark-skinned patients when visual inspection is difficult. Be sure to use the back of the hand, which is more sensitive than the fingertips to temperature changes. Good lighting is important. Use a bright flashlight during the night shift and when checking under braces.

Observe for developing pressure areas   Signs indicative of too much or prolonged pressure include:

- Reddened areas (reactive hyperemia due to rushing of the blood into an area that has been deprived of good circulation is the first sign of a pressure area)
- Localized warmth (identified by palpation)
- Hardened areas (identified by palpation)
- Localized areas of edema or blistering
- Bluish discoloration
- Small open or ulcerated areas

Note any scrapes, cuts, or bruising that would render a particular area more susceptible to skin breakdown.

Inspect weight-bearing bony prominences
As soft tissue pressure is greatest over bony prominences that support body weight, changes in body position change the areas endangered. It is important to recognize the areas of the body that will need special attention for skin care. Figure 15–1 illustrates areas most susceptible to pressure formation in the supine, side-lying, prone, and sitting positions.

Additional assessment is necessary when a patient is wearing a variety of immobilization devices or splints. Examine the skin carefully where the orthotic device exerts the greatest pressure on the skin. Table 15–2 summarizes pressure points exerted by a variety of orthoses.

Assessment of circulatory status

Spinal cord injury impairs autonomic nervous system function. Disturbed vasomotor control and decreased tone in paralyzed muscles impair circulatory return to the heart. Sluggish venous return is then overcome by gravitational forces, leading to dependent or orthostatic edema. Edema interferes with cellular nutrition, which decreases skin flexibility and elasticity and increases susceptibility to pressure.

Skin breakdown can occur at any time; however, the most dangerous period is immediately after injury during spinal shock. Loss of vasomotor control, especially in the lower limbs, leads to pooling of blood, which causes tissue hypoxia. As hypotension is common with paralysis, capillary flow pressure becomes extremely low. Light pressure or slight trauma that would not normally cause problems will do so at this time.

Assessment of nutritional status

Following spinal cord injury a number of factors can threaten nutritional status. Malnutrition and significant weight loss are common during the critical period. Trauma imposes stress, which dramatically increases energy requirements when the patient is least able to cope. Later in the rehabilitation process, anorexia, dehydration, or repeated infections may result in poor nutritional status. Protein deficiency is considered to be a significant factor in pressure sore development. A negative nitrogen

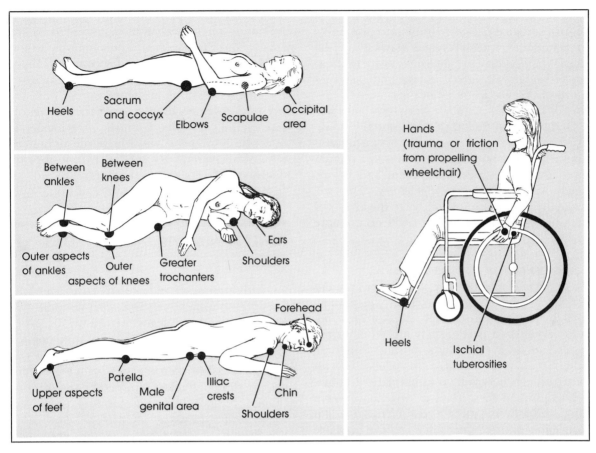

FIGURE 15–1 ■ Points on the body susceptible to pressure vary when different positions are assumed.

TABLE 15–2 ■ PRESSURE POINTS CREATED BY COMMONLY USED ORTHOTIC DEVICES

Halo-Thoracic Brace
- Pin sites and skin underneath circumference of Halo-ring
- Shoulders (especially top)
- Underarms
- Rib cage
- All edges of the brace and underneath the side buckle area

Cervical Brace
- Occiput
- Chin and jaw line
- Underarms
- Sternum
- Spine
- Underneath all edges of brace, straps, and buckles

Thoracic Brace
- Upper trunk and underarms
- Iliac crests
- Spine
- Underneath edges of brace, buckles, and straps

Hand Splints
- Palms
- Wrist bones
- Underneath straps and buckles

Calipers or "Mock-Up" Leg Braces (Collaborate with physiotherapist to observe)
- Groin area
- Hinge sites
- Heels and toes (tend to curl up in shoes)

balance signals that protein catabolism is out of control. Vitamin C is also thought to play a role in maintaining flexibility and elasticity of the skin. When cellular metabolism is decreased, tissue resistance is lowered, and the body becomes more susceptible to forces of pressure.

Observation during general illness

The febrile state associated with infection is known to increase oxygen demands at a cellular level. Failure to meet nutritional and caloric needs will cause cellular deficiency. This will make the body more susceptible to the effects of pressure and skin breakdown will occur more easily.

Assessment of functional skills

Assessment of functional skills and patient knowledge and attitudes are closely related factors. Inspection and care of the skin must become an integral part of daily life, whether patients can do it themselves or must supervise others in doing so. Nurses must collaborate with occupational therapists to assess patients' abilities to position themselves in bed, control arm and hand movements to adjust mirrors for skin inspection, and acquire skills to relieve pressure while positioned in the bed and wheelchair.

Psychosocial Factors

There has been little recognition of the relationship between psychosocial factors and pressure sores, but the patient's ability to maintain the integrity of the skin does not appear to be directly related to the level of injury. This suggests that psychosocial rather than mechanical variables play an important part in independent care of the skin.

One study revealed that maintaining the integrity of the skin was not so much a function of mechanical aids, intellect, or achievement as of patient attitudes (Anderson and Andberg 1979). Quadriplegic patients who accepted responsibility for skin care and achieved satisfaction from activities in life were less likely to lose days from treatment of pressure sores than paraplegic patients who did not accept responsibility. Acceptance of responsibility for one's body has

been viewed as a prerequisite for adaptation to the many physical changes spinal cord injury entails, and this certainly seems to apply to the incidence of pressure sores (Treischmann 1980: 80).

Further research is needed to find ways for nurses to enhance compliance with essential skin care regimes. Judging from the high incidence of pressure sores following discharge (as high as 80% of all patients (Gosnell 1973)), it appears that many efforts are currently misdirected.

GENERAL NURSING INTERVENTIONS

Although acute management is largely the nurse's responsibility, the patient, the nurse, and all interdisciplinary team members must work closely together to achieve the fundamental goals of skin care. For example, during the early stages a social worker interviewing a wheelchair patient should remind him or her regularly to change position. *Encouragement of the patient and/or family to assume the eventual onus of responsibility is the key factor to continuing success.* This is often difficult to achieve. Most nurses, at some point or another, have seen the horrible sight of large, open, weeping sores caused by neglect. Most patients have not; so it is difficult for them to comprehend the serious implications of poor skin care. Nevertheless, it is realistic to provide a sound background of knowledge, for skin care must become an important daily routine.

Relief from Pressure while Patient Is in Bed

Numerous regimes have come and gone, but such time-honored and proven nursing techniques as regular turning and bridging of bony prominences remain significant in prevention and treatment of pressure sores (King 1981: 243). Bridging refers to supporting body weight so that a free space is created between a bony prominence and the bed. For example, a pillow may be placed under the thighs of prone patients and another under the lower legs to bridge the knee. Remember and encourage

PROCEDURE 15–1 ■ METHOD TO PROVIDE WHEELCHAIR PRESSURE RELIEF (TWO ASSISTANTS)

Purpose

The purpose of a two-assistant lift is to provide relief for dependent quadriplegic patients.

Action

(First assistant)

1. Tip wheelchair back to an angle of 30 degrees.

(Second assistant)

2. Grasp patient's foot and knee, keeping leg straight.

3. Externally rotate hip and raise leg until the ischial tuberosity clears the cushion.

4. Hold for 10 to 15 sec.

5. Repeat with other leg.

6. Repeat procedure every 15 to 30 min while the patient is up.

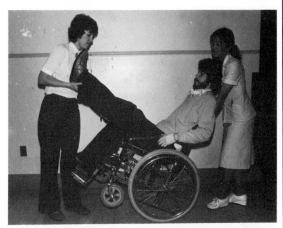

others to focus on turning and correct positioning as the key. Forget massages, powders, and creams, and concentrate on relieving the cause—pressure.

Turn patients regularly to relieve pressures of body weight: every two hours throughout the 24-hour period of initial bedrest. Minor position changes more frequently are extremely valuable and an effective comfort measure. Schedule turns from side to side. Patients will be on their backs frequently enough for bathing, catheterizations, and other procedures. As vertebral healing, physical activity, and skin tolerance increase, turning frequency and positioning can be modified to meet individual needs.

Position correctly to disperse pressure of body weight and maintain correct body alignment. Support extremities to follow the body contour to avoid edema and muscle stretching or contracting. Be sure to protect bony prominences that are bearing body weight. Commonly used and easily available devices include pillows, foam padding, and footboards. Correct positioning for patients immobilized in bed has been described in Chapter 14.

Relief from Pressure while Patient Is in Wheelchair

As soon as patients get up in a chair, they are taught to lift the weight off their buttocks to provide relief from pressure. They may perform the movement independently by pushing themselves up with their arms (commonly known as *wheelchair pushups*) or by leaning over one side of the chair and then the other. Until pressure reliefs become "automatic," remind and encourage patients to establish their own routine every 15 minutes.

If patients are dependent for pressure reliefs, lifts must be performed by assistants. There are three basic methods outlined in Procedures 15–1, 15–2, and 15–3.

Protecting Patient from Injury to Skin

Moving patients carefully

To avoid shearing and friction forces, always use lifting movements rather than dragging movements. Remove your watch and any jew-

PROCEDURE 15–2 ■ METHOD TO PROVIDE A WHEELCHAIR PRESSURE RELIEF (ONE ASSISTANT)

Purpose

The purpose of a one-assistant lift is to provide pressure relief for patients who need help.

Action	Rationale
1. Lock the castor wheel in forward position.	This safely stabilizes and balances wheelchair.
2. Ensure that patient is sitting well back in the chair seat.	This prevents patient from tipping forward and losing balance.
3. Place a pillow on patient's knees (optional).	The pillow is needed for Halo-thoracic brace to rest on.
4. Stand in front of patient.	
5. Lean patient forward. Place hands under buttocks.	This ensures that weight is on the cushion.
6. Maintain position for 30 to 60 sec.	
7. Repeat procedure every 15 to 30 min while patient is up.	

elry. Support body weight with palms of the hands, not the fingertips. Always secure tubing and prevent it from touching the skin. Always inspect the sheets and sheepskin for any folds or wrinkles. Do not use linen if laundering has made it rough.

Transferring patients safely

To avoid falls or any possible bumping or scraping to the skin should patients slip during transfer, always get adequate help and use good body mechanics. Know the exact degree of assistance the patient requires. Avoid using trousers to lift a dependent patient; this puts pressure on the groin area. Use a two-person transfer if necessary. Check brakes on the bed and chair and remove obstacles such as foot plates or grab rails. If the patient's bare skin will come into contact with a transfer board, the board can be lightly powdered to reduce friction. The toilet seat may also be powdered.

Protecting patients from mechanical hazards

To avoid trauma to the skin constantly check all equipment for mechanical safety. For example, a broken buckle on a brace may cut the skin.

One of the most dangerous problems for patients with spinal cord injuries is the lack of sensory warning mechanisms to alert them to extremes in temperature and other skin trauma. To avoid burning the skin, never use hot water bottles, heat lamps, or other heat appliances. Also avoid ice packs. The patient must be taught to avoid numerous hazards, such as carrying hot liquid in a cup between the legs while in a wheelchair or even sitting too close to a car heater.

Most important items for quadriplegic patients are *pusher mitts*. These are leather strips fitted to the palms of the hands to protect the skin while propelling the wheelchair. See Figure 15–2.

Assisting Patient with Inspection of Skin

Skin inspection is one of the first crucial skills a patient must achieve. Assessment skills must be taught to detect any developing pressure areas. If this is not physically possible, the totally dependent patient must learn to direct others with this care. When the patient has a good knowledge base, cooperation will likely improve.

The Anderson and Andberg study (1979) revealed that the people with quadriplegia who actually performed skin inspection independently had fewer pressure sores than people with paraplegia who depended on others. This

PROCEDURE 15–3 ■ METHOD TO PROVIDE PROLONGED WHEELCHAIR PRESSURE RELIEF

Purpose

The purpose of procedure is to tip wheelchair back onto the bed to provide a convenient, prolonged pressure relief. This position is useful in the early stages when patients are building general physical tolerance. The energy it would take to transfer in and out of bed for a short rest can be reserved for some other activity.

Action	Rationale
1. Lower bed fully and apply brakes.	This safely secures bed at a compatible height with wheelchair.
2. Place two pillows on opposite side of bed for patient to rest head.	
3. Back wheelchair close to edge of bed.	
4. Tip chair back onto handles and *secure wheelchair brakes*.	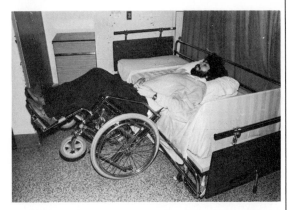
5. For quadriplegic patients, support each arm with pillows.	This protects skin, prevents gravitational edema, and avoids shoulder and neck pain by supporting weight of the arms.
6. This position can be maintained up to 2 hr.	

emphasizes the fact that patient involvement is crucial to successful care.

The patient must be turned within the first few hours after injury. Patient education should begin at this moment. A simple explanation can be: "We are going to turn you now to relieve the pressure on your back and keep up your circulation. You may have heard of bedsores; this is how they are prevented." Actually, many patients are curious to know why they must be turned, a procedure they often view as uncomfortable or inconvenient at best. This is an opportune time to introduce and reinforce the rationale behind pressure relief. (Note the terminology of *pressure* is emphasized.)

A mirror is an important aid to independence. A long-handled or adapted plexiglass mirror is needed. In collaboration with the occupational therapist nurses will teach patients a

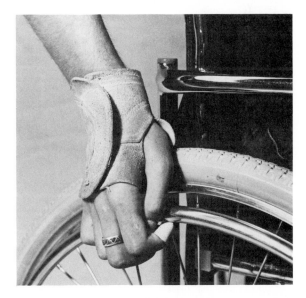

FIGURE 15–2 ■ A quadriplegic patient uses pusher mitts to protect his hands.

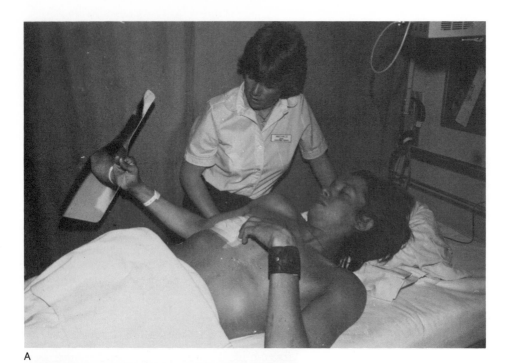

A

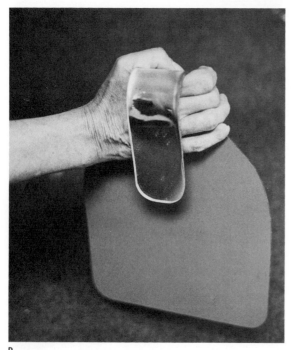

B

FIGURE 15–3 ■ (A) A patient is taught how to inspect his skin using a mirror. (B) The Plexiglas mirror can be bent so that a person with limited hand function can grasp it easily.

variety of side-lying positions for checking their skin. See Figure 15–3. Arm placement and hand function must be considered. Additional mirrors strategically placed on the wall or bed may be needed.

Provide partial or total assistance to patients in braces. Braces do not allow free access to see some parts of the skin, especially the back and buttocks; so the nurse must aid in checking these areas. In the early stages of the paraplegic treatment program, patients are not allowed excessive trunk rotation, so viewing the back is discouraged until later in the program. Encourage independence when movements are no longer restricted.

Assisting Patient to Increase Skin Tolerance

Although lifelong care is needed to protect the skin from pressure and other forces, skin tolerance can be increased. Skin tolerance is developed by gradually increasing the amount of time spent in one position followed by skin inspection to evaluate the process. For example, after any given length of time up in the wheelchair the skin should blanch when touched and pinkness or redness should disappear in 15 minutes or so. If it does, increase the time up by 15 minutes and repeat the process. If the skin does not clear, keep the patient off the area and instruct or perform pressure relief maneuvers more frequently when next up. The same principles apply to the turning schedule, especially increasing tolerance to the desirable prone position.

Assisting Patient with General Cleanliness, Personal Hygiene, and Appearance

People's appearance generally reflects the state of their health, both mental and physical. Attending to personal care and giving encouragement for the smallest signs of interest in appearance can be the patient's first steps toward increasing self-esteem, accepting responsibility for his or her own body, and eventually achieving independence.

Bathing

Bathing is refreshing and promotes normal skin functioning by removing contaminants and dead skin. Establish frequency according to need by considering general skin type, age, amount of exercise, body odor, and habits before injury. For example, patients with quadriplegia experience profuse sweating above the level of lesion, which may necessitate more frequent bathing, and active patients engaged in strenuous physical therapy will require daily showering to prevent body odor. Provide daily care to face, hands, underarms, and the groin area. Also be sure to clean and dry the skin following bowel or bladder procedures. This usually involves turning the patient, as the perineum is best exposed in the supine position and the buttocks (which must be separated) in the side-lying position. Promptly attend to the patient who is incontinent.

To minimize excessive drying and skin irritation generally select a mild soap without perfume or detergents; use tepid (not hot) water; and allow skin to "toughen" naturally. Do not apply lotions or alcohol rubs routinely. Applications of creams or lotions is necessary only if the

skin becomes dry and scaly (to prevent cracking or bleeding). Be especially careful in checking the lower limbs, where skin tends to become dry due to autonomic nervous system dysfunction and lack of sweat production.

Moisture softens the skin, so wet skin is more susceptible to breakdown. Always dry the patient thoroughly, especially between the toes and in the groin area. Remember that plastic-backed or waterproof pads trap moisture and heat. If absolutely necessary one pad correctly placed is far superior to several misplaced. These will become bunched up underneath the patient, which should be avoided. If the patient is sweating profusely, as is common with quadriplegia (due to autonomic nervous system dysfunction), terry towels placed about the neck and shoulders will help absorb the moisture. Complete linen changes may be needed with each two-hourly turn.

Tub bathing should begin as soon as possible. One extremely valuable aid for early care is a combination *bath stretcher-tub unit*. The model described here, and illustrated in Figure 15–4, was originally designed in Sweden to bathe dependent patients. It is particularly well suited for patients with spinal cord injuries, because spinal immobility can be maintained. The unit consists of three major components: a portable stretcher base; a stretcher platform; and a large tub with a submergible support structure that receives the stretcher platform. The patient is transferred to the portable stretcher unit at the bedside (a three-person lift is used) and transported to the tub. The stretcher platform is then locked into position and rolled onto the support structure in the tub. As the patient is lowered, the head of the stretcher automatically elevates 30 degrees. This feature is good for the patient in a Halo device. For a patient with a thoracolumbar fracture, who must remain flat, the stretcher may be swung around so that the feet are elevated or a spray attachment can be used. Pneumatic controls allow for ease of operation by one staff member. Other valuable features of this unit include: water temperature control, a disinfectant spray device, and soft waterproof padding for the stretcher.

It is important to remember that independent skills for washing can be introduced very

FIGURE 15–4 ■ A combination bath stretcher-tub unit: (Top) The mobile stretcher is wheeled to the bedside to receive the patient and then returned to the tub. (Middle) The platform is separated from the mobile base, moved over the tub, and anchored on a submergible frame. (Bottom) The stretcher platform is lowered into the tub by pneumatic controls. The head of the stretcher automatically elevates as the platform is lowered.

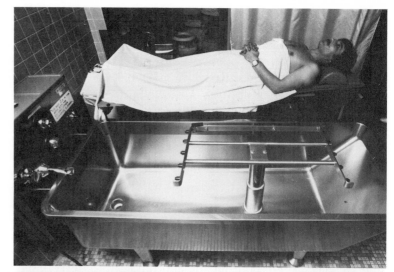

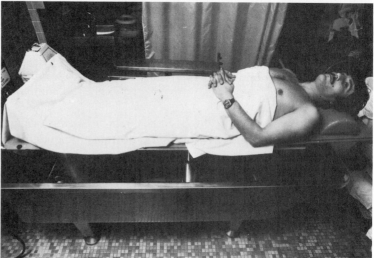

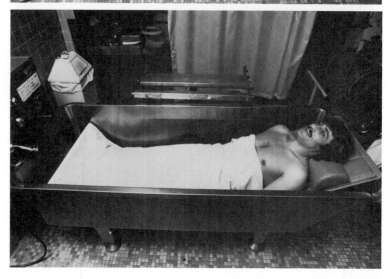

early. Once specific activity orders have been outlined by the physician—mainly the degree of elevation in bed and type of movements and transfers allowed—closely collaborate with the occupational therapist to begin a self-care regime. Generally the occupational therapist will be responsible for assessing the patient's physical potential, establishing realistic goals, advising on positioning that will allow the patient the greatest ease, selecting appropriate aids, and initiating progressions in self-care skills. It is then important for the nurse to integrate the skills into daily care, reinforce the lessons of the occupational therapist, monitor patient response, and communicate any problems to the occupational therapist. Warn the patient about excessively hot water causing burns to desensitized skin, and always have the patient test temperature beforehand. A temperature control device on a shower control is a handy item (especially during training when patients are learning skills to control hand and arm movements).

For the patient with a thoracic or lumbar injury, upper extremity washing can be introduced while on bedrest as soon as the patient is physically stable. Bathing in a stretcher-tub unit is usually permissible as soon as any surgical incisions are healed. Lower extremity washing can be introduced when the patient is allowed to sit at 45 to 60 degrees in bed. Place pillows under the knees to avoid a pulling strain on the back. As wheelchair sitting tolerance increases, the patient can be taught to transfer to a shower chair for hygiene care. When long sitting is allowed and the patient is capable of performing good lifting maneuvers, transfers to an ordinary bathtub can begin. See Figure 15–5.

For the patient with a *cervical injury,* upper extremity washing can be introduced when the patient is comfortable sitting at 45 degrees in bed. Use a bath mitt. Collaborate with the occupational therapist to use other aids and adapt positioning for individual needs. Lower extremity washing may be possible when the patient is able to balance well in long sitting.

Patients wearing the Halo device remain fairly dependent for washing skills. A device such as the bath stretcher-tub unit provides the greatest ease. It is possible to wash under the thoracic vest by immobilizing the patient in the supine or side-lying position and gently loosing the side buckles. See Chapter 14 for this procedure and further discussion of care for patients wearing the Halo-thoracic brace.

Following removal of the Halo device, the patient protected with a cervical brace can safely begin transfers to the shower chair. Be sure to use a safety strap to protect balance. Such aids as soap-on-a-rope to place around the neck and a long-handled bath sponge are helpful.

Throughout the mobilization program many bathing activities can only be performed with the added protection of a brace. When leather portions of the brace get wet they obviously cannot be worn for the remainder of the day. Former patients can be encouraged to return orthotic devices they no longer require. These make perfect bathing braces for an equipment pool!

Grooming

Attending to personal appearance contributes significantly to a patient's self-image and comfort. Clean hair, a fresh shave, or a touch of makeup can mean a lot to the dependent patient. Close collaboration with the occupational therapist is essential to promote independence in grooming.

For the patient with a *thoracic or lumbar injury,* grooming skills such as brushing teeth and combing hair can be encouraged while the patient is prone on the Stryker frame. As soon as patients can tolerate short periods up in the wheelchair they should be encouraged to complete all grooming activities at the sink. A lowered mirror, tilted forward, will help.

For the patient with a *cervical injury,* grooming skills can be introduced just after the Halo-brace is applied and the patient is comfortable sitting at 60 degrees in bed. When the patient is up in the wheelchair, and is comfortable in that position for an hour or more, grooming can be done at the sink. See Figure 15–6. When assisting patients, be sure to place them in a comfortable position free from interference from the bed or wheelchair. Individualized adaptive aids may include a padded toothbrush, comb, or hair brush or a pocket splint to fit these items. Generally, an electric razor, perhaps with an adaptive holder, is easiest.

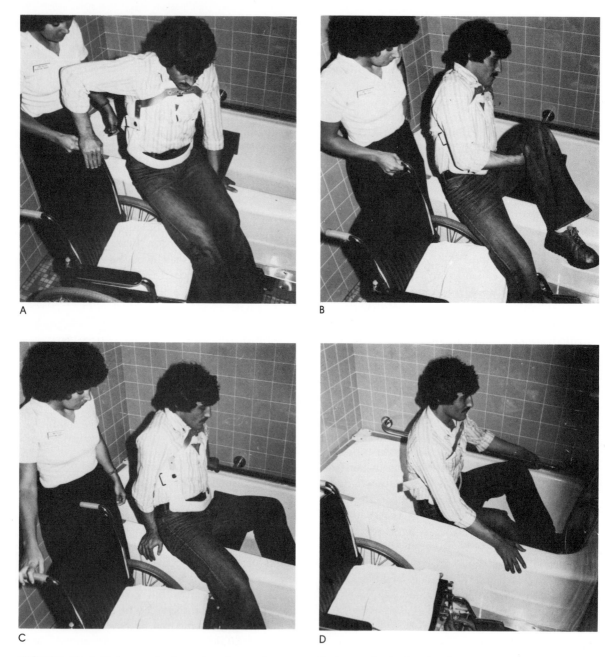

FIGURE 15–5 ■ A paraplegic patient is taught to transfer into a bathtub of a similar height to those used in most homes. Aids, such as a bath seat, may be needed.

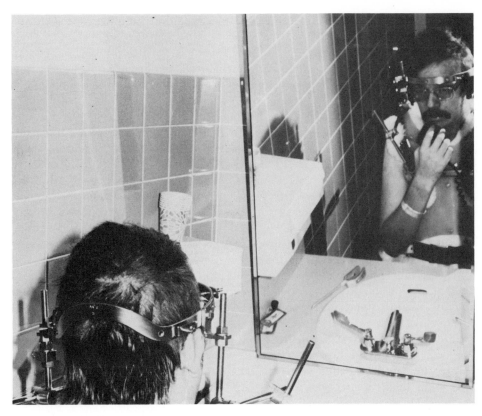

FIGURE 15–6 ■ A quadriplegic person attending to personal hygiene while still in the Halo apparatus.

Maintaining *dental hygiene* can be awkward for the dependent patient. If the patient is on bedrest take measures to prevent aspiration. Use the side-lying position; elevate or raise the head of the bed, if possible, and have a suction apparatus at hand. If the patient has difficulty expelling the debris into a kidney basin, continuous suction applied to the dependent side of the mouth can be used. Sometimes a tooth brush curved like a dental instrument, with a smaller brush area, is easier to maneuver. (These are available at most drug and department stores.) Use toothpaste and water sparingly; the mechanical action of brushing is more important. Flossing will help to remove plaque. Naturally, dental hygiene is much easier if the patient is able to sit up.

Hair care

The hair should be washed weekly or as before injury. To avoid excessive drying use a pH balanced commercial shampoo. If the patient has tong sites or pin sites use an antibacterial liquid soap. Clean sites using sterile procedure immediately after washing hair. (Review Procedures 14–2 and 14–4.) Weekly hair washing significantly minimizes risk of infection at insertion sites.

Foot care

The lack of normal wear and tear on patients with lower extremity paralysis can lead to excessive accumulation of hardened skin on the feet and hardened, thickened toenails. Cracks, cuts, calluses, and long toenails can lead to additional problems. Generally soaking the feet or wrapping them in a warm, moist towel for 20 minutes once a week is sufficient to soften the skin. Gentle rubbing with a wash cloth will remove the hardened skin. Dry feet well and massage with a lanolin-based cream. Carefully trim toenails straight across, preferably with clippers. (Clippers are a little easier to control should a spasm suddenly occur.)

Feet are also vulnerable to injury from bumping or dragging movements during transfer activity. It is important for the patient to wear shoes for added protection. A correct fit is essential to avoid pressure areas. Shoes often have to be purchased one size larger than normal to compensate for gravitational edema. Inexpensive tennis shoes are a good choice initially.

Be aware that feet are also prone to burns from hot water and car heaters. Feet must always be included in general skin inspection.

Feminine hygiene

Perineal care is a very important part of personal care for comfort and prevention of skin breakdown and bladder infections. The following information is partially based on the *Virginia Spinal Cord Injury Care and Teaching Manual* (1980) and Ford and Duckworth (1974).

Daily care should include washing the outer perineum, labia, and area between the thighs with mild soap, rinsing well, and drying thoroughly. Perineal care should be done each morning and evening and after evacuation of urine or feces. This may be performed in bed (turn the patient to the side to separate the buttocks and clean the anal area) or on a toilet or commode. Teach the patient always to wash from front to back to prevent vaginal contamination from the rectal area.

Excoriation of the perineal area may be caused by frequent use of antiseptic solutions used with an intermittent catheterization regime. To care for a woman on an intermittent catheterization program, clean with normal saline or sterile water, according to skin tolerance. Avoid harsher solutions. Squeeze excess cleaning solution out of cotton balls. This prevents the solution collecting in the gluteal crease and causing irritation. Turn the patient and dry area thoroughly following procedure. A woman with an indwelling catheter should move the leg bag from one side to the other daily to avoid pressure on the labia minora.

A local infection, such as vaginitis or urethritis, may also cause skin irritation. Specific systemic or topical medication should be ordered by the physician to control the cause. Mild vinegar

douching works well to curb mild but persistent vaginitis.

Tampons or sanitary pads may be used depending on personal preference, comfort, and ease with which a patient can independently insert tampons or place pads. Tampons are generally preferred for cleanliness. Tampons that come with a smooth plastic applicator are easier to insert. The patient will also find this maneuver easier when on the toilet. Tampons do create additional pressure on the bladder, so their use may be delayed during bladder training.

Sanitary pads with double adhesive strips that stick to the underpants are best. A pad may be placed in the crotch of the underpants before pulling them up. A crotch flap, with a Velcro closure, made in a pair of stretchy underpants from leg opening to leg opening may be useful to some patients. Many women cannot tolerate the bulk and dampness of a normal sanitary pad. Larger dressings or commercial disposable diapers may be helpful to distribute the pressure and moisture.

Tampons or pads should be changed at least every four hours. During the menstrual cycle, the entire perineal area including the gluteal crease must be observed. Assist the woman to perform this task with a mirror.

Independent and even general management of the menstrual period may become a major problem for the quadriplegic woman, especially if she has a heavy flow. Menstruation can be controlled through medication (birth control pills taken on a daily basis), or surgical intervention may be sought to eliminate menstruation entirely.

Clothing

Help the patient choose appropriate and attractive clothing. Soft, loose-fitting clothes of wash and wear fabrics are ideal. Ill-fitting clothing can cause pressure areas and edema. Cotton underwear is most absorbent. Avoid all nylon clothes as they tend to hold perspiration against the skin. Avoid large seams, buttons, or snaps on the sides of clothing. Brightly colored warm-up suits are a convenient choice during early rehabilitation. Blouses and shirts can be loose fitting or cut to fit around the bars of the Halo device. Dressing skills are discussed in Chapter 16.

Maintaining Adequate Nutritional Status

Collaborate with the nutritional team, dietitian, and physician to provide optimal nutrition. A high-protein, adjusted calorie diet is needed initially to replace weight loss often encountered during the critical period and to prevent protein deficiency or anemia. Caloric intake must be continually adjusted to suit activity. Vitamin and iron supplements are often given to promote general physical health following trauma. Maintain a fluid intake of 2000 to 3000 mL/day (adjusted to bladder management requirements) to prevent dehydration.

Promoting Systemic Circulation

In addition to regular turning and correct positioning, take measures to promote systemic circulation. Cardiopulmonary function must be adequate to ensure cellular oxygenation and nutrition. In general, nursing interventions to prevent or control postural hypotension and gravitational edema, such as passive and active range of motion exercises, graded mobility programs, and application of elastic stockings and abdominal binders, will improve systemic circulation and thus contribute to good skin care.

Selecting Devices to Assist with Pressure Relief

There are three main classifications of devices used in the prevention and management of pressures sores: devices that assist with turning; devices that alter pressure intermittently; and devices that minimize pressure (King 1981).

Turning devices particularly suited for early care of patients with spinal cord injuries are the Wedge-Stryker turning frame and the Stoke-Eggerton electrical turning and tilting bed (see Chapter 14). Both beds make it possible to maintain spinal immobility while enhancing ease of skin care.

Numerous elaborate and sophisticated devices may be used to alter pressure intermittently and minimize or equalize pressure. Flotation systems using air, water, or foam have made significant contributions to lowering or reducing external pressure so it is less than capillary pressure. Devices such as the air support system or the Rancho flotation MUD bed are mostly used for actual management of advanced or multiple pressure areas or for postsurgical treatment. These devices and others are well introduced and summarized by King (1981). As this chapter focuses on prevention, however, the more simple, practical, and economical devices (also suitable for home use) will be presented. Above all remember that *devices may reduce pressure but do not eliminate the need for turning and positioning, or, when used in the wheelchair do not eliminate the clinical practice of pressure relief maneuvers.*

Mattresses and mattress coverings

Synthetic sheepskin is a popular, practical, and convenient aid. Synthetic sheepskin, preferably the full length of the bed, helps distribute pressure evenly, prevent shearing forces, reduce friction, eliminate wrinkles, dissipate heat, and absorb moisture. Synthetic sheepskin must be laundered regularly—about every three days as it absorbs body perspiration, or more frequently if it becomes soiled with urine or fecal material. Strong detergents, hot water, or harsh drying cycles will harden and mat this material. To avoid trauma to the skin the product must then be discarded. Often special arrangements with the hospital laundry will help avoid this problem. Some patients tend to develop contact dermatitis, especially in hot weather, when using sheepskin. A soft cotton or flannelette sheet placed on top of the sheepskin may be helpful. A simple foam sheet (polyurethane), 2 inches thick, can also help distribute body weight and reduce pressure.

As previously mentioned, a number of simple fluidized flotation systems are also available. For example, commercial camper air mattresses filled with water to 60% to 70% of capacity have been used successfully as inexpensive pressure-dispersing devices (Kijeck and Jordan 1979).

Even simple devices may be needed only for special circumstances—for example, if the flu or some other temporary ailment will confine the patient to bed for a few days. If a patient is at additional risk because of malnourishment or other secondary factors, then certainly more

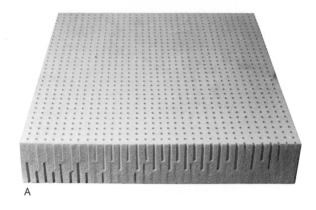

A

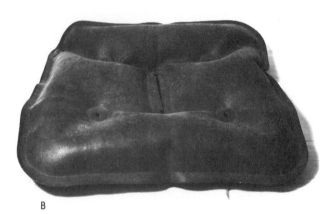

B

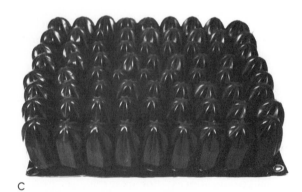

C

FIGURE 15–7 ■ The most widely used cushions are: (A) A foam rubber cushion. (B) An air inflatable cushion. (C) The ROHO cushion.

sophisticated flotation devices should be considered to help prevent skin problems.

Wheelchair cushions

The selection of a wheelchair cushion is of major importance to patients with spinal cord injuries. Many kinds are available, but no single type is clearly superior in relieving pressure for all patients (Garber et al. 1978; Fisher et al. 1978; and DeLateur et al. 1976).

Basically wheelchair cushions are dense blocks of polyurethane foam, air-inflatable bladders, flotation devices, or gel pads. See Figure 15–7 for some examples of cushions. A variety of soft fabric, plastic, or vinyl covers are used to facilitate sliding movements during transfers and to protect the cushion.

- Foam rubber cushions are widely used and recommended as a long-term serviceable choice to reduce pressure. However, dangerously high pressures may still exist over bony prominences. Individually measured and cut cushions allow weight to shift away from bony prominences. Foam cushions deteriorate over a short period of time and must be replaced about once a year.
- Air-inflatable cushions may be a simple air-inflated bladder, such as the Bye-Bye Decubiti cushion, or individually air-filled bladders secured to a single base, such as the ROHO Dry Flotation cushion, which looks like an egg carton. Although some patients find these cushions lighter to manage, the somewhat unstable surface may cause balance problems, especially when transferring.
- Flotation cushions filled with water, air, or foam are another alternative. Water flotation cushions have a lower temperature than air or foam ones. This may be an advantage, particularly in hot climates, as excessive heat is thought to render the skin more susceptible to soft tissue breakdown (Fisher et al. 1978).
- Gel pads are most successfully used by patients with paraplegia as they are heavy to move around. The tendency to sink also makes them more difficult to transfer from. They may be used in the wheelchair and then transferred to the bed to relieve pressure on the buttocks.

The nurse's responsibility in choosing wheelchair cushions varies greatly. Generally the physical therapist and occupational therapist are most involved. Pressure clinics in rehabilitation centers are slowly evolving to deal with this major problem.

More research on cushions is needed. One difficulty is collecting objective data of the *overall* distribution of pressure, not just pressure over bony prominences. The Rehabilitation Engineering Center in Texas has developed a pressure evaluation pad for use in the clinical setting, so better information may be available soon. (Garber et al. 1978)

Providing Psychological Support and Health Education

A more holistic approach to skin care and prevention of pressure sores includes assessment and promotion of desirable patient knowledge, skills, and attitudes. This type of nursing intervention helps avoid the "recipe approach to a specific procedure" (Mikulic 1980), which has met with such limited success in the past. Try to promote feelings of self-worth and self-esteem and enhance learning by applying principles outlined in Chapters 6 through 8.

Many centers have formalized educational classes on etiology, skin inspection, and the importance of relieving pressure in a variety of positions. Integrating behavioral modification and operant conditioning into the nursing process has also been advocated in an attempt to promote patient compliance with well-known preventive measures to avoid skin breakdown.

SPECIFIC NURSING INTERVENTIONS FOR MANAGEMENT OF PRESSURE AREAS

If any of the danger signs from pressure have already developed, immediately implement further preventive measures to reverse the underlying cause. As pressure sores are *always* caused by pressure, first relieve the pressure and then eliminate the sore. The following recommendations (Goldfinger and Hanak 1981 and *Virginia Manual* 1980) are used to deal with a newly developed pressure area (a reddened area that may progress to a partial thickness ulceration limited to the epidermis but with inflammatory reaction affecting all underlying soft tissue).

Goals of care

- To identify patients that run additional risks of developing pressure areas
- To recognize a pressure area immediately
- To relieve pressure on an affected area
- To identify and eliminate the cause
- To prevent secondary infection
- To help the patient implement measures to prevent recurrence

Nursing Interventions

1. Practice preventive measures on a priority basis. For example, the critically ill patient who may be hypoxic or malnourished and in spinal shock will require more frequent turning and skin inspection than stable patients who have increased their skin tolerance. A patient who has just returned from an initial weekend pass may need additional help to assess and care for any potential skin problems caused by the different environment and different routines. See Table 15–1.

2. Note any reddened areas that do not completely subside within 30 minutes following relief of pressure; blisters; open areas in the skin; scalds; and rashes or excoriated areas. Bony prominences that are most susceptible to pressure sores include:

- *The sacrum:* caused by prolonged periods in the supine position without a position change.
- *The ischeal tuberosities:* caused by lack of adequate pressure relief maneuvers when up in the wheelchair or by setting the foot plates on the wheelchair too high. Even with frequent pressure reliefs, sores will occur with foot plates set too high.
- *The coccyx* (over the tailbone on tip of the spine): caused by slouching or slipping in a sitting position in bed or wheelchair.
- *The trochanter:* caused by prolonged side-lying. Possibly adductor spasms of the legs can cause shearing forces on the hips. An individualized apparatus to spread the knees may be needed.

- *The knee* (sores on the sides or front of the knee): caused by prolonged side-lying without pillows between the knees or possibly proning without bridging the knee. Presence of adductor spasm may necessitate extra padding between the knees to separate and protect skin surfaces.
- *The heel* (sores on the back or sides of the heel): caused by prolonged supine and side-lying positioning without adequate padding. Leg spasms can pull heels into the bed or foot straps on the wheelchair. Sheepskin heel protectors may reduce friction forces but may also be difficult to keep in place; positioning a protective strap behind the calves may eliminate the need for a foot strap and prevent injury if legs spasm backward. Ill-fitting shoes can also cause pressure sores. In general the feet are most affected by any slowed circulation such as edema.

3. Relieve the pressure by not having the patient sit or lie on the affected area. This may mean returning the patient to bed for several days and limiting therapy activities or independent activities such as dressing or transferring. The patient may be mobilized on a stretcher. Anticipate relieving pressure for 48 to 72 hours for a closed reddened area and for from 10 to 14 days should necrosis occur. *Do not discontinue pressure relief positioning until redness has completely subsided.* Be sure to schedule position changes every two hours so other areas will not be subject to excessive pressure. If the patient has multiple pressure areas the use of bridging or selection of devices that equalize pressure may be needed. These devices may also be needed if secondary factors contribute to further risk of skin breakdown. Depending on the severity of breakdown specific treatments may be needed to promote healing as follows:

- *A small intact area of warmth and redness.* To reduce inflammation and swelling, rotate an ice cube over the area until it melts. Avoid ice packs that can actually "burn" the area. To protect the skin from contaminants or friction a product called Op-Site™* may be used. It is a semipermeable synthetic membrane that allows underlying skin to "breathe" while protecting it from invading moisture and bacteria. *Do not use* if the sore is weeping or open. It will trap debris and promote bacterial growth.
- *A small broken area surrounded by pink tissue.* Clean a shallow or superficial open area every four hours with regular hydrogen peroxide (H_2O_2) diluted with normal saline. This has an antiseptic effect and may improve local circulation. Dry the area by leaving it open to the air as much as possible. The area may be exposed to a stream of low-pressure oxygen (from regular wall outlet) every few hours. A light, sterile gauze dressing may be used if the area is draining. Do not use adhesive tape on desensitized skin. Secure dressing with lightweight paper or nonallergic tape.
- *An infected superficial area.* If the pressure area remains superficial but discoloration or drainage occurs, the area is probably infected. Obtain a specimen for culture and sensitivity and collaborate with the physician for further management. Systemic antibiotics are usually reserved for serious complications such as cellulitis or septicemia. Selected topical antibiotics may be ordered. At this point the door is opened to enormous selection of controversial treatments. Many agents appear to have merit but lack support of conclusive research.

However, the principle of debridement of necrotic tissue is basic to healing. The body's natural defense mechanism for removal of wound debris is activated about six hours after injury. Enzymes released by white blood cells destroy necrotic tissue. Natural debridement may be adequate for healing an ulcerated area given adequate pressure relief (Kijeck and Jordan 1979). Early debridement techniques are limited to mechanical or biochemical means.

A debridement effect can be created by allowing simple normal saline dressings to dry and then gently peeling them off. Irritant solutions may be used for bacteriostatic activity and mechanical removal of necrotic tissue. Be sure to protect the surrounding skin with a barrier cream. Wet dressings may be applied for 20 minutes every four hours. If the dressings are kept continually wet, keeping them in place will be difficult, particularly on desensitized skin.

---

* Smith and Nephew, Inc., 2100 52nd Ave. Lachine, Quebec, Canada H 8T245.

These measures are effective for healing a newly developed pressure sore. Additional measures are simply not necessary.

4. Should a *blister* form do not break it. A route for invading bacteria will be established. Continue to relieve pressure and keep the surrounding skin clean and dry.
5. Should a *burn* or *scald* occur, immediately administer first aid treatment of cold water for 20 minutes. Do not apply creams or lotions. Contact the physician. Normal saline baths, given once or twice daily, are effective for treating scalds. (Be sure to clean the tub thoroughly before and after each bath to prevent spread of infection.) Scalds frequently occur on the lap where contamination from urine or feces can easily cause infection. If skin irritation is severe, a more frequent intermittent catheterization program or an indwelling catheter to control incontinence may have to be resumed temporarily.
6. Should a *cleft sore in the gluteal crease* occur, eliminate shearing forces by maintaining bedrest, encouraging prone positioning, or modifying transfer procedure with additional assistance to avoid "spreading" of the gluteal area. This is mostly a problem when transferring and positioning the patient on a toilet. Again prevent contamination from urine and feces.

See Table 15–3 for a summary of the preceding six interventions.

7. Assess and take steps to minimize secondary factors such as malnutrition, edema, or psychological depression.
8. Reestablish mobility and rebuild skin tolerance gradually. Remember any area that has previously broken down is potentially unstable.
9. Assess patient knowledge and provide education as indicated to avoid recurrence.
10. Evaluate nursing care with objective data. Use tracings of actual sore size on graph recordings, photographs, or an instrument to measure perimeter and calculate area of the wound if necessary. Effectiveness of treatment can be evaluated according to level of outcome reached:

- Skin normal color without evidence of increased temperature, redness, or drainage
- Underlying cause eliminated
- Patient able to verbalize principles of good skin

care and demonstrate responsibility for supervising or performing skin inspection and providing adequate relief from pressure.

SELF-CARE SKILLS

The onus of responsibility for care of the skin and personal hygiene must ultimately be accepted by the patient. Once the patient has accepted this responsibility self-care skills can be taught with relative ease. However, even when varying degrees of adjustment to disability may block learning, it is still important for the nurse to include the patient and explain the rationale supporting skin care. Continually assuming full responsibility for skin care without patient education fosters the patient's feelings of helplessness, which is actually detrimental.

Basically patient education must include information on how pressure sores develop; how and when to inspect the skin; and how and when to perform pressure relief maneuvers, including turning and correct positioning in bed or in the wheelchair. In addition the patient should be taught the importance of general skin cleanliness, good personal hygiene, eating correctly, and maintaining good general circulation. Numerous hazards (such as those given in Table 15–4) and unexpected situations will occur, especially outside a rehabilitation setting. But the excellent creative literature currently written for patients can help them cope with such hazards and situations. For additional information, refer to the reference material at the end of the chapter.

The Patient with Paraplegia

The patient with paraplegia is physically capable of becoming totally independent in all aspects of skin care, although during the first six months after injury considerable assistance may be required. Orthopedic thoracolumbar appliances and prevention of spinal rotation often hamper maneuvers needed for skin inspection and care.

TABLE 15–3 ■ MANAGEMENT OF A NEWLY DEVELOPED PRESSURE AREA*

Type	Intervention
Reddened area (skin intact)	Relieve pressure until redness subsides; remove cause of pressure; apply ice cube for edema; use Op-site for protection from friction; rebuild skin tolerance
Small open area surrounded by pink tissue	Clean with hydrogen peroxide and normal saline solution; dry area, possibly with stream of oxygen; light gauze dressing (optional)
Infected superficial area (area discolored or draining)	Culture and sensitivity test; topical antibiotics as ordered by physician (optional); debridement with normal saline dressings, which are allowed to dry before removal; possible wet dressings (with irritant solutions) for 20 min every 4 hr
Blister	Do not break; relieve pressure until healed
Burn or scald	Administer first aid treatment of cold water (do not apply lotions or creams); follow with saline dressings or saline baths as ordered by physician; prevent contamination from urine or feces
Cleft sore in gluteal crease	Maintain bedrest to eliminate shearing forces; modify transfer procedure with lifting as opposed to sliding techniques; prevent contamination from urine or feces

* Note: Treatment of all newly developed pressure areas requires relief from pressure until symptoms subside; assessment and treatment of contributing secondary factors; and rebuilding skin tolerance.

The Patient with Quadriplegia

The physical activity involved in maintaining skin integrity becomes much more complex for the patient with quadriplegia. However, each patient should be encouraged to perform or direct others to inspect and care for the skin. This would include maneuvers to provide pressure relief and protect the skin from injury (such as safety factors to consider when transferring).

Independence in daily activities depends on the patient's desire and level of lesion. Many patients with quadriplegia can manage grooming skills with adaptive aids. Such things as foot care or shampooing are more complex and assistance may be required. For bathing, many patients require extensive bathroom alterations to build shower facilities that are wheelchair accessible.

LONG-TERM IMPLICATIONS

When assessing a patient who has been paralyzed for some time, keep in mind that freedom from skin breakdown is a realistic goal that can be achieved.

The community health nurse will no doubt be called in to deal with a pressure sore that already exists. A thorough history taking and assessment of current physical status as outlined will be needed to manage the problem efficiently. Based on the assessment assist the patient to continue with current preventive measures, provide appropriate intervention, or refer the patient to other resources.

TABLE 15–4 ■ COMMON HAZARDS ENCOUNTERED IN THE HOME THAT CAUSE PRESSURE OR TRAUMA TO THE SKIN

- Tight-fitting jeans!
- Objects in pockets
- Rough bed linen; fitted percale sheets are more durable; flannelette sheets tend to become rough with repeated laundering
- Pressure on elbows from dressing; elbow pads are a good idea
- Spasms causing shearing forces; especially susceptible are ankles and heels
- Burns on feet from hot water dripping into the bath tub
- No regulating device on taps to control sudden increase in hot water that causes burns
- No insulation around exposed sink pipes draining hot water that also causes burns
- Elevating the head of the bed for watching television resulting in unrelieved pressure on buttocks

Treating a pressure sore in the home must also encompass both physical and psychological aspects of care. If the patient is the homemaker, necessary bedrest may impose considerable difficulties. Support may be needed in the form of homemaking, child care, or other services. However, pressure relief is the primary goal; without it, the extent of the sore will increase and it will not heal, no matter what other treatment is used (King 1981).

Advanced pressure sore management is difficult with any patient. The additional risks run by patients with spinal cord injuries mount up very quickly. Even before surgical intervention the wound must be debrided and free from infection; underlying conditions such as malnourishment must be reversed; and spasticity, if present, must be controlled.

Self-destructive tendencies may be another issue to deal with. Pressure sores may become life threatening. Their effects on self-image, body image, family and social relationships, sexuality, and vocational potential are difficult to quantify, but the cost is evident (Kijeck and Jordon 1979).

SELECTED REFERENCES

Anderson, T., and Andberg, M. 1979. Psychosocial factors associated with pressure sores. *Archives of Physical Medicine and Rehabilitation* 60 (Aug.): 341–346. *Research reveals that psychological factors of assuming responsibility for skin care and satisfaction with the activities of life, not purely mechanical or physical risk factors, are related to the incidence of pressure sores.*

Burke, D., and Murray, D. 1975. *Handbook of Spinal Cord Medicine.* London and Basingstoke: Macmillan Press, Chapter 8. *Concise review of pressure sores; pathophysiology and treatment.*

DeLateur, B., et al. 1976. Wheelchair cushions designed to prevent pressure sores: an evaluation. *Archives of Physical Medicine and Rehabilitation* 57 (Mar.): 129–135. *A physiological comparison of several wheelchair cushions indicate that the clinical practice of weight-bearing relief is essential to combat reactive hyperemia, regardless of the cushion used.*

Fisher, M.; Szymke, T.; and Kosiak, M. 1978. Wheelchair cushion effects on skin temperature. *Archives of Physical Medicine and Rehabilitation* 59 (Feb.): 68–72. *Examines skin temperature as a contributing factor to skin breakdown, which requires further research; reveals that skin temperatures significantly increased with foam rubber cushions and significantly decreased with hydrocushions.*

Ford, J., and Duckworth, B. 1974. *Physical Management for the Quadriplegic Patient.* Philadelphia: F. A. Davis. *Provides information for practical management of feminine hygiene in long-term care.*

Garber, S.; Krouskop, T.; and Carter, R. 1978. A system for clinically evaluating wheelchair pressure-relief cushions. *American Journal of Occupational Therapy* 32 (9): 565–570. *Report on a pressure evaluation pad to determine pressure distribution when the patient is seated in a wheelchair.*

Goldfinger, G., and Hanak, M. 1981. *Spinal Cord Injury: a Guide for Care.* New York Regional Spinal Cord Injury System. *Designed for patient and family health education, the section on skin care presents information on danger signs, protective and preventive measures, foot care, turning and positioning, protective equipment, and care of superficial breakdown areas.*

Gosnell, D. 1973. An assessment tool to identify pressure sores. *Nursing Research* 22 (1): 55–59. *Evaluation of a simple, versatile assessment tool rating mental status, continence, mobility, activity, and nutrition to identify high-risk patients.*

Guttman, L. 1976. *Spinal Cord Injuries Comprehensive Management and Research.* 2d ed. London: Blackwell Scientific Publications. *A classic, multifaceted reference text on spinal cord injuries. Includes historical background information; general statistics; legal aspects; detailed anatomy and neuropathology of cord trauma and resultant effects on all body systems; regeneration; fractures and dislocations, gunshot injuries, and stab wounds; and neurophysiological and clinical management aspects including pressure sores. Extensive bibliography.*

Guyton, A. 1976. *Textbook of Medical Physiology.* 5th ed. Philadelphia: W. B. Saunders. *Classic text detailing neuroanatomy and physiology, including that of the integumentary system.*

Kavcheck-Keyes, M. 1977. Treating decubitus ulcers using four proven steps. *Nursing '77,* October, pp. 44–45. *Basic steps describing relief of pressure, ulcer debriding, wound treatment, and optimal nutrition.*

Kijeck, J., and Jordan, M. 1979. Nursing strategies: prevention and treatment of the pressure ulcer. In *Current Perspectives in Rehabilitation Nursing.* Eds. R. Murray and J. Kijeck. St. Louis: C. V. Mosby, pp. 84–96. *Focus on identification of risk factors and preventive measures; briefly reviews methods of resolving any infection and wound hygiene.*

King, R. 1981. Assessment and management of soft tissue pressure. In *Comprehensive Rehabilitation Nursing.* Eds. N. Martin, N. Holt, and D. Hicks. New York: McGraw-Hill, pp. 242–268. *Outstanding in-depth review of current theory and practice with direction for future research. Highly recommended.*

King, R.; Boyink, M.; and Keenan, M., Eds. *Rehabilitation Guide.* Medical Rehabilitation Research and Training Center No. 20. Chicago: Northwest University and Rehabilitation Institute of Chicago. *Detailed presentation designed for patient and family education; includes illustrated guide to positioning, explanation of pressure sore development, and management of other skin problems such as minor burns, ingrown toenails, bruises, and rashes.*

Mikulic, M. 1980. Treatment of pressure ulcers. *American Journal of Nursing* 80 (6): 1125–1128. *A comprehensive overview of approaches to prevention and treatment; focuses on the need for further research. Extensive bibliography citing specific treatments. Highly recommended.*

Miller, M., and Sachs, M. 1974. *About Bedsores.* Philadelphia: J. B. Lippincott. *Skillfully conveys basic concepts essential for preventing and treating pressure sores; includes full-color laboratory photographs to show the effects of pressure and shearing forces. Suitable also for patient and family education. Highly recommended.*

Spence, A., and Mason, E. 1979. *Human Anatomy and Physiology.* 2d ed. Menlo Park, Calif: Benjamin/Cummings. *Presents an in-depth coverage of both anatomy and physiology, and deals with the integumentary system in Chapter 5.*

Thomas, E. 1977. Nursing care of the patient with spinal cord injury. In *The Total Care of Spinal Cord Injuries.* Eds. D. Pierce and V. Nickel. Boston: Little, Brown, pp. 249–298. *Focus on prevention; includes helpful chart on common safety hazards and preventive measures in the home, car, when walking, and when outdoors.*

Treishmann, R. 1980. *Spinal Cord Injuries, Psychological, Social and Vocational Adjustment.* New York: Pergamon Press, pp. 79–81. *Information correlating personality characteristics and decubitus ulcer incidence.*

Virginia Spinal Cord Injury Care and Teaching Manual. 1980. The Virginia Spinal Cord Injury System, University of Virginia Center and Virginia Dept. of Rehabilitation Services, Woodrow Wilson Rehabilitation Center, Box W-279, Fisherville, Va. 22939. *Clear and concise illustrated overview of preventive measures for pressure sores. Treatment guidelines for a Grade 1 pressure sore recommended.*

SUPPLEMENTAL READING

Ferguson-Pell, M., et al. 1980. Pressure sore prevention for the wheelchair-bound spinal injury patient. *International Journal of Paraplegia* 18(1): 42–51. *Review of 600 patients attending a wheelchair cushion fitting clinic. This concept seems to be a good preventive measure against pressure sores.*

Green, B., et al. 1980. Kinetic nursing for acute spinal cord injury patients. *International Journal of Paraplegia* 18(3): 181–5. *Review of 105 patients treated on a Roto-Rest Mark I hospital bed. This bed places the patient in perpetual motion while immobilizing the spine. Common complications were reduced.*

Norris, W. C.; Noble, C. E.; and Strickland, S. B. 1981. *Spinal Injury Learning Series.* Jackson, Miss: University Press of Mississippi. *Educational program purchased on a fee-for-service basis; currently offers education on bowel, bladder, and skin care with plans to expand and continually update content.*

Richards, J. 1981. Pressure ulcers in spinal cord injury: psychosocial correlates. *Model Systems' Spinal Cord Injury Digest* 3(Summer): 11–27. *Article examines the role of the patient in the process of pressure sore prevention; specifically those psychological and emotional characteristics that allow patients to ignore instructions on prevention of pressure sores. Describes some behavioral approaches that have shown promise.*

Young, J., and Burns, P. 1981. Pressure sores and the spinal cord injured: Part I. *Model Systems' Spinal Cord Injury Digest* 3(Fall): 9–23. *Information on pressure sores occurring during the initial acute period. Data for 4758 cases injured from 1975 to 1980 were reported to the National Spinal Cord Injury Data Research Center by the 14 regional spinal cord injury systems.*

Young, J. and Burns, P. 1981. Pressure sores and the spinal cord injured: Part II. *Model Systems' Spinal Cord Injury Digest* 3(Winter): 11–26. *Second part of statistical survey of pressure sores occurring throughout the system with emphasis on pressure sores that develop over the years after discharge. Recommends a comprehensive pressure sore prevention program, which should include meticulous nursing care in specialized spinal cord injury units, patient/family education, behavioral modification, training, bioengineering, and ongoing surveillance.*

Film

Preventing Pressure Sores. Prepared by 3M wound management systems from the book *About Bedsores* (Miller and Sachs 1974). Available from 3M Center, St. Paul, Minn, 55101.

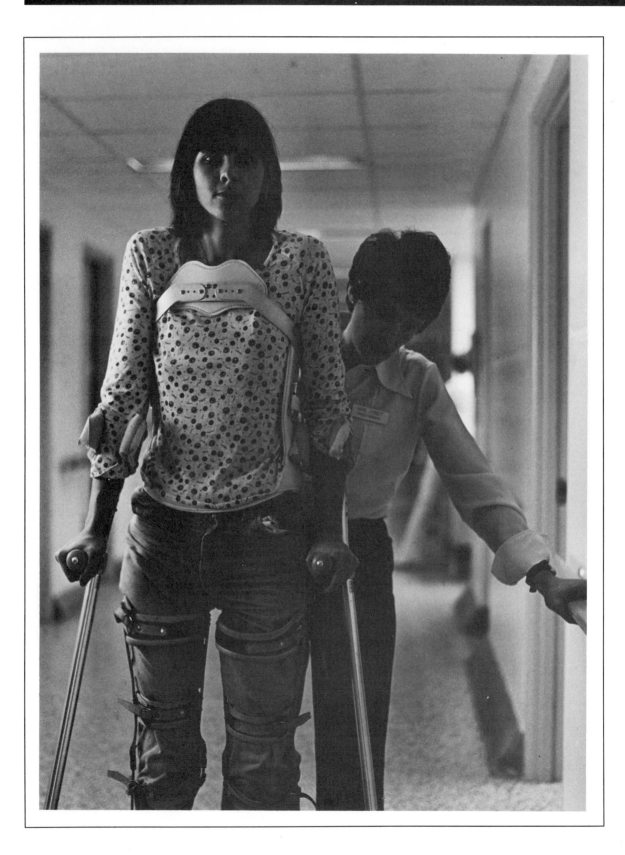

Chapter 16

Resuming Physical Activity and Achieving Independence*

CHAPTER OUTLINE

* This chapter was developed with assistance from Susan Laughlin, B.S.R., former Senior Occupational Therapist; and Dierdre Webster, B.S.R., former Senior Physical Therapist; Acute Spinal Cord Injury Unit, Shaughnessy Hospital, Vancouver, B.C.

OBJECTIVES

- To identify health care goals for resuming physical activity and achieving independence
- To reveal the potential nurse's role in reactivation
- To explain the relationship between physiological and psychological loss following spinal cord injury
- To describe the importance of the patient's history as it relates to physical activity
- To explain the significance of detailed muscle testing, joint range of motion, muscle tone, sensation, body build, and coordination in relation to functional activities
- To discuss roles of the nurse, physical therapist, and occupational therapist for promoting physical activity and patient independence
- To describe philosophy of promoting self-care activities
- To define activities of daily living (ADL)
- To outline general functional expectations for the patient with paraplegia, quadriplegia, and an incomplete injury
- To reinforce teaching of self-care skills
- To describe long-term implications associated with loss of physical capabilities following spinal cord injury

GOALS OF HEALTH CARE

As all patients with spinal cord injuries suffer from some loss of strength and ability to move, an exercise program is essential to ensure that they regain maximum possible muscle function. Exercise is supplemented by nursing measures such as correct positioning, turning, and provision of psychological support and encouragement. As the rehabilitation process evolves, physical capabilities are developed into the finer skills involved with personal care. The physical therapists and occupational therapists select and teach appropriate activities and work closely with nurses to maintain safety and comfort while allowing patients to use the skills they have learned. Later in rehabilitation, this process may involve other disciplines, such as remedial gymnasts and recreational personnel to help broaden the scope of treatment to include group performance and community living skills.

Greater recognition is being given to the concept that fostering independence is as much the nurse's responsibility as the therapist's. For rehabilitation to be effective, techniques must be incorporated into daily patient activities and thus into daily nursing care. The ready availability of therapists in patient's rooms during this time promotes application of functional activities and enhances sharing of professional expertise. This interaction is invaluable, especially to nurses involved in the early postinjury period.

To gain maximum benefits from therapeutic programs that focus on development of functional living skills for community life, preventive and restorative measures must begin within hours after injury. The goals of such exercise and physical activity programs are:

- To prevent physical deterioration by maintaining joint range of motion and avoiding muscle contractures or strains
- To promote optimal function by strengthening existing muscles and facilitating potential redevelopment of weak muscles

- To minimize patient discomfort, pain, and spasm
- To develop a self-care program that patients can realistically manage or teach others how to perform
- To teach patients to understand the rationale of their treatment; to develop a positive attitude and to set their own goals; to learn the skills required to function at their maximum level of independence; and to teach others how to assist them when necessary
- To assist the disabled person with home renovations when necessary
- To help patients use community resources for assistance with personal care; homemaking services; and vocational, social, and recreational pursuits

ASSESSMENT

Changes in Physical Capabilities After Spinal Cord Injury

Physical capabilities depend on the integrated functions of the nervous and musculoskeletal systems, modified by individual interests, desires, and inherent coordinative abilities. Following spinal cord injury, physiological damage is obvious and devastating. The patient must cope not only with motor and sensory loss, but also with skeletal immobilization and physical exhaustion in response to the initial trauma. Generally, the higher the level of lesion, the more profound the physical effects. Psychological factors associated with dramatic body image changes, compounded by accompanying physical fatigue, can suppress motivation considerably, and *motivation* is a key factor in resuming physical activity and achieving independence.

History

General health before injury
Patients who enjoyed good health, were well nourished, controlled their body weight, and exercised regularly before the injury can tolerate a planned activity program with greater stamina and more endurance. It is especially important to note any preexisting cardiopulmonary complications, which may be overt or subtle in nature. The amount of fatigue on exertion will dictate modifications in the activity program.

Age
Muscle mass, strength, and coordination diminish in the course of normal aging. The older patient will probably tolerate less physical activity at a slower rate. The effects of aging must be assessed, however, not assumed.

Preexisting neuromuscular or skeletal conditions
Conditions such as arthritis are particularly common in older patients. Skeletal afflictions, such as ankylosing spondylitis, that may have predisposed the patient to cord damage will limit many physical activities and necessitate program modifications.

Associated injuries
Patients with multiple injuries will need a very specialized activity program. The most difficult problems arise when there are associated head injuries, which may render the patient hemiplegic or unable to cooperate.

Preinjury personality
It is imperative to assess the patient's preinjury personality. This information, obtained from an interdisciplinary perspective, will help the team understand how patients think and feel and will adapt to a physical activity program:

- Does the patient like himself or herself?
- Does the patient adapt easily?
- How has the patient previously dealt with challenges?
- Is the patient easily frustrated?
- Is the patient a private person?
- Is the patient very body conscious?
- Does the patient like a direct approach?
- Does the patient like to be independent?
- Are there influential social or cultural expectations?

All these questions need to be answered; the information collected will help the health care team develop an individualized approach to self-care and problem solving.

Psychological Status

The emotions experienced during psychological adjustment to disability profoundly affect the patient's willingness to cooperate and readiness to learn. During the process of adjustment to loss, it often takes many long hours to break the cycles of depression, anger, and denial that inhibit motivation and prevent patients from totally involving themselves in planning and implementing a specific program. Emotional reactions tend to heighten when skills practiced since early childhood must be relearned. Patients with quadriplegia, for example, require tremendous energy and concentration to accomplish the simplest everyday task such as brushing teeth. Under these circumstances it is easy to become frustrated.

These feelings are normal reactions to an abnormal situation, and it requires an interdisciplinary team effort to help patients deal with them. Once patients have adjusted to inevitable physical limitations, they learn alternative methods to gain mobility and independence with relative ease.

A supportive family is another significant factor in successful reactivation. Such a family can help meet the patient's needs for love, belonging, and hope for the future, and it is encouraging when they take an active role in the patient's therapy programs. Other families may need more guidance in the form of gentle explanations of how and why the patient needs their support. Cultural expectations of members' roles also make a difference. The patients that do most poorly are generally those with no family support.

Although the family is significant, if it is not a viable resource, most persons belong to some other social network that can be tapped. Close friends can also help find ways of achieving rehabilitative goals. All resources must be creatively assessed to determine how they can be useful.

Physical Examination

In-depth assessment of neuromuscular and skeletal function involves close collaboration, primarily of the physician, the physical therapist, and the occupational therapist. Initially physicians and therapists are involved with detailed assessment to establish sound baseline data and further delineate diagnosis. Assessment is an ongoing process used to evaluate any change in neurological status, to monitor the patient's progress toward the goals of treatment, and to evaluate functional outcome of treatments. For this ongoing assessment the physical therapist and occupational therapist use similar skills and techniques but focus on different aspects of physical activity and self-care. Whereas physical therapy focuses on gross motor activities (see Figure 16–1), occupational therapy is concerned with finer movements (see Figure 16–2), especially for the quadriplegic patient, whose upper extremity function is vital to achieve independent living skills.

Although the nurse may not be directly responsible for the assessment, it is important to know the general terminology to improve communication with therapists, to appreciate the significance of their findings, and to understand implications for nursing care.

Assessment of muscle strength

Manual muscle testing can determine the degree of weakness, loss, or return of muscle function. This skill involves isolating a muscle's function and then grading the weakness or strength present. (See Table 5–2 for a manual grading system and Table 5–3 for further assessment of motor function.) Accurate and serial manual muscle testing monitors progression or regression of a patient's function. As spinal shock passes, manual muscle testing for motor strength becomes more difficult (if not impossible) to evaluate due to spasticity affecting movements. The *quality* of controlled movements, not the *quantity* of strength or movement, evolves as the main issue (Schneider 1981). Detailed sensory testing is then relied on to detect any changes in the neurological level.

Evaluation of muscle function can also be achieved by monitoring the degree of electrical activity present or absent in a muscle–nerve complex. This procedure is called *electromyelography* (EMG) and is often used to aid in diagnosis.

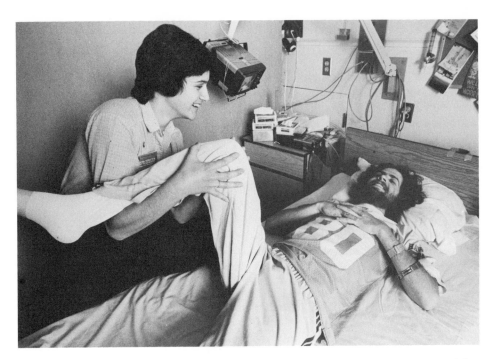

FIGURE 16–1 ■ A physical therapist facilitates gross motor activity.

Assessment of range of motion

All joints are assessed for any restriction in movement. Both *passive* movements (with the examiner moving the joint) and *active* movements (accomplished by patient strength alone) are measured. It is important to retain joint flexibility, increase muscle strength in nonparalyzed muscles, and prevent contractures in paralyzed muscles that will lead to loss of function.

The nurse must be aware of the causes of limitations in range of motion—particularly *pain* and *spasticity*—to modify movements encountered during general nursing care. The amount of pain the patient experiences often determines the amount of physical activity possible. During the acute stage only pain-free activity is usually attempted. The presence of pain and the degree of spasticity will affect the choice of positioning, the method of transfer, and the ability of the patient to perform active movements such as are involved with dressing or eating activities.

Assessment of muscle tone

Following spinal cord injury, muscles may become spastic (hypertonic) or flaccid (hypo-

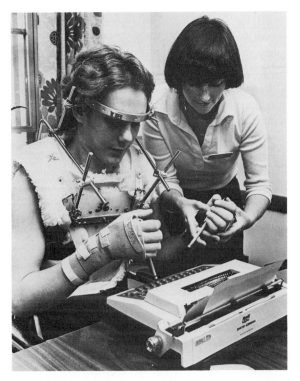

FIGURE 16–2 ■ An occupational therapist develops potential fine motor activity.

tonic) depending on the level of cord lesion and the time elapsed since injury. The state of spinal shock, in which all reflex activity below the level of lesion is suppressed, usually lasts for several weeks or months after injury. Reflex activity is recorded as normal, hyperactive, or absent. After reflex activity returns, most patients develop some degree of spasticity, which will vary with each patient. (The pathology and further assessment techniques involved with flaccid and spastic paralysis have been described in Chapter 5.) The effect of changes in muscle tone on functional movements, balance, and body posture in various recumbent and sitting positions is of vital importance to a rehabilitation program.

Assessment of sensation

Gross sensory testing is completed initially and repeated at intervals throughout the rehabilitation process to detect any improvement or deterioration in neurological function. Sensation is often illustrated schematically on diagrams (as shown in Table 5–3). Sensation is described as normal, impaired, or absent; the description also includes information on levels of:

- Pain (appreciation of pinprick and application of deep pressure)
- Temperature (appreciation of hot and cold sensation)
- Touch (appreciation of light palpation of the examiner's hand)
- Vibration sense (awareness of vibrating object placed on the skin)
- Position sense (appreciation of where limbs are in space)

When the position sense of the joints is absent, a mirror or prism glasses will help the patient perform or attempt active exercises.

Assessment of body build and coordination

Good body awareness is a definite advantage for the paralyzed patient. When it comes to moving their bodies in new ways, especially in transfers, it becomes obvious which patients are well coordinated and which are not. Overweight or tall, thin people often have problems moving their bodies in various situations.

GENERAL INTERVENTIONS

The nurse can do much to enhance the value of therapeutic sessions by promoting general health measures, particularly to minimize fatigue and pain. The condition of the patient's chest will directly determine how much physical activity the patient will tolerate. In addition to vigorous chest treatments, turning, positioning, regular breathing exercises, and encouragement to stop smoking will improve ventilation and general circulation. Moreover, the well-rested and well-nourished patient who is free from bouts of constipation or bladder infections will sustain higher energy levels and tolerate more physical exertion. It is also helpful if the patient is free of pain, so nurses should administer needed analgesics so that peak periods of pain relief will coincide with exercise times. Therapists should be informed of any changes in the patient's general condition, such as a physical setback or emotional upset, and any changes in routine schedules.

Continuity of care requires continuous communication of information, evaluation, and determination of appropriate approaches. Regular interdisciplinary team meetings, including the patient and family, are most valuable. Most importantly, everyone must understand the terminology in use. In addition to verbal communication and the medical record, one helpful tool is the use of a large interdisciplinary care plan (Kardex) where therapists can update information directly for nursing purposes. (Review Figure 4–2.) Instructional bedside charts may also clarify the necessary detailed information flow.

Maintaining Joint Range of Motion

Exercises are performed to maintain or restore full joint range of motion, prevent muscle contractures, and stimulate the circulation. If joints do not receive adequate motion daily, stiffness and contractures will develop that interfere with functional ability. For example, shoulder stiffness decreases arm movement needed for eating and makes positioning more difficult for wheelchair transfers.

Exercises are commonly *active* (done alone), *assisted* (patient needs help) or *passive* (patient is unable to participate).

The amount of range is determined by the structure of the joint and the length and tension of the muscle surrounding the joint. Range of movement is not the same for everyone, but depends on factors such as age, body build, and the limitations imposed by disease. Modifications in treatment will also be made according to the level of the fracture and the presence of pain.

Frequency of exercises will depend on the current status of joint flexibility, spasticity, and pain. (Range of motion exercises help decrease spasticity and prevent pain associated with contractures.) As mobility, strength, and independent skills increase, the need for range of motion exercises generally decreases.

The physical therapist is responsible for maintaining the full range of movement of all joints. If further range of movement exercises are to be performed by the nursing staff, the precautions and specific treatment required should be demonstrated by the physical therapist. The exercises outlined in Table 16–1 have been specifically selected to use as an *adjunct* to physical therapy treatment and do not include a complete selection of range of motion exercises.

During the acute stage the therapist performs range of motion exercises twice a day to maintain and restore muscle and joint function. Range of motion exercises should then be performed by the nursing staff, as needed, to make the patient comfortable, ensure a frequent change of position, and prevent circulatory stasis. These exercises require more skill than is commonly realized, and collaboration with the physical therapist is essential. Avoid any movements that produce pain. Move only one extremity at a time. Do not force any movement. If a spasm occurs retain a firm hold and wait until the spasm diminishes. For patients with lumbar fractures, do not flex the hip with the leg straight and do not flex the hip more than 90 degrees. (Pain may restrict flexion to 30 degrees at first.) These movements put a strain on the fracture.

Gradual Mobilization

Mobilization is introduced on a gradual basis to minimize the effects of postural hypotension and to carefully evaluate stress on the fracture site.

Adjustment to the upright position can be especially traumatic for patients with quadriplegia. Nursing care measures to minimize the effects of postural hypotension, to assist venous return, and to deal with hypotensive episodes are described in Chapter 10.

When the patient can tolerate the upright position the physical therapist will assess the patient's readiness to transfer and will perform the initial maneuver. This will occur when the patient is able to sit upright in bed for 30 to 60 minutes or can tolerate daily sessions on the tilt table for a week or so without feeling faint or dizzy. See Figure 16–3.

Throughout this process of mobilization, close collaboration with the physician is necessary to evaluate spinal immobilization and stability. Methods of monitoring skeletal healing have been discussed in Chapter 14. For the first seven to ten days after injury there will be a certain amount of pain at the injury site due to fractured bones, torn ligaments, and local muscle spasm. However, any severe, shooting pain or prolonged discomfort on return to bed may indicate the spine is not stable enough to withstand the added stress of movement. The patient should remain in bed until the physician has evaluated the situation.

Muscle-Strengthening Activities

Not only can spinal cord injury result in total loss of muscle power, but disuse can severely weaken muscles that remain intact. An individualized physical therapy program should be planned immediately on admission to develop functional mobility, that is, practical ways of getting around on an everyday basis. Treatment goals are to preserve strength and range of motion and to facilitate return of all weak but potentially active muscle groups. To compensate for lost muscle power, existing muscles must be

TABLE 16–1 ■ SELECTED PASSIVE RANGE OF MOTION EXERCISES

To maintain the comfort of the patient, it is important that the joints be moved either before or after each turn. The most practical method combines the movements of flexion, extension, abduction, adduction, and rotation. The exercise will be assisted or passive, depending on the patient's muscle strength. Use a firm but comfortable grip. Support the limbs at the joints. Perform the movement smoothly and rhythmically. Repeat three to five times every two hours.

Upper Limb Exercise

Support the patient at the wrist and above the elbow. Start with the arm down and out to the side, with the elbow straight and the palm down. Move it to place the palm on the opposite shoulder. Return to starting position.

Lower Limb Exercise

Support the patient under the knee and at the sole of the foot. Start with leg straight and in abduction. Flex the knee and the hip, move the leg up and across to place the heel on the opposite knee, and return it to the starting position.

Circulatory Exercise

To maintain adequate circulation, foot-pumping exercises should be performed during each shift. Grasp the patient above the ankle and around the sole of the foot. Keep the knee straight so that the calf muscle is stretched. Perform a firm up and down movement of the foot in a pedaling action. Repeat 40 to 50 times every eight hours.

---

strengthened to their maximum in order to achieve potential mobility and independence skills.

A *full physical therapy program* commences when the patient can tolerate being up most of the day. There are no restrictions on activity other than that of avoiding pain. All exercise is directed toward functional activities. Skills such as pressure relief maneuvers, transfers, and wheelchair management are examples of functional activities. See Figure 16–4. Prior to this the patient will undertake a *partial physical therapy program*. This is a program of varying degrees of limited activity depending on patient tolerance to mobilization and restrictions of movement necessary to reduce stress on the healing fracture site.

To promote functional exercise such as eating, transferring, and other self-care tasks the nurse must be familiar with the general treatment programs and the specific restrictions for each patient. This information should always be taken into account when supervising, assisting, moving, or positioning patients during nursing care. The therapist should inform the nurse of any changes in neuromuscular function and of progressions in treatment.

Active muscle-strengthening exercises are performed daily, progress gradually, and in-clude general activities, mat activities, gait training, and swimming.

General activities

In the early stages, particularly while the patient is in bed, the amount of activity directly depends on the amount of patient pain and fatigue. Some examples of general activities included in a physical therapy program are:

- Manual assistance or resistance, allowing the therapist to grade and control the movement
- Slings and springs to eliminate the effect of gravity and allow the patient to move a limb independently, even when it is very weak (Figure 16–5)
- Weights and pulleys to provide resistant arm exercises to improve and maintain normal strength and assist circulation (Figure 16–6)
- Biofeedback (visual and auditory signals), which informs patients of the amount of muscle activity they are producing (See Figure 16–7)

Mat activities

The purpose of mat work is to develop strength, balance, and coordination in preparation for other activities, such as transferring and dressing. Depending on the level of lesion, patients learn to balance in a sitting position, lift the

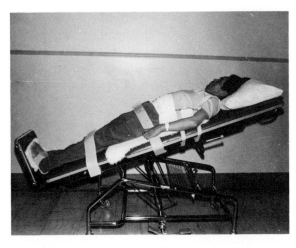

FIGURE 16–3 ■ The tilt table is used to help a patient gradually build up tolerance to the upright position.

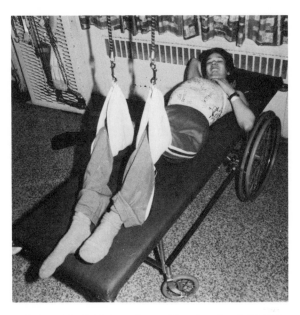

FIGURE 16–5 ■ A patient with a low level of paraplegia exercises with slings and springs. Note the self-wheeling stretcher used for early mobilization.

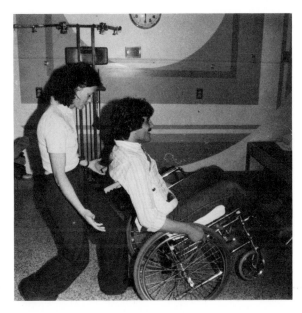

FIGURE 16–4 ■ A paraplegic patient is first taught how to balance the chair on rear wheels in preparation to perform a functional activity such as descending a curb.

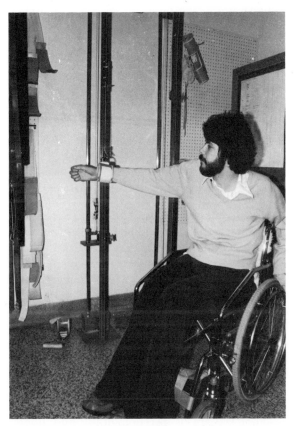

FIGURE 16–6 ■ A quadriplegic patient uses wall pulleys for arm-strengthening exercises.

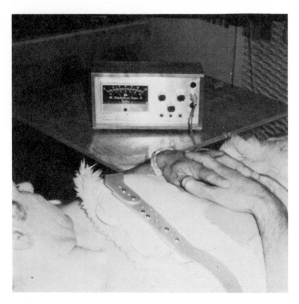

FIGURE 16–7 ■ A patient uses biofeedback techniques for incentive during exercise.

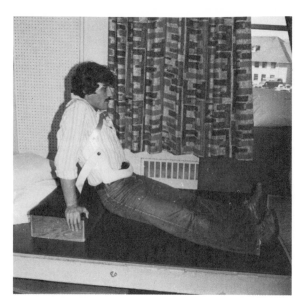

FIGURE 16–8 ■ A paraplegic patient performs a "box lift" during mat activities to prepare for functional activities.

buttocks to move around on the bed, roll over, get up into a sitting position from lying positions, and return to the wheelchair from the floor. See Figure 16–8. Once the patient is up in a wheelchair, particular emphasis is placed on balance, strength, and coordination, which promote achievement of transfers; wheelchair management; and, for some, gait training at a very early stage.

Gait training

Selected patients with low paraplegia and some pelvic control may achieve ambulation with the aid of crutches and long leg braces that provide rigid support to the knees and ankles. Braces may be modified later to suit individual needs, and crutches may or may not be needed. See Figure 16–9. Whether to use this method of ambulation depends largely on patient motivation and preference, because it consumes a great deal of energy. Many patients prefer to combine methods of mobilization, using crutch walking for some occasions and the wheelchair for others.

Swimming

Pool therapy is psychologically and physically very beneficial to patients with all levels of lesions. It is included in the treatment program

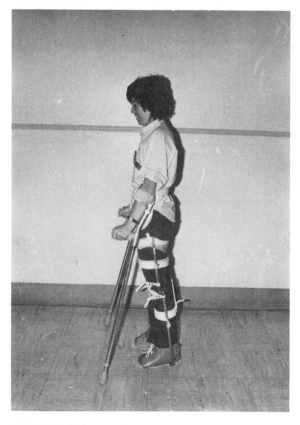

FIGURE 16–9 ■ Gait training with long leg braces and arm crutches is possible for selected patients with low paraplegia.

depending on the patient's desire, bowel and bladder management, and orthopedic stability.

Transfer Activities

When spinal stability allows, therapists are very much involved with assessing the patient's readiness for transfer activities, performing initial transfers, teaching appropriate techniques, and selecting a wheelchair with various accessories and mobility aids. The nurse then becomes active in performing, assisting, or supervising these transfers on a day-to-day basis.

To ensure safety and promote independence as the patient gains strength, sitting tolerance, and vertebral column stability, the nurse must be aware of the exact amount and kind of assistance the patient requires. The patient, the family, the nurse, and the therapist must understand the methods of transfer and terminology used to describe these maneuvers. As the patient progresses, the nurse's role changes to encourage independence and withdraw any assistance that is not really needed. Patients with physical potential will naturally progress from dependent to assisted, to supervised, and finally to independent transfers.

Dependent transfer

In dependent transfer the patient will need total assistance. This method usually requires two assistants and is usually necessary for a quadriplegic patient in a Halo-brace, or any other patient who is difficult to move, such as obese patients or patients with multiple injuries.

Assisted transfer

An assisted transfer is designed to allow patients to perform the maximum amount of the activity that they can on their own. Be prepared to assist and protect at all stages of the procedure. The method is the same as with the dependent transfer except that only one assistant is required. The patient generally uses a transfer board, and the footrests remain down in place.

Supervised transfer

A supervised transfer requires only minimal or standby assistance. Stand in front of the patient. Help with balance if necessary, and ensure

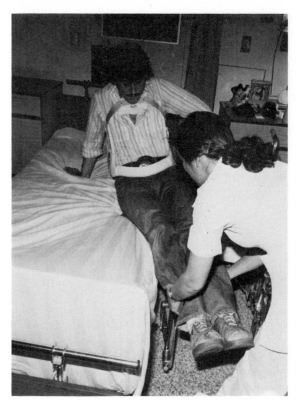

FIGURE 16-10 ■ A paraplegic patient is supervised during a transfer.

that the feet do not strike the chair as the patient puts them on the foot pedals. Help the patient lift the hips and slide into the chair as necessary. When returning to bed if long sitting is not allowed, or is difficult, have the patient transfer the buttocks to the bed first, then lift the legs onto the bed while lowering the trunk. See Figure 16-10.

Independent transfer

In an independent transfer the patient does not require any assistance. The patient with paraplegia learns to transfer from wheelchair to bed, toilet, car, bath, and the floor and back independently. The patient usually accomplishes this within four to six weeks of being allowed up. The quadriplegic patient will require assistance with all transfers, at least until the Halo-brace is removed; then achievement of independence depends largely on level of injury sustained.

Clinical proficiency at performing transfers requires formalized instruction followed by su-

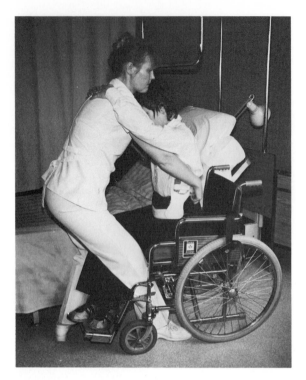

FIGURE 16–11 ■ A nurse uses correct body mechanics; good posture with knees bent to absorb stress of patient's weight.

pervised practice sessions. Important aspects include skillful application of good body mechanics (see Figure 16–11), knowledge of transfer movements, and familiarization with the wheelchair and its accessories. (Features of the wheelchair are presented in Table 16–2.) The key points involved in general transfer techniques and alternative methods of transfer are discussed in Procedure 16–1.

To transfer a quadriplegic patient in a Halo apparatus generally requires two assistants. Procedures 16–2 outlines this dependent transfer. Procedure 16–3 shows how a transfer method for a quadriplegic person is simplified once spinal stability is achieved and spinal orthoses are removed (an assisted transfer). The use of standard mechanical lifts is discouraged, especially during the acute stage, because of the undue curving pressure exerted on various parts of the spine. It is very difficult to prevent the lift from contact with the metal apparatus on the Halo-brace. Any pressure on these bars will loosen the orthoses.

To ensure safety as well as ease, many transfer techniques must be adapted to differing situations. Additional assistants may be needed when transferring a patient in a small, confined area, as from wheelchair to toilet; when transferring a wet patient from the shower chair to the bed; or when transferring a fatigued patient from the toilet to the wheelchair after bowel disimpaction. Adaptations must also be made to accommodate differing size, weight, and coordination of both patient and assistant.

Correct Position for Patient in Wheelchair

The correct position of a patient in a wheelchair ensures a balanced position without slumped posture. Correction of position may be necessary immediately following a transfer or when spasms or gravitational forces have caused the patient to slip forward in the chair. After securing the brakes and positioning and locking the small front wheels, several maneuvers can be used:

• An average patient requires one assistant behind the wheelchair. The patient should cross arms over the pubic bone, and the assistant's hands should pass under the patient's axilla and cross over the patient's hands. Lean the patient forward, squeeze the thorax, and pull back.
• The heavier patient may require one assistant in front. Grasp the patient's feet and knees between your own. Lean the patient's trunk forward, then simultaneously lift the patient's hips, and push with your knees.
• The very heavy patient or a patient with a Halo-brace may require two assistants. While the patient leans forward, the front assistant grasps the patient and on the count of three, pushes on the patient's knees, while the back assistant lifts and slides the hips back. See Figure 16–12.

Wheelchair Management Skills

As soon as patients are up, the physical therapist begins to teach them how to perform, or teach others to perform, wheelchair management skills. Individual programs are based largely on physical potential associated with level of injury sustained. Education includes basic maneuvers to wheel and position chair, negotiate obstacles, and handle the removable parts of the chair. Some patients will be able to perform advanced activities such as balancing a chair on the back wheels (wheelie) in order to ascend and descend ramps or curbs. All patients and family members will be taught dependent activities such as movement up and down stairs. Progress will include learning to cope with rougher ground and slopes out of doors. Formal instruction will be given to the patient and family by the physical therapist in preparation for day and weekend passes. However, all members of the staff should be familiar with the techniques involved, so that they can reinforce the teaching process and assist patients when necessary, especially during evenings and weekends. Table 16–3 presents some commonly encountered maneuvers. See also Figure 16–13.

Assisting Quadriplegic Patients with Upper Extremity Activities

All care is directed toward maintaining a functional position of the hand and arm. See Figure 16–14. A functional position is one that will be useful for daily activities, such as holding and drinking from a cup. See Figure 16–15. A functional hand is essential for *all* self-care activities for the patient with quadriplegia.

Components of care required for upper extremities include correct positioning of hands, elbows, and shoulders; adequate range of motion exercises; and usually hand splinting to prevent contractures and deformities (see Figure 16–16). The occupational therapist is very much involved in assessing hand and arm function; providing appropriate hand splints and teaching method of application; and developing appropriate self-care techniques, which are then taught to the patient, staff, and family. The nurse assumes a large responsibility for maintaining correct positioning, providing adequate exercise, and applying and caring for splints on a day-to-day basis during the early stages.

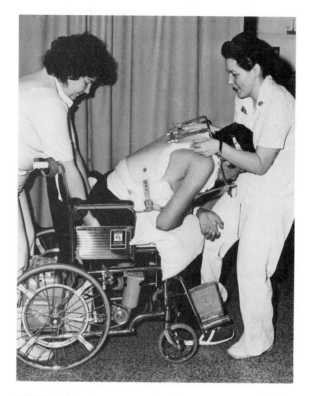

FIGURE 16–12 ■ Two assistants correct the slumped positon of a patient in the wheelchair.

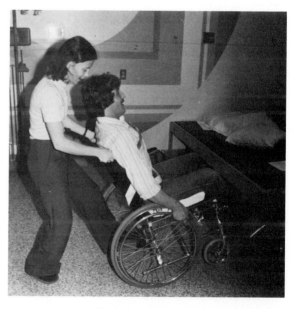

FIGURE 16–13 ■ An assistant achieves a "balanced position" of the wheelchair by stepping on the tipping lever—a basic management skill.

TABLE 16–2 ■ FEATURES OF THE WHEELCHAIR

Throughout the acute period, take extreme care to assess all aspects of a person's needs in preparation for selecting a wheelchair for permanent use. A wide variety of design variables and accessories are currently available. Prescribing a wheelchair is beyond the scope of nursing practice, but a general knowledge of selection and accessories is helpful.

"Comfort in sitting is most important for those who spend a substantial part of each day in a wheelchair. The chair, therefore, must be the right size and style and be equipped with the right accessories. The use for which the wheelchair is required must also be a factor. Mobility in this wheelchair must provide the best for the user in order to give the most speed, maneuverability, ease of operation, good postural appearance and in order to ensure that the product has good wearing qualities" (Ford 1980:5).

Wheelchairs with standard or lightweight frames are a good choice for the active user. Rear tires and front castors made of hard rubber are generally accepted as best for indoor use and are easily maintained. Pneumatic tires may be desirable for a smoother ride outdoors.

Drive rims to propel the wheelchair are located on the outside of the large rear wheels. To make wheeling the chair easier for quadriplegic people, projections or knobs can be installed on the rims to provide a point to push against (A). Projections are often used as a temporary measure while strength is rebuilding. A special "pusher" mitt is used by some to gain more friction and to protect the skin of the hand.

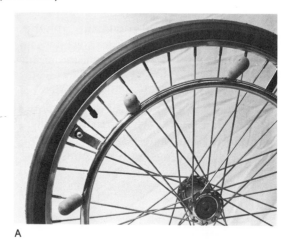

A

Swing away detachable legrests are helpful for transfer maneuverability. Wheelchair armrests are also removable to facilitate lateral transferring. Armrests are also available in varying heights and widths. Removable desk arms, which are the most popular, allow proximity to the table or desk without being removed. A paraplegic person who does not require arm support, for example, may well prefer the smaller, sloping wrap-around version (B).

For wheelchair sports, elaborate and custom designs incorporate such features as extremely low backs, deeper seats, sloping side arms, different axle positions to throw more weight on the rear wheels, antitipping devices, and roll bars to prevent the footplates from gouging floors.

Electrically driven wheelchairs for dependent people are discussed in Chapter 17.

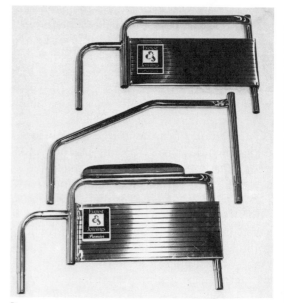

B

(Table continues)

TABLE 16–2 ■ (*continued*)

Wheelchair seats and backs are available in varying lengths and widths. For the quadriplegic person, the back height must be low enough to allow free scapular movement, which is necessary for wheeling efficiency, but be high enough to provide adequate stability for the back. People with high cervical cord injuries may need back extensions for head and neck support (**C**).

Some of the more commonly used accessories include castor locks to stabilize a stationary chair for lateral transfers (**D**); heel loops on each footplate to prevent the feet from slipping backward (**E**); H-straps to fit across and behind the legs to prevent the legs from falling backward (**F**) (often caused by spasms); seatbelts for trunk stability (**G**); and carrying pouches attached to the wheelchair back for keeping various items handy.

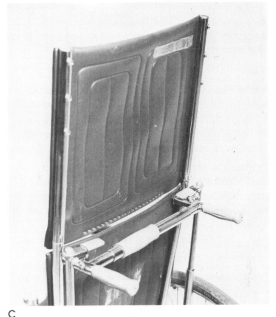

C

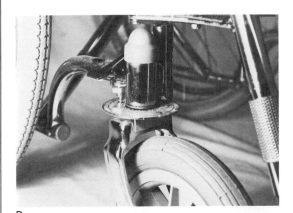

D

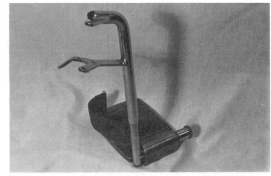

E

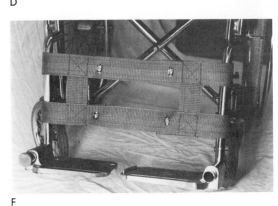

F

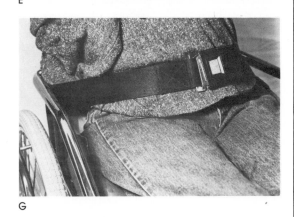

G

Source: J. Ford, *Wheelchair Handbook. A Guide to Selection, Cushions, Accessories and Maintenance,* copyright Canada, 1980 by G. F. Strong Rehabilitation Center, Vancouver, B.C., Canada.

PROCEDURE 16–1 ■ KEY POINTS IN GENERAL TRANSFER TECHNIQUES

Purpose

The purpose of this procedure is to give key points in transfer techniques and to point out alternative methods suited for the patient with paraplegia or quadriplegia.

Action

Transfers make use of *sliding* or *lifting* techniques. A situation in which lifting techniques are necessary is transferring a patient (without protective clothing) to a commode or shower chair. These techniques may also be used in combination.

1. Prepare the patient by explaining the planned moves in advance; during transfer give short, clear directions of what to do next. To time moves, indicate when ready and perform moves together on the count of three.

2. On completion of transfer it is very important to clarify any areas of difficulty or concern.

3. During the early stages it may be necessary to *ease* patients to the sitting position.
- Roll patient on side (optional) and then raise the head of the bed 45 degrees.
- Pull the patient forward and up to sitting position by slipping hands under patient's arms and placing over the scapula (A).

Rationale

Sliding techniques are generally used during the early stages or when patients are unable to help with body movements; *lifting* techniques are taught as patient becomes more independent in transfers; they also provide additional protection to the skin.

This allows the patient to understand moves and be able to instruct others in the future.

This will help them to accommodate to the upright position and minimize discomfort.

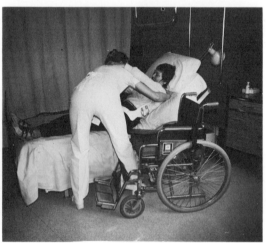

A

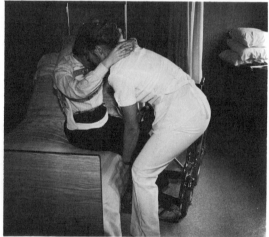

B

- Use your body weight to get patient's body in line.
- Simultaneously guide feet over edge of bed (B).
- When patient has a cervical injury, avoid pulling on the hands, arms, or shoulders.

4. It is important that the patient is dressed appropriately. Avoid pants with rigid seams or those that are

This gives long leverage and good mechanical advantage.
Pulling forces applied too soon will stress the cervical spine and cause pain.

It is necessary to protect the skin.

PROCEDURE 16–1 ■ (continued)

Action	Rationale
tight fitting, especially jeans. Running suits are ideal attire for early mobilization. It is possible to grasp patient's clothing to assist with sliding transfers, but *never* pull up on clothing to lift the patient. It is also important for patient to wear socks and shoes to provide additional protection for the feet when transferring (C).	Pulling on pants can bruise the perineal area, create a split in the cleft of the buttocks, or blister or chafe the skin.
Flat shoes with nonskid soles are a good choice.	A size larger than normal may be necessary if gravitational edema is a problem.
5. Ensure that wheelchair is placed correctly in relation to bed.	This will eliminate unnecessary movement and lifting.
• When getting patient out of bed, back wheelchair in alongside bed so that the front edge of chair is level with patient's hips.	
• When returning patient to bed, back wheelchair alongside bed and position front edge of the chair two thirds up from foot of bed. Adjust bed height so it is the same as wheelchair height.	This places patient's buttocks in correct position for lying down.
6. *Lock the bed brakes.* One feature that is particularly helpful on a regular hospital bed is the addition of small legs that come in contact with the floor only when the bed is adjusted to the lowest position. It is possible to remove the wheels from some beds. Always check mechanical safety of beds.	This will eliminate any movement of the bed when patient's weight is shifted. This offers maximum security as the weight of the bed is off the wheels.

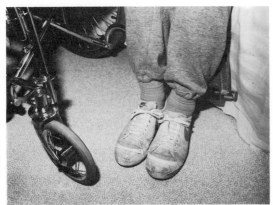

C

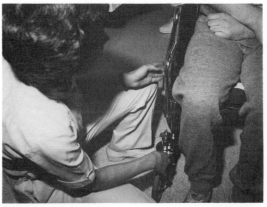

D

Action	Rationale
7. Set small front wheels of wheelchair facing forward to lengthen base of the chair and secure castor locks to maintain this position. *Lock the wheelchair brakes* (D).	This will stabilize wheelchair.
8. It is necessary to support the chest and buttocks and/or knees and feet.	This ensures security of patient with paralyzed trunk musculature and/or paralyzed lower extremities.
• Slide buttocks forward so that feet easily touch the floor.	This ensures that body weight is over the center of gravity. *(Procedure continues)*

PROCEDURE 16–1 ■ KEY POINTS IN GENERAL TRANSFER TECHNIQUES (*continued*)

Action	Rationale
• Stabilize patient's feet and knees to prevent their sliding out of position. This is achieved by gripping your feet and knees on either side of the patient's. If this feels awkward, secure the lower extremities between your outer leg and the bed (E).	This will control paralyzed lower extremities.

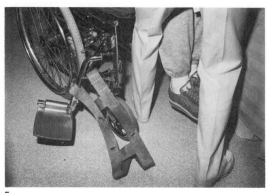

E

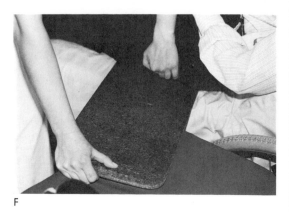

F

9. Protect the patient's buttocks from contact with wheel rim. With armrest removed, a protective device can be fitted to cover top of wheel.	
10. If a straight transfer board is to be used, a 10-inch × 28-inch (with rounded corners to protect the skin) is a good size for maximum support (F).	Make sure patient is well forward to avoid bumping the rim.

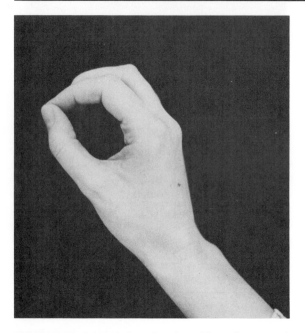

FIGURE 16–14 ■ A functional position of a normal hand.

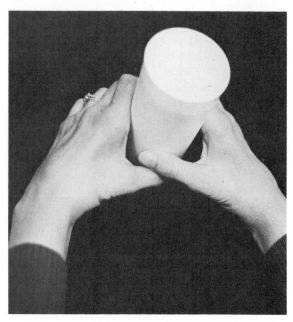

FIGURE 16–15 ■ A functional hand position for the person with quadriplegia.

PROCEDURE 16–2 ■ TRANSFERRING A QUADRIPLEGIC PATIENT WITH A HALO-BRACE

Part A: From the Bed to the Wheelchair

To prepare the patient for transfer:

A Slide the patient toward the edge of the bed.

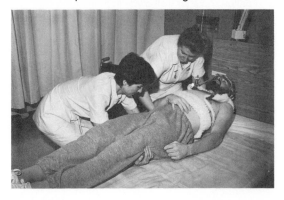

B Position the transfer board.

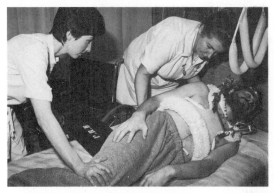

C Position board to be free of wheel rim.

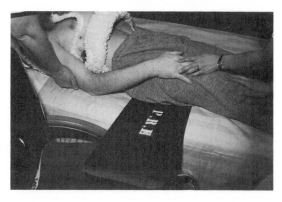

D Ease to a well-balanced sitting position.

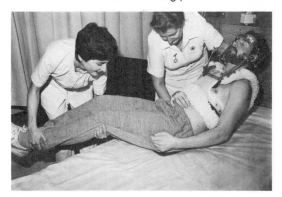

E For this taller person, place the feet directly on the floor for stability; otherwise feet may be balanced on footplate.

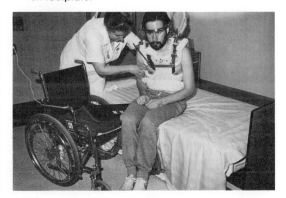

(Procedure continues)

Part A: From the Bed to the Wheelchair

To transfer the patient:

The assistant *at the front* simply stabilizes the patient's trunk and knees and guides the patient to the chair. Do not *lift*. This is the key to the success of this tranfer technique. The assistant *at the back* gently lifts the patient's buttocks along the transfer board to the chair.

F   Position the patient's body weight well forward to provide good mechanical advantage.

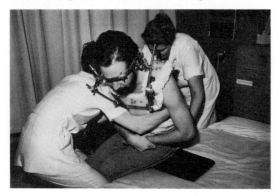

G   Position shoulder well away from the Halo bars to protect both patient and self.

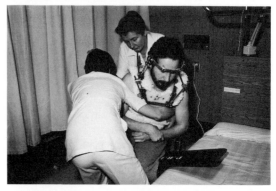

H   Remove the transfer board.

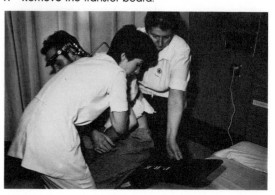

Part B: From the Wheelchair Back to Bed

To prepare the patient for transfer:

A   Place the wheelchair at the correct angle to the bed.

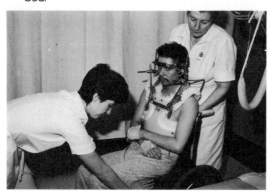

B   Position the transfer board while helping the patient lean to the opposite side of the chair.

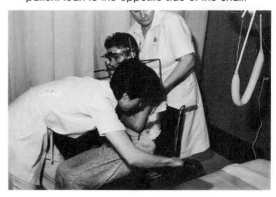

(Procedure continues)

Part B: From the Wheelchair Back to Bed

C   Stabilize the patient in the sitting position.

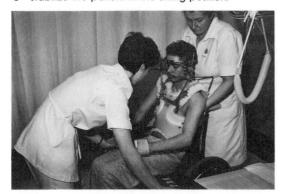

To transfer the patient:

D   The front assistant *guides*, but does not lift, the patient's torso.

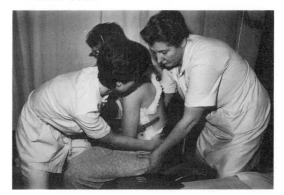

E   Lean well away from the Halo bars.

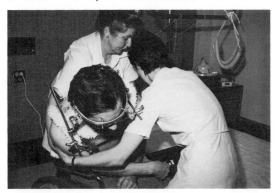

F   The assistant at the back, having the mechanical advantage, lifts the patient's buttocks along the transfer board.

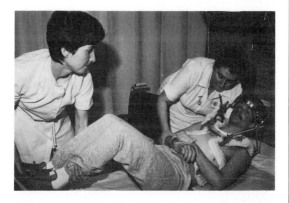

G and H   Together ease the patient to the recumbent position.

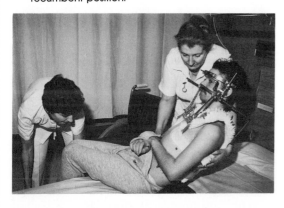

Prepared under the direction of Jack Ford, Director of Remedial Gymnastics; G. F. Strong Rehabilitation Centre, Vancouver, B.C.

PROCEDURE 16–3 ■ TRANSFERRING A QUADRIPLEGIC PERSON FROM THE WHEELCHAIR TO BED

To prepare the patient for transfer:
Ensure that the bed and chair are stabilized (the front castors of the wheelchair are locked into position) and that the chair is angled in the correct position to the bed.

A   Using good body mechanics, ease the patient to the front of the wheelchair.

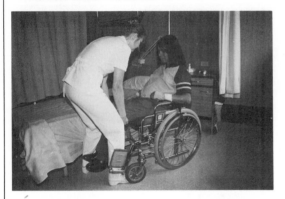

B   Position the transfer board

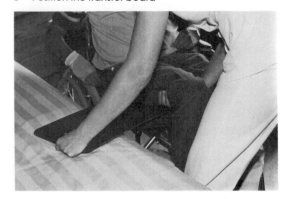

C   Position the shorter person's feet on the footplate; stabilize the patient's knees between your own; bend the patient with a stabilized spine completely forward to displace much of the patient's weight forward and gain mechanical advantage.

D   Lift and guide the patient's buttocks to the bed.
E   Achieve a balanced position before easing the patient to the recumbent position.

These technqiues can be simply reversed to transfer the person from the bed to the wheelchair.

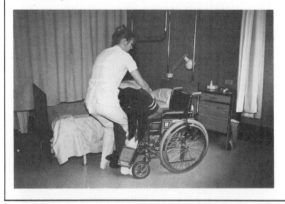

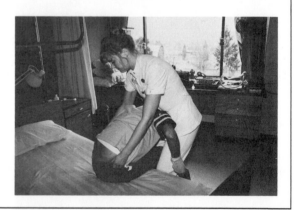

As rehabilitation progresses, the nurse's role changes to encourage independence and withdraw any assistance that is not really needed. As the patient is able to participate more in self-care activities, muscles are strengthened and range of motion is maintained without specific exercises and exact positioning becomes less important. Again, the patient, the nurse, the family, and the therapist must understand the terminology used to describe activities and be aware of the exact amount of assistance required by the patient.

Positioning and range of motion exercises

Positioning and range of motion exercises are combined, since they must supplement each other if the overall program is to be successful. Specific positioning of the upper extremities while the patient is on an immobilization bed is

TABLE 16–3 ■ WHEELCHAIR MANAGEMENT SKILLS

- **Tilting the Chair Backward**

  Grasp the handles. Keep close to body. Place one foot on the tipping lever. Tilt the chair back until in a balanced position.

- **Mounting Curbs**

  Back the chair to within one foot of the curb. Tilt the chair back by stepping on the tipping lever. Pull the chair up the curb and wheel it back so that the front castors will be on the sidewalk when the chair is lowered. Alternatively, tilt the wheelchair back and place small wheels up on curb; simultaneously, roll the chair forward and lift up onto the curb.

- **Descending Curbs**

  Facing the roadway, tip the chair back to balance on its back wheels. Roll the chair slowly over the curb and push forward before lowering the front castors. To maintain the patient's balance, support the front of the patient with one hand while lowering the front castors.

- **Wheeling Over Rough Ground**

  When negotiating rough or soft ground, tilt the chair back onto the two rear wheels. If the terrain is very difficult, it will be easier to pull the chair backward in the tipped position. In this position, the person in the chair is more secure and less likely to fall out.

- **Wheeling Down Slopes**

  Steep slopes may require that the chair be wheeled down the hill backward. If wheeling down forward, ensure the patient's balance in the chair with one hand over the patient's shoulder. If the slope levels abruptly, care must be taken not to snag the footrests when wheeling forward.

- **Ascending Stairs**

  Tilt the chair back until balanced. Place one foot on the first step and one on the second. Pull the chair up the first step. Keep your arms straight. Mount the next step before proceeding. The patient can assist the lift by grasping the wheel rims and coordinating the pulling action, timing the "ready–lift" at each step.

- **Descending Stairs**

  The same positions are used as for ascending stairs. Until confident, two assistants should be used. The front helper must be prepared to hold the chair if necessary, but don't attempt to lift, as the balance of the chair will be disrupted.

- **Lifting the Wheelchair into a Car**

  To fold the chair, fold the footrests up and pull up on the seat. Secure brakes and tip the chair so that you can reach the far side. Grasp the spokes below the axle at the front of the frame. Rock back, balancing chair on thighs. Hold armrests close to body. Swing and lift chair into trunk.

described in Chapter 14. Specific measures are needed for patients with quadriplegia.

To the quadriplegic patient, wrist and thumb joint mobility are extremely important movements required for self-care. For example, a flexible wrist is important for transfers. Patients can only support their weight when their shoulders and arms are extended in external rotation, the elbows are locked, and the wrists are bent backward. Bending the wrist backward creates *tenodesis*. Tenodesis is the natural bending inward (flexion) of the fingers when the wrist is extended or bent backward. See Figure 16–17A. To simulate this action, cock your right wrist back with your left hand. If your right hand is relaxed, your fingers will automatically curl inward. Tenodesis is a key movement because it can be used to pick up objects when finger move-

ment is absent. The hand must be trained to assume this position. Contractures of the fingers are actually encouraged. To assist tenodesis the web space between the thumb and first two fingers must be maintained to enhance the grasp motion with the thumb in opposition. To release the grasp, patients simply relax the wrist. See Figure 16–17B.

The occupational therapist is responsible for maintaining full range of motion in the hand. If additional exercises are needed they will likely consist of bending the wrist forward, straightening each joint, spreading the fingers apart, and bringing them together; rotating the thumb toward the little finger (grasp the thumb at the base rather than the tip and pull away from the palm); and extending the wrist backward with fingers bent (never straighten the fingers when the wrist is extended as it will weaken tenodesis).

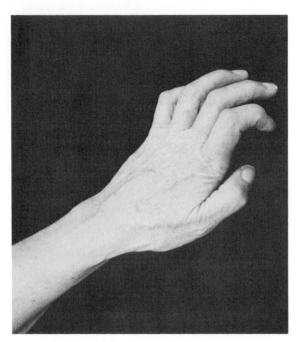

FIGURE 16–16 ■ A nonfunctional contracted hand results from lack of positioning and inadequate exercise. Note the tight flexion of the thumb; the web space is lost. This person would be unable to pick up a cup as pictured in Figure 16–15.

Splinting

If there is partial or total paralysis of the hand, temporary splints are needed and should be applied within 48 hours of injury. Generally splints should be worn all night and whenever the patient is resting to maintain a functional or, for the high quadriplegic patient, a cosmetic position. Splints stabilize flail joints and prevent contractures causing deformity. These are referred to as *static* or *positioning splints*.

During the early stages the nurse's role involves correct application of positioning splints and meticulous care of the skin. Regardless of what type of splint is used, the nurse must check the skin for reddened areas every two hours and alert the occupational therapist if adjustments are necessary. Red marks most often occur when splints have been improperly applied or have slipped. Mark the corresponding area on the splint and reapply correctly. Remove splints if red marks persist and position the hand with a foam roll until the splint can be modified by the occupational therapist.

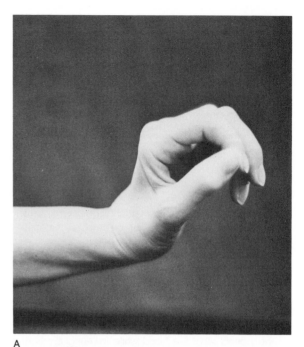

A

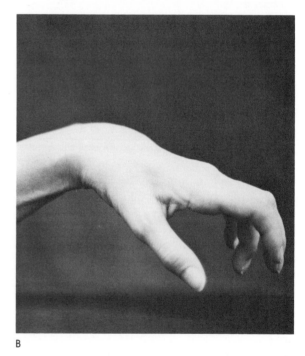

B

FIGURE 16–17 ■ (A) Tenodesis, the natural flexion of the fingers when the wrist is extended, is a valuable maneuver that enables quadriplegic patients to pick up objects when finger movement is absent. The hand must be trained to assume this position. (B) When the flexible wrist is relaxed, the fingers open.

When hand swelling subsides, the occupational therapist will design and fabricate an appropriate permanent positioning splint. Such splints are made from thermal plastic (molded directly on the patient for precise fit) or padded metal supports. Generally *opponens* splints are used to keep the thumb in opposition to the first two fingers, maintain the web space, and slightly flex the fingers. Depending on wrist movement *short* or *long* opponens splints may be used; the long opponens splint is necessary to support a flaccid wrist; the short opponens splint is used when there is good wrist movement. See Figure 16–18. Splints may be removed for range of motion exercises, hygiene, wheelchair activities, or, as directed by the occupational therapist. Positioning splints are worn all night.

As the patient progresses *dynamic splints* may be used to enhance a pincher grasp and actually assist the patient with independent activities. The thumb is used as a stable post, and the first two fingers act together to oppose the thumb. This allows the patient to pick up, hold, and release light objects in a limited but useful way (Fishwick and Sellers 1979). The power of the pincher grasp is directly related to the strength of the wrist extensor muscles. The purpose of dynamic splinting is to convert the motion or ability to flex the wrist into activation of the orthoses to support the pincher grasp. See Figure 16–19. Dynamic splints may range from a simple short opponens splint, used when the patient has good wrist extensor movement, to externally powered hand splints, which may be activated by shoulder movements when wrist extensor movement is absent. Quadriplegic patients with minimal neurological deficit may not need an orthosis; others may use an orthosis as a muscle-training device and then remove it; some may need an orthosis as a permanent functional aid.

Mobile arm supports may be needed for patients who have weak shoulder muscles and cannot place their arms appropriately to allow hand function. Once trunk position and stability are achieved, antigravity support is provided to the shoulder and elbow. In other words the weight of the upper arm is so supported as to permit sideways movement of the arm and hand function. Mobile arm supports may be metal structures attached to the wheelchair (commonly

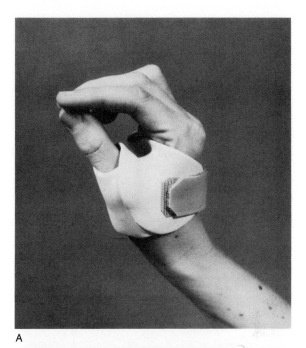

A

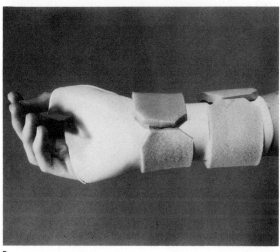

B

FIGURE 16–18 ■ (A) A short opponens splint maintains the thumb in opposition to preserve a functional hand position. Good wrist movement is needed. (B) A long opponens splint is used for the same purpose when wrist movement is weak or absent.

called *balanced forearm orthoses* or overhead suspension slings; see Figure 16–20). They can be used in conjunction with a variety of splints or clip-on utensils so the patient can perform such tasks as eating. Sometimes they are used purely as exercise devices.

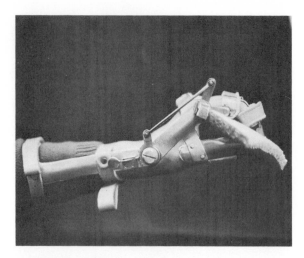

FIGURE 16–19 ■ A dynamic splint converts the ability to flex the wrist into activation of the splint to enhance the pincher grasp for functional activities.

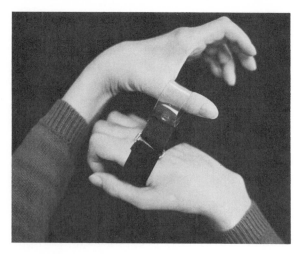

FIGURE 16–21 ■ A quadriplegic woman applies her own Palmer cuff.

Dynamic splints are applied during daily activities. They are not worn during the night.

Nurses are often responsible for correct application, checking the underlying skin, and conveniently placing additional equipment, for example, adjusting table height, arranging meal tray, cutting food up, and so on.

In addition, one commonly used aid is the universal Palmer cuff, into which an object such as a pencil or utensil may be inserted. A quadriplegic person may learn to apply this aid independently. See Figure 16–21.

The occupational therapist will introduce any new orthosis to the patient and will closely supervise its use until the patient becomes somewhat comfortable with the new equipment. It is important for nurses to understand the benefits of orthoses to encourage and support patients using them. Observe the patient's frustration levels or tolerance of orthoses used, and communicate any areas of concern to the occupational therapist.

Dressing

Dressing skills are most complex and involve both fine and gross motor coordination. Complete dressing cannot be achieved until spinal stability occurs and the patient can bend the trunk freely.

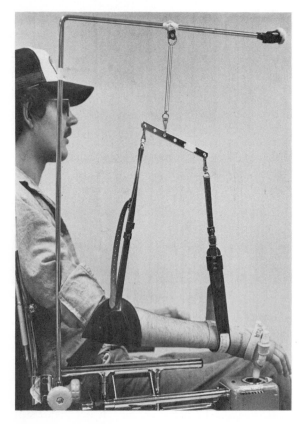

FIGURE 16–20 ■ A quadriplegic patient maneuvers an electric wheelchair with the aid of a mobile arm support. The nurse may be responsible for setting up this or similar devices when the patient uses them for such tasks as eating.

Lower extremity dressing is a very difficult task. Often the patient cannot totally complete all the dressing skills and therefore needs help when tired or unable. See Figure 16–22.

Upper extremity dressing is possible as soon as thoracic or lumbar injured patients can comfortably roll from side to side. This eventually includes donning a brace. Lower extremity dressing can begin when long sitting is allowed. Dressing is then most easily achieved in bed. Long-handled adaptive aids such as a dressing stick, sock aid, or shoehorn may be needed.

Upper extremity dressing for the cervical injured patient can begin when the Halo device is removed; otherwise it is too difficult to maneuver clothing over the brace. Lower extremity dressing can begin when patients can roll themselves over in bed and help with pulling on clothing. Mat activities in physical therapy help improve rolling ability and sitting balance before dressing skills are taught. When the patient improves with sitting balance during mat activities and progresses to long sitting in bed at 90 degrees, such activities as donning socks and shoes and pulling clothing up from feet can be introduced. The bed can eventually be lowered as dressing skills improve. Adaptive clothing and aids such as button hooks, zipper rings, and long-handled aids to reach feet are usually needed. Overhead loops may also be necessary to assist in lifting body weight.

If the patient begins undressing in the wheelchair and uses a transfer board to return to bed, the board should be powdered lightly and covered with a towel to protect the bare skin.

Caring for Patients with Spasticity

Following the passing of spinal shock, muscles regain tone and may become hypertonic, and often spasticity, due to upper motor neuron damage, will occur. These involuntary movements, which may be sustained (tonic) or intermittent like a "jumping" movement (clonic), are caused by an increased or abnormal amount of reflex activity below the level of injury.

The average time for the appearance of spasticity is six to ten weeks after injury (Burke and Murray 1975). Usually reflex excitability is

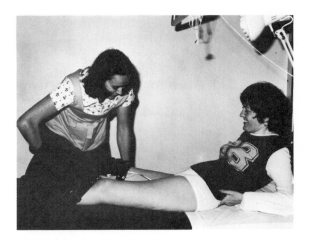

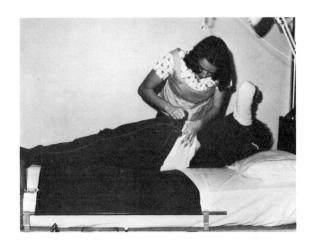

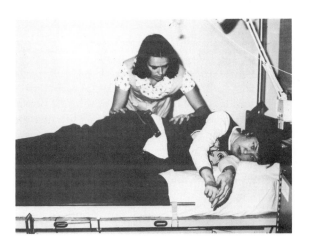

FIGURE 16–22 ■ A nurse helps a quadriplegic woman with lower extremity dressing. Having the patient roll from side to side is the easiest way.

at a maximum about two years after injury and gradually diminishes. Those with incomplete lesions may have more severe spasticity than those with complete injuries. Almost all patients with cervical injuries experience spasticity. A certain amount of spasm may be useful to help with patient movements and maintain muscle tone, but severe spasms can interfere with progress and cause damage, such as muscle and joint contractures, or lead to skin breakdown.

Basically spasticity occurs in flexion or extension patterns. If spasms interfere with dressing, transfers, or bowel and bladder care, try to position the patient to break the spasm pattern. For example, flex hips and knees to avoid extension or place the patient in a flexion position in the wheelchair to prevent back extension. Curl toes downward to stop the feet from jumping on the foot pedals of the wheelchair. Also avoid uneven pressure on limbs, such as pushing the foot hard against the footboard, which will cause clonus (jerking movements).

Always try to keep the patient calm, as spasticity is related to anxiety levels. Fatigue or emotional exhaustion will aggravate this condition. It is also important not to interpret spasticity erroneously as return of function. Be sure to explain the causes and difference between spasms and voluntary movement to the patient.

Full range of motion exercises to joints twice daily will minimize the effects of spasticity. The therapist will combine these exercises with passive stretching of spastic muscles and, possibly, applications of hot or cold treatments. Collaborate with the therapist to select the exact passive exercises and frequency needed. Continually observe for contractures, joint damage, or stiffening and maintain correct positioning. If possible, encourage proning to counteract hip flexion contractures.

Administer antispasmodic drugs as ordered. Observe pattern and frequency that needed (prn) medications are requested, and be aware that addiction can occur.

Be alert for factors that contribute to spasticity. An irritating focus below the level of lesion will increase spasms. The causes are most commonly related to the urinary system (infection, stones, and fistula); the intestinal system (flatus, impaction); and the integumentary system (wound infection, ingrown toenails, and pressure sores). Chronic spasticity is discussed later in this chapter.

SELF-CARE SKILLS

Physical independence in daily life is something able-bodied people take for granted, and the loss of this freedom can be devastating. Patients with spinal cord injuries suffer this loss initially because of their lack of mobility and inability to take care of their personal needs. This personal care, described as activities of daily living (ADL), includes all the things we do every day for ourselves. These include eating, dressing, grooming, hygiene, attending to bowel and bladder needs, and enjoying nonspoken communication skills, such as writing, reading, or even typing. Functional living skills, then, become one of the most important measures of a patient's rehabilitation. In fact, the entire health care team looks to these levels of performance in helping the patient define goals for the future (Ritt and McColey 1981). To survive in this hectic, independent world, people with spinal cord injuries must learn to get themselves up and ready to face the world at school, work, or during leisure hours.

Following assessment, therapists collaborate with the patient to design a self-care program. In the beginning the goals are most often the therapist's goals, because patients have little specific idea of their potential. Expertise developed by therapists has made it possible to outline functional expectations and establish realistic goals for groups of patients with similar disabilities. Table 16–4 summarizes expectations for potential functional status as related to the neurological level of lesion sustained. As the rehabilitation process evolves, goals are modified to become more specific to each individual. There is also a natural progression from simpler skills, such as eating and developing sitting balance, to more complex skills, such as dressing. Therapists and nurses must use continual assessment and flexible problem solving to meet individual needs.

The emphasis of self-care is on continual encouragement to learn and take responsibility for the body and its new and different ways of functioning. By virtue of their continual patient contact, nurses are in a unique position to reinforce all therapeutic activities (Heustis 1979) and make a valuable contribution to developing this independence. Nursing actions reflect the nurse's understanding of and commitment to the entire philosophy of rehabilitation, be it in the intensive care unit or on a recreational outing. However, this ideal isn't always easy for nurses to put into practice. One conflict that must constantly be overcome is the urge to assist a struggling patient with a particular skill. This is contrary to the ingrained (but not always appropriate) image of the nurse as a "helper."

Another major conflict arises between nursing "efficiency" and patient goals. Obviously it takes longer to supervise a patient with an activity such as eating than it does to perform the task yourself. However, nothing can be more detrimental to patients than not letting them contribute to their care, regardless of how slowly it is accomplished. Sometimes we are not creative enough to allow patients these opportunities. Naturally in any given situation, each nurse must consider the constraints and limitations of time and other priorities of patient care that may interfere with patient goals. It is important to remember that these conflicts are not unique to nursing. Similar situations occur with all team members. Making therapists aware of problems may not only help solve them but also contribute to better interdisciplinary relationships.

To help the patient achieve potential functional living skills, the nurse must be familiar with general treatment programs; individual patient goals; adaptive equipment available; and the specific adaptations for each patient. This is important because the nurse must decide or inquire what assistance the patient may need. Detailed information must be readily available. Direct communication involving the patient, the nurse, and the therapist during daily activities facilitates thorough communication. Obviously this is not always possible. One efficient way to

ensure continuity of care is the use of bedside charts that can be easily updated. An example is shown in Table 16–5. It is important for the nurse to carry over self-care activities into the evenings and weekends. Families often visit at these times. Their participation is encouraged, but they need education about the amount and kind of assistance that would be most helpful to the patient.

The Patient with Paraplegia

Patients with paraplegia are potentially physically capable of becoming independent in all self-care activities without the use of aids or specialized equipment. They can perform transfers independently, and selected patients with low paraplegia can master walking with the aid of leg braces and crutches. These patients can achieve independence within two or three months.

The Patient with Quadriplegia

The level of injury sustained dramatically affects the quadriplegic patient's ability to perform functional living skills. For example, a patient with quadriplegia at the C_4 level is totally dependent on others for all personal care needs, whereas a patient with quadriplegia at the C_5 level can, by using adaptive aids, become independent with personal care and operate a regular wheelchair. This may mean the difference between requiring a personal attendant and living unassisted.

Patients with high quadriplegia have C_{1-4} neurological involvement and are severely disabled. These patients are dependent for all their personal care needs and will require an electric wheelchair, environmental controls, and possibly respiratory support all or part of the time. The unique problems of the patient with high quadriplegia are discussed in Chapter 17.

Patients with low quadriplegia have C_{5-8} neurological involvement and have suffered loss of hand function. With adaptive aids and teaching, however, they can become independent with many aspects of their personal care within three to six months.

	Neurological Status	
Neurological Level of Lesion[1]	Motor Ability	Sensory Appreciation[2]
Part A: Levels of Quadraplegia		
C_{1-4}	Limited movement of head and neck C_{1-3} and some shoulder cap and diaphragm control (C_4) 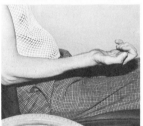	Limited sensation to head, neck (C_{1-2}), and shoulder caps (C_{3-4}) 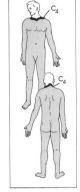
C_5	Full head, neck, shoulder, and diaphragm control *Add:* Some elbow flexion 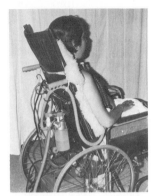	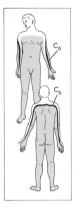Full head, neck, and shoulder cap sensation *Add:* Upper chest and back and lateral aspect of upper arm
C_6	*Add:* Some wrist extension (tenodesis) 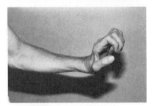	*Add:* Sensation to the lateral aspects of forearm to include the thumb and first finger
C_7	Full elbow flexion *Add:* Elbow extension, wrist flexion, and some finger control 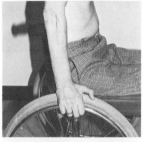 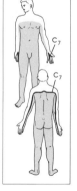	*Add:* Sensation to the second finger 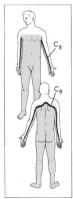
C_8-T_1	Moderate to full arm and wrist control *Add:* Moderate to full finger control 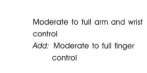 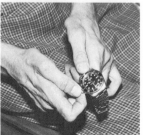	*Add:* Sensation to all the hand (C_8) and the medial aspects of the upper and lower arm (T_1)

(Table continues)

456

TABLE 16–4 ■ (*continued*)

Functional Ability[3]						
Eating and Grooming	Dressing	Bathing	Bowel and Bladder Care	Transfers	Mobility	Nonverbal Communication
Part A: Levels of Quadraplegia						
Dependent on an assistant	Dependent on assistant	Dependent on assistant	Dependent on assistant	Dependent on assistant	Requires electric wheelchair with breath, head, or shoulder controls. Likely dependent on a portable respiratory support system all or part of the time	Independent with environmental controls[4]
Independent with aids[5] and setup[6]	Requires major assistance with aids	Requires wheelchair shower with major assistance	Requires major assistance with some aids and raised toilet seat	Major assistance required: variable with type of transfer	Requires electric wheelchair with adapted hand control and/or manual wheelchair wheel rim projections	Independent with aids and setup
Independent with aids	Requires minor assistance with aids	Independent in wheelchair shower with aids	Independent with aids and raised toilet seat	Minor assistance required: variable with type of transfer	Independent in manual wheelchair	Independent with aids
Independent with or without aids	Independent with aids	Independent in wheelchair shower or tub with bath board and aids	Independent with aids and raised toilet seat	Independent with aids in all transfers	Independent in manual wheelchair	Independent with or without aids
Independent	Independent	Independent in tub with bath board and aids	Independent with aids and raised toilet seat	Independent with aids	Independent in manual wheelchair	Independent

(*Table continues*)

TABLE 16-4 ■ POTENTIAL FUNCTIONAL STATUS AS CORRELATED WITH NEUROLOGICAL LEVEL OF INJURY

	Neurological Status		
Neurological Level of Lesion[1]	Motor Ability	Sensory Appreciation[2]	

Part B: Levels of Paraplegia

T_{2-12}	Full upper extremity control *Add:* Limited to full trunk control	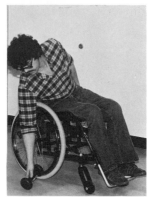	Full arm sensation *Add:* Partial trunk sensation to the level of the injury	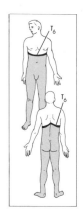
L_{1-5}	Full trunk control *Add:* Some hip (L_{1-3}), knee (L_{3-4}), and ankle (L_{4-5}) control and foot movement (L_5)	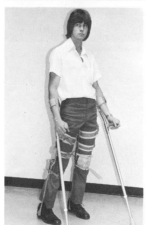	Full trunk sensation to the anterior upper leg (L_{1-3}), anterior/posterior and lateral aspects of the lower leg and dorsum of foot (L_{4-5})	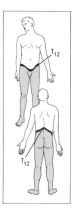
S_{1-5}	Moderate to full leg control *Add:* Some foot control (Disability can still be severe because of bowel, bladder, and sexual dysfunction)	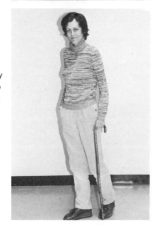	Sensation to the lateral aspect of the dorsum and the sole of foot (S_1); posterior aspect of the upper leg (S_2); sacral area (S_{2-5})	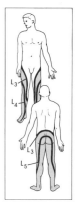

(Table continues)

1. The neurological level of lesion refers to the last normal functioning neurological level, not to the orthopedic fracture site: that is, a C_{5-6} level of injury means that the C_5 nerve root is normal and there is partial functioning of the C_6 nerve root. Many people with spinal cord injuries will have a mixed neurological picture.

2. For this chart *sensory appreciation* is defined as the ability to appreciate light touch, deep touch, pain, and temperature.

3. *Functional ability* depends on many variables other than neurological status. The most significant ones are:
   • Motivation • Body build/strength/age • Sociocultural status • Preexisting medical condition(s) • Amount of motor and sensory sparing • Spasticity

TABLE 16—4 ■ (continued)

Functional Ability[3]						
Eating and Grooming	Dressing	Bathing	Bowel and Bladder Care	Transfers	Mobility	Nonverbal Communication
Part B: Levels of Paraplegia						
Independent	Independent	Independent	Independent with aids and with or without raised toilet seat	Independent	Independent in manual wheelchair	Independent
Independent	Independent	Independent	Independent with or without aids	Independent	Optional use of long leg braces	Independent
Independent	Independent	Independent	Independent with or without aids	Independent	Independent with or without short leg braces	Independent

4. *Environmental controls:* Technological equipment enabling a person to control various needs in the environment by the use of electrical devices and computer systems, for example, lights, phone, television, and a door lock. A person accomplishes this by a single or dual control switch that can be adapted for use with different body parts such as the shoulder, head, chin, or tongue.

5. *Aid:* A specially fabricated piece of adapted equipment or an altered version of an item already in use. Each aid is designed to meet the needs of an individual person and situation. Most aids are prescribed and fitted by the occupational therapist. (Examples are seen throughout the book.)

6. *Setup:* Assembly or preparation of any or all of the items required by the person to accomplish a given task.

Prepared by Acute Spinal Cord Injury Unit, Shaughnessy Hospital, Vancouver, B.C. Photography by G. F. Strong Rehabilitation Center.

TABLE 16–5 ■ SELF-CARE STATUS*

		OCCUPATIONAL THERAPIST:
		PHYSICAL THERAPIST:
		SPEECH PATHOLOGIST:
NAME:		**DATE:**
SPECIAL ATTENTION:		**SPLINTING:**
		BRACING:
		OTHER:

✔ **DEPENDENT**   × **MAJOR ASSIST**   ＊ **MINOR ASSIST**   □ **SUPERVISION**   ○ **INDEPENDENT**

EATING		
GROOMING		
BATH/SHOWER		
DRESSING — UPPER / LOWER		
TRANSFERS		
MOBILITY — BED / W/C / WALK		
COMMUNICATION		

*This bedside chart has a plastic cover designed to be used with a grease pencil to facilitate continual updating.

The Patient with an Incomplete Injury

Patients with an incomplete lesion at any level have some involvement that affects their level of functioning including personal care. Some incompletely injured patients can be severely disabled. For example, patients with a central cord lesion may have no hand function but be able to walk. The length of time to become independent varies.

LONG-TERM IMPLICATIONS

When assessing a patient who has been paralyzed for some time, keep in mind that most active patients are at least relatively free from limited joint range of motion; muscle contractures; pain; and spasticity. Research also indicates that the majority of patients sustain the level of functional living skills reached during rehabilitation, with a few exceptions involving personal preference, such as chaneling energies away from self-care activities into intellectual pursuits (Rogers and Figone 1980).

Two major complications limiting mobility and independence are chronic pain and severe spasticity.

Chronic Pain

It is beyond the scope of this text to deal with the far-reaching physiological and psychological aspects of chronic pain. However, it is important to realize that *total* loss of all sensation below the level of lesion is almost nonexistent and that the sensations that do remain are mostly unpleasant and may follow bizarre patterns. Sensations of numbness, tingling, burning, or stabbing are referred to as *paresthesia* and are believed to be related to cord scarring or possibly nerve root entrapment. Severe pain seems to be most troublesome for patients with cauda equina injuries. Pain may also occur secondary to complications of late spinal instability.

It is important to make sure that muscle or joint contractures are not the source of pain. These may be treated conservatively with physical therapy or surgically with a number of orthopedic operations.

For a true chronic pain syndrome, drugs generally meet with little success and dependency occurs quickly. Some patients have successfully used meditation as an alternative to drugs. For intractable incapacitating pain, ascending sensory tracts can be cut surgically with such procedures as a rhizotomy or cordotomy.

Based on the principle that electric currents interrupt or disturb ascending pain sensations, spinal implants placed on the posterior cord (dorsal columns) have offered varying degrees of pain relief. The risks of surgical insertion and the ever-present threat of infection limit the use of this procedure, however. More recently the noninvasive use of electrical stimulators, primarily the transcutaneous nerve stimulator, applied directly to the skin over the painful area holds considerable promise for the future. Individuals can carry small battery-operated devices for convenient use to relieve pain symptoms.

The use of biofeedback is a more holistic approach to the treatment of chronic pain. Techniques work indirectly as a form of relaxation to break a habitual pain–tension–anxiety cycle. When biofeedback techniques indicate that affected muscles are becoming tense, the person is alerted to concentrate on relaxation techniques. In this way thought processes reeducate muscles. Biofeedback also holds promise for the future, particularly because techniques are not addictive, are nonchemical, and are noninvasive.

Chronic Spasticity

A certain degree of spasticity can be anticipated following upper motor neuron damage to the spinal cord. However, excessive spasticity is inevitably associated with contractures and loss of functional mobility if unchecked. For example, if flexor muscles in the arm are continually in spasm and not counteracted by extensor muscles because they are impaired, the flexor muscles involved will eventually shorten and limit shoulder, elbow, and hand function. Positioning and transfers will be more difficult.

The three major approaches currently used singly or in combination are pharmacologic, surgical, and physical. Physical therapy, alone or in combination with the other methods, remains the most practical and fruitful form of treatment (Bishop 1977). Preventive and conservative measures have been previously described. For extreme spasticity problems that incapacitate the patient, there are several neurosurgical procedures to create a lower motor neuron lesion. These procedures actually cut or interrupt reflex arcs, causing a flaccid paralysis. The simplest of these procedures is a *neurectomy*, which interrupts a peripheral nerve supplying a localized area. Surgical procedures to nerve roots (such as *rhizotomy*) or to the spinal cord (such as *myelotomy*) are considered more drastic measures to relieve extremity spasms. These procedures are considered most carefully because of associated bowel, bladder, and sexual functioning changes and loss of any preserved sensation.

To deal with the complex problems of chronic pain and spasticity, a community health nurse must be able to recognize the onset and realize the potential dangers involved if the problems are not minimized. Appropriate intervention would be referral to a skilled rehabilitative physician or follow-up services from a rehabilitation center. Then it is most important that support services in the home be established as needed.

Functional Living Skills

Throughout treatment during hospitalization, it is important to plan with the patient's home situation and desires in mind. This encompasses such things as vocational and avocational assessments and home assessments. This process can extend itself to involve a number of community agencies, such as worker's compensation board, insurance companies providing third-party payment, and employment services.

To begin with, architectural barriers in the

home must be assessed. Physical alterations or the installation of equipment may be necessary to allow maximum wheelchair independence while minimizing effort and ensuring safety. Temporary adaption is best when the patient is going home only for short passes. It is important that families receive expert advice before initiating any costly permanent alterations.

Next, the availability of community resources must be explored. Sometimes geographical location is a problem, and families relocate because of alternative opportunities.

Educational and employment background must also be considered. Can programs be modified to meet the patient's possible future requirements?

A most valuable asset is driver training for the disabled person. For convenience and safety a number of modifications can be made to regular vehicles that will enable even the patient with quadriplegia to drive. Hand controls are used to accelerate and brake, steering aids are available,

and many vans can be equipped with electrical ramps for ease in entry. For many patients with paraplegia, driver training can commence within a few weeks after injury, thus enabling greater and earlier mobility in outpatient services offered. The inherent benefits not only to the disabled population but to society at large appear obvious. The ability to drive safely enables the individual to enter the normal world for vocational, social, and recreational aspirations (Kent et al. 1979).

A nurse in the community setting must be able to comprehend the potential capabilities of clients to help them decide what they want to do and what they are capable of doing. Appropriate consultation and referral are often needed to differentiate between altered functional living skills as a personal choice and inactivity and decreased ability to care for oneself as a result of unresolved physical or psychological problems.

SELECTED REFERENCES

Bishop, B. 1977. Spasticity: its pathology and management, Part IV. Current and projected treatment procedures for spasticity. *Physical Therapy* 57 (4): 396–400. *Cites advantages and disadvantages of pharmacologic, surgical, and physical procedures with comments on future directions for management.*

Burke, D., and Murray, D. 1975. *Handbook of Spinal Cord Medicine.* London and Basingstoke: MacMillan Press Ltd., Chapter 11. *Introductory presentation of physiology and treatment of spasticity.*

Fishwick, G., and Sellers, J. 1979. Occupational therapy for patients with cervical cord injury. In *Total Management of Spinal Cord Injuries.* Eds. D. Pierce and V. Nickel. Boston: Little, Brown, pp. 205–224. *In-depth presentation of upper extremity splinting; philosophies, advantages, disadvantages, and practical application.*

Ford, J. 1980. *Wheelchair Handbook: A Guide to Selection, Cushions, Accessories and Maintenance.* G. F. Strong Rehabilitation Center, Vancouver, Canada. *A concise, liberally illustrated guide for rehabilitation professionals.*

Heustis, D. 1979. Physical therapy in rehabilitation. In *Current Perspectives in Rehabilitation Nursing.* Eds. R. Murray and J. Kijeck. St. Louis: C. V. Mosby, pp. 187–192. *Discusses the role of the physical therapist and approaches to mobility and self-care.*

Kent, H., et al. 1979. A driver training program for the disabled. *Archives of Physical Medicine and Rehabilitation* 60 (June): 273–276. *Report on results of a driver training program; includes recommendations for "van modifiers," eligibility requirements, and functional and general health assessment.*

Klose, K., and Goldberg, M. 1980. Neurological change following spinal cord injury: an assessment technique and preliminary results. *Spinal Cord Injury Digest* 2 (Summer): 35–42. *Description of a quantitative tool: the University of Miami Neurospinal Index (UMNI). The UMNI consists of two subscales: the Sensory and Motor scales. Scale scores are indicators of overall spinal cord functional capacity within the sensory and motor modalities.*

Krenzel, J., and Rohrer, L. 1977. *Paraplegic and Quadriplegic Individuals.* Handbook of care for nurses. Chicago, Ill: National Paraplegia (Spinal Cord Injury) Foundation. *Overview of initial and later rehabilitative care; both physical and emotional adjustments are addressed.*

Ritt, B., and McColey, J. 1981. Functional living skills. In *Comprehensive Rehabilitation Nursing*. Eds. N. Martin, N. Holt, and D. Hicks. New York: McGraw-Hill, pp. 298–340. *Examines self-care areas of positioning, feeding, hygiene, dressing, bathing, and toileting in general and specifically for people with spinal cord injuries.*

Rogers, J., and Figone, J. 1980. Traumatic quadriplegia: follow-up study of self-care skills. *Archives of Physical Medicine and Rehabilitation* 61 (July): 316–320. *Report on a study to assess the use of self-care skills learned during formal rehabilitation and of orthotic devices provided once community living was resumed; examines areas most sensitive to change and suggests modifications to current therapy.*

Schneider, F. 1981. Physical therapy assessment. In *Comprehensive Rehabilitation Nursing*. Eds. N. Martin, N. Holt, and D. Hicks. New York: McGraw-Hill, pp. 269–297. *Detailed musculoskeletal, neurological, cardiopulmonary, and functional assessment; includes numerous samples of charts and forms used in physical therapy.*

SUPPLEMENTAL READING

Basmajian, J. 1977. Biofeedback: the clinical tool behind the catchword. *Association of Rehabilitation Nurses Journal* 2 (Sept.–Oct.): 10, 14, 22. *Introductory overview; includes definitions, historical development, myths, and clinical application.*

Breines, E. 1979. Occupational therapy: It's more than fun and games. *Journal of Practical Nursing* 29 (Feb.): 16–17. *Focuses on role of the licensed practical/vocational nurse in collaboration with occupational therapy.*

Delaney, J. 1980. Medical treatment of spasticity. *Current Problems in Surgery* 17(4): 245–248. *Outlines commonly used drugs for treatment of spasticity. The exact neurophysiology of spasticity remains unclear.*

Ford, J., and Duckworth, B. 1976(a). Moving a dependent patient safely, comfortably. Part 1—positioning. *Nursing '76* 6(1): 27–36 *Photostory of a variety of techniques and when to use them.*

Ford, J., and Duckworth, B. 1976(b). Moving a dependent patient safely, comfortably. Part 2—transferring. *Nursing '76* 6(2): 58–65. *Photostory of techniques to choose from depending on the patient's size and disability and your size and capability; focuses on bed and toilet transfers.*

Fordyce, W., et al. 1973. Operant conditioning in the treatment of chronic pain. *Archives of Physical Medicine and Rehabilitation* 54: 399–408. *Analysis of a successful alternative for some to cope with chronic pain.*

Gunley, P. 1981. From regeneration to prosthesis: research on spinal cord injury. *Journal of the American Medical Association* 245(13): 1293–1297. *Review of current American research in regeneration, old and new therapies, and prostheses. Concise and clear.*

Halstead, L., Willems, E., and Frey, C. 1979. Spinal cord injury: time out of bed during rehabilitation. *Archives of Physical Medicine and Rehabilitation* 60 (Dec.): 590–595. *Report on quantitative monitoring of patient activity patterns described in relation to clinical and functional outcomes; a new strategy for evaluating physical and psychological health in rehabilitation.*

Hansen, A. 1976. Towards independence for paraplegics. *The Canadian Nurse*, December, pp. 24–31. *Overview of early rehabilitation; focuses on mobility and self-care skills.*

Richards, J., et al. 1980. Psycho-social aspects of chronic pain in spinal cord injury. *Pain* 8(3): 355–65. *A study done of 356 patients with spinal cord injuries to determine and analyze differences between those who reported chronic pain and those who did not.*

Stauffer, E., Hoffer, M., and Nickel, V. 1978. Ambulation in thoracic paraplegia. *Journal of Bone and Joint Surgery* 60(6): 823–824. *Presents criteria to be met if walking with crutches and braces is going to be a realistic functional goal.*

Wilson, D., McKenzie, M., and Barbar, L. 1980. *Spinal Cord Injury: A Treatment Guide for Occupational Therapists*. Thorofare, N.J.: Charles B. Slack. *Reference resource presenting general guidelines for treatment of people with traumatic spinal cord injury.*

Wittmeyer, M., and Stolov, W. 1978. Educating wheelchair patients on home architectural barriers. *American Journal of Occupational Therapy* 32(9): 557–564. *Report on a visual instructional module and checklist to help patients identify architectural barriers when selecting a residence. Helpful bibliography.*

Wolf, S. 1979. EMG biofeedback applications in physical rehabilitation: an overview. *Physiotherapy Canada* 31(2): 65–71. *In-depth review of specific biofeedback techniques with emphasis on use with neuromuscular rather than musculoskeletal dysfunction, including spinal cord injury.*

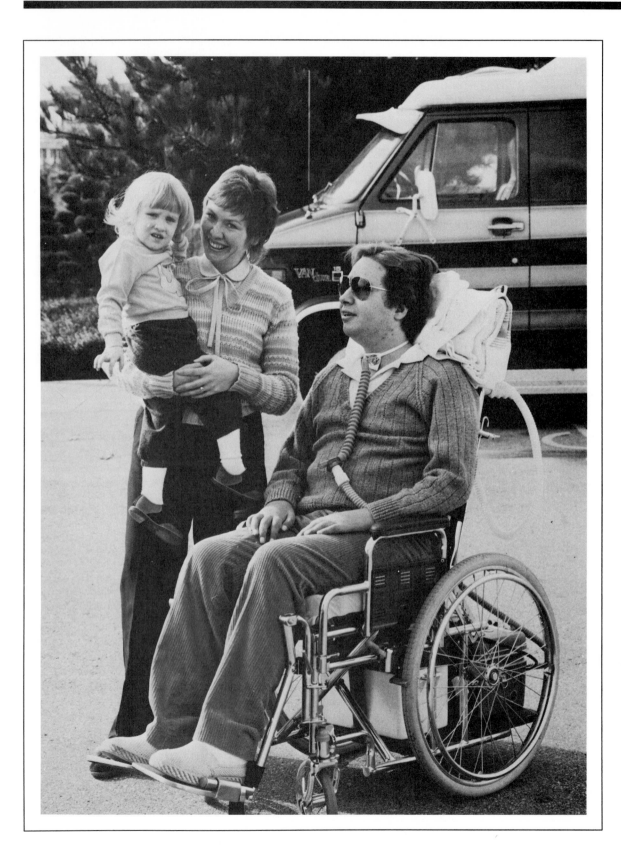

Chapter 17

High Cervical Cord Injury: Respiratory Quadriplegia*

CHAPTER OUTLINE

---

* This chapter was developed with the assistance of Linda MacNutt, M.S.W., and Gail Roche, R.N., Head Nurse, Pearson Hospital, Vancouver, B.C. The residents with respiratory quadriplegia also added valuable insights.

OBJECTIVES

- To define health care goals
- To discuss the significant role of the family, the health care profession, and society in relation to the individual with respiratory quadriplegia
- To describe helpful nursing interventions during the process of psychosocial adjustment to disability
- To discuss the importance of personal feelings toward respiratory quadriplegia; to

reveal how emotional reactions can influence nursing intervention; and to identify appropriate assistance for coping with these influences

- To describe interventions that promote optimal respiratory function
- To describe methods to reestablish mobility and promote independence
- To demonstrate support of and participation in initiating new rehabilitation options

GOALS OF HEALTH CARE

In the recent past a severe injury at the high cervical cord level was invariably fatal. But this situation is changing. People with high-level spinal cord injuries are surviving and the severity of residual disability poses awesome challenges to the patient, the family, the health care profession, and society as a whole.

It must be remembered that patients with respiratory quadriplegia are only a very small part of the spinal cord injured population, and very little is known about them. As the population itself grows, needs are being defined and changed as more information is gathered and shared. One concept is becoming increasingly clear: a psychosocial health model of care promotes self-esteem, acceptance, and self-actualization, all of which are essential to a meaningful life.

Consequently, a rehabilitation philosophy that not only emphasizes expert medical intervention but also encourages an interdisciplinary holistic approach to health care will better support and maintain positive and growth-oriented interactions between people with respiratory quadriplegia and their environment. This chapter attempts to examine potential psychological and physical needs of people with respiratory

quadriplegia and to suggest ways in which a nurse can participate with the health care team to meet those needs.

In addition to meeting the needs encountered with the classic profile of quadriplegia, the goals of the health care team are:

- To gain a full perspective of the meaning of respiratory quadriplegia and then to act in the patient's interest to enhance the quality of life
- To develop a positive attitude toward rehabilitation, despite the severe physical disability respiratory quadriplegia causes
- To provide optimal respiratory care to those requiring permanent respiratory support
- To accept and create new ways of increasing mobility and independence

PHYSICAL CONSEQUENCES OF RESPIRATORY QUADRIPLEGIA

Following emergency care and stabilization of the patient's general condition, detailed neurological examination is essential to understand the patient's potential abilities and to establish clearer rehabilitation goals. In addition to the classic profile of quadriplegia, people with respiratory quadriplegia will experience variable losses of sensation and motor control of the head and neck area, depending on the level of injury. In terms of functional neurological levels Stauffer and Bell (1978) describe two distinct classifications: *respiratory quadriplegia* and *respiratory pentaplegia.*

To understand the diagnosis clearly it is important to remember how terminology is used to describe the level of injury. If a patient is diagnosed as having a C_3 quadriplegia, this means the C_3 neurological level of the third cervical cord segment and root is *intact,* while the fourth is not. In other words C_3 is the last neurological level to function normally.

The spinal respiratory center is located primarily at the C_4 level of the cord but receives some innervation from C_3 and C_5. Through the phrenic nerve outflow the spinal respiratory center innervates the diaphragm, the main muscle of breathing. When the diaphragm is nonfunctional, the patient will need permanent respiratory support. As described and illustrated in Chapter 9 the accessory muscles of breathing are also innervated by the cervical cord (C_{2-7}) and refer to the sternocleidomastoid, which also receives innervation from the spinal accessory (cranial) nerve, and scalenus muscles located in the neck and upper chest. By strengthening and retraining these muscles, patients with respiratory quadriplegia can achieve some periods off the respirator.

Following traumatic cervical cord injury a patient with C_4 quadriplegia is expected to establish voluntary control of breathing, albeit at a subnormal capacity. However, if the lesion is higher (and complete), this is not possible.

A patient with *respiratory quadriplegia* has a C_2 or C_3 functional level and will have full sensation of the head and upper neck and some neck control. This eventually enables patients to balance the head, which helps maintain an upright position in the wheelchair and allows various mouthstick activities. Most importantly, partial preservation of the accessory muscles of breathing offers potential to develop tolerance for being off the respirator for a few hours.

The patient with a C_1 functional level is described as having *respiratory pentaplegia.* Little or no sensation or motor control of the head and neck is preserved except for the "face mask" area. Without neck control patients cannot balance the head and will have difficulty maintaining an upright position in the wheelchair without external support. Without some accessory muscles of breathing, there is little or no potential for developing tolerance for being off the respirator.

Most cord injuries extend several segments above and below the main traumatic area, and therefore damage may extend into the brain stem where the nuclei of the lower cranial nerves are located. This can cause sensory and motor impairment of the face and, most importantly, the swallowing muscles. This type of deficit may be temporary—particularly if caused by cord edema—or permanent. Assessment and treatment then become highly individualized to prevent aspiration and to provide nutritional requirements.

Maintaining physical functions for patients with high-level cord injuries incorporates similar principles to promoting health and managing the effects of disability for other patients with spinal cord injuries. For example, optimal bowel and bladder elimination requires the specific skills outlined to manage dysfunctions caused by upper motor neuron lesions. Nursing care measures to maintain the skeletal and integumentary systems are also similar.

PSYCHOSOCIAL IMPLICATIONS OF RESPIRATORY QUADRIPLEGIA

While advancements in early care and assessment have evolved with rapidity, solution for the looming issues surrounding the quality of life have not. In general the present lack of rehabilitation opportunities for patients with respiratory quadriplegia is comparable to the limited opportunities available for patients with quadriplegia 30 years ago. The magnitude of medical, psychosocial, and vocational problems has rendered the traditional medical model of care inadequate to meet these unique needs. As a result, providing direct psychosocial support encompasses some very broad issues.

The onset of injury resulting in respiratory quadriplegia may be defined as a crisis. It is a

■ *RESPIRATORY QUADRIPLEGIA*   *Some Reflections on Its Meaning*

From the injured person's point of view

I am a person with respiratory quadriplegia. I am this way against my will, for the risks I took in life did not prepare me for this. Perhaps nothing could.

So here I am, I cannot move my arms or legs. I cannot dress or feed myself. I cannot talk with my hands anymore, and I can no longer run in joy or anger. I have lost the pleasure of feeling someone touch my body or being able to reach out to hold another with my arms. Please forgive my anger; it is not always directed at you.

A machine helps me breathe and orders me to measure my speech to its respirations. I hate the machine, for it reminds me of what I have, but I need the machine, for it reminds me that I am.

I will learn to change from my previous life-style, but it does take time. It takes so long even to read again. Jog five miles and you know how I feel after turning pages with a mouthstick. Sometimes I need to be pushed a little or encouraged to try new things, but I must be able to feel some control, for I have already lost so much. Let me talk a little about my fears and my exhaustion as well as about my goals. Sometimes I need to cry. This is a risk. And sometimes I need to laugh and see others laugh. Always I need to teach others about myself; at times I am very tired of it all.

So here I am. I am alive. I laugh and cry just like you. I am not ill but a person with a disability. Just like you I have good days, bad days, feelings, and ideas. I also have dreams and hopes. This bed and chair is not my life. Most of my body's numb, but I can still feel my heart, my hair, my face, perhaps my neck. I have not lost the pleasure of feeling someone stroke my face or of offering pleasure to another with my lips, my face. In a way I'm born again. I'm learning new ways to talk and do, for myself and for others. With practice I am not so tired, and new tasks soon become routine.

And so, here I am. It is not something I can ever accept completely but I can acknowledge myself in this situation and learn to cope. And I must always have hope. Please remember that.

From another's point of view

I know someone who has respiratory quadriplegia. At first I am afraid that this could happen to me. How would I cope, what would I do? I'm not sure how to act or what to say. I feel sorry for you and am afraid of my pity, for I suspect you do not need it.

I must learn to listen to a sentence often interrupted by a machine and wonder if I say the right or the wrong thing. But is there a right or wrong thing, maybe I should just talk? This machine, it doesn't talk, yet it means so much. I need to know about it, so I need not feel so afraid.

Sometimes I forget the energy it takes to read or get out of bed and I grow impatient. When I am tired or have many things to do it is easy to forget to show a willingness for little things. I forget you cannot use your arms and legs as I can and that you probably still remember when you could. Sometimes I forget how much you risk when you explore new things and I need to remember my own fears and how I cope.

Feeding and dressing an alert adult is, at first, strange to me. I'm not sure how to make it a comfortable experience. Perhaps my own awkward feelings make it the same for you. Thank you when you gently let me know how you feel.

(Box continues)

■ *RESPIRATORY QUADRIPLEGIA (continued)*

I am confused when you are angry and I'm not sure why. How can I make myself remember that it may not be me you are angry at but your situation? Maybe we can talk about it, or perhaps you just need to be left alone for a while.

After a time I see beyond your disability, for you are just a person after all. In many ways you manage your life and I needn't try to tell you how. You have the same rights to privacy and respect as any other person I know. We can, perhaps, share our ideas and perceptions. Doing so, I must watch you struggle to find your balance between dependence and independence and wonder when to speak my mind or to step aside. Later we can laugh, when it's a little easier. Above all I must remember that just because you require so much care it does not mean you are ill.

How much you have taught me about life and about myself. Your struggles and failures teach me about my own. I think now that there are no such things as failures but only experiences to build on. Thank you for that.

Compiled from a series of encounters by Linda MacNutt, M.S.W.

---

traumatic event that requires solutions, invariably new, in relation to the individual's previous life experience. Consequently there is severe disruption of living patterns accompanied by tension and distress that results in a reorganization of the life situation. In the case of the person with respiratory quadriplegia the crisis revolves around extreme and traumatic physical injury with subsequent implications for the individual, family, health care, and community systems.

It is unrealistic to expect injured people and their families to resolve all the implications of the disability during formal rehabilitation; implications vary from the acute care fear of death and disability to the long-term struggle to achieve mobility and other skills that expose individuals and families to social barriers. As individual goals are determined, challenged, and met, personal growth occurs. This personal and rehabilitative growth leads to psychosocial adjustment.

The Patient

It must be emphasized that psychosocial adjustment to the crisis of respiratory quadriplegia occurs over a very long time. It is unrealistic to expect that vast identity changes imposed by severe disability be incorporated too quickly, especially considering that the concept of self begins to develop in early childhood. Burnham and Werner (1978–79) describe disturbances in formal thought or cognition caused by the traumatic physical and emotional injury as significant factors in slowing the adjustment process for the person with respiratory quadriplegia. It is also logical that the inability to communicate (when a cuffed tracheostomy tube is necessary during the early months) may retard the expression of emotional factors inherent in the adjustment process.

As time progresses patients begin to realize the impact of severe disability. Major consequences include changes in body image, methods of communication, locus of control, and personal roles.

Body image

Patients must develop a new body image, for they can no longer define themselves in preinjury terms. One patient felt his feeling of success in life was due to his physical prowess in sports and had difficulty thinking of what to do to feel good about himself again. Another described a feeling that her head and body were split. She thought of herself only as a head and felt disgust with her paralyzed limbs.

Patients must also adjust their body image to include mechanical aids. Reidentification in this existential sense is difficult indeed. The electric wheelchair and the respirator become extensions of the self in relation to mobility and life itself. There is often inner turmoil in the relationship between the individual and machines (Burnham and Werner 1978–79).

Methods of communication

Patients with high-level injuries must discard many original methods of communication. They can no longer use their hands to express themselves in speech, or touch another when words are not enough. They must now describe rather than point out objects, find new releases for powerful emotions, and try to find words instead of the actions previously used for communication.

Locus of control

Severely injured people no longer have the same control over their bodies they once had. They can no longer feed or dress themselves or attend to their intimate personal hygiene; therefore, they must accept the help of others in addition to instructing others in their care. Even a slight element of choice becomes very significant, because it reestablishes some measure of control. Being able to decide what to eat first (peas or carrots) and what time to bathe are important choices to physically dependent people even if they seem mundane to us.

Personal roles

The process of identification with new roles will probably be influenced by the individual's perception of the sick and disabled roles. Due to the initial life and death situation in acute care, injured people are indeed ill and intensive medical skill and nursing care are required to keep them alive. But there is danger of stabilizing in the sick role on a long-term basis. Illness may be preferable to disability as it may sustain a belief in cure and lack of acknowledgment of the disability. One patient stated that he half believed he would be cured when transferred from acute care, simply because leaving the hospital *should* have meant that he was cured.

Patients will have to reexamine vocational opportunities and reassess dreams or ideals within the limitations of severe disability. After injury recreational pastimes will likely change from the more concrete (action oriented) to the more abstract (watching television, listening to the radio, reading, drawing). Such activities will often require the use of the electronic environmental controls. Ironically, while intellectual or abstract pursuits are gradually emphasized, access to life experiences is reduced.

The Family

Psychosocial implications have meaning for the family as a whole as well as for each member of that system. Implications for the family are closely related to those experienced by the patient. As time progresses family members, too, begin to understand the injury's full consequences.

Perceptions of the disabled family member

The family must change their perceptions of the injured person in relation to vocational, recreational, and social relationships. Dreams, hopes, and expectations for a child, sibling, or spouse are not given up easily. It is difficult to perceive them as incapable of walking or even feeding themselves again. In addition, the person's inability to breathe without a respirator can generate fear of death, fear of the machine, and fear of inability to handle potential emergencies.

Family roles

The tasks at the onset of injury usually mean some family members leave jobs and/or home towns to spend much of their time at the hospital. This is not usually a permanent change and after acute hospitalization the family returns to its initial tasks while at the same time assuming the additional patient care tasks. Role strain through such task reorganization is common. For example, conflict arises when a parent is trying to help a son or daughter toward independence while the demands of physical care almost force overprotective relationships.

Considerable adjustment must also be made when a spouse (more often the husband) is in-

I was injured in a diving accident four years ago. My family all reacted in different ways, each coinciding with their various personalities. Dad was the strongest one holding the family together, always being positive around me, but breaking down many times outside the hospital—I found out months later. However, I believe it was a healthy and necessary reaction at the time. Mom and my two sisters reacted in a similar way by showing compassion, understanding, and patience throughout my good and bad times. My oldest brother, then and now, finds it harder to cope and adjust to my situation— always waiting to wake up and find things back to normal. My youngest brother was affected the least because of his age and easy-going nature.

Some of my closest friends stood by me and handled the situation as well as could be expected, maybe a little awkwardly at first. Others I never did see again. Some of the ones I least expected to come in have become my closest friends. You sure learn who your friends are. Without my family and friends there is no predicting what might have been.

jured. There is a frequent need to adjust, possibly to reverse roles, and to learn new ways of communicating feelings and needs. Financial resources may be severely strained, especially as vocational opportunities for people with respiratory quadriplegia are presently limited.

With regard to family power structures, the disabled individual may be viewed as developing into a power figure due to the mechanistic tasks of personal care and all the attention that it requires. Power can also be centered around the individual's ability to manipulate the family's well-being. For example, a depressed attitude can affect the family mood and motivate people to meet the disabled person's idiosyncratic needs.

The Nurse

Caring for a respiratory quadriplegic patient in any acute or long-term care setting is stressful in the sense that professional and personal attitudes and values become an important part of the therapeutic environment.

All practitioners experience another's disability only indirectly and their perceptions are fixed with personal and professional attitudes. Inevitably a question asked when faced with the realities of respiratory quadriplegia is, "Could I live as Joe must live now?" Severe disability such as this is often questioned because people identify with the patient and have difficulty anticipating any quality of life remaining. How often have feelings been expressed by saying, "If this ever happens to me, someone pull the plug"? But as one patient explains, "The shock of being told I would never move again was devastating. I wanted to die and if I could have reached my (respirator) hose I would have pulled it out. Now, although I feel it sometimes doesn't matter one way or the other, when my air goes off, I fight for it."

Be reassured that people with respiratory quadriplegia and their families eventually can cope and do enjoy life. The several personal viewpoints throughout this chapter reveal that life still offers purpose. As Burnham and Werner (1978–79) describe, eventually low moments do not seem to override the will to live for people with respiratory quadriplegia. Private definitions of personal purpose, such as fulfilling the responsibilities of parenthood, reflect a driving force much stronger than the search for physical sustenance. Too often we underestimate the resilience of the human race.

Patients and families rely on health care professionals to look objectively beyond the immediate crisis at hand. If we don't, who will? Consequently, it is important to view the family over a long period of time so as not to take on their feelings of crisis and devastation in the immediate situation. The nurse must share with other team members the role of expert practitioner; counselor; advocate; educator; coordinator; and planner to ensure as many opportunities as possible for a full and positive future for people with respiratory quadriplegia and their families.

Society

It is apparent that adaptation is not the patient's responsibility alone, for society as a whole helps create the problems to which the individual must adapt. As many disabled people emphasize, much of the disability associated with physical impairment is a result of social conditions and values rather than limitations imposed by physical incapacities (Mechanic 1961).

The individual, the family, and health care professionals are all part of society. General values and beliefs in society will help define each group's attitudes toward disability. What are some of these values or norms that encourage us to define disability as a problem for society? One of them is our society's value of beauty (Goffman 1961). Since one of our criteria for beauty is physical wholeness, we tend to view the severely disabled as not beautiful and therefore pitiable or even contemptible.

Another important value held by our society is that of independence or self-reliance. This emphasis may make injured people less inclined to want or accept help. But people with respiratory quadriplegia have no choices, they depend on help in all aspects of daily care and must try to seek self-reliance in other things. It is important to remember that their need for help does not mean they are sick or not self-directing.

Our society also values productivity. Visible contributions, particularly work, are interpreted as accomplishment, and who we are (self-concept) is often measured by what we can do. People who do not "contribute" are often viewed as a burden to society, for their maintenance is a great financial cost, and often the disabled person is relegated to second-class citizenship and the "helpless" role is transformed into the "useless" role. Society continually wrestles with justifying substantial financial expenditures to gain limited results. One cannot deny that the constant care required by people with respiratory quadriplegia is costly. Unfortunately such a cost–benefit analysis does not always measure the less tangible accomplishments of the individual and the need to ensure a high quality for the life that is saved.

Severely disabled people may be encouraged to act "normal," but they face social contra-dictions. Stigma, limited employment opportunities, lack of technological aids, lack of transportation, and architectural barriers are some examples.

These factors isolate the severely disabled person, which limits stimulating contact with other human beings and minimizes the potential for enhancing inner personal resources. Respiratory quadriplegia therefore is a problem that cannot be separated from society. Adaptation to disability is a joint responsibility, because society as a whole helps define disability.

HELPING PEOPLE ADAPT TO RESPIRATORY QUADRIPLEGIA

Promoting Psychosocial Adjustment

To promote psychosocial adjustment it is fundamental to apply the concept that basic physical needs must be met before psychological growth can flourish. It is profoundly important for the nurse to become comfortable with the needed specialized equipment in order to help create a relaxed environment conducive to meaningful communication. In reality, preparation of numerous staff members just to meet the exceptional *physical* needs of the respiratory quadriplegic patient is frequently a major problem.

Principles of psychological support were described in Chapter 6. Outlined assessment techniques and suggestions for coping with emotional reactions and behavioral crises (including personal feelings) very much apply when caring for the patient with respiratory dependency in addition to a spinal cord injury.

Dealing with depression
As the life-threatening impact of trauma subsides, the realization of the implications of disability become clearer. Inevitably feelings of helplessness and hopelessness prevail. Expressed feelings such as "Why did they save me? I'm of no use to myself or anyone else. Let me die" are often heard.

■ *PERSONAL VIEWPOINT*

I was injured on the uneven parallel bars while practicing for the gymnastics team one day after school. I was 16 years old at the time and a sophomore in high school. Shortly thereafter, my family moved to Houston, Texas, so that I could go to the Texas Institute for Rehabilitation and Research (TIRR). (We had been living in Shreveport, Louisiana.) Since I was a C_{1-2} injury, a respirator has been required at all times. At first, I was on an MA-1. The first side of the phrenic pacemaker was implanted in December 1970—about 2 years after my injury, which occurred in April 1968. The following year, the other side was implanted, and I began to gain time using them. I still used a Bantam respirator on my wheelchair for several years.

I graduated from Captain Shreve High School with my class in 1970. My family took me back to Shreveport especially for that event. Then I applied to Rice University, where I graduated in 1977 with a B.A. in liberal arts (sociology, political science, and English). I started University of Houston College of Law in 1976 (one year before my official graduation from Rice), and graduated in 1980. I took the July 1980 Bar Exam and was licensed in November 1980. I am currently running my own business (a women's store) and plan eventually to start my own law practice.

Looking back, it is difficult to express what kinds of things the nurses did that were helpful, or were not helpful, because so much depends on personal qualities. Perhaps above all, don't let the families of newly injured persons feel as though the care required for a person with respiratory quadriplegia is impossible for them to learn. Even though this may seem to infringe on your professional training, stress to all concerned that everything you do for the respiratory

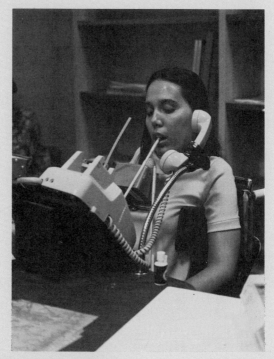

Kathleen DeSilva

quadriplegic person can eventually be successfully learned and performed by family and friends. Also, allow as much visiting time as possible; hospital hours should be bent when a person's mental outlook needs strength and support from those who are closest.

My mother took care of me while I lived at home with help from my younger brothers and sisters who would do such things as turn pages, wash my face and hair, and change television channels. Both my parents attended class at Rice with me. I stayed in a room that was built on to the house. Then we moved to a new house where the study was my bedroom.

When my mother had her seventh child, we hired someone to come in part-time during the day. Otherwise, my parents did all my care. (I have a wonderful family and consider myself very fortunate in this respect.)

(Box continues)

■ *PERSONAL VIEWPOINT (continued)*

The events leading to my moving out were very sudden and unexpected. My mother died in 1974 when the baby was a year and a half old. I went into (TIRR) for back surgery and during the months of recuperation, my father and I decided that the best thing was for me to find a private attendant and move into my own apartment. My parents and I had discussed this before, but now it was almost a necessity.

I advertised and interviewed for two months and finally hired a young woman in her twenties just before Christmas. She trained at TIRR for about two weeks and then we moved into an apartment. It was quite a memorable experience! I have been living in the community now for seven years and presently live in a complex where a group of disabled individuals share attendant services and van pooling. I still have a private attendant as well because of my breathing status.

I also have some advice on hiring an attendant:

- Look for someone who is "willing to learn" about your care. I have had more success with persons who have had no medical experience at all. Those who have tend to think that they know what is best for you. You are the best judge of that and you know your care better than anyone. It is your responsibility to teach it.
- Advertise in newspapers, community papers, church bulletins, college papers, bulletin boards, university placement centers.
- Consider a roommate who is also an attendant. You can offer room, board, and perhaps a small salary. This is especially true with someone who is nonprofessional or working through school.
- Ask your friends for help on weekends or evenings so your attendant can have time off. You would be surprised at how eager your friends are to help, but they don't know how until you tell them.
- Be persistent! It takes time to find a good attendant and sometimes you have to go through several bad ones. Chalk it up to experience; you will inevitably learn something from each one.

Here is a list of a few memorable experiences:

- Swimming in my father's pool on a floating lounge chair
- A three-week trip from Texas to Michigan in a van with my roommate–attendant
- Camping on a friend's land in a tent with no running water
- A weekend flight to my ten-year high school reunion in Shreveport
- A convention at the beach with an upstairs meeting room and no elevator

Kathleen De Silva
Houston, Texas

Several people with respiratory quadriplegia described these and other similar statements in retrospect as ways of expressing the desperate fear of the unknown future. They were seeking *reassurance*. They needed to know that life would improve and that they were still important, valuable people who deserved to keep on living.

How can the nurse respond? The people mentioned above repeatedly emphasized the need to respond positively, but realistically, without false hope. In order to do so the nurse must reflect a positive inner attitude, which is developed by gaining an awareness of the life-styles now possible. If a patient is grasping for some positive feedback on what the future will hold, the nurse who is totally unfamiliar with what is possible will create even more negative feelings.

Be reassured that a warm, caring, and honest relationship provides a sound baseline, despite probable feelings of personal helplessness. Sit down and encourage the patient to talk about feelings and past and present experiences; perhaps share some of your own. Guard against responses that block communication. When talking about a death wish, statements such as, "Don't be silly," "What a ridiculous thing to say," "I know how you feel and would want to die too," or "You owe it to your family and friends to live," communicate a lack of sensitivity and tend to cause further alienation.

It is also important not to give false hope. False hope prolongs recovery and aggravates suffering. Once the prognosis has been disclosed by the physician, a consistent team approach to statements and questions is vital.

To be optimistic and realistic, at the same time, try to focus on how a particular part of the present situation will improve. Perhaps it means removal of a stomach tube, ability to sit up, a portable respirator, a new wheelchair, or ability to take a college course. It is surprising how an awkward response from the nurse can be interpreted as false hope. For example, a young respiratory quadriplegic boy and his parents were discussing his return to school in time for graduation. When they looked to the nurse for approval, the nurse "simply didn't have the heart" to initiate a discussion on why this activity would not be possible. Instead the nurse smiled and quickly left the room. Avoiding the subject created more uncertainty, which allowed unrealistic expectations to grow. In some situations it may not be appropriate to explore a subject further at the time, but be sure to refer your concerns to counseling professionals of the health team.

Do not hesitate to seek guidance and support from counseling professionals. Especially in the acute stage, the patient tends to develop a more intimate relationship with selected nurses giving direct care.

The adjustment process is a lengthy one and progress is slow. It is important to keep expectations realistic and compatible with the person's preinjury personality. A person's failure to achieve goals can lead to many unresolved frustrations to say nothing of discouragement for all concerned.

Patient and family health education

Patient and family health education facilitates the adjustment process. The general educational approach described in Chapter 8 will help acquaint the patient and family with the extent and meaning of the disability and effect attitudinal and behavioral changes in patients and families so that they will assume an active role in the management of disability and maintenance of optimal health. Despite the individual's illness and the recent crisis, the acute care nurse can apply the principles previously described to begin developing a positive attitude toward future health care. Understandably, patients may not be fully ready to learn specific care measures for some time.

In addition to the physical tasks at hand, the patient and possibly the family must develop an effective approach for directing others in various aspects of personal care. Incorporating the expertise of counseling professionals into educational programs could help the patient and family develop skills in supervising and relating to others. In essence, the patient and family are assuming a new role as educators themselves. If the nurse introduces this concept successfully, and if all concerned view the introduction of new staff members as an opportunity to enact these new roles, rehabilitation will become more flexible and less stressful.

When patients begin to apply their knowledge and take initiative in participating or supervising their daily care they demonstrate an acceptance of responsibility for their bodies and daily lives (Burnham and Werner 1978–79). Regulating fluid and dietary intake, or supervising inspection and implementation of measures to prevent skin breakdown are some examples of such responsibilities.

Long-term planning can help patients exercise control over the environment, thereby enhancing feelings of self-worth. Involvement in making business and financial decisions, planning modifications to the home environment, and beginning to fulfill the role of a parent or son or daughter are good opportunities.

The dependency created by respiratory quadriplegia places a great deal of responsibility on the family. Therefore, it is extremely important to develop a sensitivity to the family's

■ *PERSONAL VIEWPOINT*

I was injured about three years ago and have respiratory quadriplegia. So many of my initial memories are vague, almost like a foggy, cloudy experience that was constantly present. My most important concern was just staying alive and not thinking as much about my paralysis as life itself, figuring I would deal with the paralysis when the time was right.

Although I am now aware of the theory that adjustment is reached in stages, for the most part my personal recollection of these stages is very blurred. I do remember becoming increasingly angry and irritable about two to three months after my accident. The feelings of fear, frustration, and anger kept building during this time because I was unable to express myself verbally. When my speech did return, coping with the situations and personalities became easier because my feelings could be ventilated, particularly by talking to my family. I never took it out on my family but mostly on those people whom I would normally have avoided but that I now couldn't avoid because of my disability.

Many different people doing personal care is hard to get used to, although I realize efficient care requires close and regular inspection of my body. Even though most of my nurses were very understanding and did all they could to help me, sensitivity levels among staff members are surprisingly different. Unfortunately, there were some bad feelings and unresolved problems because of

my unique situation and their inexperience. But I did have a couple of [primary care] nurses that in my eyes could do no wrong, which made the trying times much easier.

I felt then, and often still do now, that all this is temporary, just too much to cope with and tomorrow I'll just walk away from it all. However, I'm able to deal with my paralysis much better now, trying to extract the positive things out of my situation. I still hope and feel that most of my movement will return, but I don't dwell on the thought. I live my life planning for the future in the state I'm in, trying to challenge myself with things that previously wouldn't have been as difficult. I get great satisfaction out of these challenges as long as I keep them in perspective by not comparing to the past.

Perhaps you are a nurse caring for someone with respiratory quadriplegia. Be reassured that yes, there is definitely a worthwhile life ahead for persons with a disability similar to mine. One is still the same person mentally and you'd be surprised at what can be accomplished if one has his mind set on it. So whatever you do, don't give up. Relax. Try to give as much hope as you can without being unrealistic. Above all do not give false hope. Everything is not going to be all right, but some things will be. Try to find out what new options are available, and feel comfortable in being honestly optimistic. After all, where there is life, there is always hope.

needs and reactions that can block learning. To gain the fullest benefits, the adjustment level of the family must complement that of the patient.

The following situation was described by a 23-year-old quadriplegic girl with respiratory dependency.

My mother became increasingly silent after my accident. Her usual reaction was to internalize feelings about problems. Later on she wouldn't

have anything to do with my care, such as emptying my leg bag, tipping my chair back, or even moving my limbs to a more comfortable position. As far as she was concerned the health professionals were there to do that sort of thing. I finally perceived the source of the problem, and with many misgivings, rightly or wrongly, our roles were temporarily reversed. I confronted her with the reality that she had a daughter who was permanently disabled, and if she wanted to keep her she must accept the fact there would be times when we would be alone together. The discussion was a turning point that cleared the air. Slowly she was able to learn about my care.

In this case opportunities for professional intervention were clearly missed. Closer liaison with counseling professionals could have helped alert the nurse to the ways in which family members dealt with problems and the kinds of behavior that would indicate the mother was having difficulty. Meanwhile, many afternoons had been wasted trying to force the mother to learn various activities for the patient's sake. The mother's angry reactions and demanding requests were confusing and frustrating to the staff, especially when the patient was coping so well. Finally the patient and her mother could have benefited from counseling support to explore their feelings and enhance the mother–daughter relationship. If the underlying problems had been recognized, professional intervention could have helped resolve these conflicts much sooner and made the educational process more effective.

Planning for Relocation

Relocation or transfer from one unit to another or one facility to another is a crisis for the patient, the family, and new staff members second only to the major crisis of the physical injury. The relocation process, then, can have a significant impact on psychosocial adjustment. The change in environments is usually great, with new staff, a new physical environment, new patients, and new programs. Difficult changes most frequently mentioned by patients are decreases in staff, different physical environment, and difficulty of separation from former primary care nurses.

Emotional reactions

Relocation may arouse many emotional reactions such as anxiety, uncertainty, and confusion. Different authors report varying degrees of frustration, a rise in tension, individual upset, disorganization of function, and feelings of overwhelming helplessness and loss of control (Rapoport 1965). At this point most individuals also experience a sense of shock and confusion. Separation from primary care nurses was especially

■ *PERSONAL VIEWPOINT*

It is an art to make people feel comfortable around you. When my family and friends visited me they gradually performed little tasks for me. As they became more confident, and I was able to react calmly, it was easy to teach them about my respirator and my care.

In terms of helping family and friends learn how to help a disabled person, it is extremely important that the individual learn as much as he can about his own care, including the equipment he depends on. It is essential that the disabled person is aware of the problems that he can encounter in his day-to-day living, and be prepared for those exigencies. In the case of a respirator-dependent person, understand the respirator, know what can go wrong with it, and know what to do when something does go wrong. This is much easier to do if the person is not totally dependent, but is able to breathe on his own for a little while, but it is even more important for the person who has no breathing to make sure that the people around him know what to do in an emergency. The onus should be on the disabled person to make sure that the people around him know what to do when the occasion arises. Even if a person is living in an institution it is important that he or she accept some responsibility for personal care.

difficult and left a sense of loss, which was increased when there was no opportunity to discuss these feelings.

The effect of relocation can also be very positive. The need to move on is very pressing for most people. They feel ready to leave the more acute care settings in spite of leaving familiar and caring people. They are, perhaps, eager to relinquish the sick role in favor of increasing freedom to come and go in a new, less structured environment.

In terms of crisis theory, if people helping to restructure a life situation emphasize succumbing features, the injured person will probably be filled with bitterness and despair, but if the possibilities for growth are emphasized, adjustment should be characterized by hope, confidence, and personality growth (Shontz 1975). Relocation, then, can serve as a catalyst to maximize positive cycles of adaptation.

Continuity of care

Planning for continuity of care is an important helping technique and a major factor in determining how well the patient and family are able to handle the move. While the value of interdisciplinary, even interagency, conferences is recognized more and more, the content—not to mention the practicality of actually having them—needs to be addressed.

As an example, let us examine the preparation and follow-up care for a patient transferring from a critical care unit to a ward setting. Typically the stay in the unit has been long, and the move is suddenly necessary because patients with more acute illnesses take priority. Often a detailed nursing care plan does accompany the patient, but it is difficult for the receiving nurse to welcome the patient; prepare the bedside environment; and select, communicate, and transcribe appropriate information all at the same time. Meanwhile, the slightest difference in a suctioning technique or a change in visiting hours can balloon into a major unpleasant issue, and the difficulties begin.

How can this situation be improved? If the nursing service as a whole, including nursing leaders and those nurses who are transferring and receiving the patient, understand the long-term goals and the magnitude of potential problems, the approach will be more unified and supportive, yet flexible. This will involve taking measures to ensure adequate information and communication with nurses at the bedside.

For example, when sharing information about the patient's individual needs, be prepared to explore even the seemingly direct statements. It is not sufficient, for example, to note that the patient requires suctioning about every two hours. Can the patient communicate the need to be suctioned? How will the suction setup differ? Are the catheters the same? Does the procedure differ? Who will be doing it? A registered nurse or a nursing assistant?

The issue of what category of staff will be performing what procedures is frequently complicated. Although suctioning a tracheotomy is not generally considered a nursing assistant's responsibility, the person with respiratory quadriplegia has unique needs. If a nursing assistant cannot perform this procedure, is it likely that opportunities for rehabilitation will be limited? For example, will outings off the ward be limited, perhaps just to sit outside? Limitations such as these can significantly prolong hospitalization.

If all members of the the nursing care team are not allowed to meet the patient's basic needs, what messages are sent to the family? What implications does this have for the nursing assistant trying to manage daily bedside care? After all, family and even friends are expected to learn these procedures eventually.

These kinds of decisions affect policy making, implications of which may extend outside the health care facility to licensing bodies. However, if individualized needs are to be met, these questions must be addressed, and well ahead of time for adequate planning.

Preparing the patient

When the team judges the patient to be medically and emotionally capable, they will initiate discussion of the potential transfer. At this point the social worker and primary nurse, in view of their daily contact, may be the appropriate persons to meet with the patient. The initiation of a formal discussion should indicate to the individual that there is the opportunity for full expression of thoughts and feelings (positive and negative) about the move.

Most patients find it difficult to be flexible at this point. Do not let the patient's rigid expectations and preference for nurses deter you from approaching the subject. This is also the time to begin termination of the primary care relationship (if the process is not already begun) and create opportunities for expression of feelings about this separation.

Discussion of goals and of probable length of stay in the new environment will help minimize vague expectations and lack of certainty associated with increasing stress. Above all it is important to focus on the fact that it is the improvement in the patient's general state of health that is making the move necessary. This improvement dictates changes in care requirements, but unless the patient and family are well prepared, the new nurse's approach is often perceived as incompetent.

The critical care nurse must help the patient and family view the anticipated changes as a positive step in the transition period toward a more homelike situation. The receiving nurse must be alert for potential problems and be prepared to demonstrate immediate confidence in spite of the different ways of doing things. It is also helpful if the patient, family, and new nurse can be open to the new role of the patient as educator in terms of individual needs.

It is reassuring for the patient and family to know that there will be a formal opportunity for discussion following relocation. It is also helpful if the original social worker or clinical nurse specialist can maintain contact during the transition period to enhance continuity.

Choosing the appropriate setting

Selecting the most appropriate setting following the critical phase is difficult. Providing safe and detailed care while increasing opportunities for independence and rehabilitation is a very real problem.

Caring for respiratory-dependent patients on a general ward setting is often an isolated experience for an institution. Therefore, staff members are often inexperienced in this kind of care. In-depth staff education is necessary but not always feasible. As a result, patients with respiratory quadriplegia sometimes experience detrimental, costly, and prolonged stays in a critical care area. When relocation does occur, it may be to a setting where rehabilitation is not the primary focus. These factors emphasize the need for development of specialized, integrated, rehabilitative services.

In preparation for discharge, either to home or a long-term care facility, the process described in Chapter 18 is relevant to people with respiratory quadriplegia.

Promoting Optimal Respiratory Function

Promoting optimal respiratory function will be a constant and life-long endeavor for people with high cervical cord injuries. Mobility and in-dependence often require the use of a portable, wheelchair-adaptable ventilator (Figure 17–1). Some people can breathe by using an internal phrenic nerve pacemaker to stimulate the diaphragm.

The health care goals for people with respiratory quadriplegia emphasize provision of adequate ventilation and lung tissue perfusion while helping them to manage lung secretions effectively.

The patient requiring prolonged mechanical ventilation requires highly specialized nursing care. Chapter 9 is primarily devoted to the critical phase of this care while this section focuses more on long-term implications. However, basic principles and skills apply to each phase of care.

To most people with respiratory quadriplegia, the portable ventilator (respirator) represents *independence* —independence made possible by a life-support system designed specifically for long-term (permanent) use. Technological sophistication is combined with the practical requirements of simplicity of operation, dependability, economy, and most importantly, *mobility.*

When caring for a patient on a portable ventilator there are several major areas of concern. The nurse must know about the portable equipment in use; be aware of the gradual transition period required to accept a portable ventilator; understand respiratory management principles (as for any patient requiring mechanical ventilation); and implement ongoing measures to prevent infection and other complications.

Portable ventilation equipment

Each ventilator-dependent patient must have: a portable ventilator (with a backup system), a portable suction unit (with a backup bedside system), and a manual ventilating (resuscitation) bag.

The portable ventilator The portable ventilator operates on room air and is designed for use with a pneumobelt (a corset structure with an inflatable bladder that is placed around the waist to act as the diaphragm) or a mouth piece or a tracheostomy. For the spinal cord injured person, a tracheostomy is used. Currently the most successful and widely used systems are the LP$_3$ (Life Products, Inc., P.O. Box 3370,

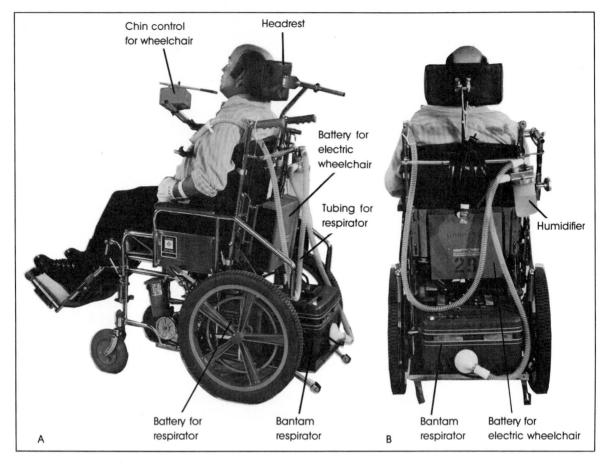

FIGURE 17–1 ■ The portable ventilator (Bantam respirator). (A) Side view. (B) Back view.

Boulder, Colo. 80303) and the Thompson Mini Lung previously referred to as the Bantam Respirator (Thompson Respiration Products, Inc., 1925 55th Street, Boulder, Colo. 80301). Throughout this section the LP_3, which is particularly suited for patients with spinal cord injuries, will be used as a model to describe principles and illustrate details for portable mechanical ventilation.

When working with a portable ventilator system it is important to be familiar with the power requirements, the operating time, indicators and controls, the mobility of the patient, the ease of positioning the ventilator, and the maintenance of the equipment.

Portable ventilators operate on a motor-driven piston, which is a time-cycled device with variable volume, pressure, and rate controls. The unit's power source is either a 110-volt AC current (wall outlet) or a 12-volt DC auto battery

(external). A limited internal battery power source is used primarily as a backup system for short periods.

The LP_3 unit automatically selects the power source available, choosing first the 110-volt AC current for an indefinite operating time, then the external battery for up to 24 hours operating time (when fully charged), and finally the internal battery for up to one hour. The unit should be plugged into a wall outlet unless the person is up and around in the wheelchair.

A crucial nursing responsibility is to ensure that the external battery is sufficiently recharged to last for the amount of operating time desired. The LP_3 incorporates a fully automatic charger to recharge and maintain a full charge whenever the unit is connected to the wall outlet (with or without the unit operating). The rule of thumb is that the charging time should be $1\frac{1}{2}$ times the operating time. To allow for 8 to 10 hours operating time the unit should be plugged into the wall outlet for 12 to 15 hours. Other units may not incorporate this feature or the feature may not be powerful enough to allow the patient as much time up as desired, so a standard heavy-duty battery charger may be needed. Whatever the system, it is essential to understand, adopt, and follow a recharging policy.

Whatever portable ventilator is in use, it is important to remember that establishing a connection to the power source only activates the motor. The hot air that blows out the ventilation holes within a few seconds is merely normal forced ventilation to keep the motor cool. Although there may be a blowing sound, to be functional the power switch must be turned to the "ON" position. The motor will then begin to pump air and establish the cycle.

A portable unit offers a simplified system of indicators and controls, which generally provides information about the volume, pressure, and rate of respirations and the power source in use. All controls of the LP_3 are easily accessible and visible on the front panel with a clear plastic shield available to prevent accidental change of control settings (Figure 17–2). The unit may be operated with the front panel facing forward or upward. The *rate* control, adjustable from 8 to 30 breaths per minute with a front panel knob, delivers the desired number of breaths per minute to the patient. The *volume* control, adjustable from 0 to 3000 mL with front panel toggle switch delivers the desired amount of air with each breath. The *pressure* control is adjustable up to 100 cm water maximum setting with a front panel knob. The LP_3 emphasizes delivery of a preset volume of air with the pressure setting acting as an integral safety device to prevent pressure buildup above a preset level. There are also audible alarms for high or low pressure and power failure. A light system indicates whether the power source currently received is from the external battery, the internal battery, or the AC wall outlet.

Portable humidification with a passive condenser is located in the patient air hose assembly in the LP_3. Active humidification with the addition of any standard in-line humidifier is also possible. Not all portable models have this vital feature.

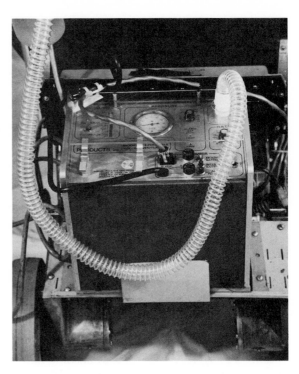

FIGURE 17–2 ■ The LP_3 portable volume ventilator.

Cleanliness and maintenance of portable ventilators is an important factor. The risk of infection from cross-contamination is greater in a hospital than at home; therefore hospital procedures are more rigid and sterilization is stressed. To prevent infection, the ventilator should be dusted and the air tubing, dust filter, and exhalation port changed every 72 hours. All equipment should then be gas sterilized.

For home use this equipment should be washed in warm water and liquid soap followed by an overnight soak in a vinegar solution (one cup vinegar to one gallon water). Tubing cared for in this manner will generally last for a year. The water level in the respirator battery should be checked weekly, and the casing may be cleaned with a little bicarbonate of soda in water as necessary.

The portable suction unit Like ventilators, portable suction units are designed to run on internal and external battery power as well as standard outlets. The Laerdal Suction Unit (Laerdal Medical Corporation, 136 Marbeldale Road, Tuckahoe, N.Y. 10707) is an example of such a device primarily designed for use as a

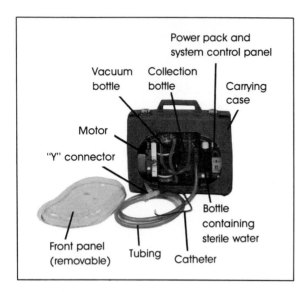

FIGURE 17–3 ■ The Laerdal suction unit.

versatile emergency aspirator in rescue vehicles (Figure 17–3). It is important to become familiar with the power source, operating time, principles of operation, and maintenance procedures.

The Laerdal unit is a high-vacuum and free airflow system well suited for tracheal suction. It consists of four main components:

1. A power pak and system control panel containing the internal batteries and power selection switch
2. The piston-driven motor pump unit, which creates a vacuum in the attached cylinder
3. A vacuum bottle, which receives the transferred vacuum and serves as a collection bottle for the aspirated material
4. A line of sunction tubing to which a Y connector and catheter can be attached.

This equipment is mounted in a carrying case, about the size of a small briefcase.

The operating time of the unit depends on battery capacity, load during practical use, and the voltage suppled. Feasible operating times (allowing for continuous suction) on fully charged (internal) batteries are:

• Half-strength power (6 V) 60–80 minutes
• Full-strength power (12 V) 35–40 minutes

A powerful suction of 600 mmHg and an airflow of 30 liters per minute is supplied on full power.

Half-strength power is generally sufficient to aspirate normal respiratory secretions.

The batteries are designed to accept a continuous charge from a wall outlet. (Batteries will not be damaged by overcharging.) Although other charging options are available, this method is most convenient and provides for maximum operation at any time. After full use batteries need 14 to 16 hours recharging time. If not in use the equipment should be checked every 30 days. Whatever systems are used, it is important to establish and follow an appropriate charging routine.

To prevent infection, the suction unit must be thoroughly cleaned after each use. Parts that have been in contact with mucus should be rinsed before sterilizing. For home use, where risk of cross-contamination is less, the unit should be cleaned in liquid soap and warm water, rinsed thoroughly, and soaked in a vinegar and water solution or boiled. It is wise to order two sets of inner parts (bottles and tubing) to allow for flexibility and convenience when cleaning. Although somewhat outdated, a foot-operated (nonbattery) suction apparatus can be useful as a backup system (Figure 17–4). Some people find it useful when traveling any distance such as on a car trip.

The manual ventilating bag The manual ventilating or resuscitation bag is a *vital* accessory for ventilator-dependent patients and must be available at all times. Choose a ventilating bag made of pliable material that is easy to compress. This will make any continued use less tiresome. Dismantle the apparatus and check to see that the one-way valve is inserted correctly to allow a free intake of air. For individual use, the appropriate-size tracheostomy adapter can be kept attached to the bag and the unit can be stored in a plastic drawstring bag easily placed on the wheelchair or kept at the bedside.

Nursing the patient requiring a portable ventilator

Preparation of the patient and equipment The purchasing and availability of specialized equipment requires a concentrated team effort to ensure skillful early planning and to cope with the socioeconomic implications. Any delay in arrival of individualized equipment can hamper the patient's progress significantly.

Prior to mobilization with portable equipment not only must the patient's general health and respiratory status be adequate, but successful management of the vertebral column injury and autonomic nervous system impairment must also be accomplished.

Once the patient has been stabilized on a volume respirator using room air (without additional oxygen), transference to a portable ventilator can begin. The patient should be free from symptomatic infection, excessive lung secretions, or other pulmonary complications, such as atelectasis or pneumonia.

Minimizing fear and anxiety is a key factor in determining acceptance of new equipment. Careful preparation, including familiarization with the new respirator equipment and possible sensations to expect, and constant reassurance during the actual process are most helpful. Consistency in assigning nurses and involvement of the patient and family members in care are essential.

Airway management Preparation and care of the airway is of constant importance. The first step is to wean the patient to a small, uncuffed tracheostomy tube more suitable for permanent use. (This is described in Chapter 9.) A Portex-plastic tube with a soft cuff is recommended for use with mechanical ventilation during acute illness. Cuffed tracheostomy tubes are necessary to prevent air leakage around the airway, particularly on expiration. Such a closed ventilation system promotes more exact control of respiration variables because expired air is channeled back through the respirator. To allow the patient to talk, however, portable ventilators specifically do not incorporate such a feature. Air is expired directly around the uncuffed tracheostomy tube, over the vocal cords, and out through the mouth and nose.

Stainless steel and hard plastic tracheostomy tubes are widely used with portable mechanical ventilators, due to ease of insertion and cleaning, less risk of infection, and durability. Also, the lining of the trachea and the skin at the tracheostomy site doesn't tend to adhere to such tubes.

The artificial airway parts include an inner and outer cannula with an obturator for insertion. An appropriate-size elbow cannula adapter then connects to the air tubing of the ventilator. See Figure 17–5. For normal use, the

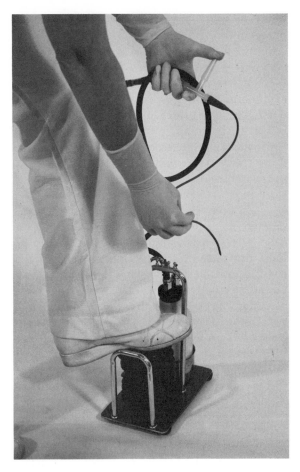

FIGURE 17–4 ■ A manually operated (foot-pump) suction apparatus.

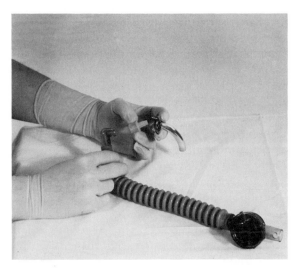

FIGURE 17–5 ■ Metal tracheostomy tube with plastic adapter to accommodate wide-bore tubing.

inner cannula remains locked in place inside the outer cannula. Once the outer cannula is secured with tie tapes, the inner cannula can be removed as needed for cleaning without changing the tracheostomy tube. Soaking the inner cannula in hydrogen peroxide will dislodge encrusted mucus. Additional cleaning with flexible cotton swabs or pipe cleaners may be necessary. Rinse thoroughly in sterile water or saline before reinserting. When the entire airway is changed the reusable tubes may be boiled or autoclaved to sterilize.

When a tracheostomy is well established, the dangerous possibility of it closing over when the tube is removed is almost nonexistent. During long-term care the actual changing of the tracheostomy tube is usually a nursing responsibility (review Procedure 9–9).

Maintaining a clear airway is vital. Minimize risk factors as described in Chapter 9. Particularly focus on the physical skills of chest assessment and manual techniques used to clear the bronchial tree (Procedures 9–1 through 9–6).

Suctioning will be practiced on a lifelong basis. Once well established on a portable ventilator, patients may simply tell you when they need to be suctioned. Frequency varies considerably from one individual to another. Very rarely would suctioning be necessary on an hourly basis unless pulmonary complications are evident.

Take care to perform suctioning correctly and gently to avoid any tracheal trauma.

Never insert a soiled catheter into the trachea. Use a fresh catheter for each session of tracheal suctioning. Select a soft, pliable catheter. Many disposable catheters are too stiff unless warmed, which is inconvenient, and rubber catheters, especially the cheaper variety, have a tendency to become brittle with repeated sterilization.

In an institutional setting disposable equipment is more convenient and probably less expensive. For home use reusable catheters may be thoroughly rinsed with tap water; boiled for five minutes, or possibly soaked in a basin with a vinegar solution (one cup vinegar to one gallon of water) as an alternative when rushed or traveling; and then placed in a dry towel for storage.

The transition period Gradual accommodation to a portable system is crucial, for both physical and psychological well-being. Initial periods on portable equipment may progressively increase from 15-minute intervals to a few hours, then gradually to permanent use. Throughout this process blood oxygen tension levels are monitored by arterial samples or ear oximetry. Serial comparison with baseline data obtained while the patient was on a larger respirator will best indicate the level of tolerance to the portable one.

Select the pressure, volume, and rate controls as ordered by the attending physician. A typical setting might be: pressure, 25 to 40 cm H_2O; rate, 10 to 12 breaths/minute; tidal volume, 1000 mL with a cuffed tube or 1400 mL with an uncuffed tube. Note the higher tidal volume settings for use with an uncuffed tube and a portable ventilation system to compensate for air escaping around the tracheostomy tube. Final adjustments of control settings may have to be altered slightly for patient comfort.

The transition period from constant observation in a critical care setting to independence on a small portable respirator requires close monitoring balanced with opportunities to gain freedom and confidence. Assessment techniques eventually rely less on sophisticated diagnostic analysis than on individual responses.

Continuing care In addition to maintaining a clear airway, continuing care focuses on recognizing respiratory insufficiency, the onset of which is often characterized by subtle signs of distress. Be alert for signs of general malaise, poor appetite, mild forgetfulness, mild confusion, grogginess on awakening, disturbed sleep, excessive dreaming (nightmares), headache, restlessness, irritability, and shortness of breath. These signs may progress to a pale or dusky color of facial skin, diminished breath sounds on air entry (which may be bilateral), respiratory noises, and poor chest expansion. Extrathoracic signs may include an increased pulse, nasal flaring, and excessive contraction of the neck and shoulders which indicates overuse of the accessory muscles or respiration. If respiratory insufficiency is unchecked, unresponsiveness, coma, and respiratory arrest are imminent.

Respiratory insufficiency can be related to trachiobronchial obstruction, commonly caused by trapped or excessive secretions associated with pulmonary infection, or possibly tracheal stenosis. Ventilator malfunction is another major cause. As Benvenuti (1979) explains,

> If ventilation is inadequate (as determined by patient response, comfort, and excursion of the chest), check the patient for mucus plugs or for increased secretions and the need for suctioning before considering the equipment as the source of the problem. Thus, it is important to know the patient well—his frequency of suctioning, the character of his secretions, and his normal breath sounds.

Assess the patient carefully to ensure adequate ventilation, particularly when changing machines or switching from wall to battery power. If the patient complains of not receiving enough air:

- Check to see if there is a free flow of air through the corrugated tubing that is attached to the tracheostomy tube. If not, the tubing may need to be replaced.
- Check the cascade gasket and make sure that the lid is secure.
- Check the exhalation valve and diaphragm for a free flow of air. The valve may not be positioned correctly or the diaphragm may be wet. Dry the diaphragm and reset it.
- If none of these actions resolves the problem—and the indicators are at the desired readings—the entire assembly should be changed.

The respirator that performs adequately on wall power may seem drained on battery power. The patient may feel there is not enough air being forced into the lungs (pressure) or that the respiratory rate is too slow. In this situation it is best to substitute another respirator until the mechanical problem can be investigated by a maintenance service.

Techniques to relearn breathing Finally, one most important feature of nursing care is to help provide opportunities for the patient with respiratory quadriplegia to relearn breathing. Although it may not be a realistic goal to become ventilator free, a certain degree of safety and psychological comfort is gained if a patient can learn to breathe for short periods independently. This may not be possible for several months after injury due to neck immobilization and spinal shock. It may never be possible, but people with respiratory quadriplegia consis-

tently emphasize how necessary it is at least to try.

There is a certain amount of confusion that exists regarding the techniques used. Glossopharyngeal breathing, or "frog breathing," is a substitute method of breathing that was perfected mainly for people with postpolio respiratory paralysis. The person is taught to use the muscles of the tongue, soft palate, fauces, pharynx, and larynx to force or swallow air into the lungs. However, this technique has not been successful for people with spinal cord injuries causing respiratory paralysis, probably due to their loss of sensation and proprioception (which postpolio victims retain).

As previously noted, strengthening the remaining accessory muscles of breathing, primarily the scalenus muscles of the neck, offers potential development of time off the respirator. Occupational and physical therapists can teach exercises that enhance neck control and head balance, and mouthstick activities are generally helpful. Weaning the patient off the ventilator is the specific activity used for respiratory muscle strengthening. A progressive weaning program gradually increases the functional vital capacity. The initial weaning period may be as short as 30 seconds for some patients. It should never be so long that the patient tires or panics. Follow the principles and parameters outlined in Chapter 9, keeping in mind that the goal of the weaning process may only be to breathe independently for a few minutes. It is important to realize that independent breathing must be practiced daily if muscle strength is to be maintained.

Phrenic nerve pacemakers

The use of phrenic nerve pacemakers is still largely in the experimental stages. Successful candidates must have an intact phrenic nerve; that is, the lower motor neurons must be preserved so the reflex arc is able to react to the electric charge of the pacemaker. This means the cord must be free from trauma at the C_4 segmental level. As this cord level corresponds with the more frequently injured C_{3-5} vertebrae, the possibility of phrenic pacing is relatively rare for people with spinal cord injuries. However, if injury is sustained at the C_{1-2} vertebrae and the C_4 segmental level is intact, the use of a pacemaker is theoretically possible. Following the passing of spinal shock, diagnostic tests to determine prognosis include fluoroscopic examination to visualize diaphragmatic excursion and transcutaneous nerve conduction studies to determine phrenic nerve response to electrical stimulation.

The phrenic nerve pacemaker works on a similar principle to that of a cardiac pacemaker; that is, an external, battery-operated transmitter–antenna unit activates internal implants. The phrenic nerve stimulator has three major components:

1. The electrode cuff, which is implanted in the neck circumventing the phrenic nerve (near its origin)
2. The receiver unit, which is secured internally in a subcutaneous pouch just below the rib cage
3. The external transmitter–antenna unit (D'Agostino and Welch 1979)

When the phrenic nerve is stimulated, the diaphragm descends, pulling air into the lungs. To activate the phrenic nerve a current flows from the transmitter to the antenna, then to the internal receiver to the electrode cuff, which stimulates the diaphragm into motion. Tolerance to full pacing for the quadriplegic patient may well take up to three months.

Nursing care measures focus on unique pre- and postoperative care, gradually establishing a pacing schedule, promoting psychological acceptance, and providing comprehensive patient and family health education. The original works of D'Agostino and Welch present a comprehensive, specialized guide for care of patients undergoing this select procedure, most often in specialized facilities.

Reestablishing Mobility and Independence

Reestablishing mobility and independence can only be accomplished by a concerned and skilled interdisciplinary team. The following information is primarily based on Dingemans and Hawn (1978–79), who describe reactivation in stages of early mobility, continuing mobility, and mobility in the community.

Early mobility

Vertebral column injuries generally require a three-month period of rigid immobilization followed by application of a supportive device to allow for adequate bony healing. During the initial postinjury period, immobilization of the cervical spine is achieved with bedrest and cervical traction. Ideally, the Halo-thoracic brace is applied within the first month when acute medical problems have been resolved and respiratory status has stabilized. If the latter criteria are not met, application of the Halo may be unsuitable, because the brace limits chest exposure and expansion. However, since resumption of the upright position is believed to be the most important factor in reducing pulmonary complications in the ventilator-dependent patient, a cervical brace may be adapted. Because this method offers less support, the patient may require a longer period of bedrest with cervical traction. If the injury is inherently stable, a hard collar with a tracheal opening is sufficient.

Once stabilization is achieved, gradual mobilization to the upright position in the wheelchair can begin. Choose a manual wheelchair with elevated legrests for initial use. Perform a three-person lift to transfer the patient.

Anticipate severe postural hypotension due to the large body area subject to autonomic nervous system impairment. Practice measures to build tolerance to the upright position. In close collaboration with therapists, initiate a program of head elevation (when possible) and passive exercises when in bed. Apply supportive elastic stockings and an abdominal binder prior to getting up. Monitor blood pressure and observe for feelings of light-headedness and fainting. If symptoms occur, return the patient to the horizontal position.

Continuing mobility

As the patient progresses with sitting up and adjusting to the portable ventilator equipment, the physical therapist and occupational therapist closely collaborate to facilitate any returning function in the neck or shoulder muscles. They devise activities that focus on body awareness and redeveloping a sense of balance and exercises to strengthen neck muscles, which will help the patient operate special equipment. In addition, they work to overcome patient fear and anxiety when being moved.

Designing transfer methods is a vital aspect when reestablishing mobility and independence. A sliding board transfer, using several assistants, is the most practical and adaptable. See Chapter 16 for recommended methods.

The electric wheelchair is a very important item to a person with respiratory quadriplegia. Dingemanns and Hawn (1978–79) emphasize the importance of collaboration between the patient and the therapist to explore and evaluate the various systems available. Several options must be considered: wheelchair controls, reclining systems, various supportive accessories to maintain body position, and ventilator adaptations.

To control the electric wheelchair a chin and tongue control system or the sip and puff breath control switch are widely used (Figure 17–6). An optic control system is also being developed, which may increase the available options.

Independently operated reclining systems are designed to offer a change in position, which shifts weight for pressure relief. A reclining position provides rest periods, which can increase activity options by increasing the time allowed out of bed and decreasing the need for attendant care. In addition custom-designed head, trunk, and extremity supports may be needed.

An electric wheelchair can also be adapted to accommodate portable ventilator equipment. The most frequent adaptation is a platform–tray located underneath the chair seat. The Falcon Reclining Respirator chair (Falcon Research & Development, 1225 South Huron, Denver, Colo. 80223) is an example of a modified chair, incorporating several of the options described.

Whatever equipment is used, it is important for the nurse to be familiar with its features. Remember that to maintain the chair in working order the battery must be adequately charged. Most models will require overnight charging to operate continuously during the day. A weekly check of the water level in the battery is also necessary.

Evolving scientific advances are rapidly increasing and expanding the scope of special

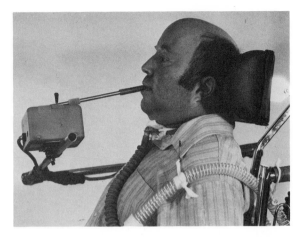

FIGURE 17–6 ■ A control system for the electric wheelchair.

equipment available to maximize freedom and privacy and decrease the need for constant attendant care. For the nurse engaged in rehabilitation of the totally physically dependent patient, consultation with skilled occupational therapists, physical therapists, and possibly bioengineers is essential. This may even involve referrals to outside health care facilities for appropriate collaboration. Equipment should be introduced as early as possible, both for physical reasons and for psychological acceptance and independence. When selecting special equipment several facts must be considered, including financial resources and environmental limitations at home, school, or work.

Environment control equipment is designed to help the patient operate or manipulate the immediate environment. Many are electronically controlled systems usually activated by light touch, a lick of the tongue, or by a sip and puff breath switch. Environmental controls may be very simple, such as a call bell, or very complex, such as computer-operated equipment.

The Enco unit is a particularly useful bedside or home item, which operates up to five pieces of equipment such as light switches, television, and so on (Figure 17–7). More sophisticated equipment, such as the Apple computer, makes it possible to play games on a television monitor and learn data processing skills. The latter is particularly valuable because

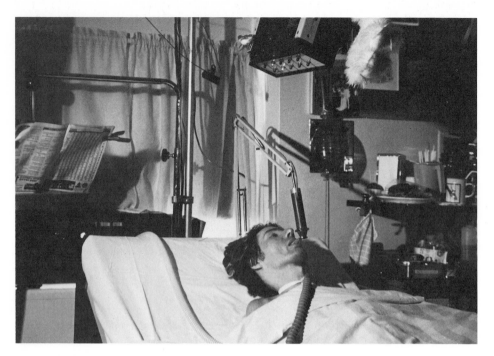

FIGURE 17–7 ■ A patient operates the Enco unit with a tongue switch.

it is a marketable employment skill. However, it should not be assumed that every patient will want or be able to use computer technology as a vocational skill.

Mobility in the community

A specially equipped van is a popular method of transportation for the person with respiratory quadriplegia. See Figure 17–8. The electric wheelchair and respirator equipment can easily be boarded and secured for travel. It is also possible to transfer the person with respiratory quadriplegia into a regular car providing adaptations for safety in travel are provided. Of course the electric wheelchair does not fold, so a manual chair is needed in this situation.

People with respiratory quadriplegia are even more hampered by architectural barriers than other spinal cord injured people. For example, even low curbs are difficult to negotiate with the cumbersome electric wheelchair. Appropriate and sophisticated equipment and independent wheelchair activity with comprehensive patient and family health education can better preprare people with respiratory quadriplegia to manage in the community and can significantly increase life-style options.

Providing Rehabilitation Opportunities

Related to, but beyond the parameters of, increasing mobility and physical independence is the consistent emphasis on the need for services with a rehabilitative element. While recognizing that physical rehabilitation is limited due to the severity of the disability, health care workers can define rehabilitation for the patient primarily in psychosocial and vocational terms. The following are some concepts that are integrated into a rehabilitative program.

1. Alteration in body image, discomfort in asking for help, and difficulties dealing with others' attitudes may constitute some problems in meeting self-esteem needs.

2. Physical exercise programs, such as physical therapy mat programs, aquatics, or hydrotherapy programs, help patients combat the feeling that the mind and body are split. The sensory experience of rolling and of being touched may help deemphasize the feeling of physical and psychological fragility and allow patients to see their bodies move again. In addition, they can consider themselves "touchable," which contributes to feelings of emotional well-being.

3. A breathing program, even one that weans the patient from the respirator for only a few minutes at a time, could provide backup support in case of mechanical breakdown. It is also thought to improve self-esteem and self-image (separation from machinery).

4. The injured individual may encounter problems with sexual–love adjustments, social effectiveness, limitations in social activities, and family adjustments or conflicts. Both individual and group counseling can provide the opportunity to share and express feelings with others in similar situations. This can reduce tension and feelings of isolation. In addition, individuals can share methods of coping and practical information, such as care and maintenance of equipment or information on current social legislation for disabled people.

5. Peer counseling can also be an effective service. It may be easier to ask for help from someone in the same situation than from a professional. The counselor may also be more sensitive to the individual's situation.

6. Stress management and human relations training might help increase social effectiveness. A stress management course developed by Garrison (1978) focuses on the teaching of relaxation to cope with undesirable responses to stress. Garrison suggests that paralyzed people imagine tensing and relaxing ineffective muscles.

7. New social communication and behavior skills can be learned and practiced. Individuals can learn to have some control in their interactions with others through verbal skills, which are extremely valuable since speech is one of the most important forms of expression left to the person with respiratory quadriplegia. This training could also help people make transition from a concrete to a more abstract form of thinking. The individual may also lack personal goals, knowledge of how to master tasks, and a sense of meaning or purpose to life. A task-centered approach to the development of realistic life goals can provide a feeling of purpose and accomplishment.

8. Recreational activities can help prevent social and intellectual isolation. Programs that help

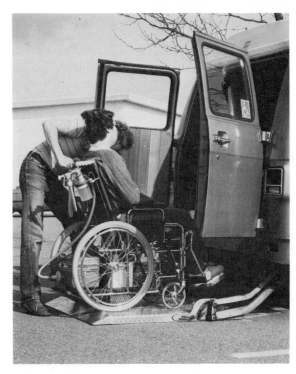

FIGURE 17–8 ■ Community mobility.

individuals learn how to play and develop hobbies or interests in accord with their physical limitations will increase the quality of life.

9. Environmental barriers such as those imposed by architecture, transportation, or lack of mobility can limit opportunities for growth. Mobility equipment, such as the wheelchair and environmental control units, are essential components of the environment. Equipment failure may cause long and frustrating periods of immobilization. Education about the use, maintenance, and repair of equipment is useful. Integration programs, such as mobility practice in the institution before going out into the community, might also be useful. For example, an obstacle course could be set up approximating community architectural barriers, such as narrow doors and crowded furniture in houses and restaurants.

10. Vocational assessment programs are set up to evaluate and explore individual occupational goals. The advent of the computer has brought new vocational possibilities. The Apple B computer, recently introduced to some individuals with respiratory quadriplegia, may help open occupational prospects in the areas of computer programming, because this machine can be operated with a mouthstick. Work with the stock market might also be handled by the individual. Consulting professionals must have a knowledge of the individual's skills and education to offer concrete, useful, and innovative program suggestions. It should be emphasized, though, that the person with respiratory quadriplegia may not be ready for training and education for some time. Individuals consistently mention the need for time to adjust to the new situation and master small tasks such as using a mouthstick before exploring vocational goals. It should also be stressed that computer operation is not the answer for everyone.

11. Trends toward deinstitutionalization continue, along with an increase in consumer participation in services. In the United States today, staggering medical costs often necessitate returning to live at home. But options are limited if the home situation is not stable, if community support systems are not adequate, or if a young person desires to free aging parents from care burdens. An example of an alternate living arrangement is a group home situation in a residential setting of the community. Such homes are managed by the disabled people themselves. This trend is explored more fully in Chapter 19.

SELECTED REFERENCES

Banting, G., et al. 1978. Depression and the A. C. U. nurse. *Nursing '78* 8(3):60–65. *Explores staff reactions of frustration and anxiety when faced with caring for a young man with long-term respiratory insufficiency in an acute care unit.*

Benvenuti, C. 1979. Independence for the quadriplegic: the Bantam respirator. *American Journal of Nursing.* 79 (5):918–920. *Describes patient teaching, maintenance for equipment, and trouble shooting; includes chart on causes, signs and symptoms, and management of respiratory distress on a portable ventilator. Highly recommended.*

Burnham, L., and Werner, G. 1978–79. The high-level tetraplegic: psychological survival and adjustment. *International Journal of Paraplegia* 16: 184–192. *Describes dependency created by respiratory quadriplegia; focuses on psychosocial adjustment in the acute and early rehabilitative period; also discusses problem areas following discharge.*

Cleveland, M. 1979. Family adaptation to the traumatic spinal cord injury of a son or daughter. *Social Work Health Care* 4 (Summer): 459–471. *Presents a case history of a family in crisis; examines the family's grief reactions and patterns of adaptation in task orientation, affection, communication, and power structures; and discusses suggestions for clinical intervention.*

D'Agostino, J., and Welch, P. 1979. The phrenic pacemaker. *Nursing '79* 9 (5):41–50. *Excellent presentation of patient selection criteria, preoperative care and preparation, implantation techniques, establishing a pacing schedule, and discharge teaching; includes anatomical drawings, photographs of equipment, and samples of bedside monitoring charts. Essential reading for nurses with patients using this device.*

Dingemans, L., and Hawn, J. 1978–79. Mobility and equipment for the ventilator-dependent tetraplegic. *International Journal of Paraplegia* 16: 175–183. *Clearly written approach to mobilize and equip the ventilator-dependent patient. Highly recommended.*

Garrison, I. 1978. Stress management training for the handicapped. *Archives of Physical Medicine and Rehabilitation* 59: 580–585. *Suggestions applicable to those with respiratory quadriplegia.*

Goffman, T. 1961. *Asylums.* New York: Anchor Books. *In-depth approach to issues surrounding long-term institutionalized care.*

Leinart, B. 1979. Attitudes of nurses toward spinal cord injury patients. *Association of Rehabilitation Nurses Journal* 4 (Jan.–Feb.): 7–9. *A comparison of attitudes of nurses working in acute, intermediate, and rehabilitation areas; stresses the importance of professional attitudes as an integral force determining the degree of success in patient adjustment to disability.*

Levin, S. 1978. Unpublished proceedings of interdisciplinary educational symposium on high-level quadriplegia. Shaughnessy Hospital, Vancouver, BC, October 26, 1978. *Interdisciplinary presentation of acute medical care, physical mobilization, equipment, environmental adaptions, and psychosocial needs and supportive care. A perspective from the Craig Rehabilitation Center, Denver, Colorado.*

Liebowitz, B. 1974. Impact of intra-institutional relocation. *The Gerontologist*, August, pp. 293–295. *General perspective on the aspects of change that affect the elderly and can be applied to severe disability.*

Mechanic, D. 1961. The concept of illness behaviour. *Journal of Chronic Disability* 15:189–194. *Explores "sick role" behaviors and how they may be unnecessarily prolonged when disability is involved.*

Rogers, J., and Figone, J. 1979. Psychosocial parameters in treating the person with quadriplegia. *American Journal of Occupational Therapy* 33 (7): 432–439. *Documents how rehabilitants envisioned a more flexible, comprehensive treatment model that would give priority to developmental status, changing life goals, interpersonal relationships, and social roles. Highly recommended.*

Sadlick, M., and Penta, F. 1975. Changing nurse attitudes toward quadriplegics through use of television. *Rehabilitation Literature* 36 (9): 274–278. *A technique for enhancing more positive attitudes toward potential patient outcomes during rehabilitation.*

Stauffer, E., and Bell, G. 1978. Traumatic respiratory quadriplegia and pentaplegia. *Orthopedic Clinics of North America* 9 (4): 1081–1089. *Explains neurological assessment for accurate and early diagnosis, skeletal injury, complications, orthotic treatment, phrenic nerve stimulation, and anticipated hospitalization time. Pediatrically oriented.*

SUPPLEMENTAL READING

Alexander, M., et al. 1979. Mechanical ventilation of patients with late stage Duchenne muscular dystrophy: management in the home. *Archives of Physical Medicine and Rehabilitation* 60: 289–292. *Related information on discharge preparation for a patient requiring portable ventilation.*

Carter, R., and Donovan, W. 1981. Reflections of impact of electrophrenic respirations in management of high quads. *Model Systems' Spinal Cord Injury Digest* 3 (Fall): 37–43. *Reviews use of electrophrenic pacemaker over a decade. Found to be useful for C_{1-2} lesions but not as useful in C_{3-4} lesions.*

Dobson, K. 1980. A second chance. *The Canadian Nurse*, June, pp. 37–40. *Reviews mechanics of portable ventilation weaning from a cuffed tracheostomy tube; and related nursing care for an ambulatory patient with chronic obstructive lung disease.*

Engstrand, J., and Stuart, B. 1979. *Patient Handbook of Self-Care Procedures.* 2d ed. Birmingham, Ala: Spain Rehabilitation Center of the University of Alabama. *An educational guide to home care of tracheostomy; includes suctioning technique; changing dressings, tapes, and tubes; and cleaning procedures.*

Gunley, P. 1981. From regeneration to prosthesis: research on spinal cord injury. *Journal of the American Medical Association* 245 (13): 1293–1297. *Review of current American research in regeneration, old and new therapies, and prosthesis. Includes latest technology report on advancements helpful to those with high quadriplegia. Concise and clear.*

Hamric, A., et al. 1976. Caring for the totally dependent patient, some traps—some guidelines. *Nursing '76*, July, pp. 38–43. *Information shared about mistakes made to help others. Provides excellent help for nurses, especially when nursing the respiratory-dependent patient is an isolated experience.*

Lieberman, J., et al. 1980. Serial phrenic nerve conduction studies in candidates for diaphragm pacing. *Archives of Physical Medicine and Rehabilitation* 61(11): 528–531. *Serial phrenic nerve studies demonstrated a pattern of function that changes with time. Before a final decision is made about phrenic nerve viability, serial studies should be carried out for at least two years after injury on nonresponsive nerves.*

Sell, G., et al. 1979. Environmental and typewriter control systems for high level quadriplegic patients: evaluation and prescription. *Archives of Physical Medicine and Rehabilitation* 60 (June): 246–252. *A technical article describing suitability of various electronic assistive devices evaluated in the occupational therapy laboratory, at the bedside, and in the home.*

Waren, C., and Inre, J. 1980. Technical service delivery: a needed complement to the rehabilitation plan. *Spinal Cord Injury Digest* 2 (Fall): 18–22., *Describes how a severely disabled individual may benefit from available technology in relation to environmental control systems.*

Young, J. 1980. Statistics on high cervical C_{1-4} spinal cord injuries. *Spinal Cord Injury Digest* 2 (Winter): 11. *Describes demographic etiology of neurological changes, mortality, use of mechanical respirators, days hospitalized and total hospital cost, attendant care, and residence during follow-up years. Statistics based on 649 persons with high quadriplegia.*

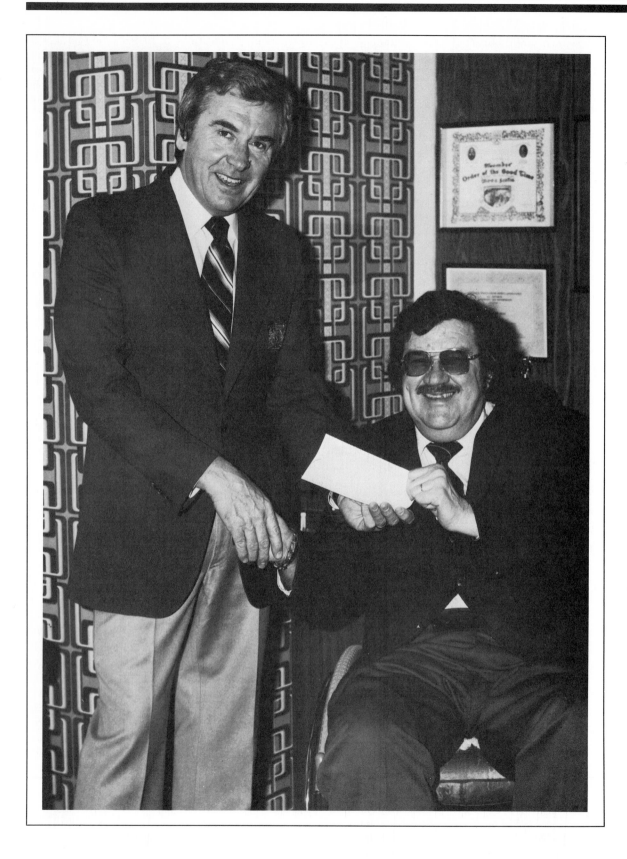

PART VI
PLANNING
FOR THE
FUTURE

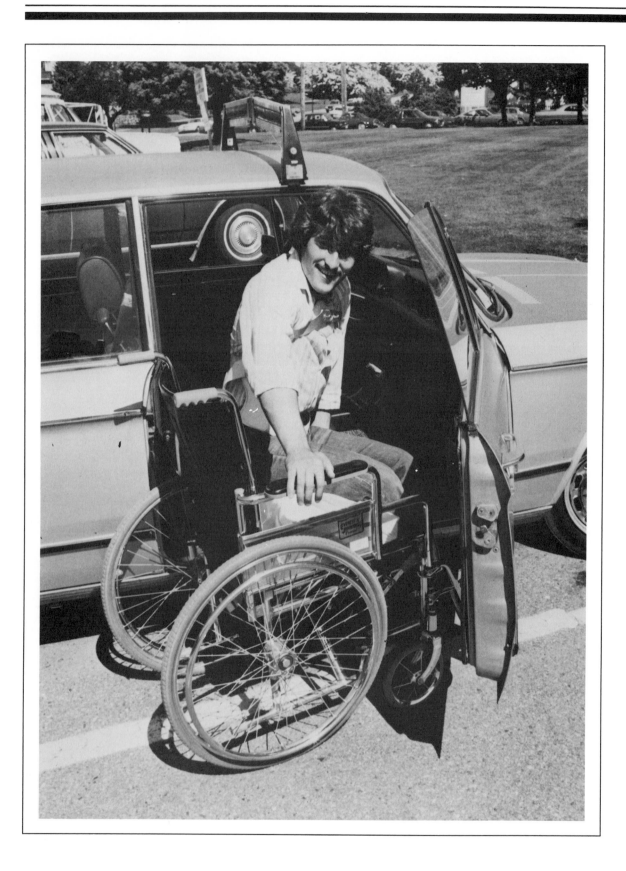

Chapter 18

The Discharge Process*

CHAPTER OUTLINE

OBJECTIVES

- To identify the goals of the discharge process
- To define the discharge process and describe factors that give direction to nursing care
- To identify concepts that have important implications for development of rehabilitation programs and community support services to facilitate the discharge process
- To discuss the application of the nursing process to discharge planning and preparation

* This chapter was developed with the assistance of Judy Little, R.N., whose experience in acute and rehabilitative settings lends valuable insight into the discharge process.

GOALS OF HEALTH CARE

Rehabilitation is defined by the National Council on Rehabilitation as "the restoration of the individual to the fullest physical, mental, social, vocational and economic capacity of which each is capable." Many must learn the physical skills necessary for independent mobility; others must engage in occupational training or retraining; and most must learn new social skills necessary to relate successfully in the community at large. Some of these skills may be learned easily, while some will require more effort and time, and others may never be performed independently, depending on the extent of injury and such factors as the extent that each desires.

To accomplish the goals of rehabilitation, patients, and their families, must undergo tremendous adjustments to cope with the effects of disability and require a great deal of support and assistance. The majority of persons enter the world of the spinal cord injured with little or no idea of what their capabilities are or how well they can adjust. They and their families will need the services of a specialized interdisciplinary team, including physician consultation and care, nursing, physical therapy, occupational therapy, and psychological, social, and vocational services during the rehabilitation process. The entire team, including the patient and family, must work together, from the time of admission throughout the rehabilitation process, toward discharge, assessing, goal setting, intervening, evaluating, problem solving, and adjusting.

There is a point in the rehabilitation process when most patients and families begin to achieve long-term goals; others reach a point when it is clear that they are no longer benefiting from the services offered. In other words, the rehabilitation process has reached its potential value or capacity; the therapeutic environment is no longer therapeutic; and it is time to separate patients and families from the institution. At this point the discharge process actively begins.

The discharge process is the final step in the rehabilitation process. It includes preparation to maintain health, to manage the effects of disability, and to reintegrate into community life. The discharge process is of intrinsic importance because it is a pivotal point on which to capitalize on the entire rehabilitation process.

The immediate and long-term rehabilitative goals of discharged patients will be determined not only by their physical abilities, but also by their social, psychological, and vocational adjustment. In order to provide for appropriate support services to this end, knowledge of a patient's progress in all aspects of rehabilitation is essential. Therefore, the nurse must participate with the health care team to achieve the following goals:

- To provide a consistent rehabilitative environment conducive to developing patient and family autonomy to facilitate the discharge process
- To focus on psychosocial adjustments to disability, in addition to assessment of physical health and independence skills, when determining readiness for discharge
- To promote optimal health care, stressing prevention and early detection of complications in relation to managing the effects of disability
- To minimize the stress of transition into the community by appropriate referral to and provision of uninterrupted health care from follow-up support services
- To complete patient and family health education to best use support services
- To assume advocacy and leadership roles in development of better resources to support disabled people in the community

FACTORS THAT AFFECT THE DISCHARGE PROCESS*

The discharge process is affected by both positive and negative factors, including those directly related to the abilities of the patient and family and those that depend more on the environment, of which the nurse is a part. Consideration of several interrelated variables will help determine the kinds of problems patients have

* This section is based on interpretations from S. MacLean, 1981.

when discharged, and the approaches that will be most effective. Important variables include the patient, the family, the environment the patient will go to following discharge, the rehabilitation program, and community services.

The Patient

Factors that influence patient concerns and responses are related to self-concept and self-esteem, time since injury, physical health, and independence skills.

Psychosocial adjustment

In the aftermath of spinal cord injury patients' and families' self-concept and self-esteem are particularly vulnerable. Extensive research concludes that successfully living with a disability depends on the value or worth (self-concept and self-esteem) people place on themselves. Psychosocial adaptation then, rather than intellectual abilities or level and completeness of injury, is the critical factor in determining rehabilitation success (Treischmann 1980).

Thompson and Lott emphasize that psychosocial redevelopment following injury is at the most critical point when the patient returns to the community. This confrontation is described as "leaving a safe environment (hospital and rehabilitation) which was controlled and which aided him in coming to terms with his new image of himself as disabled" and "returning to an environment which is not controlled and in which he last functioned as able bodied. Therefore the stages . . . through which he has passed *must be further reprocessed*" (1980:42).

While there are theoretical and descriptive differences between the various interpretations of adjustment to disability, one notable similarity is that adaptation to such a loss is a process that occurs over time. There is a point in the rehabilitation process that patients are discharged; while physical rehabilitation may be complete, mental, social, and vocational adjustments will likely not be. Good physical restoration does not guarantee good emotional adjustment. As a result, patients being discharged have different problems and require different approaches, largely depending on psychosocial adjustment to injury.

Physical health and independence

A current assessment of neurological, orthopedic, respiratory, cardiovascular, nutritional, urological, gastrointestinal, and integumentary systems status and rehabilitative skills is necessary to determine physical health and degree of independence. The discharge decision requires a global view of each patient's situation in addition to demonstrated progress in specific areas.

Team members and the patient will work together closely to evaluate the skills, knowledge, and attitudes that are necessary to manage the implications of disability in the following basic areas:

- Physical activity, including use of mobility aids (which need to be prescribed and evaluated)
- Activities of daily living, such as dressing and grooming
- Nutritional habits and management of bowel and bladder routines
- Care of the skin and prevention of skin breakdown
- Care of the respiratory, circulatory, and musculoskeletal systems

Principles of management of all body systems and how needs have changed following spinal cord injury are addressed throughout this text. This information will provide the nurse with the knowledge necessary to teach the patient and family what they need to know, including how to minimize risk factors, prevent complications, perform or supervise personal care, care for equipment, obtain supplies, and respond appropriately to problem situations. Sections on potential complications, self-care, and long-term implications in the previous chapters are relevant to discharge planning.

Comprehensive physical assessment cannot be completed in isolation from psychological considerations. Poor mental health will lower resistance to physical stress. For example, if depression is manifested in poor nutritional habits or drug or alcohol abuse, the details of physical care quickly become dangerously neglected. Thus, comprehensive physical assessment is a crucial step in the discharge process.

The learning process

Patients with spinal cord injuries are subjected to a myriad of psychosocial influences at the same time that they are expected to engage in the complex learning process that constitutes a rehabilitation program. Nurses can help by providing psychosocial support and assisting with sexual adjustments, which in turn will promote openness to learning (see Chapters 6 and 7).

Throughout the rehabilitation period, continuous assessment is closely related to ongoing evaluation to determine if learning has occurred. In addition to guidelines for implementation of a health education program, Chapter 8 explores how to evaluate progress. The success of comprehensive patient and family health education is of the essence in the discharge process.

The Family

The impact of disability on families and on family roles is an important variable influencing discharge planning. Immediately following a spinal cord injury, an individual is sick, and the rules and norms of the "sick role" apply. Generally families are supportive during this period, and problems do not become clear until the extent of the disability is known. Families will grieve, and at the same time they must assess and reorganize family objectives and goals to accommodate a disabled family member. Role conflicts may arise if expectations of the disabled person differ among family members. A common conflict can be seen when, for example, a capable husband and father returns home after being in the hospital for a long time. His wife, now used to paying the bills and managing the household in general, may have difficulty in resharing that role. Failure to return to preinjury roles and responsibilities, or at least similar ones, can be devastating for the injured person. Family attitudes and capabilities related to managing the effects of disability are of paramount importance. Care tasks can significantly interfere with the quality of relationships over time. To minimize future problems, it is vital to assess both individual and family concerns during discharge planning with insight.

The Environment Following Discharge

The environment the patient chooses following injury is an essential consideration when planning discharge. It must be the most comfortable and easiest place for adjustment possible. This is where the person will come to "get away from it all," to relax and be happy, to live.

Good preparation for living in that setting is essential. Poor or nonexistent renovations and adjustments in the home can cause tremendous problems at a time when the person is going through one of the most difficult periods of adjustment to injury. A patient going to another institution may need a great deal of psychological preparation, such as personal visits there and visits from staff and perhaps other patients, to establish a good knowledge of what to expect there.

Significant others play an important role in the discharge setting selected. For the most part families must be involved in discharge preparations with the patient. The strength and desire on the part of patient and family to make discharge living arrangements will help determine how actively the health care team must be involved. For some, the issues concerning attendant care are of paramount importance to create a desirable discharge environment. Often people with spinal cord injuries have never been employers, and they need to learn still another new role to cope with unfamiliar living arrangements.

The Rehabilitation Program

The rehabilitation environment is important throughout the entire program. It must be an environment where individuals are active participants in making decisions about their care to the extent they are able and are encouraged to solve problems for themselves. It must also be one where individuals are allowed to grieve their loss, and where they can learn how to stop being patients and start being real people again.

In relation to the discharge process, it helps immensely if all staff members are encouraged to have a comfortable attitude of encouraging learning and fostering patient independence and autonomy. For professionals in the rehabilitation setting to work effectively, they must work together and strive toward a good knowledge and understanding of all the aspects that influence and assist patients and families in good rehabilitation and thus preparation for discharge. The physical environment must also be conducive to learning and using the skills appropriate to long-term needs and plans of patients and families. Factors in a rehabilitation program that facilitate the discharge process and promote easier patient and family adjustment include:

- Early determination of ultimate patient and family goals and how best to achieve them
- Early understanding by patient and family of the institution and how it functions best
- Continuous assessment and provision of necessary changes in individualized rehabilitation programs for patients and families
- Encouragement of activities outside the rehabilitation center before discharge
- Support of socialization skills in the new role facing a disabled person
- Completion of comprehensive patient and family health education, and, for some, sessions on hiring, firing, and promoting harmonious working relationships with an attendant
- Provision for independent living situations within the care unit
- Encouragement to use transitional living centers
- Good coordination with follow-up services for patients and families
- Good communication and working relationships with resources in the community
- Involvement of the rehabilitation center in developing community facilities and resources to meet growing and changing health care demands of disabled persons in the community

Therapeutic excursions and leaves

Adjustment to living with the stresses imposed by spinal cord injury requires a gradual exposure to community situations outside the spinal cord injury care unit. Therapeutic passes and excursions into the community, prior to discharge, are considered an essential element of a total management program. [*Guidelines* 1981:11]

Experiencing early reintegration into the community enhances readiness for discharge and minimizes fears of the outside world from building. Valuable opportunities for resocialization have been facilitated by the advent of day and weekend passes early in the program. With careful planning soon after admission, an excursion into the community may be possible within two to four weeks after injury. For example, even when neither patient nor family is able to perform an intermittent catheterization technique to the desired degree of competency, all may benefit from a short outing planned between procedures.

In preparation for day and weekend leaves the nurse must collaborate with the interdisciplinary team to ensure the patient's general physical and mental health is stable. The nurse must also be satisfied that safety needs will be provided for and that the patient and escort are capable, responsible, and well informed about the patient's needs. Figures 18–1 and 18–2 are examples of basic pass checklists to prepare for day and then weekend leaves. Note that the activity tolerance suggested in these lists ensures the patient comfort and guards against excess fatigue.

It is helpful to encourage these experiences, otherwise patients are not exposed to real-life situations and do not have opportunities to find out what they can or cannot cope with. Passes frequently provide an incentive for learning based on the concept that adults tend to view education as a means to overcome a problem at hand (Knowles 1972). For example, incontinence in the rehabilitation center is one thing, when a quick change of the track suit will solve the not so obvious problem; it is quite another if good clothes become obviously wet in front of friends. The situation may encourage the patient to learn more about drinking patterns and bladder control or condom application. If this situation is not experienced until after discharge, however, the patient will not have access to the same resources to solve the problem. Unfortunately, the situation is more likely to cause social isolation; the person may simply be too afraid to risk going out.

The nurse must be sensitive to the patient's response on return from a pass. Patients experience the realities of disability outside the rehabilitation environment, so emotional reactions, particularly behavioral outbursts, typically occur when they return. Nurses must look beyond the behavior at hand and explore the cause if their interventions are to be both timely and meaningful.

DAY PASS CHECKLIST

MEDICAL NURSING EDUCATION	PATIENT	ESCORT	PROBLEMS
1. MEDICATIONS			
(a) Name			
(b) Dosage			
(c) Time			
(d) Purpose			
(e) Precautions			
2. DIET			
(a) Fluids			
(b) Precautions			
3. SKIN CARE - PRECAUTIONS			
(a) Smoking			
(b) Car heaters			
(c) Weather			
(d) Plumbing			
(e) Hot liquids			
4. BLADDER CARE			
(a) Catheter schedule			
(b) Expression			
(c) Application of condom			
(d) Care of drainage system			
(e) Hygiene			
5. BOWEL CARE			
(a) Hygiene			
6. EMERGENCY SITUATIONS			
(a) Autonomic dysreflexia			
(b) Ward telephone numbers			
(c) Emergency facilities			

PHYSIOTHERAPY EDUCATION	PATIENT	ESCORT	PROBLEMS
1. SITTING TOLERANCE 3 Hours			
2. SKIN CARE			
(a) Weight Shift			
(b) Transfer Precautions			
3. TRANSFERS			
OCCUPATIONAL THERAPY EDUCATION			
1. ACCESSIBILITY			
EQUIPMENT CHECKLIST			
Transfer board			
Eating aids			
Additional clothing			
Bladder equipment			
Bowel equipment			
Medications			

FIGURE 18–1 ■ Day pass checklist. (Courtesy of Acute Spinal Cord Injury Unit; Shaughnessy Hospital, Vancouver, B.C.)

Assessment following passes might deal with practical questions such as:

- Was the patient able to instruct others when unable to do something?
- How did the family respond to the patient's new role or to their new role as attendants?
- What precautions were taken against incontinence when on pass, and how was it dealt with if it did occur?
- Did the patient take the initiative to check the accessibility of a building before going there?
- How did the patient deal with physical barriers in the community?

Patients who live a substantial distance from a rehabilitation center can use a vacation leave to check out the physical environment of the home; try managing daily care; identify problems; and, on returning to the rehabilitation center, join the interdisciplinary team in solving problems before discharge.

Community Follow-Up Services

Related follow-up services for disabled people in the community aid in the discharge process. Although tremendous progress has been made in the past decade with development of these resources, today more people with greater degrees of disability survive spinal cord injury, and more people return to the community sooner after injury. This trend creates the need for and emphasizes the lack of appropriate ongoing health services currently available in most communities. This situation is not unique to people with spinal cord injuries; it is part of a major health and economic concern: how best to develop resources to meet the ever-increasing needs of those requiring long-term health care.

Existing health care services are available in the community from a variety of sources. However, the experience of varied rehabilitation centers confirms that unless supported by special-

WEEKEND CHECKLIST

EDUCATION - ADDITIONAL TO DAY PASS CHECKLIST			
NURSING	**PATIENT**	**ESCORT**	**PROBLEMS**
1. SKIN CARE			
(a) Positioning			
(b) Inspection			
(c) Common pressure areas			
(d) Abrasions			
(e) Night turns			
2. BLADDER			
(a) Self-catheterization			
(b) Signs and symptoms of infection			
3. BOWEL CARE			
PHYSIOTHERAPY			
1. ACTIVITY TOLERANCE　　6 Hours			
2. TRANSFERS			
(a) Bed			
(b) Toilet			
(c) Car			
OCCUPATIONAL THERAPY			
1. BRACING			
(a) Splint regime			
(b) Application and care of brace			
2. ACCOMMODATION OR HOME ASSESSMENT			
SEXUAL COUNSELING			

WEEKEND CHECKLIST

EQUIPMENT CHECKLIST
1. BLADDER AND BOWEL EQUIPMENT
(a) Catheter Supplies
(b) Condom
(c) Urinal
2. MEDICATIONS
(a) Suppository
3. BED EQUIPMENT
(a) Sheepskin
(b) Pillows
4. ADDITIONAL CLOTHING
5. WHEELCHAIR ACCESSORIES
6. EATING AIDS
7. GROOMING AIDS
8. DRESSING AIDS
9. SPLINTS - BRACES
10. BATHROOM AIDS

FIGURE 18–2 ■ Weekend pass checklist. (Courtesy of Acute Spinal Cord Injury Unit; Shaughnessy Hospital, Vancouver, B.C.)

ized liaison and educational activities, referrals are less than ideal. While health care professionals in the community may lack expertise in recognizing and dealing with the uniqueness and severity of the problems encountered by people with spinal cord injuries, those in rehabilitation centers may have little or no idea of the problems faced in the community. This situation is especially pronounced when the rehabilitation center is in a large city and the patient is from a distant rural community.

Nurses, particularly in the expanded role, are in a good position to be effective educators and liaisons between rehabilitation and community professionals. For example, there is a Nurse Practitioner Continuity of Care Clinic in the Regional Spinal Cord Injury Care System of Southern California designed to manage health care needs of those patients who have been discharged. These nurses contribute immensely to cost-effective health maintenance and prevention and to more effective use of professionals' time in several specific areas of referral (Murphy and Pautsch 1981).

The sharing of expertise between rehabilitation and community professionals promotes a system of follow-up services with a preventive, rather than a crisis intervention, focus. It is realized that an informed resource person close at hand is in a better position to prevent a problem situation from becoming a crisis situation. (Treischmann 1980).

The first year of community living is usually the most traumatic for injured persons and their families, so support and encouragement without their dependence is of great value. It has been found most helpful to provide follow-up contact at frequent intervals in the first year: that is, at one month, three months, six months, and one year after discharge and then annually as necessary. The objective is to maintain telephone or personal contact—more frequently for patients considered to be at risk of developing complications—to detect any problems early, and to mobilize available resources as a preventive measure.

To expand traditional rehabilitative opportunities, the concept of transitional living programs is meeting with growing success. These programs provide "halfway homes" and support services to ease adjustment to community living.

Transitional living programs are explained further in Chapter 19.

THE NURSING PROCESS AND DISCHARGE PLANNING

It is logical that psychological and social adjustments are not complete when patients are discharged from a rehabilitation center. They continue to need help in accepting an altered reality, learning new roles, and coping with the many tasks necessary to manage the effects of disability. Nurses can help ensure that positive adjustment continues after discharge by skillfully applying the nursing process to discharge planning. The nursing process includes assessing patients' progress at intervals throughout the rehabilitation process; determining readiness for discharge; identifying problems as patients prepare for discharge; and planning and evaluating interventions.

Assessment

It is important to have established criteria to assess progress through the rehabilitation process. The nurse must participate with the interdisciplinary team to determine:

- How well patients understand their condition
- Where patients are in the adjustment process
- How well patients perform independence skills or, when appropriate, instruct others to perform them
- How much responsibility patients demonstrate in maintaining health and managing the effects of disability
- Whether patients are ready to learn new roles

Independence, mobility, and self-care skills are used to determine progress in physical aspects of rehabilitation. Social and psychological adjustments are more difficult to assess and criteria for doing so are less clearly established. Assessments of the patients' understanding of their condition and adjustment to disability are left very much to professional judgment but are reflected in such things as:

- How well they manage their skills both in the rehabilitation setting and on excursions and leaves
- How they interact with peers, professionals, and family
- How they teach others to assist with their care
- How much interest they take in various aspects of their rehabilitation

Meaningful communication and expert coordination are essential throughout the discharge process. The nurse must be aware of each team member's plans and progress and communicate to others a nursing perspective on patient and family progress toward discharge. Figure 18–3 provides a guideline to facilitate interdisciplinary assessment in which psychosocial readiness is described. Other categories include medical status of readiness, functional readiness, readiness in communication skills, and expressed readiness for future living patterns.

Goal Setting

Goal setting is a progressive or building step of the nursing process, but in relation to discharge planning it is more a *reassessment* and *refining* of long-term goals for patients and, when appropriate, families. This step evaluates and gives direction to the progress of rehabilitation toward discharge.

The long-term goals set on admission are based on professionals' knowledge of physical potentials related to the level and extent of injury and on the patient's plans for the future. These goals may need some adjustment. For example, a young quadriplegic woman planned to return home to live with her family. When she realized how independent she could be with some attendant care, however, she decided to share accommodations with a friend. Unfortunately, conflicts can arise among family members in such situations. For example, a 23-year-old quadriplegic man wanted to live on his own, while his family felt he should stay at home where his mother could care for him. The family had modified their home to accommodate their son's special needs, and he felt trapped. Careful reassessment of both individual and family goals during discharge planning can help prevent such problems.

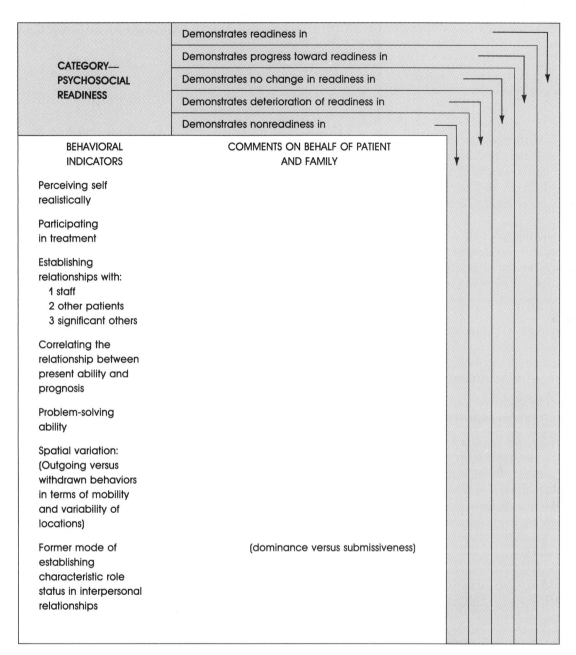

CATEGORY—PSYCHOSOCIAL READINESS	Demonstrates readiness in
	Demonstrates progress toward readiness in
	Demonstrates no change in readiness in
	Demonstrates deterioration of readiness in
	Demonstrates nonreadiness in

BEHAVIORAL INDICATORS	COMMENTS ON BEHALF OF PATIENT AND FAMILY
Perceiving self realistically	
Participating in treatment	
Establishing relationships with: 1 staff 2 other patients 3 significant others	
Correlating the relationship between present ability and prognosis	
Problem-solving ability	
Spatial variation: (Outgoing versus withdrawn behaviors in terms of mobility and variability of locations)	
Former mode of establishing characteristic role status in interpersonal relationships	(dominance versus submissiveness)

FIGURE 18–3 ■ An interdisciplinary tool for assessing patients' psychosocial readiness for discharge in the rehabilitation setting. (From A. Fenwick, *Journal of Advanced Nursing*, Vol. 4, p. 15, 1979. Reprinted with permission of Blackwell Scientific Publications, Ltd)

Interventions

During preparation for discharge nursing interventions will relate to assessment and to reassessed and refined goals and will, of necessity, vary with the emotional and physical state of the patient. Skilled interventions help patients and families reduce the uncertainties they face when patients return to the community and promote healthful living.

Interventions that ease the patient's transition to home and community life include:

- Encouraging early community excursions and leaves
- Helping the patient and family adapt various procedures done in hospital so that they can be done at home
- Assisting in home renovation planning
- Gathering equipment and supplies, predicting how long they will last, and providing information on where and how to get more (Remember the first month after discharge is often the most difficult, and patients may take little interest in securing supplies they might run out of)
- Completing patient and family health education and, on discharge, being sure patient has written materials to refer to in the future. A patient *workbook* is particularly useful.
- Reviewing information on community resources
- Encouraging continuation of leisure activities enjoyed in the rehabilitation program and facilitating contact with leisure and interest groups in the community when possible

Interventions to assist with medical aspects of health care include:

- Providing for regular medical follow-up of patient, more frequently for those considered at risk; ideally patient and family will become established with a family practitioner and community health services near their home
- Reviewing the preventive aspects of follow-up care, focusing on early detection of possible complications
- Arranging for nursing support services within the home
- Participating in training of an attendant if necessary

The nurse and patient can complete a discharge and follow-up summary (see Figure 18–4) to facilitate ongoing care by providing current and concise information to community health care workers. The form cannot be used in isolation but must be supported by liaison and educational services from the rehabilitation center and personal or telephone contact if indicated. Patients must agree to the release of the information, and it is generally in their best interests to encourage them to do so.

It is important to alert those in the community of potential medical and social problems,

---

■ *PERSONAL VIEWPOINT*

A 32-year-old, self-employed, quadriplegic businessman is preparing for discharge from the rehabilitation center. He understands his disability and how to care for himself and takes responsibility for the care he must get. He can afford and wishes to live in an apartment of his own. He will need an attendant for most of his personal care, housecleaning, and meal preparation. Unfortunately he is a difficult man to care for, and since most nurses dislike doing so, there is a real possibility that he may not be able to survive in the community.

To help him prepare for living in the setting he chooses, nursing and interdisciplinary interventions in the discharge process may include:

- Helping him understand the present and, possibly, future problem
- Explaining the difficulty in finding good attendants and providing guidelines on securing and retaining them
- Encouraging him to learn to work with attendants in the rehabilitation setting and developing his ability to accept constructive criticism from health care professionals
- Helping him find, hire, and train an attendant while he is still in the rehabilitation setting

---

many of which are related to inactivity. Often people with paraplegia, who are capable of independence with personal care and mobility and therefore do not require physical assistance from others, become more isolated than those with quadriplegia. As a preventive measure, health care professionals promote activity for all people with spinal cord injuries.

As options increase, it is important for the nurse to be aware of the type, quality, and availablility of continuing care resources. Knowledge of current resources will profoundly affect the discharge decision. The nurse must participate with the patient, family, and other health care professionals to determine the degree of risk to the patient and relate this risk factor to the intensity of follow-up services required.

Needs for supervision will vary, but most patients will require some assistance. Those who are having difficulty with adjustment will require help commensurate with their ability to be responsible for their own care. Those who have developed more adaptive behaviors may require help in learning new roles.

Knowledge of the ways that patients learn new roles provides direction for planning interventions that will facilitate successful enactment of the new roles. Regular visits by a community health nurse to help plan appropriate sequencing of activities of increasing social difficulty and contact with a peer and professional counselor will help provide support through this phase of psychosocial adjustment. These interventions and similar beliefs have expanded the concept of rehabilitation, which today includes transitional living centers; formal development of specific community resources; self-help groups; and supportive social movements.

Evaluation

Evaluation is essential to determine the effectiveness of predischarge assessment and planning. The outcome of rehabilitation will eventually be determined by patients' ability to maintain optimal health, manage the effects of disability, adapt to an altered reality, and develop skills that will allow them to live in a community of nondisabled people.

Follow-up services are used for evaluation, not only to assist the individual patient and family, but also to incorporate feedback mechanisms to give future directions to the discharge process. See Figure 18–5. Evaluation methods currently in use include home visits, telephone contact, questionnaires, comparison of discharge summary forms to current status, follow-up clinics, and liaison activities.

Current research indicates that many problems face the patient and family during the transition to community living. One area that nurses in particular must focus on is the effect of phys-

ical care tasks on family relationships. For example, a middle-aged quadriplegic man returned home having his wife perform his bowel care every other day. Both partners disliked this experience but coped with it at first. After a while they found they argued a lot on bowel care days and soon found themselves not speaking to each other on those days at all. Eventually the couple separated and the wife told the nurse that the "distasteful event" of bowel care was a major causative factor.

Evaluation of this story and others like it suggests that more sensitivity in discharge planning or follow-up care might have prevented such a drastic outcome. The age factor itself suggests that the couple might have a more limited capacity to adjust and adapt to new situations and that the added physical tasks might impose a particularly heavy fatigue factor. The nurse must look beyond the procedure at hand and examine role implications. In this situation, was there a role conflict when the wife was expected to be an attendant and partner at the same time? Could the wife have managed bowel care with less stigma if aids were used? Would attendant care have relieved the source of stress and helped preserve the relationship? Nurses must be forewarned that bowel and bladder care precipitates some very complex family issues.

LONG-TERM IMPLICATIONS

Involving the patient, the family, health care professionals, and community resources in comprehensive discharge planning and preparation can smooth the patient's transition to successful community living. Fragmented discharge planning and preparation can hinder or even prevent this transition.

The responsibility for continuing health care falls mainly on the patient and the family. However, it is the responsibility of health care professionals to establish and develop necessary community support services. The nurse is in a unique position to comprehend and participate in this multifaceted concept and to help people with spinal cord injuries return to the community as persons of independence and worth.

DISCHARGE AND FOLLOW-UP SUMMARY

PATIENT _____   D.O.B. _____   SEX _____   MARITAL STATUS _____

ADDRESS _____   PHONE NO. _____

DIAGNOSIS _____   DATE OF OCCURRENCE _____   ADMISSION DATE _____

DISCHARGED TO _____   DISCHARGE DATE _____

FOLLOW-UP COORDINATOR _____   CENTER DOCTOR _____   FAMILY DOCTOR _____

ON THE PATIENT'S AUTHORIZATION, THIS SUMMARY HAS BEEN SENT TO PUBLIC HEALTH UNIT _____

REFERRAL TO HOME CARE   yes ___   no ___   LONG-TERM CARE APPLICATION COMPLETED   yes ___   no ___

AMBULATORY: TOTALLY ☐   PARTIALLY ☐   WHEELCHAIR ONLY ☐

SELF-CARE: INDEPENDENT ☐   PARTIALLY DEPENDENT WITH SUPERVISION ☐

PARTIALLY DEPENDENT WITH ASSISTANCE ☐

TOTALLY DEPENDENT ☐

comments:

special needs for grooming

safety measures recommended

patient able to instruct others in his/her care?   yes ___   no ___
family or attendant has been instructed in patient's care?   yes ___   no ___
if yes, give name and relationship to patient

SEEN BY	YES	NO
P.T.		
O.T.		
GYM		
SPEECH		
SOCIAL		
VOCATIONAL		
PSYCHOLOGY		
SEXUAL HEALTH CARE		
DIETARY		

TRANSFERS	DEP.	ASSIST.	INDEP.
BED TO W/C			
W/C TO TOILET			

TRANSFERS	DEP.	ASSIST.	INDEP.
W/C TO BATH			
W/C TO CAR			

SKIN (nutrition, circulation)

BOWELS (times per week)

BLADDER

SPECIAL SENSES

speech

hearing

vision

comprehension and memory

perceptual problems

ALLERGIES

EQUIPMENT PROVIDED	
WHEELCHAIR	
BRACES	
CRUTCHES	
CANES	
WALKER	
CUSHION	
BED	
MATTRESS	
NYLON SHEET	
OVERHEAD BAR	
BATH SEAT	
TRANSFER BOARD	
COMMODE	
RAISED TOILET SEAT	
URINARY SUPPLIES	
ACTIVITY AIDS	
ORTHOSIS	
PROSTHESIS	
OTHERS (specify)	

MEDICATIONS

HOME EXERCISE PROGRAM GIVEN TO PATIENT BY _____ DEPT.

EXERCISE PROGRAM RECOMMENDED

PATIENT'S STRENGTHS (interests)

SPECIAL CONCERNS OR INTERESTS TO BE PURSUED BY COMMUNITY HEALTH NURSE

OTHER REMARKS

_____   _____
form completed by   date

_____

A U T H O R I Z A T I O N

I AGREE THAT A COPY OF THIS DISCHARGE AND FOLLOW-UP

SUMMARY BE SENT TO THE PUBLIC HEALTH UNIT, IN ADDITION

TO THE COPY BEING FORWARDED TO MY DOCTOR-DR. _____

_____   _____
patient   date

_____   _____
witness   date

FIGURE 18–4 ■ Discharge and follow-up summary sheet. (Courtesy of G. F. Strong Rehabilitation Centre, Vancouver, B.C.)

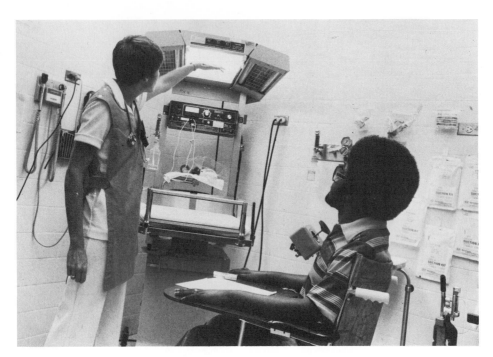

FIGURE 18–5 ■ A nurse participates in a specialized follow-up clinic at a rehabilitation center.

SELECTED REFERENCES

Fenwick, A. 1979. An interdisciplinary tool for assessing patient's readiness for discharge in the rehabilitation setting. *Journal of Advanced Nursing* 4: 9–21. *Describes rationale, establishment, and evolution of a tool to determine readiness for discharge; reviews current perspectives of measurement in rehabilitation and desirability of interdisciplinary planning.*

Guidelines for facility categorization and standards of care: spinal cord injury. 1981. American Spinal Injury Association and American Spinal Injury Association Foundation, 250 E. Superior Street, Room 619, Chicago, Ill 60611. *Clearly presents purposes and requirements of the major components of care: emergency medical services, trauma centers, specialized acute care and rehabilitation facilities, and follow-up community care.*

Knowles, M. 1972. *The Modern Practice of Adult Education.* New York: Association Press. *Classic text on principles and methods of adult learning.*

MacLean, S. 1981. The discharge process and spinal cord injured patients. Unpublished material. University of British Columbia, Vancouver, B.C.

An examination of how theoretical considerations affected three quadriplegia patient's during preparation for discharge.

Murphy, M., and Pautsch, H. 1981. An approach to spinal cord injury. *Spinal Cord Injury Digest* 3 (Spring): 11–14. *Describes a nurse practitioner care clinic operating at Rancho Los Amigos five days a week. The clinic saw all patients one year after discharge for annual evaluations and also treated episodic illnesses.*

Shontz, F. 1975. *The Psychological Aspects of Physical Illness and Disability.* New York: Macmillan. *Superior background reading; explores cyclical adjustment to disability.*

Thompson, D., and Lott, J. 1980. Psychosocial redevelopment of spinal cord injured persons. *Spinal Cord Injury Digest* 2 (Winter): 6. *Describes the psychosocial aspects of treatment, rehabilitation, and community environment and how these relate to reprocessing of Erikson's life span development stages.*

Treischmann, R. 1980. *Spinal Cord Injuries, Psychological, Social and Vocational Adjustment.* New York: Pergamon Press. *Only existing work exclusively devoted to the psychosocial impact of spinal cord injuries on persons and their families. Includes an exhaustive critique of the literature with a view to dispelling myths and stimulating research to develop future strategies; focuses on the discharge process.*

SUPPLEMENTAL READING

Archer, S., and Fleshman, R. 1979. *Community Health Nursing.* 2d ed. North Scituate, Mass: Duxbury Press. *Explores current health care concepts at work in the community; includes helpful sections on working with families and how economics, politics, and the health insurance industry, among other controversial issues, affect community nursing activities and services.*

Better, S., et al. 1979. Complications among spinal cord injury patients following discharge. *Association of Rehabilitation Nurses Journal* 4 (Mar.–Apr.): 8–10. *Explores and documents medical, psychosocial, financial, mechanical, and architectural problems encountered by a home health team.*

Bowich, E., and Warner, B. 1980. What makes a caring community. *Spinal Cord Injury Digest* 2 (Spring): 25–30. *Plea to accept disabled persons back into the mainstream of community life. Discusses absence of barriers, physical facilities, social support systems, and responsibility of the client.*

Dinsdale, S., et al. 1981. Community based monitoring for spinal man. *Canadian Journal of Public Health* 72 (May–June): 195–198. *Compares an innovative community-based system for providing post-discharge follow-up of patients to the traditional hospital-centered program.*

El Ghatit, A., et al. 1980. Training apartment in community for spinal cord injured patients: a model. *Archives of Physical and Medical Rehabilitation* 61(2): 90–92. *Describes a training apartment in the community as a successful predischarge strategy to regain confidence and independence.*

Garfunkel, M., and Goldfinger, G. Undated. *Living with Spinal Cord Injury—Questions and Answers for Patients, Families and Friends.* New York University Medical Center, New York Regional Spinal Cord Injury System, 400 E. 34 St., New York, NY 10016. *Readable question/answer format, for example: Is financial assistance available after spinal cord injury? Can spinal cord injured persons work or go to school? Focuses on life after rehabilitation. Creative photography reinforces positive attitudes communicated.*

Getchel, N. 1974. Health program maintenance by males with spinal cord injury. *Communicating*

Nursing Research 7: 63–77. *Examines assessment of educational background, knowledge of condition, number of self-initiated activities, number of significant others in the home environment, and extent of injury (paraplegia versus quadriplegia) in the rehabilitation setting to predict success after discharge.*

King, R.; Boyink, M.; and Keenan, M. 1977. *Rehabilitation Guide.* Medical Rehabilitation Research and Training Center No. 20. Chicago: Northwest University and Rehabilitation Institute of Chicago. *Section on going home offers practical advice for determining and ordering quantities of medical supplies and equipment; emphasizes need for follow-up care.*

Martin, N.; Holt, N.; and Hicks, D., eds. 1980. *Comprehensive Rehabilitation Nursing.* New York: McGraw-Hill, pt. 4. *Addresses multifaceted challenges that affect the nurse and the discharge process: planning, vocational rehabilitation, resocialization, the environment, and the insurance industry as a support structure. Includes a wonderful personal account of a quadriplegic executive returning to work.*

Rogers, J., and Figone, J. 1978. The avocational pursuits of rehabilitants with traumatic quadriplegia. *American Journal of Occupational Therapy* 32 (9): 571–576. *Documents how rehabilitants envisioned a more flexible, comprehensive treatment model that would give priority to developmental status, changing life goals, interpersonal relationships, and social roles.*

Smith, N., and Meyer, A. 1981. Personal care attendants: key to living independently. *Rehabilitation Literature* 42 (9–10): 258–265. *Focuses on preparation of people with spinal cord injuries to interact effectively with people who are caring for them.*

Vivian, J., and Mitchell, C. 1981. Southwest regional outreach follow-up care program. *Spinal Cord Injury Digest* 3 (Spring): 35–39. *Describes outreach clinics for follow-up care established by spinal cord injury center treatment team in patients' home communities. The treatment team worked with local physicians and allied health and vocational representatives with emphasis on training and education.*

Watson, P. 1979. Rehabilitation legislation of the seventies and the severely disabled. *Association of Rehabilitation Nurses Journal,* May–June, pp. 4–11. *Outstanding review of current relative legislation. Extensively rsearched references and bibliography.*

Young, J., and Northup, N. 1980. Spinal cord injury system involvement in follow-up medical care. *Spinal Cord Injury Digest* 2 (Fall): 9–14. *Reports the combined experiences of regional model spinal cord injury centers in providing ongoing medical care.*

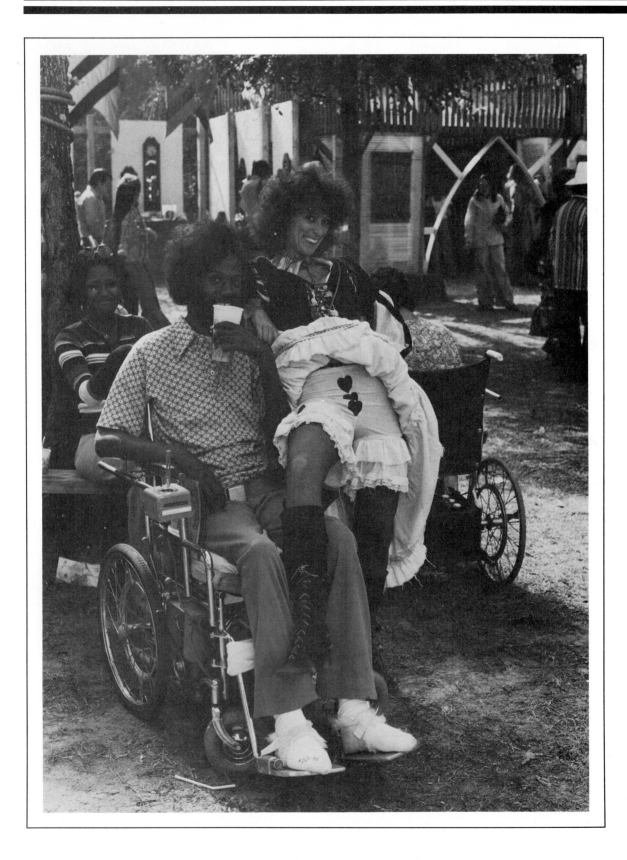

Chapter 19

Is There Life
After Rehabilitation?

Lex Frieden, Ph.D, M.S.P.

OBJECTIVES

- To provide some perspective on the positive outcomes of rehabilitation
- To present some ways, in addition to providing optimal professional care, in which nurses can promote those positive outcomes for people with spinal cord injuries

LIFE GOALS

Whether they express it or not, people with spinal cord injuries begin to wonder about the outcome of their predicament almost from the point of injury. Their expectations of the future and the goals they set for themselves are shaped by a wide range of variables. First impressions may be affected by the extent and nature of information they are given about their injury, the reactions of family members, and previous experiences with and attitudes toward persons with similar injuries.

In most cases, the first questions people deal with are those of survival: Yes, no, and, if yes, how? Patients continue to ask these questions, if only of themselves, long after they begin the rehabilitation process. The answers they give themselves may change many times during the course of rehabilitation, and their answers are largely determined by what they learn and how they are treated.

Early patient expectations of outcome may be unrealistic and extreme. They may range from the fear of forever being a "vegetable," confined to bed, and in need of 24-hour professional care, to a belief in complete recovery with no serious consequences. Patients develop more realistic expectations as individual circumstances become known and as the educational function of rehabilitation takes effect. Patients who are treated as adults, given responsibility, and taught to manage their own care are likely not only to be more realistic about their disabilities, but also to experience a significantly higher quality of life following rehabilitation.

The expectations, hopes, and goals of people with spinal cord injuries often change following discharge from the hospital or rehabilitation center. These changes occur for at least several reasons. Individuals may experience some functional return; gain additional strength in residual muscle function; increase their stamina and tolerance; make personal and environmental adaptations; learn new ways of doing things; and acquire new adaptive equipment.

Some changes may lead to the reestablishment of a positive self-image and expanded options for living. Other changes effected by life beyond the protective walls of the institution may damage self-image, narrow expectations, and restrict options. Old friends may stop by once and never come again. Other friends and family members may pamper, patronize, and pity. The realities of economic and environmental barriers may be overwhelming. People with spinal cord injuries may have physical setbacks and complications. Bowel and bladder accidents, pressure sores, and infections that persist may become overbearing.

All the changes that occur following discharge necessitate constant reassessment of individual options, expectations, and goals. For this reason, many centers have established follow-up programs to keep in touch with patients after discharge and provide support during the crucial stages of adjustment and readaptation to community life. Although these programs are generally limited by insufficient funding, they do constitute an important part of the overall rehabilitation process.

The question is often asked, "What are the long-term goals of individuals with spinal cord injuries?" More than likely, the answer is that their goals are generally the same as anyone else's. Most people want to have a family, a home, a car, a job, and social and recreational opportunities.

Some professionals, friends, and family members have, in the past, discouraged people with spinal cord injuries from adopting or seeking these goals. Many injured people have been led to believe that these were impossible, unrealistic goals and that they should be satisfied and happy just to be alive. In fact, the general public's expectations of life for people with spinal cord injuries were weighed on a different scale of normality from their own. What was considered a normal life-style for the general population was not considered normal for people with spinal cord injuries. As a result of these attitudes, many people with spinal cord injuries restricted their goals and lowered their expectations. Sometimes hope for a better life was buried so deeply that it disappeared.

THE CONCEPT OF INDEPENDENT LIVING

During the late 1960s and early 1970s, a new concept of rehabilitation and quality of life began to be expressed by people with spinal cord injuries and other disabilities. This concept, called independent living, was at first a sort of reaction to repression. Some disabled people felt their lives were unnecessarily restricted by their disabilities. They acknowledged that the barriers to independence were increased by disability, but they believed that the barriers could be overcome. They felt that supportive programs could be established and environmental accommo-

dations could be made that would allow them to seek the goals open to the general public. They rejected the notion that they should be confined to institutional care; the assumption that they had fewer rights than nondisabled people; and the idea that the government's obligation to them was limited because of their disability.

These people began to assert themselves in public forums. They organized and formed lobbying groups; they claimed equal rights as citizens to public services like transportation, housing, education, and employment; and they claimed the right to vote. Although most of these rights were not denied intentionally or directly, they were indirectly denied by virtue of the fact that public transportation, housing, schools, businesses, public offices, and polling places were generally inaccessible.

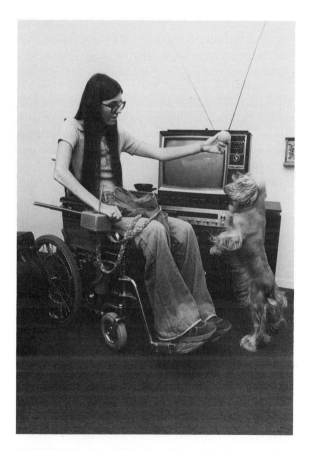 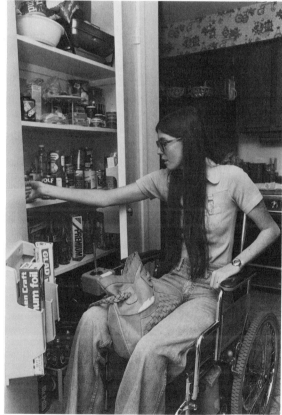

FIGURE 19–1 ■ Adjusting: Terry Ensign participates in a transitional living program, which provides a homelike environment in which to apply rehabilitative skills.

From the concept of independence, a movement emerged to overcome the barriers to a higher quality of life for disabled people. This movement was joined by disabled people, family members, friends, neighbors, people throughout society, professionals, politicians, and policy makers. The movement led to:

- New laws asserting the equality and protecting the rights of disabled people
- New or adapted accommodations making housing, transportation, public places, schools, and job sites accessible to people with disabilities
- New, more positive attitudes by the general public toward people with disabilities, and by disabled people toward themselves
- Perhaps most important, new opportunities for severely disabled people, including those with spinal cord injuries, to seek independence, to enjoy the benefits of their labors, and to enjoy the quality of life that society offers

As a result of the independent living movement and the changes that have occurred during the past few years, people with spinal cord injuries may now realistically seek goals that once were limited to people without disabilities. In fact, the limits imposed by spinal cord injury may be less important in determining the achievement of goals than are certain other demographic and socioeconomic variables that are not related to disability. Many patients now go directly from the rehabilitation center to independent living arrangements in the community; others do so after a temporary respite with their families; and still others do so after participating in extended vocational rehabilitation or transitional living programs.

BARRIERS TO INDEPENDENCE

The principal barriers to achieving goals of independence for spinal cord injured people may be categorized in three groups:

1. *Environmental barriers* that are beyond the immediate control of the individual. They are exemplified by curbs, steps, and narrow doorways.

2. *Personal barriers* that are directly related to and controlled by the individual. Personal barriers are negative attitudes, low self-esteem, poor self-image, feelings of dependence, unreasonable insecurity, unwillingness to take risks, preoccupation with cure, lack of ability to organize and plan, and unnecessarily limited expectations and goals.

3. *Economic barriers* that are related to inability to purchase needed equipment, supplies, and services. Economic barriers may restrict the possible solutions to both environmental and personal barriers.

Ways to Overcome Barriers

There are now more ways to overcome the barriers to independence than ever before. To overcome environmental barriers, one may purchase or make adaptive equipment and devices. For example, people with high-level quadriplegia may purchase electrically powered wheelchairs controlled by slight movements of the chin or by sipping and puffing into a straw. Also available are sophisticated remote control devices and primitive robots. In addition to customized, individual solutions, there are solutions of a broader, more systematic scale. These include mass transportation vehicles made accessible by widening doorways, expanding seating areas, and installing ramps or lifts, and communitywide efforts to install ramps on curbs and provide access to both public and private buildings. Solutions like these to environmental barriers are now widespread, and continued advocacy efforts are leading to more solutions of this nature each day.

There are also several possible solutions to personal barriers. Rehabilitation counselors, psychologists, social workers, and other professionals can help a person analyze and overcome personal barriers. Peer counselors may share information, serve as role models, and provide necessary support. Family members and friends can give encouragement and help. Finally, self-determination, self-encouragement, self-control, and simply the passage of time may help the disabled person overcome personal barriers. On a broader scale, constructive attitudes and expectations of the general public and positive portrayals of disabled people by the media may also help overcome personal barriers.

Economic barriers may be the most difficult to overcome and the most important, since they can affect solutions to the other two types of barriers. Most people depend on private and public insurance, private and public aid, or their own ability to earn money in order to overcome economic barriers. Independence costs more for people with spinal cord injuries than it does for nondisabled people, because, in addition to the normal expenses of housing, transportation, food, clothing, and routine medical care, people with spinal cord injuries often have expenses for adaptive equipment, medical supplies, and attendant care. The economic barriers to their independence are frequently complicated by the fact that in order to be independent, one needs a job, but in order to have a job, one needs to be reasonably independent.

Individual solutions to economic barriers are typified by a person who receives housing subsidies to help pay for housing, vocational rehabilitation agency grants or subsidies to help pay for educational or work-related expenses, welfare or human service agency subsidies to help pay for attendant care expenses, and work income or Social Security disability insurance payments to cover other expenses. More general solutions to overcoming economic barriers may be legislated in the form of a nationalized health insurance program, a nationwide attendant care or home health care program, or the establishment of a nationwide system for purchase and distribution of equipment and devices for disabled people.

Independent living programs

Independent living programs, which have been established since the independent living movement began and subscribe to the tenets of the independent living philosophy, are located in at least one community in every state of the United States. Altogether, there are now more than 170 independent living programs in the United States and as many as 50 more through-

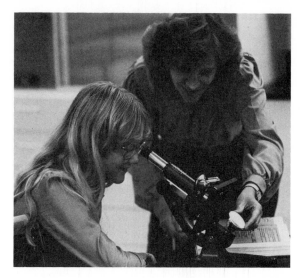

FIGURE 19–2 ■ Learning: Stacy Norman resumes her high school education.

out the world. These community-based programs are unique, because they are generally run by or managed in large part by disabled people themselves. They provide a variety of services including housing referral, attendant care referral, information about goods and services provided by other agencies, peer counseling, transportation, equipment repair, independent living skills training, and advocacy. (See Table 19–1.) Their goal is to assist severely disabled people by increasing self-determination and minimizing unnecessary dependence on others.

A particular type of independent living program, the *transitional living program,* has proven to be exceptionally effective in helping people with spinal cord injuries acquire the information and skills they need in order to establish an independent life-style following rehabilitation. Transitional programs include support services to provide opportunities for practical application of newly acquired skills in such areas as personal and attendant care; health care; homemaking; financial management; getting around in the community; seeking accommodations and employment; time management; interpersonal development; and so on. Most importantly, these programs encourage individuals to make their own decisions and be responsible for their own lives.

TABLE 19–1 ■ INDEPENDENT LIVING PROGRAMS: FOUR PRIMARY VARIATIONS

Conceptually, an *independent living program* is generic—the most broadly defined term relating to organizations working with disabled individuals who wish to live independently. Several different kinds of programs providing services that foster independent living have been identified: independent living center, independent living residential program, and independent living transitional program.

What kinds of features an independent living program has will depend on the needs of the clients served, the availability of existing community resources, the physical and social makeup of the community, and the goals of the program itself.

Independent Living Program	Independent Living Center	Independent Living Residential Program	Independent Living Transitional Program
Community based	Community based	Community based	Community based
Consumer involved	Consumer controlled	Consumer involved	Consumer involved
	Nonresidential		Goal oriented
	Nonprofit		Time linked
Provides/coordinates:	Provides/coordinates:	Provides/coordinates:	Provides/coordinates:
Housing	Housing	Housing	Skills training in independent living
Attendant Care	Attendant care	Shared attendant services	Other services
Information	Peer counseling	Transportation	
Other services	Financial/legal advocacy	Other services	
	Community awareness and barrier removal programs		
	Other services		

Reprinted from Lex Frieden, Laurel Richards, Jean Cole, and David Bailey. "A glossary for independent living." *ILRU Sourcebook: A Technical Assistance Manual on Independent Living.* Houston: The Institute For Rehabilitation and Research (TIRR), 1979.

There are many community agencies, organizations, and groups working to help overcome the barriers to independence posed by disability. A system of vocational rehabilitation agencies exists throughout the United States. These agencies, funded principally by the federal government, provide educational/vocational counseling and other services to assist disabled people in finding, getting, and keeping employment. They pay for some medical treatment, education and training, equipment, supplies, transportation, attendant care, and other services for eligible clients. Located in every state, these agencies have counselors working in most rehabilitation centers and most large communities.

Community support services

In addition to the networks of vocational rehabilitation and independent living programs, many other public and private service organizations throughout the United States provide vital primary care and support services to aid disabled people in their communities. These organizations include medical and vocational rehabilitation centers, voluntary organizations such

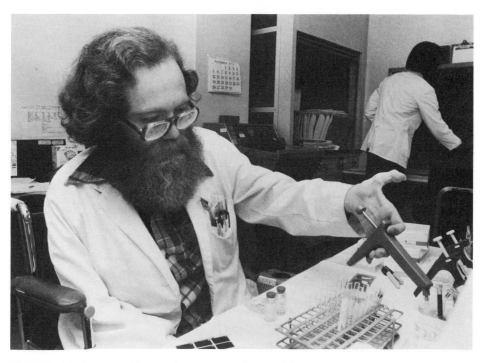

FIGURE 19–3 ■ Working: Bob Henry works as a laboratory technician.

as Goodwill and Easter Seal societies, and home health care agencies like the Visiting Nurses Association. Parallel development of similar organizations exist in Canada and most other Western countries.

Perhaps more important to those who are well adjusted to living in the community are advocacy organizations and social and recreational groups.

Advocacy organizations

Advocacy organizations assist people with disabilities in either of two principal ways:

1. They may function as case advocates, representing and advising the individual on matters related to specific benefits, programs, or civil rights.

2. They may function as class or systems advocates, representing the needs and interests of all people with spinal cord injuries or other disabilities or any other specifically defined group.

Advocacy organizations play an important role in our sociopolitical system by representing peo-

ple who either cannot or choose not to represent themselves.

On a national level in the United States, the advocacy organizations that seem to be most effective in representing disabled people are those with memberships made up mostly of disabled people. These include the American Coalition of Citizens with Disabilities, the Paralyzed Veterans of America, and the National Spinal Cord Injury Association. The latter two focus on issues affecting people with spinal cord injuries. In addition to their advocacy work, these organizations provide other services such as counseling, information, and referral. Besides their national offices, each of these groups has chapters organized at state and local levels.

In addition to these consumer-oriented groups, several organizations of professionals in the field of rehabilitation are active advocates. These groups include the American Congress of Rehabilitation Medicine, the Association of Rehabilitation Nurses, the National Rehabilitation Counselor Association, and the American Spinal Injury Association. Each of these organizations has been effective in lobbying for progressive legislation to benefit disabled people and in

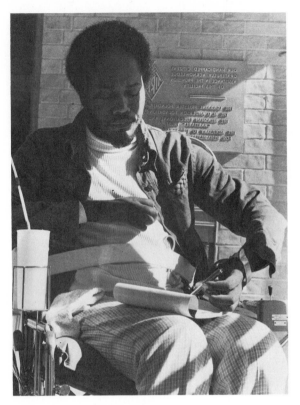

FIGURE 19–4 ■ Helping: Charles Harrison participates in community activities.

speaking out for improvements in the health care, social service, and rehabilitation systems at many levels. In particular, the American Spinal Injury Association has begun to provide an important forum for the exchange of information and ideas related to the care and treatment of people with spinal cord injuries.

Social and recreational groups

Besides advocacy organizations, social and recreational groups may provide valuable peer support and opportunities for meaningful involvement with other disabled and nondisabled people. These groups are usually locally organized according to the interests of people in their own communities. They may focus on such diverse activities as handicrafts, square dancing, sailing, hunting, basketball, and tennis. Recently, national sports and recreational organizations have become popular. These groups, such as the National Wheelchair Basketball As-

sociation, the National Wheelchair Tennis Association, and the National Wheelchair Pilots Association, organize local, regional, and national competitions and exhibitions to match skills and promote positive attitudes toward their associations and the people they represent.

In addition to finding needed support and camaraderie among organizations of and for disabled people, people with spinal cord injuries often discover that they are accepted into nonsegregated community groups such as civic clubs, garden clubs, and neighborhood circles. Many disabled people feel that their participation in common organizations such as these fosters better understanding and attitudes of the general public toward people with disabilities. These groups may be just as supportive and, perhaps, more effective in breaking down barriers to independence than those made up mostly of people with disabilities.

THE NURSE'S ROLE

At this point, it is appropriate to consider the nurse's role in life after rehabilitation. Actually, this begins during the early stages of comprehensive rehabilitation. The extent to which a person has a good outcome following rehabilitation directly depends on the quality of care provided during the entire rehabilitation process and on the expectations, attitudes, and self-image shaped during this initial stage of life after injury.

Following discharge from the rehabilitation center, the individual may require in-home follow-up, occasional outpatient clinic visits, and routine checkups. Obviously, nurses may be involved in each of these activities, and in this way, may be instrumental in helping the individual readapt to life in the mainstream. Even beyond the point of direct contact with the individual, nurses may be helpful in promoting more positive attitudes toward people with disabilities.

There are many important ways by which nurses can affect the quality of life of people with spinal cord injuries in addition to those involving direct nursing care:

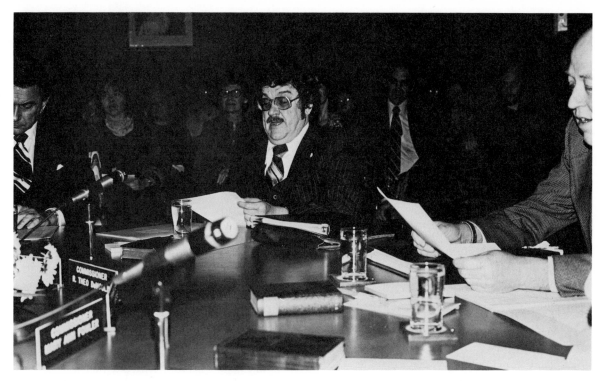

FIGURE 19–5 ■ Leading: Doug Mowat, an elected official, conducts a public forum.

• They can help prevent spinal cord injury by developing pragmatic educational and legislative programs to make driving, sports, and other activities safer.
• They can participate in research on minimizing the effects of spinal cord injury.
• They can lobby for improved health care for disabled people, for more and better rehabilitation facilities and programs, for improved follow-up and home care programs, and for more comprehensive payment mechanisms to meet the additional expenses caused by disability.
• They can join consumer groups or professional organizations to work toward more access for people with disabilities and for laws preventing discrimination and inappropriate institutionalization.
• They can support the development of new independent living programs by seeking funding for these programs at local, state, and national levels.

CONCLUSIONS

It may be difficult for nurses and other professionals to remember that people with spinal cord injuries are capable of living productive, rewarding lives in spite of the severity of their disabilities. There is no doubt, anymore, that people with spinal cord injuries can lead comparatively normal lives in their communities following rehabilitation and may, in fact, be just as productive and just as active after their injuries as they were before. People with spinal cord injuries are now doing things they were not expected to do a few years ago, such as having children, working as farmers, being auto mechanics, and holding elective offices. Even the biggest barriers—lack of knowledge and negative attitudes—have begun to disappear. Independence for these people is a realistic, achievable goal.

SUGGESTED RESOURCES FOR THE U.S.

Periodicals—Consumer Oriented

Achievement: The National Voice of the Disabled
    C. J. Lampos, Ed.
    Boosters of Achievement, Inc.
    925 N. E. 122nd Street
    N. Miami, Florida 33161

Accent on Living
    Raymond C. Cheever, Ed. & Pub.
    Cheever Publishing, Inc.
    Gillum Road & High Drive
    P.O. Box 700, Bloomington, Illinois 61701

*Rehabilitation Gazette: International Journal of
Independent Living for the Disabled*
    Gini & Joe Laurie, Eds.
    4502 Maryland Ave.
    St. Louis, Missouri 63108

Paraplegia News
    Cliff Crase, Ed. & Pub.
    5201 N. 19th Ave., Suite 111 (PVA)
    Phoenix, Arizona 85015

Books

Handicapping America
    Frank G. Bowe
    Harper & Row
    10 East 53rd Street
    New York, New York 10022
    1978

New Options
    Jean A. Cole, Jane C. Sperry, Mary Ann Board,
        Lex Frieden
    The Institute for Rehabilitation and Research
    1333 Moursund Ave.
    Houston, Texas 77030
    1979

Access: The Guide to a Better Life for Disabled Americans
    Lilly Bruck
    Random House
    201 East 50th Street
    New York, New York 10022
    1978

Rehab Sourcebook
    Esther Erving, Ed.
    Sourcebook Publications
    P.O. Box 1586
    Winter Park, Florida 32790
    1982

The Source Book for the Disabled
    Glorya Hale, Ed.
    Paddington Press Ltd.
    Distributed by Grosset & Dunlap
    51 Madison Ave.
    New York, New York 10010
    1979

*The Unexpected Minority: Handicapped Children in
America*
    John Gliedman, William Roth
    Harcourt Brace Jovanovich
    757 Third Ave.
    New York, New York 10017

*Design for Independent Living: The Environment and
Physically Disabled People*
    Raymond Lifchez, Barbara Winslow
    Whitney Library of Design
    An Imprint of Watson-Guptill Publications
    1515 Broadway
    New York, New York 10036
    1979

Independent Living in America
    Nancy Crewe and Irving Zola, Eds.
    Jossey-Bass Inc., Pub.
    433 California Street
    San Francisco, California 94104
    In Press

Films

Changes
    Barry Corbett, Prod.
    Access Incorporated
    177 S. Lookout Mountain Road
    Golden, Colorado 80401
    16 mm, 28 minutes

Outside
    Barry Corbett, Prod.
    Access Incorporated
    177 S. Lookout Mountain Road
    Golden, Colorado 80401
    16 mm, 28 minutes

A Different Approach
South Bay Mayors' Committee
2409 N. Sepulveda Blvd., #202
Manhattan Beach, California 90266
16 mm, 21 minutes

National Wheelchair Tennis Association
3855 Birch Street
Newport Beach, California 92660

National Wheelchair Pilots Association
11018 102nd Avenue, North
Largo, Florida 33540

Organizations—Consumer Oriented

American Coalition of Citizens with Disabilities
1200 15th Street, N.W., #201
Washington, D.C. 20005

Paralyzed Veterans of America
4350 East-West Highway, #900
Washington, D.C. 20014

National Spinal Cord Injury Association
369 Elliot Street
Newton Falls, Massachusetts 02164

National Wheelchair Basketball Association
110 Seaton Bldg.
University of Kentucky
Lexington, Kentucky 40506

Organizations—Professionally Oriented

American Congress of Rehabilitation Medicine
30 N. Michigan
Chicago, Illinois 60602

Association of Rehabilitation Nurses
2506 Grosse Point Road
Evanston, Illinois 60201

National Rehabilitation Counselor Association
633 S. Washington Street
Alexandria, Virginia 22314

American Spinal Injury Association
250 E. Superior Street
Chicago, Illinois 60611

Appendix

A Glossary for Independent Living

This selected glossary presents definitions of terms relating to independent living and kinds of independent living programs. Obviously, it is neither exhaustive nor comprehensive, especially since new terms are being created to describe new circumstances. However, there is a need to standardize the meanings of several key terms so that rehabilitation service providers, consumers, and others will have a common frame of reference.

The definitions in the glossary were developed after a review of the relevant literature by the ILRU staff. The project's national advisory committee played a major role in this effort through group discussion of concepts and through written comments on early drafts of the definitions.

Reprinted from Lex Frieden, Laurel Richards, Jean Cole, and David Bailey. "A glossary for independent living." *ILRU Sourcebook: A Technical Assistance Manual on Independent Living.* Houston: The Institute for Rehabilitation and Research (TIRR), 1979.

INDEPENDENT LIVING ■ Control over one's life based on the choice of acceptable options that minimize reliance on others in making decisions and in performing everyday activities. This includes managing one's affairs, participating in day-to-day life in the community, fulfilling a range of social roles, and making decisions that lead to self-determination and the minimization of physical or psychological dependence on others.

Discussion

Independence is a relative concept that each individual defines personally. Similarly, the concept of independent living is quite broad, subsuming many levels of functional independence.

Some severely disabled people view these varying levels of functioning as important distinctions of independence. For instance, certain activities not central to personal control of one's destiny or the day-to-day management of one's life are considered to be the essence of living independently. Some individuals perceive physical activities such as dressing oneself to be important examples of their ability to live independently. On the other hand, others view any extra time and energy spent dressing themselves as time and energy that could be spent more profitably at work. In fact, whether one performs these particular activities oneself or relies on the assistance of others has little to do with the amount of control one exercises over one's own life.

Independent living is not dependent on programs that foster functional independence. Instead it is based on the individual's ability to choose and achieve a desired life-style and to function freely in society.

It should be stressed that not every person will be capable of achieving total independence in the sense described here. Some persons may not be able to or may not choose to exercise self-determination in certain matters. In such cases, the person may opt for or be restricted to a kind of modified independent living, limited independent living, or semi-independent living.

INDEPENDENT LIVING MOVEMENT ■ The process of translating into reality the theory that, given appropriate supportive services, accessible environments, and pertinent information and skills, severely disabled individuals may actively participate in all aspects of society.

Discussion

For years, some severely disabled individuals have lived comparatively independent lives by finding or making barrier-free residences and by securing attendant care, transportation, and other supportive services on an individual basis. In spite of these self-styled arrangements, programmatic and broadscale efforts to facilitate independent living were stifled by restrictive statutes, regulations, and an inadequate allocation of resources.

Historically, the independent living movement has been characterized by a great amount of consumer involvement and consumer control. Also, the movement has been associated with expanding noninstitutional residential alternatives for severely disabled individuals.

Independent living programs have always been seen as sources of specific information and referral. Developments in independent living probably reflect a lack of coordination of services that already exist in the community and gaps in the community-level service delivery system.

With the arrival of federal funds to support the development of independent living programs on a large-scale basis, many more programs designed to facilitate independent living by severely disabled people are likely to emerge in the near future.

Presently, approximately 35 programs may be classified as independent living programs. If one includes progressive group home projects, halfway houses, and other personal adjustment and mobility-training programs in this census, there may be as many as 100 to 200.

INDEPENDENT LIVING PROGRAM ■ A community-based program that has substantial consumer involvement and provides directly or coordinates indirectly through referral those services necessary to assist severely disabled individuals to increase self-determination and to minimize unnecessary dependence on others.

Services that an independent living program must provide or coordinate through referral are housing; attendant care, readers, and/or interpreters; and information about goods and services relevant to independent living. Other services that are either provided or coordinated by independent living programs include transportation provision or registry, peer counseling, advocacy or political action, independent living skills training, equipment maintenance and repair, and social–recreational services.

Note: Custodial care facilities and primary medical care facilities are specifically excluded from the definition of an independent living program.

Discussion

Independent living programs differ from one another in at least six primary areas: the *service setting* may range from residential to nonresidential; the *service delivery method* may range from direct to indirect, or a combination of both; the *helping style* may range from nonhandicapped to consumer; the *vocational emphasis* may range from primary to incidental; the *goal orientation* may range from transitional to ongoing; and the *disability type served* may range from single to many.

What kinds of features an independent living program has will depend on the needs of the clients served, the availability of existing community resources, the physical and social makeup of the community, and the goals of the program itself.

Conceptually, *independent living program* is generic—the most broadly defined term relating to organizations working with disabled individuals who wish to live independently. Several different kinds of independent living programs with specified purposes have been identified. Some of these are independent living centers, independent living residential programs, independent living transitional programs, and independent living service providers. Table 19–1 illustrates the relationships between these elements.

INDEPENDENT LIVING CENTER ■ A

community-based, nonprofit, nonresidential program that is controlled by the disabled consumers it serves, provides directly or coordinates indirectly through referral those services that assist severely disabled individuals to increase personal self-determination and to minimize unnecessary dependence on others. The minimum set of services that are provided by an independent living center are housing assistance; attendant care, readers and/or interpre-ters; peer counseling, financial and legal advocacy; and community awareness and barrier removal programs.

INDEPENDENT LIVING RESIDENTIAL PROGRAM ■ A live-in independent living program that provides directly or coordinates through referral shared attendant services and transportation. Related services that increase personal self-determination and minimize unnecessary dependence on others may be provided.

INDEPENDENT LIVING TRANSITIONAL PROGRAM ■ An independent living program that facilitates the movement of severely disabled people from comparatively dependent living situations to comparatively independent living situations. The primary service provided by these programs is skill training in such areas as attendant management, financial management, consumer affairs, mobility, educational–vocational opportunities, medical needs, living arrangements, social skills, time management, functional skills, sexuality, and so forth. Additional services may be provided. Transitional programs are usually goal oriented and/or time linked.

INDEPENDENT LIVING SERVICES PROVIDER ■ An organization that provides several discrete services that can be used to increase an individual's ability or opportunities to live independently. For example, a medical rehabilitation facility may provide outpatient services designed to maintain the physical health of a person who lives independently in the community. However, if the center does not provide or coordinate a full set of services including transportation, attendant care, and so forth, it would be an independent living service provider rather than an independent living program. While an independent living service provider does not meet the criteria necessary to be classified as an independent living program, the services it provides may be used or coordinated by an independent living program.

INDEX